ORTHOPAEDIC ANATOMY AND SURGICAL APPROACHES

Orthopaedic Anatomy and Surgical Approaches

FREDERICK W. RECKLING, M.D.
Professor and Chairman
Division of Orthopaedic Surgery
University of Kansas Medical Center
Kansas City, Kansas

JoANN B. RECKLING, R.N., M.N.,
M.A. PHILOSOPHY
School of Nursing
University of Kansas
Kansas City, Kansas

MELVIN P. MOHN, PH.D.
Professor Emeritus
Department of Anatomy and Cell Biology
University of Kansas Medical Center
Kansas City, Kansas

With an Historical Overview by Leonard F. Peltier
and Foreword by D. Kay Clawson

ILLUSTRATED BY LARRY P. HOWELL

Mosby
Year Book

St. Louis   Baltimore   Boston   Chicago   London   Philadelphia   Sydney   Toronto

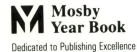

Dedicated to Publishing Excellence

Sponsoring Editor: James D. Ryan
Associate Director, Manuscript Services: Fran Perveiler
Production Project Coordinator: Karen Halm
Proofroom Supervisor: Barbara M. Kelly

q
RD 705
O75
1990

Mosby-Year Book, Inc.
11830 Westline Industrial Drive
St. Louis, MO 63146

1 2 3 4 5 6 7 8 9 0 V C 94 93 92 91 90

Library of Congress Cataloging-in-Publication Data

Orthopaedic anatomy and surgical approaches/[edited by] Frederick W.
  Reckling, JoAnn B. Reckling, Melvin P. Mohn.
    p.   cm.
  Includes bibliographical references.
  Includes index.
  ISBN 0-8151-7120-X
  1. Orthopedic surgery.   2. Musculoskeletal system—Anatomy.
I. Reckling, Frederick W.   II. Reckling, JoAnn B.   III. Mohn, M. P.
(Melvin P.)
  [DNLM: 1. Musculoskeletal System—anatomy &
  histology.
2. Orthopedics.   WE 168 07623]   90-12694
RD705.075 1990   CIP
617.3—dc20
DNLM/DLC
for Library of Congress

This book is dedicated to our patients, medical students, and residents, past and present. The former are our inspiration, the latter our stimulation as we try to answer their probing questions and teach them orthopaedic anatomy and the safe, effective method of carrying out orthopaedic approaches.

CONTRIBUTORS

MARC A. ASHER, M.D.
Professor of Surgery (Orthopaedics)
University of Kansas Medical Center
Kansas City, Kansas

GOPAL JAYARAMAN, PH.D.
Professor of Biomechanics
Michigan Technological University
Houghton, Michigan

DAVID P. KRAKER, M.D.
Assistant Professor of Surgery (Orthopaedics)
University of Kansas Medical Center
Kansas City, Kansas

MELVIN P. MOHN, PH.D.
Professor Emeritus
Department of Anatomy and Cell Biology
University of Kansas Medical Center
Kansas City, Kansas

PASQUALE X. MONTESANO, M.D.
Assistant Professor
Department of Orthopaedic Surgery
University of California at Davis
Sacramento, California

STEPHEN W. MUNNS, M.D.
Assistant Professor of Surgery (Orthopaedics)
Associate Professor, School of Allied Health
University of Kansas Medical Center
Director, University of Kansas Sports Medicine Institute
Kansas City, Kansas

JAMES R. NEFF, M.D.
Professor of Surgery (Orthopaedics) and Pathology
University of Kansas Medical Center
Kansas City, Kansas

BRAD W. OLNEY, M.D.
Assistant Professor of Surgery (Orthopaedics)
University of Kansas Medical Center
Kansas City, Kansas

LEONARD F. PELTIER, M.D., PH.D.
Professor Emeritus of Surgery (Orthopaedics)
Division of Orthopaedic Surgery
Acting Chairman of Department of Surgery
University of Arizona Medical Center
Tucson, Arizona

FREDERICK W. RECKLING, M.D.
Professor and Chairman
Division of Orthopaedic Surgery
University of Kansas Medical Center
Kansas City, Kansas

GEORGE A. RICHARDSON, M.D.
Assistant Professor of Surgery (Orthopaedics)
Chief, Hand Service
University of Kansas Medical Center
Kansas City, Kansas

CHARLES E. RHOADES, M.D.
Assistant Clinical Professor of Surgery (Orthopaedics)
University of Kansas Medical Center
Kansas City, Kansas
Associate Professor
Department of Orthopaedic Surgery
University of Missouri-Kansas City School of Medicine
Kansas City, Missouri

JAMES H. WHITAKER, M.D.
Clinical Assistant Professor of Surgery (Orthopaedics)
University of Kansas Medical Center
Kansas City, Kansas
Clinical Assistant Professor
Department of Orthopaedic Surgery
University of Missouri-Kansas City School of Medicine
Kansas City, Missouri

GREGORY A. WOODS, M.D.
Team Physician, Fort Hays State University
Chairman, Department of Orthopaedics
Hadley and St. Anthony Hospitals
Hays, Kansas

FOREWORD

The primary role of the academic community is the creation of new knowledge and the dissemination of current knowledge in a manner that can be understood by the student, and readily applied by the practitioner. Human morbid anatomy has been well described and recorded in numerous atlases and texts, with little added, since the 17th Century. Following the introduction of anesthesia in 1847, surgical anatomy was born as practitioners found reason to operate on the living, preserving function of nerves, vessels, muscles and joints. Surgical approaches are continually being modified, with some classics surviving without change, while others are improved. Additionally, as technology improves, areas of the body such as the spine and pelvis are further explored and better understood. The addition of fiberoptics has added a new dimension for visualizing normal and abnormal anatomy. Approaches to arthroscopic visualization of joints are being developed and modified.

The authors of this book, with a total of more than 135 years as orthopaedic teachers and practitioners, and 46 years of teaching gross anatomy, have created a text that combines basic musculoskeletal anatomy with common orthopaedic approaches.

The book is illustrated with superb drawings, including cross-sectional presentations, to allow the student to quickly refresh his/her memory of the anatomy before moving on to descriptions of common surgical approaches, while being reminded of the pitfalls beneath the scalpel that await the unsuspecting surgeon. If these presentations do not satisfy the reader, each chapter includes a selected bibliography, combining classic historic treatises with modern articles detailing approaches and orthopaedic procedures.

The book is in keeping with the rich orthopaedic traditions of the University of Kansas Medical Center. The chapter on historical perspectives of orthopaedic anatomy by Peltier is, in itself, worth the price of the book.

All students and practitioners must be lifetime learners. Yet the explosion of new knowledge makes it difficult to keep one's status current while remembering what one has learned from the past. The textbook by the Recklings and Mohn is one step toward making this task easier.

D. Kay Clawson, M.D.
Executive Vice Chancellor
University of Kansas
Kansas City, Kansas

PREFACE

Human anatomy doesn't change, but its surgical relevance does. Advancements in surgical technology have given the modern orthopaedic surgeon the opportunity to intervene in anatomic areas (e.g., the anterior aspect of the upper and lower cervical spine and anterior cervical-thoracic junction, the entire bony pelvis) thought not to be safely approachable a few years ago. However, these advancements cannot be translated into help for our patients unless they are carried out in a safe manner, avoiding injury to important anatomic structures. This textbook was written to enable the surgeon to review regional anatomy and correlate it with standard operative approaches. The actual surgical procedures or techniques are not emphasized; instead, the focus is upon "the road to get there." The authors claim no originality in developing or describing the operative approaches, but have synthesized and modified standard surgical approaches designed to facilitate the accomplishment of a specific task. Obviously, all the possible surgical approaches cannot be presented in a single text. The approaches included have been those effectively utilized by the authors in their many years of surgical practice.

One of the editors (M.P.M.) has directed the gross anatomy teaching effort for medical and postgraduate students at the University of Kansas Medical Center for 25 years. In addition to his contributions to the anatomical material presented in this text, he has assisted in the preparation and carefully scrutinized the surgeons' contributions. As in any descriptive textbook, the artist's ability to interpret and synthesize ideas and to reproduce them visually is crucial. In this text, the illustrations include modification and redrawing of standard anatomical material and surgical approaches found in the literature, as well as drawings based on direct operating room observation and cadaver dissections.

Following a brief chapter on the historical perspective of orthopaedic anatomy and surgical approaches, the book is organized into four additional parts: upper limb; spine; pelvis and lower limb; and anatomy and musculoskeletal oncology. The upper limb, spine, and pelvis and lower limb are introduced by a brief discussion of function and biomechanics. Each chapter begins with a description of the regional anatomy, commencing with the skeletal structures, followed by ligaments, muscles, vessels, and nerves.

The surgical approaches are presented following the anatomical descriptions. In keeping with modern orthopaedic practice, arthroscopic portal anatomy of the shoulder, elbow, wrist, knee, and ankle is included. Anterior and posterior approaches to the cervical and thoracolumbosacral spine are presented in detail. Extensile exposures to the pelvis and acetabulum are described in depth. The chapter on anatomic considerations of biopsy and orthopaedic oncological management is particularly pertinent in view of current emphasis on limb salvage procedures in attempts to cure patients with the least amount of morbidity and long-term disability.

As is the case in any endeavor, there are many people who have functioned "behind the scenes" in making this publication possible. We are indebted to our radiology consultants, John Bramble, M.D., Norman Martin, M.D., and Mark Murphey, M.D.; Richard Lark, the director of our research laboratory; and our secretaries, Elizabeth Brown, Jan Brunks, Beth Chu, Betty Moore, Jana Parrett, Kathy Reinke, Karry Schweiger, Diana Shortino, and Odulia Sites. We are also indebted to the Mosby-Year Book, Inc., staff and in particular, Karen Halm, Project Coordinator, Fran Perveiler, Assistant Director, Manuscript Services, and especially to the Executive Editor, James D. Ryan, who has been so kind and understanding of the time required to see the book to fruition.

FREDERICK W. RECKLING, M.D.
JoANN B. RECKLING, R.N., M.N., M.A. PHILOSOPHY
MELVIN P. MOHN, PH.D.

CONTENTS

PART I

Historical Overview

Historical Perspective of Orthopaedic Anatomy and Surgical Approaches

Leonard F. Peltier, M.D., Ph.D.

IN SEARCH OF AN ORTHOPAEDIC ANATOMY

Though we owe a huge debt to the fathers of medicine, in the field of anatomy their major legacy lies in the area of terminology. Hippocrates[1] was the first to mention specific muscles by name, i.e., the masseter and temporalis. To Herophilus of Alexandria, the father of anatomy, we owe the terms prostate and duodenum.[2] Galen wrote a short book on the bones, usually known by its Latin title, *De ossibus ad tirones (On bones for beginners)*. It was written about A.D. 180 and is the only anatomical work surviving from antiquity that was based on human material.[3] Galen introduced terms such as epiphysis, apophysis, symphysis, diarthrosis, synarthrosis, ginglymoid, sphenoid, bregma, zygoma, odontoid, thorax, acromion, carpus, metacarpus, phalanges, and many others. Galen wrote another book, *On the anatomy of muscles,* in which he described about 300 different muscles, most of them quite accurately. However, his myologic nomenclature was deficient.[4] From the Arabs, we have retained the terms nucha, cephalic, retina, saphenous, and sesamoid.[5] Succeeding generations of anatomists gradually added to the anatomical nomenclature during the middle ages.

The scientific study of anatomy began with Andreas Vesalius (1514–1564), a Belgian surgeon educated at Louvain, Paris, and Padua. In 1537 he became professor of anatomy at Padua, where he reformed the teaching of anatomy by displacing the prosectors and demonstrators, and performing the dissections himself. In 1543, his great work, *De Fabrica corporis humani (On the fabric of the human body)*, was published in Basel.[6] In this work, which marks the beginning of the Renaissance of science, he introduced the terms atlas, alveolus, choanae, corpus callosum, incus, and mitral valve. Though Vesalius was a humanist and his work was motivated toward a greater understanding of man as a work of the great Creator, he could not as a surgeon completely overlook the real practical value of a thorough knowledge of anatomy.

The work of Vesalius was rapidly disseminated throughout Europe, with at least 25 editions of the *Fabrica* appearing between 1543 and 1782. In addition to this, his work was widely plagiarized by other authors, including Ambroise Pare.[7] This increased the number of individuals able to appreciate Vesalius, since Pare wrote in the French vernacular rather than in Latin.

The first book devoted entirely to surgical anatomy was published in 1672 by Bernardino Genga.[8] Genga was a professor of anatomy and surgery in Rome. He emphasized in his teaching the importance of Harvey's discovery of the circulation of blood. He published a second book[9] on anatomy for artists, which was outstanding.

The bones remained an especially popular subject for students because they were easily obtained from graveyards and charnel houses and preserved easily. William Cheselden[10] (1688–1752), a London surgeon, wrote a book on anatomy for his students. His book was used for many years, passing through 13 editions. In addition, he published a remarkable work on the anatomy of the bones, the illustrations for which were drawn through the camera obscura to gain precision. *Osteographia, or the anatomy of the bones,*[11] is considered to be the best product of the 18th-century anatomists. In addition to the bones of the normal child and adult, there are some drawings of diseased bones and animal bones.

One of Cheselden's students, Alexander M. Monroe (1697–1767) became professor of anatomy and surgery in Edinburgh. He also published a popular book on the bones, *The Anatomy of the Human Bones,* in 1726. This was translated into French by Jean Joseph Sue and published in a sumptuous folio edition of two volumes, the second of which contains the copper plates of bones of both the adult and foetus.[12]

The surgical procedures that were carried out prior to the beginning of the 19th century were very simple and straightforward. They consisted primarily of the drainage of abscesses, treatment of open and closed fractures, amputations, excision of the breast, removal of bladder calculi, and couching for cataracts. No procedure required a great deal of anatomical knowledge for success. It was not until operations became more extensive and sophisticated that the study of surgical anatomy became a reality. Even then the description and depiction of anatomy was subordinate to the operative procedure. Dupuytren's monograph on lithotomy[13] is one exception, the plates conveying a great deal of pertinent anatomical material. There are other exceptions as well. However, it is quite difficult to find a line of demarcation between surgical anatomy per se and the description of surgical procedures.

The first elective operation that can be called an orthopaedic procedure was subcutaneous tenotomy, first carried out by Delpech in 1816 and popularized by Stromeyer and Little 15 years later. Initially applied to the tight heel cord, subcutaneous tenotomy and myotomy were quickly adapted to a wide variety of tight muscles and tendons. Subcutaneous osteotomy followed. The introduction of anesthesia in 1847 permitted more extensive elective orthopaedic procedures, but until the introduction of antiseptic surgical precautions by Lister in 1865 such operations were accompanied by a substantial risk of infection. As a result, orthopaedic surgery did not become a major surgical specialty until the last quarter of the 19th century.

Between 1852 and 1859, the Russian surgeon Pirogov[14] published an atlas of cross-sectional anatomy, which was of enormous help in understanding the anatomical relationships of structures in the trunk and extremities. For many years cross-sectional anatomy was taught as a part of general courses of gross anatomy, but was dropped as the curriculum became crowded. The introduction of computed tomography and magnetic resonance imaging scanning technics and their cross-sectional reconstructions has changed this completely. This type of anatomical orientation has become an invaluable tool for the orthopaedic surgeon.

Theodor Kocher[15] (1872–1917) of Bern, in his book on operative surgery, developed the concept of approaching the deep structures by using the neutral zones between muscles supplied by different nerves to minimize the damage.[16] This important consideration has affected the development of operative approaches, particularly in the extremities, ever since.

The publication on December 28, 1895 of the discovery of x-rays by Roentgen was immediately exploited by physicians of all kinds. X-ray films of the skeleton were made very early, since the bones had the highest density and could be visualized better than the less dense soft tissues. Such pictures revealed the presence of numerous anomalous small bones, such as commonly occur in the foot, whose presence and significance had barely been appreciated. These films also showed that some "anomalous" bones in the wrist were not anomalies at all, but rather fragments of nonunited fractures of the navicular. The structure of the skeleton, as visualized by x-ray film, has given orthopaedic surgeons an additional fund of knowledge regarding the anatomy of the bones.

There have been an enormous number of works of varying thrust and quality on topographic anatomy, regional anatomy, surgical anatomy and operative surgery. Such publications have been of great help to generations of surgeons, including orthopaedists. Only one, however, has introduced a concept as valuable as Kocher's principle of approaching the deep structures through neutral zones. That is the little book by Arnold K. Henry (1886–1962) titled *Extensile Exposure Applied to Limb Surgery.*[17] His principle is simplicity itself in concept: "Exposure that will vie effectively with the 'great arsenal of chance' must be a match for every shift, and therefore have a range, extensile, like the tongue of the chameleon to reach where it requires."[18] The amount of useful information packed into its 171 pages and 127 figures is a fine example of clear and concise communication. If there is an orthopaedic anatomy, Henry's book typifies what it should be. Not tied to one operation or technique, it is useful for all. By utilizing the principles espoused in his monograph, anatomy comes to the aid of the surgeon rather than being his antagonist.

Has our search for an orthopaedic anatomy been successful? The roots of our specialty are deep, and we share them with all of surgery. We have drawn valuable material from many traditions and techniques. A few basic principles have been established. Yes, there is an orthopaedic anatomy.

REFERENCES

1. Hippocrates: *The Genuine Works of Hippocrates* (translated from the Greek by Francis Adams). Baltimore, Williams & Wilkins Co, 1939, p 222.
2. Singer C: *A Short History of Anatomy and Physiology from the Greeks to Harvey*, ed 2. New York, Dover Publications, Inc, 1957, p 29.
3. Singer C: Galen's elementary course on the bones. *Proc R Soc Med* 1952; 45:767–776.
4. Singer: *A Short History of Anatomy*, pp 53–57.
5. Singer: *A Short History of Anatomy*, pp 79–80.
6. Vesalius A: *De humani corporis fabrica libri septem*, Basel, Ioannis Oporini, 1543.
7. Singer: *A Short History of Anatomy*, pp 134–135.
8. Genga B: *Anatomia chirurgica*, Rome, A Ercole, 1672.
9. Genga B: *Anatomia per uso et intelligenza del disegno ricercata non solo su gl'ossi, e muscoli del corpo humano*. Rome, G J de Rossi, 1691.
10. Cheselden W: *The anatomy of the human body*, London, N Cliff & D Jackson, 1713.
11. Cheselden W: *Osteographia, or the anatomy of the bones*. London, 1733.
12. Monroe A: *Traite d'Osteologie, ou l'on a ajoute des planches en taille-douce qui representent tous les os de l'adulte et du foetus, avec leurs explications* (translated by Jean Joseph Sue). Paris, Guillaume Cavelier, 1759.
13. Dupuytren G: *Operation de la pierre d'apres un methode nouvelle*, Bruxelles, H Dumont, 1834.
14. Pirogov NI: *Anatome topographica sectionibus per corpus humanum congelatum triplici directione ductis illustrata*. Petropoli, J Trey, 1852–1859.
15. Kocher T: *Chirurgische Operationslehre*, Jena, G Fischer, 1892.
16. Kocher T: *Text-Book of Operative Surgery*, ed 3 (translated by Stiles HJ, Paul CB). New York, Macmillan Publishing Co, 1911, p 277.
17. Henry AK: *Extensile Exposure Applied to Limb Surgery*. Edinburgh, E & S Livingstone, Ltd, 1945.
18. Henry AK: *Extensile Exposure*, p vii.

PART II

Upper Limb

Overview

Frederick W. Reckling, M.D.

The upper extremity is composed of several complex components, which must function synchronously to allow humans to use this prehensile limb with maximum efficiency. It can be considered a series of rigid links or interconnected lever arms powered by muscles that allow the use of the end organ (hand) to accomplish a specific task such as grasp, pinch, pull, or release.

To perform a specific task the hand must be positioned at the appropriate point in space. The shoulder permits the hand to be placed anywhere on the surface of an imaginary sphere that represents the full excursion of shoulder motion with the elbow in extension.

The arm is a site for the origin and insertion of muscles (Figs II–1 and II–2) that power the limb and a conduit for the essential neurovascular structures. The primary function of the elbow is to adjust the height and length of the limb to reach any point within the sphere of shoulder motion. It also sup-

plies an axis for the forearm lever and functions as a weight-bearing joint in people who use an assistive device for ambulation.

The forearm rotates to place the hand in the most effective operating position. Once the hand is located, the muscles of the forearm act to apply or resist forces.

The wrist joint is the site for major postural change between the arm beam and the working hand piece. It has a multiarticulated architecture that creates a potentially wide range of motion.

The hand is a complex, multipurpose organ. As a prehensile organ the hand can grasp with forces exceeding 45 kg as well as hold and manipulate a delicate thread. As a sense organ for touch, the hand is an extension of the brain to provide information about the environment. The hand is also an important organ for expression and nonverbal communication.

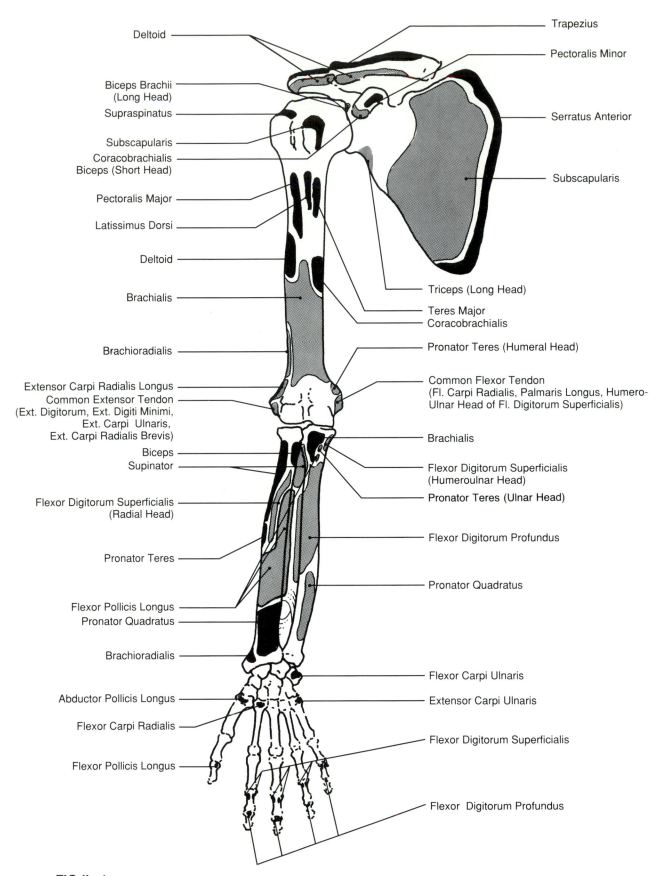

FIG II−1.
Origin *(gray shaded areas)* and insertion *(dark areas)* sites of muscles of the upper limb (anterior view).

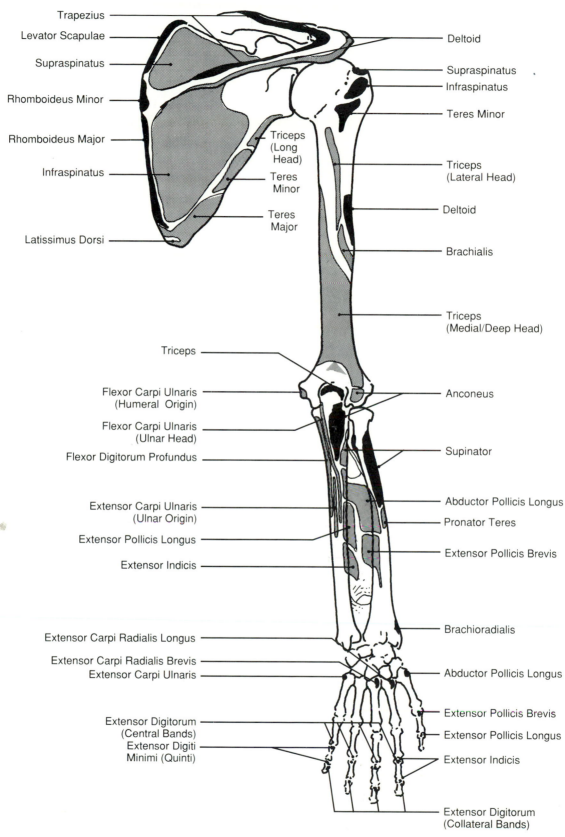

FIG II–2.
Origin *(gray shaded areas)* and insertion *(dark areas)* sites of muscles of the upper limb (posterior view).

2

Shoulder

Frederick W. Reckling, M.D.

Stephen W. Munns, M.D.

Gregory A. Woods, M.D.

ANATOMIC FEATURES OF THE SHOULDER REGION

The shoulder is where the arm joins the trunk of the body. Through precise, coordinated movements, it allows humans to use the prehensile extremity at a maximum level of efficiency.

Bony Anatomy

The skeletal features of the shoulder are the clavicle, scapula, proximal humerus, and sternum (Fig 2–1). The S-shaped clavicle has a large medial end, which articulates with the sternum, and a flat lateral end, which articulates with the acromion of the scapula. The scapula is a flat triangular bone with three borders: superior, medial, and lateral. The lateral border has an expanded end referred to as the glenoid, whose lateral surface, or glenoid fossa, articulates with the head of the humerus. A hooked projection known as the coracoid process (raven's beak) extends forward from the neck of the scapula near the glenoid. The dorsal surface of the scapula displays a transverse ridge, or spine, which separates the suprascapular and infrascapular regions. The spine ends laterally in an expanded acromion process. The ventral surface of the scapula is smooth and slightly concave. The scapula glides along the thorax during shoulder motion, and this area is considered the scapulothoracic joint. It is not a true diarthrodial joint, but it is an important com-

ponent of shoulder function. The proximal end, or head, of the humerus articulates with the glenoid fossa of the scapula. There are two prominences known as the greater and lesser tubercles (tuberosities) on the anterior surface of the upper end of the humerus. They are separated by the intertubercular, or bicipital, groove, through which the tendon of the long head of the biceps travels.

Sternoclavicular Joint

The sternoclavicular joint is formed by the articulation of the medial end of the clavicle with the manubrium portion of the sternum and the superior surface of the first costal cartilage (Fig 2–2). The articular surfaces are separated by an intraarticular fibrocartilaginous disc. The entire joint is isolated by a capsule, which is reinforced in front and behind by the anterior and posterior sternoclavicular ligaments. The joint is also strengthened by two accessory ligaments, the interclavicular and costoclavicular. The latter is the most substantial supporting structure of the sternoclavicular joint. The important structures on the anterior and superior aspects of this joint are the upper fibers of the pectoralis major, the sternal head of the sternocleidomastoid muscle and, in close proximity, the clavicular head of the same muscle. The anterior and external jugular veins disappear beneath the medial and lateral borders of the sternocleidomastoid muscle, respectively.

Posterior to the medial 2.5 cm of the clavicle, from superficial to deep, are the attachments of the

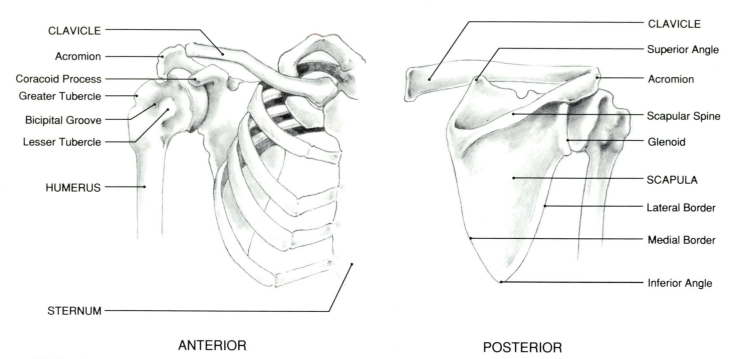

FIG 2–1.
Skeletal features of the shoulder.

sternohyoid and sternothyroid muscles, which separate the bone from the innominate vein, phrenic nerve, internal thoracic artery, pleura, and lung (Fig 2–3). When it is necessary to approach the sternoclavicular joint surgically, a straight or slightly curved incision is made directly over the joint anteri-

orly. The periosteum and heads of the sternocleidomastoid muscles are then carefully dissected off subperiosteally. The right sternoclavicular joint is related posteriorly to the innominate artery. The left sternoclavicular joint is in close relationship to the subclavian vein. These structures are at risk when

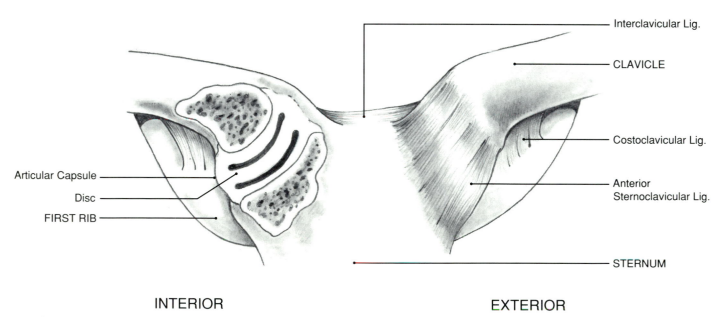

FIG 2–2.
The sternoclavicular joints (interior and exterior aspects).

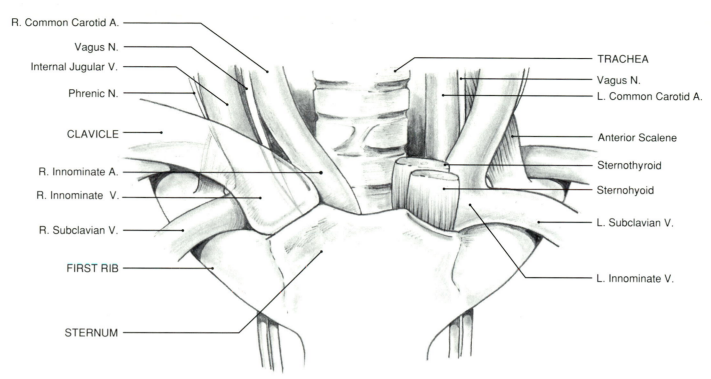

R. Common Carotid A.

Vagus N.

Internal Jugular V.

Phrenic N.

CLAVICLE

R. Innominate A.

R. Innominate V.

R. Subclavian V.

FIRST RIB

STERNUM

TRACHEA

Vagus N.

L. Common Carotid A.

Anterior Scalene

Sternothyroid

Sternohyoid

L. Subclavian V.

L. Innominate V.

FIG 2–3.
Relationships of neurovascular structures to the sternoclavicular joints. (*Note:* left clavicle removed to reveal underlying structures; right sternohyoid and sternothyroid muscles are not shown.)

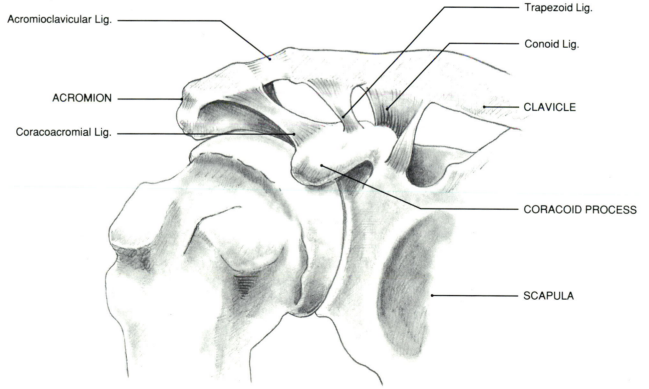

Acromioclavicular Lig.

ACROMION

Coracoacromial Lig.

Trapezoid Lig.

Conoid Lig.

CLAVICLE

CORACOID PROCESS

SCAPULA

FIG 2–4.
Acromioclavicular joint and surrounding structures (anterior view).

the sternoclavicular joints are manipulated or surgically approached.

Acromioclavicular Joint

The acromioclavicular joint is a diarthrodial joint formed by the articulation of the lateral end of the clavicle and the acromion (Fig 2–4). The capsule is weak but the joint is strengthened by the coracoclavicular ligaments (conoid and trapezoid), which extend from the upper surface of the coracoid process to the inferior aspect of the lateral end of the clavicle. The coracoclavicular ligaments constitute the most important structural support of the acromioclavicular joint. Complete dislocations of the acromioclavicular joint cannot occur without some damage to the coracoclavicular ligaments.

Glenohumeral Joint

The glenohumeral joint is the articulation of the relatively large humeral head with the small, slightly concave surface of the glenoid cavity of the scapula (Figs 2–4 and 2–5). The glenoid cavity is deepened somewhat by a fibrocartilaginous structure, known as the labrum, around its periphery. Superiorly, the joint is protected by the coracoid process, the acromion, and the coracoacromial ligament that connects them. The capsule is also reinforced anteriorly by three ill defined but important glenohumeral ligaments (superior, middle, and inferior). The inferior glenohumeral ligament is the most important structure in preventing dislocation of the glenohumeral joint when the shoulder is abducted and externally rotated.

The long head of the biceps (Fig 2–6) arises by a

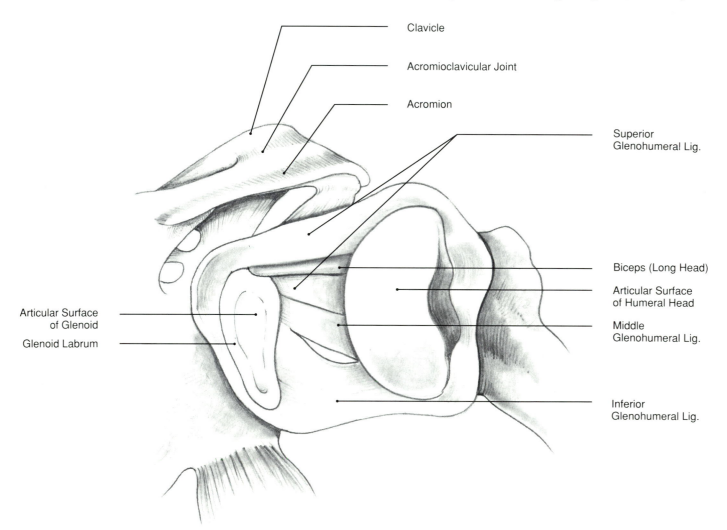

FIG 2–5.
Posterior view of glenohumeral joint. Note anterior glenohumeral ligaments as seen from the posterior aspect of the shoulder.

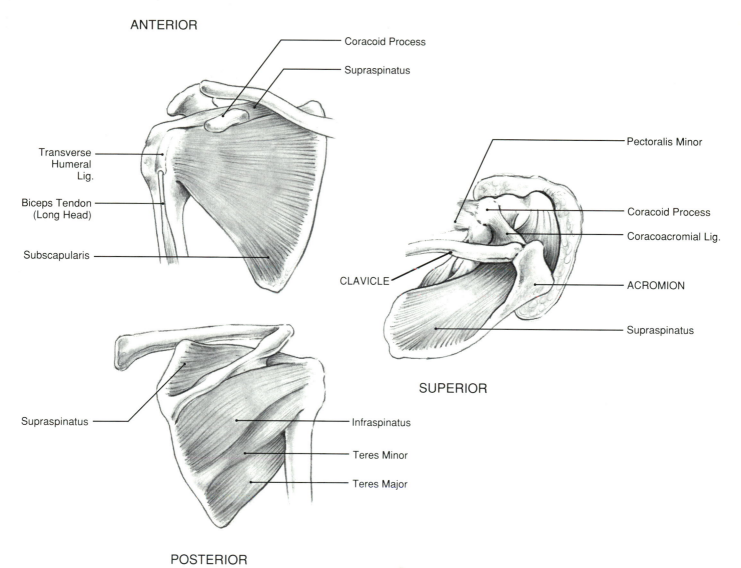

ANTERIOR

Coracoid Process

Supraspinatus

Transverse Humeral Lig.

Biceps Tendon (Long Head)

Subscapularis

Pectoralis Minor

Coracoid Process

Coracoacromial Lig.

CLAVICLE

ACROMION

Supraspinatus

SUPERIOR

Supraspinatus

Infraspinatus

Teres Minor

Teres Major

POSTERIOR

FIG 2–6.
Long head of the biceps tendon and components of the rotator cuff (musculotendinous cuff derived from the subscapularis, supraspinatus, infraspinatus and teres minor muscles, which cover the glenohumeral joint before inserting on the humeral head).

tendon from the supraglenoid tubercle. It traverses the glenohumeral joint until it enters the intertubercular groove of the humerus. From there it continues to be covered with synovium for a short distance. The tendon is held in the groove by the lateral margin of the joint capsule and the insertion of the pectoralis major on the lateral lip of the intertubercular groove. The biceps tendon is also held in the groove by the transverse humeral ligament, which forms the roof of the groove.

Rotator Cuff

All but the inferior portion of the glenohumeral joint is covered by a musculotendinous cuff known collectively as the rotator cuff (see Fig 2–6). This is one of the essential components of the force-couple that is the mechanism for active elevation of the arm. These tendons are continuations of the subscapularis, supraspinatus, infraspinatus, and teres minor muscles. The anterior portion of the cuff is derived from the subscapularis muscle, which inserts on the lesser tuberosity of the humerus. The supraspinatus tendon inserts superiorly, and the tendons of the infraspinatus and teres minor posteriorly. These latter three tendons insert on the greater tuberosity of the humerus. The subscapularis muscle is innervated by the upper and lower subscapularis nerves from the posterior cord of the brachial plexus. The supraspinatus and infraspinatus muscles are innervated by the suprascapular nerve, and the teres minor by the axillary nerve.

Muscles and Related Structures

In addition to the deep muscles of the shoulder region (the rotator cuff), the glenohumeral joint is virtually covered anteriorly, laterally, and posteriorly by the deltoid muscle (Fig 2–7). The deltoid arises from the acromion process and spine of the scapula and the distal third of the clavicle. It inserts on a prominence on the lateral aspect of the humerus. At its anteromedial border, the deltoid muscle lies against the lateral border of the clavicular portion of the pectoralis major muscle. The deltoid is a powerful abductor of the humerus. It also aids in flexion and extension of the glenohumeral joint when the humerus is abducted. It is innervated by the axillary nerve.

The trapezius muscle inserts on the medial aspect of the same bony surfaces that give rise to the deltoid (lateral third of the clavicle, acromion, and scapular spine). The trapezius suspends the shoulder girdle. It is a powerful elevator of the shoulder and assists in rotation of the scapula on the chest wall. It is innervated by the spinal accessory nerve

and branches of the third and fourth cervical nerves.

Deep to the deltoid muscle is the subacromial bursa. This bursa is very large. It lies on the deep surface of the deltoid and extends beneath the acromial arch and coracoacromial ligament as far medially as the root of the coracoid process.

The pectoralis major muscle arises from the medial portion of the clavicle, the anterior surface of the sternum, the upper ribs, and the external oblique aponeurosis. It inserts by a flat trilaminar tendon into the lateral lip of the humerus. The pectoralis major flexes and adducts the humerus and to some extent internally rotates the arm. It is innervated by the medial and lateral pectoral nerves.

The pectoralis minor is a thin, triangular muscle that arises from the outer surfaces of the third through fifth ribs. It inserts into the medial border of the superior surface of the coracoid process of the scapula. The pectoralis minor pulls the scapula medially and downward on the chest wall. It is innervated by the medial pectoral nerve.

The latissimus dorsi and teres major form the posterior axillary wall. The tendon of the latissimus dorsi winds around that of the teres major to insert into the floor of the intertubercular groove of the humerus. The teres major inserts into the medial lip of the intertubercular groove. The latissimus dorsi

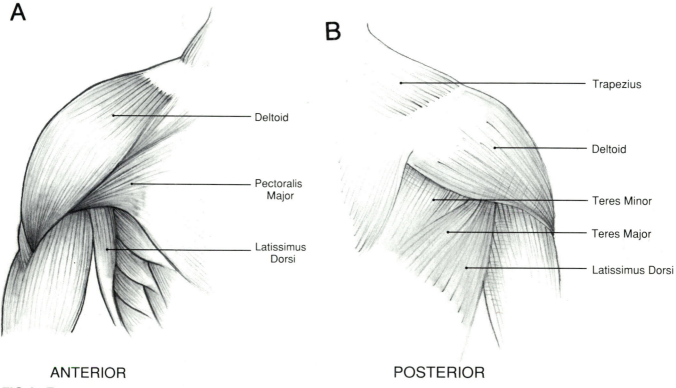

A

Deltoid

Pectoralis Major

Latissimus Dorsi

ANTERIOR

B

Trapezius

Deltoid

Teres Minor

Teres Major

Latissimus Dorsi

POSTERIOR

FIG 2–7.
Shoulder musculature. **A,** anterior view. **B,** posterior view.

pulls the arm down and back and rotates it medially. This muscle is innervated by the thoracodorsal nerve. The teres major adducts and medially rotates the arm. It is innervated by the lower subscapular nerve, a branch of the posterior cord of the brachial plexus.

An important landmark, the cephalic vein, lies in the groove between the deltoid and pectoralis major muscles. As the vein passes upward, it occupies a progressively deeper level and pierces the clavipectoral fascia to join the axillary vein (Fig 2–8). When the shoulder is surgically approached from the anterior aspect, the cephalic vein must be dealt with appropriately.

Coracoid Process and Its Relationship to Underlying Structures

The coracoid process (Fig 2–9) lies under the cover of the anterior deltoid and is easily exposed by development of the deltopectoral groove. The short

head of the biceps and the coracobrachialis muscles, innervated by the musculocutaneous nerve, arise from the coracoid, and the pectoralis minor muscle inserts on it. Medial and deep to the coracoid process lie the branches and cords of the brachial plexus and the great vessels; caution should be used when this area is approached.

Quadrangular Space

The quadrangular space is found in the postero-inferior aspect of the shoulder (Fig 2–10). The boundaries of this important area, through which pass the axillary nerve and posterior humeral circumflex artery are laterally, the shaft of the humerus; inferiorly, the teres major; medially, the long head of the triceps; and superiorly, the subscapularis in front and the teres minor behind.

Triangular Space

The triangular space (see Fig 2–10) is medial to the quadrangular space. Its boundaries are formed

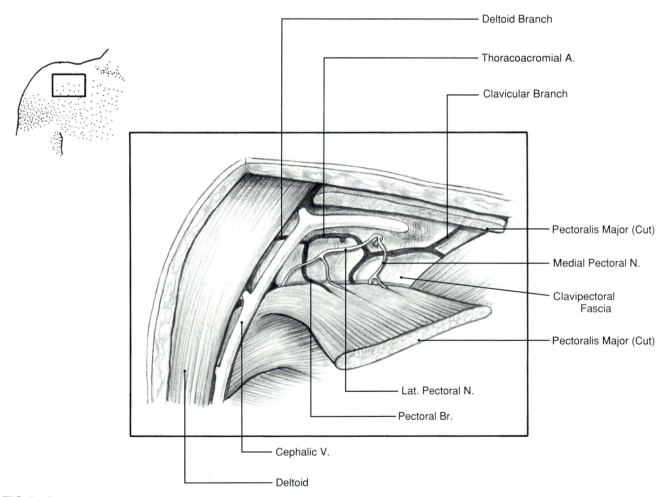

FIG 2–8.
The cephalic vein (landmark of the deltopectoral interval) and thoracoacromial artery and branches.

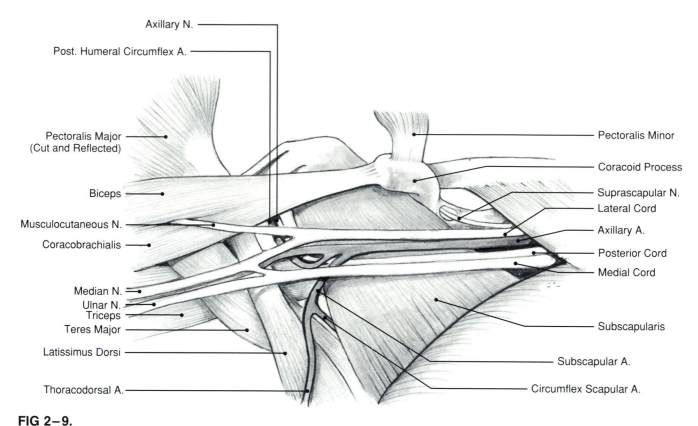

FIG 2–9.
The relationship of the coracoid process to underlying neurovascular structures. (Deltoid has been removed and pectoralis major reflected.)

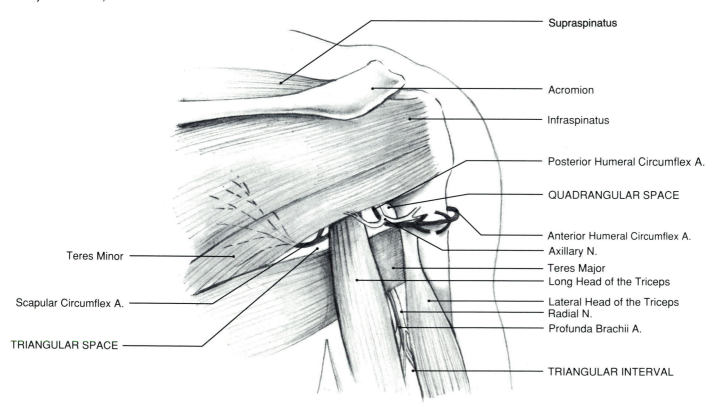

FIG 2–10.
The quadrangular space (contents: axillary nerve and posterior humeral circumflex artery), triangular space (contents: scapular circumflex artery), and triangular interval (contents: radial nerve and profunda brachii artery).

by the teres major below, the subscapularis (anteriorly) and teres minor (posteriorly) above, and the long head of the triceps laterally. The anterior part of the triangular space transmits the scapular circumflex artery. The artery does not pass posteriorly through this space; instead it turns around the lateral border of the scapula deep to the teres minor.

There is an area distal to the inferior border of the teres major between the long and lateral heads of the triceps that is known as the triangular interval. This interval contains the radial nerve and the profunda brachii artery.

Arteries

The arteries that are at risk and must be protected or avoided in surgical approaches to the shoulder include the axillary artery and its branches (particularly the thoracoacromial and the anterior and posterior humeral circumflex) and the suprascapular artery (Fig 2–11).

The axillary artery begins at the lateral border of the first rib as the continuation of the subclavian artery and ends at the inferior border of the teres major muscle. It then becomes the brachial artery and passes into the arm. During its course through the axilla, the axillary artery passes posterior to the pectoralis minor muscle. The axillary artery can be thought of as being divided into three parts, according to its relationship to the pectoralis minor. The first part is medial to this muscle, the second part lies beneath it, and the third part is lateral to it. Although there is considerable variation, the first part usually gives rise to the superior thoracic artery, which does not supply the shoulder joint. The thoracoacromial and lateral thoracic arteries arise from the second part beneath the pectoralis minor muscle. The subscapular artery and the anterior and posterior humeral circumflex arteries arise from the third part of the axillary artery.

The thoracoacromial artery arises by a short trunk from the second part of the axillary artery. It

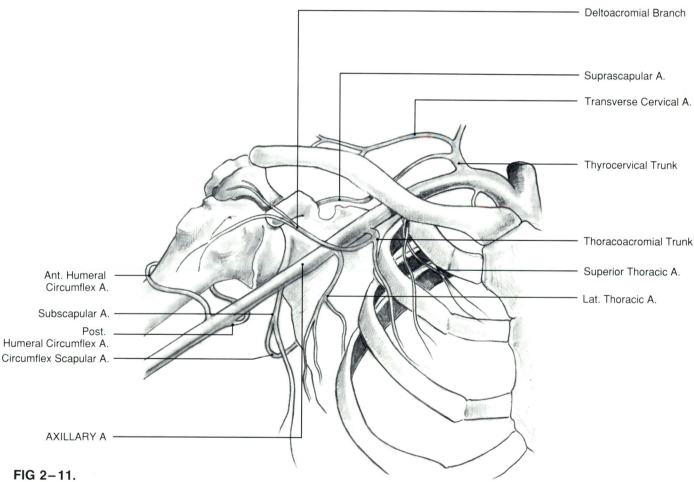

FIG 2–11.
The axillary artery and its branches.

winds around the upper border of the pectoralis minor to pierce the costocoracoid membrane (the part of the clavipectoral fascia above the pectoralis minor), after which it divides into numerous branches (see Fig 2–8). Several large pectoral branches of the thoracoacromial artery course downward between the pectoralis major and minor, where they anastomose with the intercostal and lateral thoracic arteries. A clavicular branch courses superiorly toward the clavicle. An acromial branch passes laterally beneath the tendon of the pectoralis minor and is often found on the inferior aspect of the coracoid process. The deltoid branch runs distally through the intermuscular interval between the deltoid and the pectoralis major. The lateral thoracic and subscapular arteries, which arise from the second and third parts of the axillary artery, respectively, supply the area of the lateral chest wall and scapular muscles.

The anterior and posterior humeral circumflex arteries arise from the third part of the axillary artery. The anterior humeral circumflex artery arises at the lower border of the subscapularis muscle and passes behind the mutual origin of the coracobrachi-

alis and short head of the biceps. This artery is found beneath the deltoid muscle on the surgical neck of the humerus, where it divides into ascending and descending branches. The larger posterior humeral circumflex artery arises near the origin of the anterior humeral circumflex artery. It passes posteriorly through the quadrangular space with the axillary nerve to wind around the surgical neck of the humerus deep to the overlying deltoid muscle.

The suprascapular artery is a branch of the thyrocervical trunk of the subclavian artery (Figs 2–11 and 2–12). It courses across the posterior triangle of the neck toward the scapula, continues laterally above the suprascapular notch, and passes around the spine of the scapula deep to the supraspinatous muscle to reach the infraspinous fossa.

Nerves

The nerve most vulnerable to injury from trauma or surgical approaches to the shoulder is the axillary (circumflex) nerve (Fig 2–13). This nerve is a branch of the posterior cord of the brachial plexus, and it

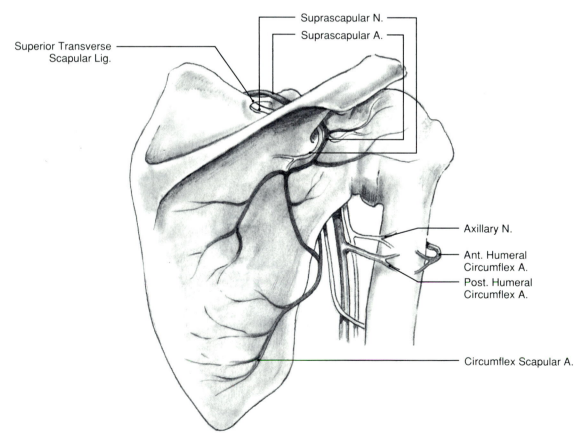

FIG 2–12.
Relationship of the suprascapular artery and nerve to the scapula.

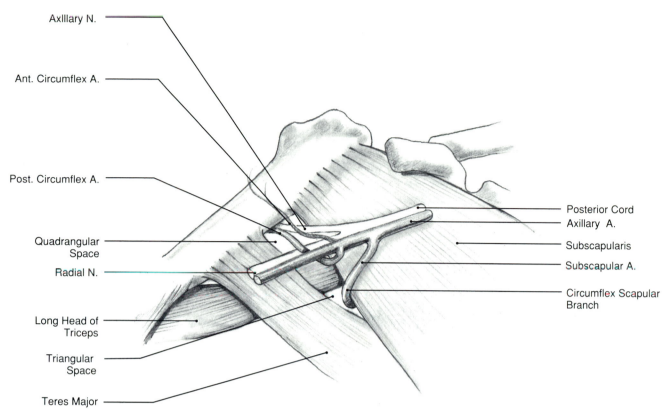

Axillary N.

Ant. Circumflex A.

Post. Circumflex A.

Quadrangular Space

Radial N.

Long Head of Triceps

Triangular Space

Teres Major

Posterior Cord
Axillary A.
Subscapularis
Subscapular A.
Circumflex Scapular Branch

FIG 2–13.
Relationship of the posterior humeral circumflex artery and axillary nerve to the subscapularis muscle.

passes inferior to the glenohumeral joint through the quadrangular space. At this point it divides into anterior and posterior branches. The posterior branch supplies motor innervation to the teres minor and the posterior portion of the deltoid muscle. The posterior branch also provides sensation to the skin over the distal two thirds of the posterior part of the deltoid region. The anterior branch supplies the anterior two thirds of the deltoid muscle and sends a few small cutaneous filaments to the skin over the distal deltoid. To avoid injury to the axillary nerve, the fibers of the deltoid muscle should not be separated for more than 5 cm distal to the acromion.

Another nerve at risk during shoulder surgery is the musculocutaneous nerve (see Fig 2–9), a branch of the lateral cord of the brachial plexus. It passes 2 cm deep to the coracoid process to supply the short head of the biceps, the coracobrachialis, and most of the brachialis muscles. It continues distally to become the lateral antebrachial cutaneous nerve, which supplies sensation to the lateral aspect of the forearm and wrist. Surgery requiring osteotomy of the coracoid process and/or retraction of the muscles it innervates can result in injury to the musculocutaneous nerve.

The suprascapular nerve (see Fig 2–12) is also vulnerable to injury during shoulder surgery. It arises from the superior trunk of the brachial plexus and takes an almost direct course across the posterior triangle of the neck. It passes through the suprascapular notch under the superior transverse scapular ligament. It then runs deep to and supplies the supraspinatus muscle. It continues around the lateral border of the root of the spine of the scapula to enter the infraspinous fossa and supply the infraspinatus muscle. Injudicious traction on the supraspinatus or infraspinatus muscle may injure this nerve.

SURGICAL APPROACHES TO THE SHOULDER REGION

Anterior Deltopectoral (Comprehensive) Approach to the Shoulder

The shoulder joint is most commonly approached surgically from the anterior aspect to deal with problems such as acromioclavicular separations, recurrent glenohumeral joint dislocations, rotator cuff tears, and impingement syndromes, as well as reconstructive procedures such as hemiarthroplasty or total joint replacement. The anterior deltopectoral groove approach is a comprehensive approach to the anterior shoulder. In some instances only part of the approach may be necessary to carry out the intended surgery.

With the patient in the "beach chair" position on the operating table, a bolster is placed between the thoracic spine and scapula on the operative side. The arm is draped free to allow manipulation during the operation. A skin incision is made over the anterior aspect of the acromioclavicular joint and carried medially along the anterior margin of the lateral one third of the clavicle. The incision is then swung inferiorly along the anteromedial margin of the deltoid muscle, a distance of 10 cm. A preferred option is a straight incision (Fig 2–14).

The deltopectoral groove is identified and developed. The cephalic vein is retracted or ligated. Branches of the thoracoacromial artery are carefully identified and protected or ligated as encountered. Removing the medial portion of the deltoid from the clavicle and retracting it laterally will allow greater exposure. Care must be taken to reattach the deltoid firmly at the conclusion of the procedure. The coracoid process of the scapula with the origins of the short head of the biceps and coracobrachialis muscles, as well as the insertion of the pectoralis minor muscle, can now be readily seen. External rotation of the humerus will expose the subscapularis tendon as it inserts on the medial lip of the bicipital groove (lesser tuberosity) of the humerus.

For greater exposure of the subscapularis tendon, the origins of the short head of the biceps and coracobrachialis can be detached from the coracoid process. The origins are then retracted medially and inferiorly (or the coracoid osteotomized with the muscles attached). When the coracoid is osteotomized and retracted, it is important to avoid injury to the musculocutaneous nerve, which enters the substance of the coracobrachialis 4 to 5 cm distal to the coracoid process. When operative procedures are carried out on the coracoid process, the neurovascular structures are much less vulnerable if the arm is adducted to the chest wall. When the arm is abducted away from the chest, the neurovascular structures lie directly under the coracoid process and are in harm's way.

Sectioning the subscapularis tendon approximately 1 cm medial to its insertion and incising the joint capsule will allow exposure of the glenohum-

eral joint. In sectioning the subscapularis tendon, care must be taken to avoid injury to the axillary nerve and circumflex vessels, which are found at the inferior margin of the subscapularis near its humeral attachment. If the exposure is limited due to the pectoralis major muscle, the muscle may be safely detached where it inserts on the lateral lip of the bicipital groove. Caution must be taken not to enter the groove itself.

Some surgeons prefer a long, straight incision, beginning at the acromioclavicular joint and extending to the deltoid tuberosity, as a modification of the anterior deltopectoral approach. This is particularly useful in performing hemiarthroplasties or total shoulder arthroplasties. The long, straight incision leaves a cosmetically more pleasing scar than the curved incision, but in some situations the exposure is restrictive. The incision begins at the acromioclavicular joint and extends distally to the deltoid tuberosity of the humerus. The interval between the deltoid and pectoralis major is then developed, just as described above, with identification and ligation of the cephalic vein and branches of the thoracoacromial artery. An advantage of this approach is that not much of the deltoid is removed from the clavicle or acromion; this lessens the problems of reattachment of the deltoid.

Superior Limb of the Anterior Deltopectoral Approach

The superior limb of the comprehensive anterior deltopectoral approach can be utilized to carry out an anterior acromioplasty (as treatment for chronic impingement syndrome of the shoulder) or to repair or reconstruct a disrupted acromioclavicular joint or rotator cuff (Fig 2–15). For anterior acromioplasty an oblique incision is made from the lateral tip of the acromion to the coracoid. The deep fascia is incised, the deltoid fibers split distally, and a small amount of deltoid muscle removed from the anterior aspect of the acromion. The coracoacromial ligament is identified and removed from its coracoid attachment. The anteroinferior aspect of the acromion is removed with a sharp osteotome to complete the acromioplasty.

If wider exposure of the acromioclavicular joint is required, the skin incision should begin at the posterior border of the joint, proceed over the top of the shoulder, and extend distally approximately 4 cm. Development of the interval between the deltoid and the pectoralis major exposes the coracoid process. It is important to protect or ligate the cephalic

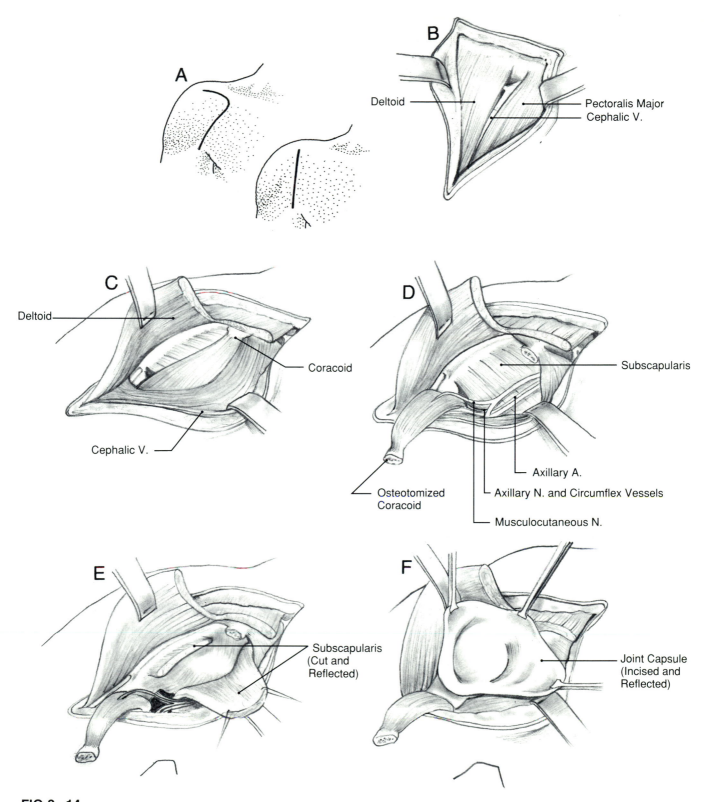

FIG 2–14.
Anterior deltopectoral (comprehensive) approach to the shoulder. **A,** curved or straight incision from the acromioclavicular joint to the medial side of the deltoid tuberosity. **B,** development of deltopectoral interval. **C,** retraction or ligation of the cephalic vein. Minimal resection of deltoid origin from clavicle. **D,** osteotomy of coracoid process and retraction with attached muscles. **E,** retraction of resected subscapularis. **F,** capsular incision allows exposure of glenohumeral joint. (Modified from Bankhart ASB: The pathology and treatment of recurrent dislocation of the shoulder-joint. *Br J Surg* 1938–1939; 26:23–29.)

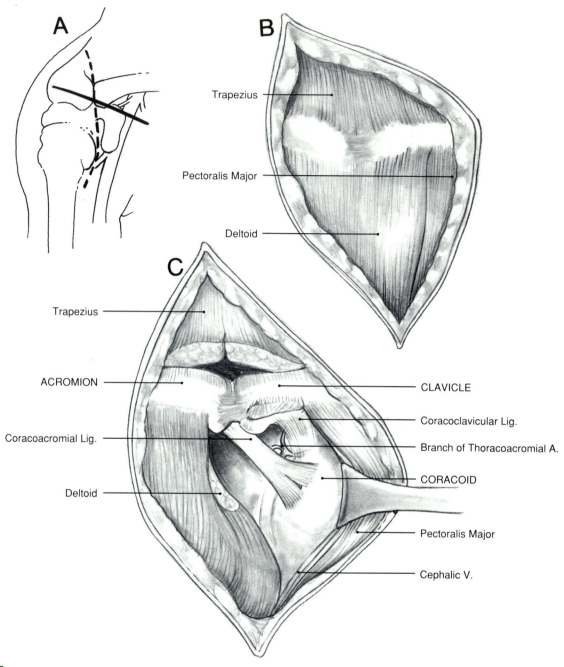

FIG 2–15.
Superior limb of anterior deltopectoral approach. **A,** skin incisions. *Solid line* = incision for anterior acromioplasty; *dashed line* = incision for acromioclavicular joint repair or reconstruction or for rotator cuff repair. **B,** subcutaneous dissection. **C,** deltoid and trapezius detachment and exposure of acromioclavicular joint and coracoacromial ligament.

vein and the branches of the thoracoacromial artery. Subperiosteal dissection of the medial 3 to 4 cm of the attachment of the deltoid and trapezius from the clavicle and acromion brings into view the coraco-clavicular ligaments (the trapezoid and conoid) and fibrous capsule of the acromioclavicular joint. Once these ligaments have been exposed, repair can be carried out by a variety of techniques. If, instead of repairing a disrupted acromioclavicular joint, the goal of surgery is to identify and repair a rotator cuff tear, excision of the distal 2 cm of the clavicle will allow wide exposure to the subacromial bursa. With removal of bursal tissue, the rotator cuff is exposed. In wound closure the deltoid must be carefully reattached to remaining structures.

Anterior Axillary Approach to the Glenohumeral Joint

Operations such as those described by Putti-Platt and Magnuson to prevent recurrent anterior dislocation of the shoulder can be performed through an anterior axillary incision, described by Leslie and Ryan (Fig 2–16). The advantages of this approach compared to the comprehensive anterior deltopectoral approach are that removal of the deltoid from the clavicle is not required, bleeding is minimal, and the appearance of the scar is more pleasing. The incision is started at the midpoint of the axillary fold over the pectoralis major muscle and carried 5 to 7 cm posteriorly and inferiorly into the axilla. The dissection is then developed subcutaneously in all directions except inferiorly.

The interval between the deltoid and pectoralis major is developed, and the cephalic vein and branches of the thoracoacromial artery are protected or ligated. To gain additional exposure the pectoralis major may be partially or totally detached from its humeral insertion. An additional option is to osteotomize the coracoid, leaving the muscles attached, or detaching the short head of the biceps and coracobrachialis from the coracoid process. The location of the musculocutaneous nerve, which lies deep to the coracoid process and enters the coracobrachialis muscle about 5 cm distal to the coracoid process, must be kept in mind. The glenohumeral joint is exposed by detaching the subscapularis near its insertion and incising the joint capsule. With this exposure, as with the comprehensive anterior approach, caution must be exercised to avoid injury to the axillary nerve and the posterior humeral circumflex artery; these enter the quadrangular space at the lower border of the subscapularis muscle.

Total Deltoid Detachment Approach

Exposure to the rotator cuff and the proximal humerus can be obtained by extending the proximal portion of the anterior comprehensive approach laterally around the acromion and medially along the spine of the scapula and detaching most or all of the deltoid muscle origin (Fig 2–17). The deltoid is carefully retracted to avoid injury to the axillary nerve. Because of the difficulty of obtaining and maintain-

ing secure reattachment of the deltoid, this approach is not commonly used.

Transacromial-Deltoid Splitting Approach

The transacromial-deltoid splitting incision described by Kessel allows full exposure of lesions of the subacromial areas, such as displaced fractures of the greater tuberosity of the humerus, tears of the rotator cuff, and painful subacromial arc (the so-called impingement syndrome). It has also been advocated for reconstructive procedures such as hemiarthroplasty and total shoulder replacement. The most appealing aspect of the approach is that the deltoid muscle origin is not disturbed, thus eliminating the problems of deltoid reattachment or dehiscence.

In this approach the skin incision, which bisects the angle formed by the clavicle and acromion, is extended 3 cm proximally and 5 cm distally from the acromion process (Fig 2–18). The trapezius proximally and the deltoid distally are split in the line of their fibers up to the acromion. Deep to the trapezius is a constant pad of yellow fat overlying the supraspinatus. Beneath the deltoid lies the subdeltoid bursa. The axillary nerve courses along the humerus, and if the dissection does not extend more than 5 cm distal to the lateral edge of the acromion, the nerve should not be jeopardized.

The incision across the acromion is developed, and flaps of periosteum and bone are raised from the superior surface of the acromion. The acromion is divided with an oscillating saw or osteotome in line with the posterior border of the clavicle. The two halves of the acromion, as well as the fibers of the trapezius and deltoid, are retracted, thus exposing the subdeltoid bursa. After the bursa is dissected, almost the entire rotator cuff can be fully visualized if the humeral head is moved about in internal and external rotation. Incision and spreading of the fibers of the rotator cuff will allow exposure of the humeral head.

The wound is closed by approximation of the osteoperiosteal flaps that were raised from the superior surface of the acromion. There is no need to repair the acromion formally. The pull of the deltoid and trapezius muscles will approximate rather than retract the suture line.

Subdeltoid Approach to the Proximal Humerus

Surgical exposure of the proximal humerus is difficult due to the overlying deltoid muscle. Divi-

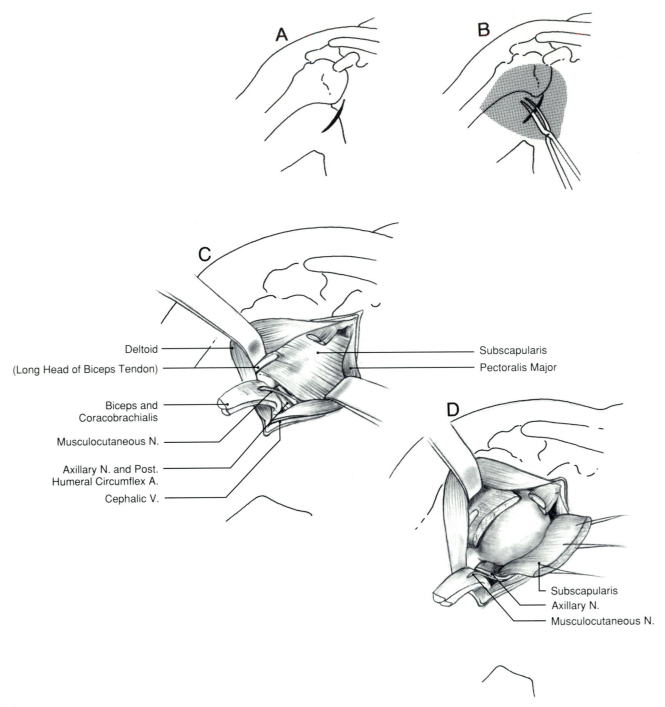

FIG 2–16.
Anterior axillary approach to the glenohumeral joint. **A,** skin incision. **B,** subcutaneous dissection. **C,** resection of tendons (short head of the biceps and coracobrachialis) from the coracoid process. **D,** resection and retraction of subscapularis. (Modified from Leslie JT, Ryan TJ: The anterior axillary incision to approach the shoulder joint. *J Bone Joint Surg* 1962; 44A:1193–1196.)

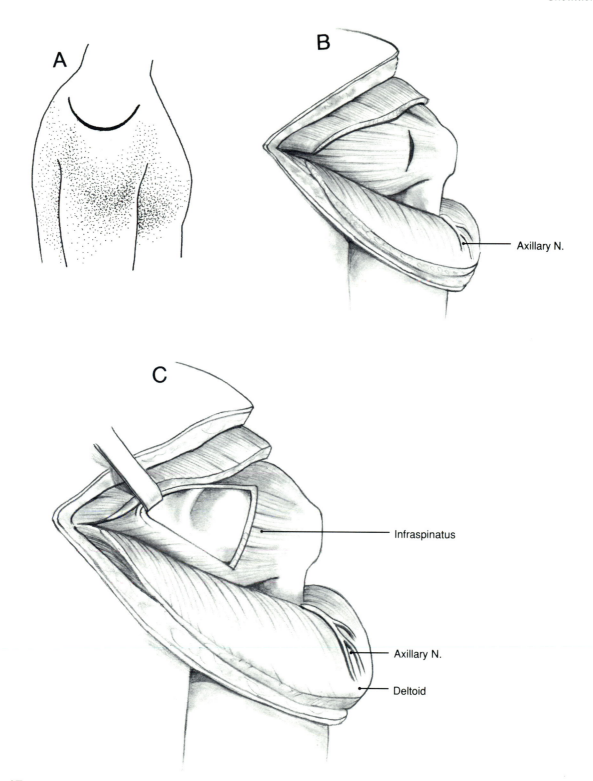

FIG 2–17.
Total deltoid detachment. **A,** skin incision. **B,** detachment of entire deltoid from clavicle, acromion, and scapular spine. **C,** incision through infraspinatus muscle to expose posterior aspect of the glenohumeral joint. Note axillary nerve. (Modified from Cubbins WR, Callahan JJ, Scuderi CS: The reduction of old or irreducible dislocations of the shoulder joint. *Surg Gynecol Obstet* 1934; 58:129–135.)

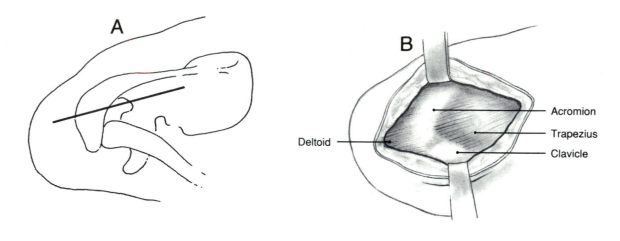

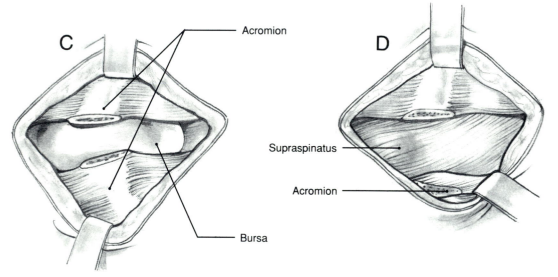

FIG 2–18.
Transacromial-deltoid splitting approach. **A,** skin incision. **B,** exposure of trapezius and deltoid. **C,** osteotomy and retraction of the acromion, exposing the subacromial bursa. **D,** bursa excised, exposing the rotator cuff (supraspinatus).

sion of the deltoid insertion at the deltoid tuberosity of the humerus and reflection the muscle proximally, can obtain excellent exposure. This approach, described by Martini, is particularly helpful in reduction and internal fixation of fractures of the proximal humerus. The skin incision consists of anterior and posterior portions, which meet at the junction of the middle and upper thirds of the humerus (Fig 2–19).

The interval between the deltoid and pectoralis major muscles is developed anteriorly, with care taken to identify and retract or ligate the cephalic vein. The deltoid insertion with a small fragment of bone is lifted from the humerus, and the posterior border of the deltoid is separated from the long and lateral heads of the triceps. The deltoid is then reflected proximally to expose the upper end of the humerus. In order to avoid injury to the axillary nerve, care must be exercised not to retract forcefully on the deltoid. At the completion of the procedure, deltoid reattachment is accomplished with a washer and screw or a few nonabsorbable sutures. The advantages of this exposure are that no muscle fibers are divided and the axillary nerve is visualized. However, the size and cosmetic appearance of the scar can be considered a disadvantage.

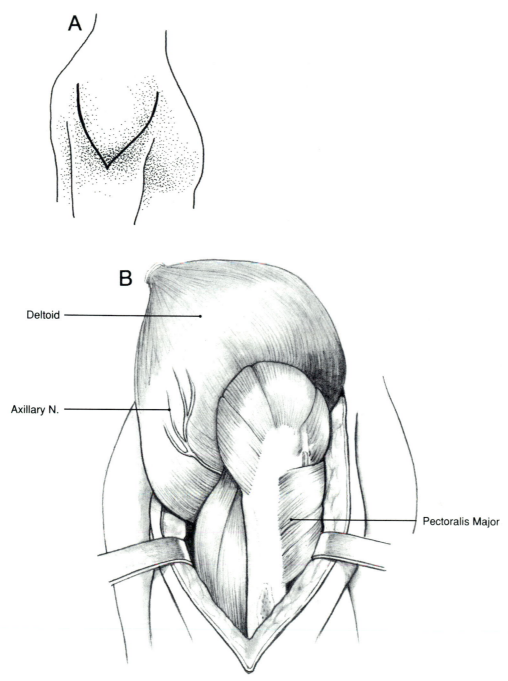

FIG 2–19.
Subdeltoid approach to the proximal humerus. **A,** skin incision. **B,** exposure of the proximal humerus by proximal retraction of the deltoid with detached portion of the deltoid tuberosity.

Comprehensive Approach to the Posterior Aspect of the Shoulder

Care must be taken in obtaining exposure of the posterior and inferior aspects of the shoulder joint, to avoid injury to the suprascapular nerve and artery (see Fig 2–12). These are vulnerable in their relation-ship to the suprascapular notch and as they course around the root of the spine of the scapula. Care must also be exercised to avoid injury to the axillary nerve and its branches as they pass through the quadrangular space and around the surgical neck of the humerus. The comprehensive approach allows adequate and safe exposure to the posterior and inferior aspects of the shoulder to deal with such problems as recurrent posterior dislocations and fractures of the posterior aspect of the glenoid.

The patient is placed in the prone or lateral decubitus position with the arm draped free. The skin incision begins at the junction of the middle and in-

ner thirds of the spine of the scapula, extends laterally along the spine of the scapula to the tip of the acromion, and then swings distally for a distance of 5 cm (Fig 2–20).

The deltoid attachment is removed subperiosteally from the spine of the scapula and posterior

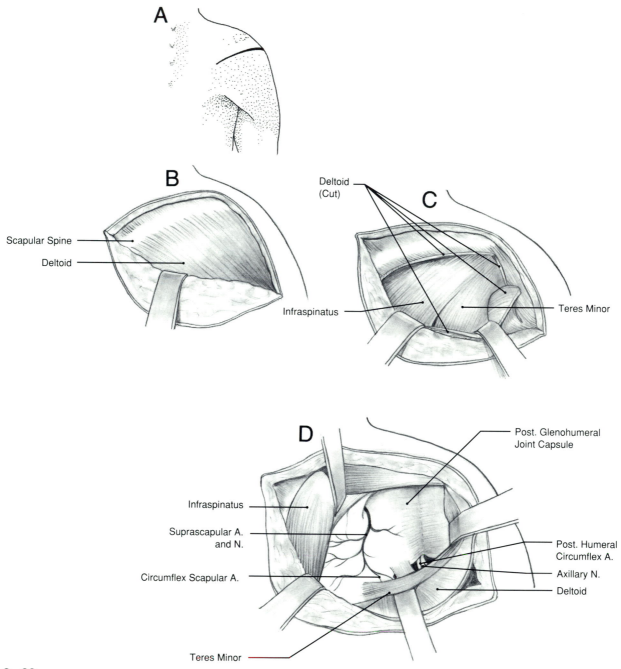

FIG 2–20.
Posterior comprehensive approach to the shoulder. **A,** skin incision. **B,** exposure of deltoid resection site. **C,** resection of the deltoid from scapular spine and acromion. The lateral edge of the deltoid is split in the direction of its fibers. Distal retraction of deltoid. **D,** development of interval between infraspinatus and teres minor muscles. (Modified from Bennett GE: Shoulder and elbow lesions of the professional baseball pitcher. *JAMA* 1941; 117:510–514.)

acromion. Laterally, the muscle fibers are split distally a distance of no more than 4 to 5 cm to avoid injury to the axillary nerve. Distal retraction of the deltoid allows visualization of the infraspinatus and teres minor. The infraspinatus and teres minor muscles are separated by blunt dissection. This is an internervous plane, therefore this maneuver avoids injury to the suprascapular nerve, which supplies the infraspinatus. Keeping the dissection above the teres minor also avoids injury to the axillary nerve, which passes through the quadrangular space, and the branches of this nerve, which supply the teres minor. Care must be taken not to dissect too far medially, or injury to the suprascapular or circumflex scapular arteries may occur. Dividing the tendinous attachment of the infraspinatus 1 cm from its insertion on the greater tuberosity of the humerus exposes the joint capsule. The joint can be entered by a vertical or transverse incision to allow inspection and operative procedures in the posterior glenoid area.

Brodsky et al. have advocated a modification of the comprehensive posterior approach to the shoulder that requires minimal, if any, deltoid muscle detachment (Fig 2–21). The patient is placed in either the prone or lateral decubitus position. The arm is draped free and abducted 90 degrees to place the deltoid muscle in a more proximal position over the humeral head. Limiting abduction to 90 degrees minimizes the possibility of traction injury to the neurovascular structures. A vertical incision is made, starting at the posterior border of the acromion and running distally for 10 cm. Proximal retraction of the deltoid muscle, when necessary, may be facilitated by releasing 2 cm of its medial attachment from the spine of the scapula.

Retraction of the deltoid muscle exposes the underlying muscles of the rotator cuff. The internervous interval is developed between the infraspinatus (supplied by the suprascapular nerve) and the teres minor (supplied by the axillary nerve). The posterior aspect of the glenohumeral joint capsule is opened. It should be remembered that the axillary nerve and posterior humeral circumflex vessels are located at the inferior border of the teres minor. Injury to these structures can be avoided if care is taken not to incise the capsule too far inferiorly.

Shoulder Disarticulation

Severe injury or disease of the upper limb may at times necessitate shoulder disarticulation (Fig 2–22).

The patient is placed in lateral decubitus position. The skin incision is begun at the coracoid process, carried distally along the anterior deltoid border to the deltoid tuberosity, and directed superiorly along the posterior border of the deltoid to the posterior axillary fold. The two ends of the incision are joined with another incision, which is made through the axilla. The deltopectoral groove is developed and the cephalic vein identified and ligated. Lateral retraction of the deltoid allows visualization and release of the pectoralis major from its humeral insertion. Detachment of the coracobrachialis and short head of the biceps from their origin on the coracoid process exposes the axillary vessels and brachial plexus. The axillary artery and vein must be doubly ligated, transected, and allowed to retract superiorly. The branches of the brachial plexus are also divided and allowed to retract. The deltoid is detached and reflected proximally, and the latissimus dorsi and teres major muscles are detached from their humeral insertions.

With the arm internally rotated the infraspinatus and teres minor muscles are divided. With the arm externally rotated the subscapularis and supraspinatus muscles are detached. After the shoulder capsule is completely opened, the triceps is detached from the infraglenoid tubercle. The long head of the biceps is detached from its origin, and the arm is removed. The severed ends of the rotator cuff muscles are sutured together. The deltoid muscle flap is reattached to the tissues inferior to the glenoid. The acromion is excised to give the shoulder a more rounded contour. Wound closure is carried out in a routine manner.

Interscapulothoracic (Forequarter) Amputation

Disease or extensive injury to the shoulder girdle may occasionally require forequarter amputation. A skin incision is made along the entire length of the clavicle anteriorly. The incision is turned posteriorly over the top of the shoulder, turned downward vertically across the spine of the scapula along its vertebral border, and then directed laterally at the inferior angle of the scapula toward the axillary fold (Fig 2–23). The two ends of the first incision are connected by a second incision, which passes anteriorly and superiorly through the axilla, extending from the posterior axillary fold to join the initial incision at the middle third of the clavicle. The cephalic vein is ligated. The pectoralis major muscle is detached from its clavicular origin. By careful dissection, the

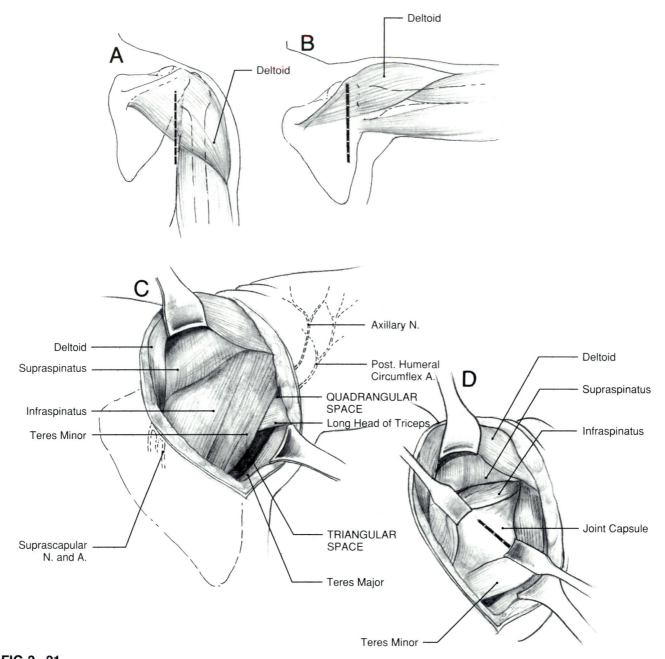

FIG 2–21.
Modified comprehensive posterior approach. **A,** skin incision *(dashed line).* Note arm at the side showing normal position of deltoid. **B,** skin incision *(dashed line)* with arm in 90 degrees of abduction. Note how deltoid is pulled proximally. **C,** underlying muscles of the rotator cuff. **D,** exposure of the joint capsule and joint capsule incision *(dashed line).* (Modified from Brodsky JW, Tullos HS, Garstman GM: Simplified posterior approach to the shoulder joint. *J Bone Joint Surg* 1987; 69A:773–774.)

tissues posterior to the clavicle are cleaned off, and the external jugular vein is ligated. The sternoclavicular and acromioclavicular capsules are incised, the coracoclavicular ligament divided, and the clavicle carefully lifted up. All adjacent soft tissues are removed. This must be done cautiously to avoid injury to the underlying structures. The pectoralis major insertion on the humerus and the pectoralis minor insertion on the coracoid process are divided. The axillary vessels, the transverse cervical and suprascapular arteries, and the branches and cords of the brachial plexus are carefully pulled down, divided, and individually ligated. They are then allowed to retract proximally. The latissimus dorsi is detached

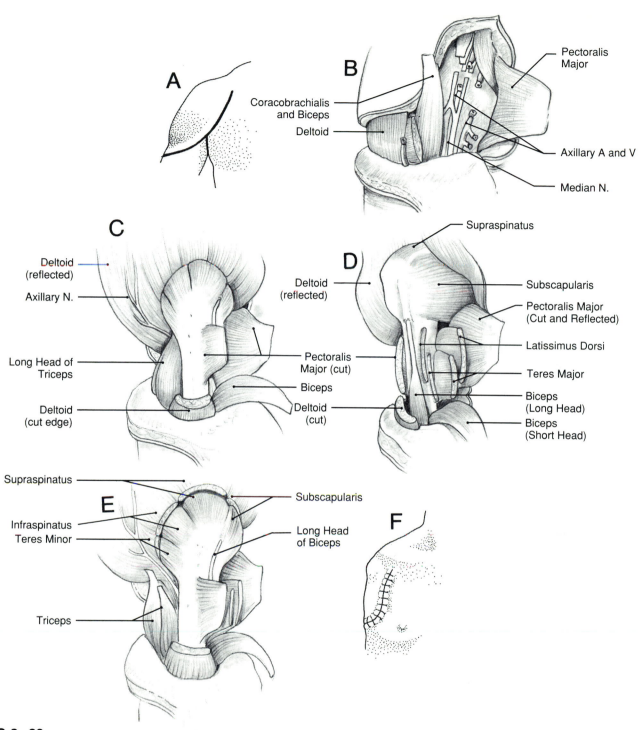

FIG 2–22.
Shoulder disarticulation. **A,** skin incision (anterior view of right shoulder). **B,** resection of coracobrachialis, short head of the biceps, and pectoralis major. Ligation and transection of the axillary vessels and transection of components of the brachial plexus. **C,** deltoid freed and retracted proximally. **D,** detachment of the teres major and latissimus dorsi from the humerus. (Note arm is externally rotated.) **E,** resection of the components of the rotator cuff and long head of the biceps. The joint capsule is then opened and the arm disarticulated. **F,** wound closure. (Redrawn from Slocum DB: *An Atlas of Amputations.* St Louis, C V Mosby Co, 1949, p 168.)

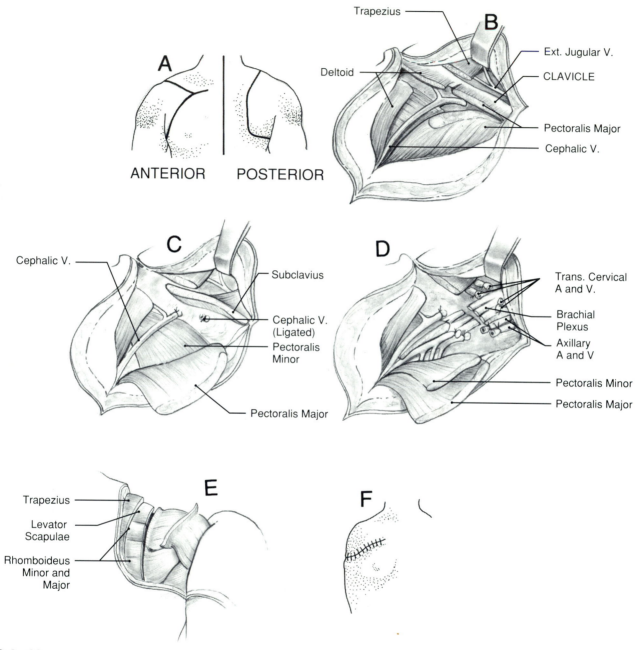

FIG 2–23.
Interscapulothoracic (Forequarter) amputation. **A,** skin incision. **B,** anterior dissection showing detachment of deltoid, pectoralis major, and trapezius from the clavicle. **C,** clavicle completely removed after subperiosteal dissection. **D,** division of the branches and cords of the brachial plexus and ligation and division of the axillary vessels. **E,** posterior dissection showing division of the muscles inserting on the medial border of the scapula. **F,** wound closure seen from the anterior view. (Modified from Slocum DB: *An Atlas of Amputations.* St Louis, C V Mosby Co, 1949, p 171.)

at its insertion, which allows the limb to be moved posteriorly. The posterior incision is deepened, and the muscles attaching the scapula to the vertebral column and rib cage are identified and divided at their scapular insertions. These muscles include the trapezius, levator scapulae, rhomboideus minor and major, and finally the serratus anterior. The posterior part of the shoulder is exposed by lifting the scapula off the thoracic wall. This completes the detachment of the arm and the scapula. The pectoralis major, trapezius, and other muscle cuffs are sutured together over the rib cage, and skin closure is carried out.

ANATOMICAL CONSIDERATIONS IN SHOULDER ARTHROSCOPY

Shoulder arthroscopy is a procedure in evolution. Although it is not intended to replace a thorough history, physical examination, and diagnostic studies (e.g., radiographs, arthrography, arthrotomography, magnetic resonance imaging), it is an important adjunct in diagnosing complex shoulder problems. In skilled hands it also offers an increasing number of alternatives in operative treatment of shoulder problems. As in the knee, shoulder arthroscopy requires in-depth understanding of the three-dimensional anatomy of the shoulder to be safely performed. Unlike the knee, the shoulder is deep to a cloak of muscle. The routine portals pass near important neurovascular structures, and the shoulder is not amenable to tourniquet application for hemostasis. Therefore, certain specialized techniques must be used to make shoulder arthroscopy safe.

The operation is performed with the patient under general anesthesia in lateral decubitus position and the shoulder slightly posterior to the perpendicular plane. Local anesthetic with epinephrine is used at intervals to control hemostasis and lessen postoperative discomfort. Ten to fifteen pounds of skin traction is applied to the forearm (with the fingers left free for neurovascular examination), with the arm held in 45 to 60 degrees of abduction and 15 to 20 degrees of forward flexion. Careful positioning of the head and arm, with frequent examination of the head and arm, is necessary to prevent traction injury. A minimum of two portals are necessary for diagnostic and surgical arthroscopy; three or more are often utilized. Considerable variation in technique, based on the surgeon's preference, is possible. When the procedure is properly performed, all intraarticular structures, along with those in the subacromial space, can be visualized.

Palpable Landmarks

With the patient appropriately positioned, the following landmarks are palpated: the acromion (tip, neck, confluence with the scapular spine, acromio-

clavicular joint), the clavicle, the coracoid process of the scapula, and the humeral head. Until the surgeon is very familiar with the technique, these landmarks should be drawn on the prepared patient's skin with a marking pencil each time the procedure is performed (Fig 2–24).

Portal Placement

Posterior Portal

This is the primary viewing portal and the safest to place first. Most of the structures to be viewed are visible from this portal. The entry site is 2 to 3 cm inferior and 1 to 2 cm medial to the posterolateral border of the acromion (Fig 2–25,A). More inferior placement may damage the axillary nerve, and more medial placement could injure the suprascapular nerve and/or vessels.

Gentle internal-external rotation of the suspended arm allows palpation of the glenohumeral joint. The entry site for the posterior portal is, in the absence of obesity or excessive muscularity, a palpable soft spot corresponding to the interval between the infraspinatus and the teres minor muscles. To palpate this site, the examiner's hand (Fig 2–26) is placed over the shoulder with the index finger on the coracoid process anteriorly and the thumb on the entry site posteriorly. The entry site is then marked with a marking pencil.

An 18-gauge spinal needle is inserted at the entry site, directed toward the coracoid process. A "pop" is usually felt as the joint is penetrated. The joint is insufflated with 40 to 50 mL of saline; proper position is confirmed by easy injection and free backflow upon removal of the syringe. Ten mL of local anesthetic with epinephrine 1:200,000 is injected for hemostasis as the needle is withdrawn. A stab wound is made at the point of the needle insertion, and the arthroscope cannula with sharp trocar is inserted through the posterior musculature, aimed toward the coracoid process. As soon as the "pop" of capsular penetration is felt, the sharp trocar is replaced by the blunt trocar and the rim of the glenoid palpated as the cannula is advanced into the joint. The arthroscope is inserted and a rapid inspection is performed. Identification of the humeral head, anterior glenoid rim, and biceps tendon orients the viewer and allows placement of the second portal anteriorly.

Anterior Portal

A second portal is essential for effective ingress and egress of irrigation fluid and any type of instru-

FIG 2–24.
With patient in lateral decubitus position, bony
landmarks are outlined on prepped patient.

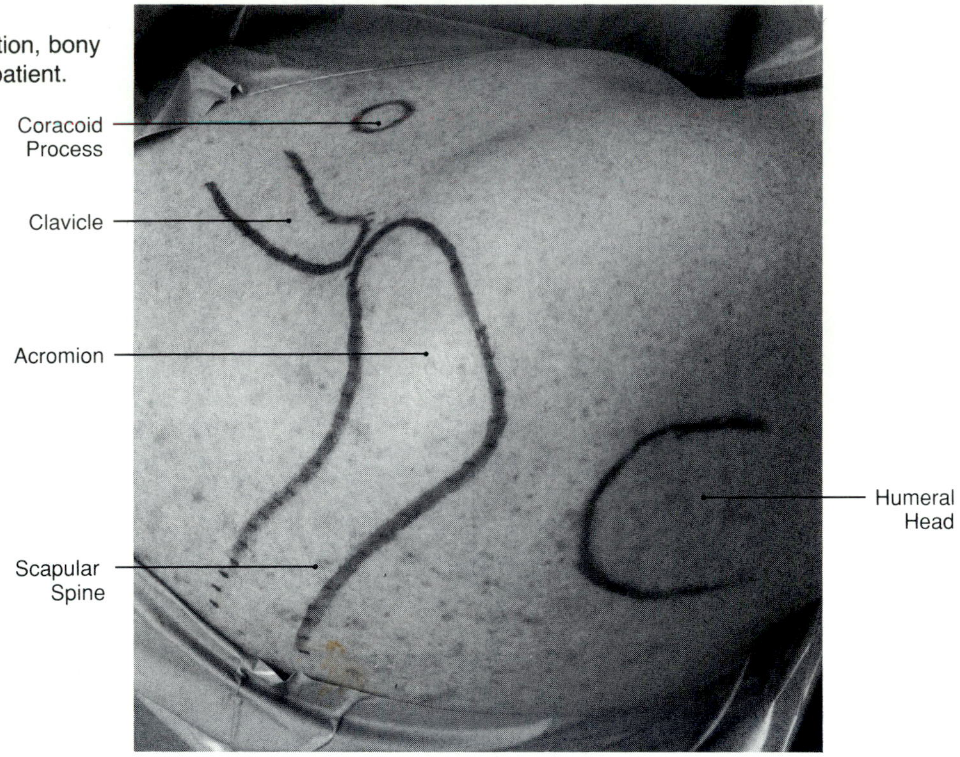

Coracoid
Process

Clavicle

Acromion

Scapular
Spine

Humeral
Head

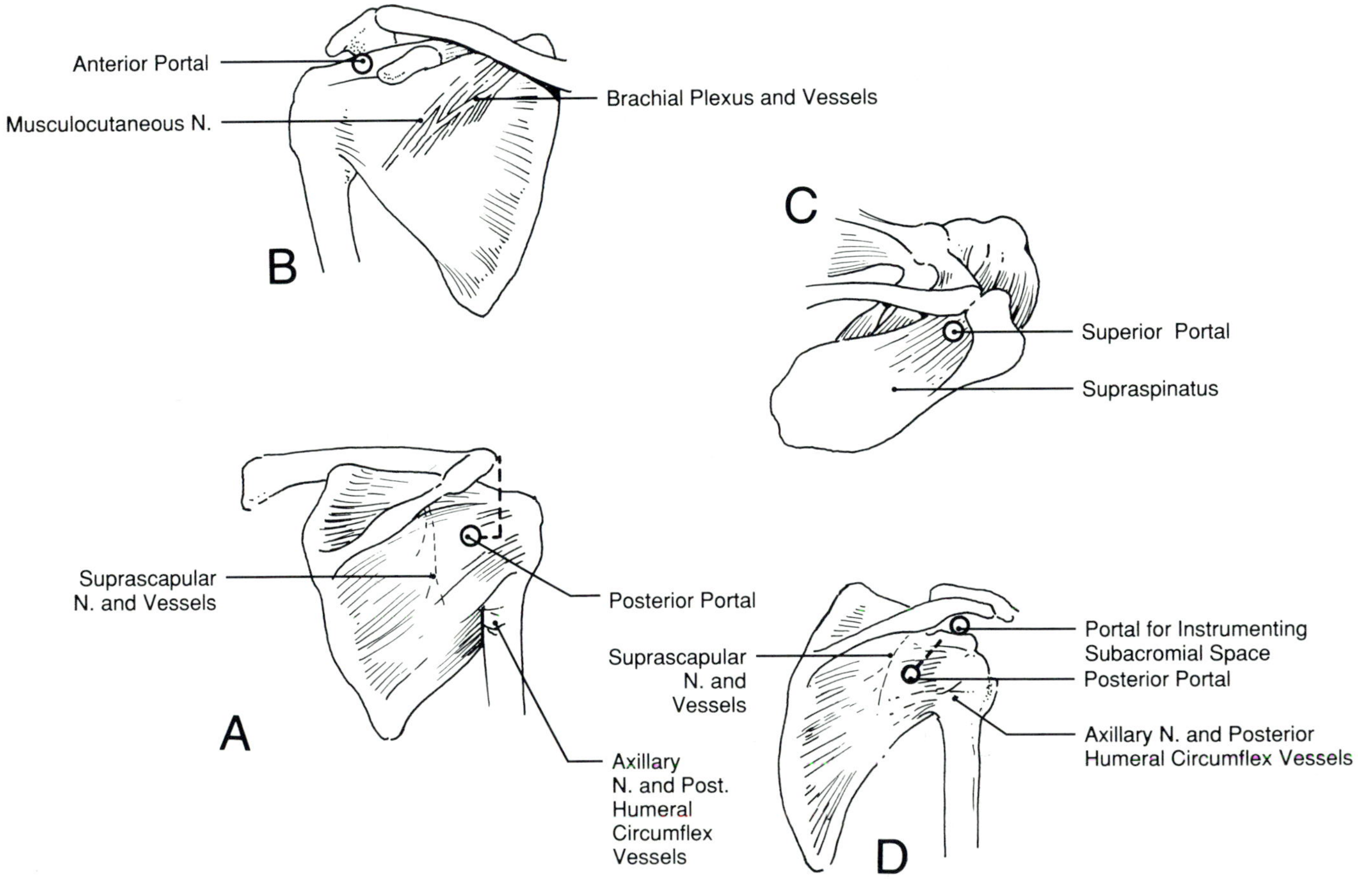

Anterior Portal

Musculocutaneous N.

Brachial Plexus and Vessels

B

C

Superior Portal

Supraspinatus

Suprascapular
N. and Vessels

Posterior Portal

Suprascapular
N. and
Vessels

Axillary
N. and Post.
Humeral
Circumflex
Vessels

A

Portal for Instrumenting
Subacromial Space
Posterior Portal

Axillary N. and Posterior
Humeral Circumflex Vessels

D

FIG 2–25.
Arthroscopy portals. Note location of brachial plexus and vessels, suprascapular nerve and vessels, and axillary nerve and
posterior humeral circumflex vessels. **A,** posterior portal. **B,** anterior portal. **C,** superior portal. **D,** portal for instrumentation of
subacromial space. Viewing arthroscope is introduced through the posterior portal and directed toward the subacromial space
(*dashed line* indicates path).

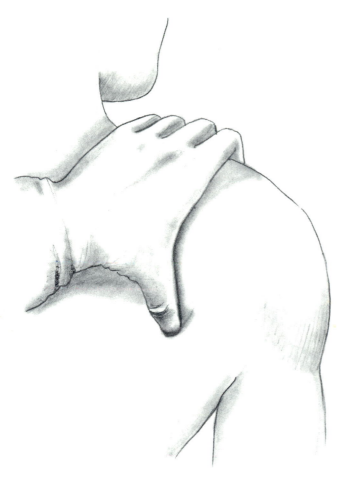

FIG 2–26.
Examiner's thumb locating entry site for posterior portal.

ternative method is to withdraw the arthroscope from its sheath after it is located anteriorly, and advance a Wissinger rod through the sheath and out anteriorly. An incision is made directly over the rod as it tents the skin. The portal can then be injected with local anesthetic with epinephrine along the rod and the 5.5 mm metal cannula advanced along the rod until it touches the arthroscope sheath. The arthroscope sheath is retracted 1 to 2 cm as the anterior cannula is simultaneously advanced. The rod is then withdrawn posteriorly and the arthroscope reinserted. The anterior sheath is now connected for proper fluid exchange or used for instrumentation. A 5.5-mm plastic operative cannula may be substituted if desired. A second anterior portal may be placed by using the first anterior portal as a landmark and passing an 18-gauge spinal needle cephalad (with the patient in lateral decubitus position) to the biceps tendon under direct visualization with the arthroscope. Placement of these portals too far medially or inferiorly may injure the musculocutaneous nerve or the neurovascular structures in the axilla.

Superior Portal

The superior portal, which passes through the muscular portion of the supraspinatus, provides a useful alternative access for fluid exchange or instrumentation. The entry site is determined by palpation of bony landmarks (the curved neck of the acromion laterally, the acromioclavicular joint anteriorly, and the acromial spine posteriorly) (see Fig 25,C). After palpation of a "soft spot" at this location, an 18-gauge spinal needle is passed into the joint. The needle is aimed approximately 20 degrees laterally and 15 degrees anteriorly. It should be visualized arthroscopically to pass just posterior to the biceps tendon origin on the glenoid. Injection of the portal and insertion of a metal cannula and trocar are then performed as described above.

With all intraarticular portals, it must be emphasized that the sharp trocar should not be advanced beyond the point of capsular penetration to avoid scuffing of intraarticular structures. To advance further, the blunt trocar must always be used. By use of the 5.5 mm metal cannulas, rotation of the arthroscope from one portal to another is easily accomplished. By placement of 4 mm rods in the desired instrumentation and arthroscope cannulas, the cannulas can then be withdrawn and switched over the rods (called "switch sticks"). This avoids the trauma of relocating the portals.

mentation; the anterior portal is routinely used for these functions. It is located approximately halfway between the coracoid process and the anterolateral border of the acromion (see Fig 2–25,B). Placement is determined by the intraarticular anatomy. A quadrangular space formed by the biceps tendon cephalad, the superior border of the subscapularis caudad, the humeral head laterally, and the anterior rim of the glenoid medially is located arthroscopically (Fig 2–27). The arthroscope is advanced into the center of this space to allow placement of the portal at the tip of the arthroscope in one of two ways. By transillumination through the anterior skin, an 18-gauge spinal needle can be advanced to the light. Its position can be checked with the arthroscope to confirm proper position. After injection of local anesthetic with epinephrine while the needle is withdrawn, a stab wound is made. A 5.5 mm metal cannula is advanced. The capsule is penetrated under direct vision with a sharp trocar and the cannula is advanced with a blunt trocar. An al-

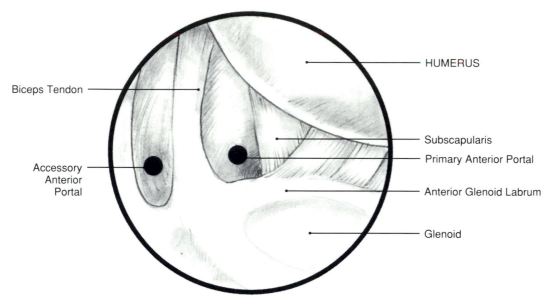

Biceps Tendon

Accessory
Anterior
Portal

HUMERUS

Subscapularis

Primary Anterior Portal

Anterior Glenoid Labrum

Glenoid

FIG 2–27.
Arthroscopic view from posterior portal.

Subacromial Bursa Examination

The subacromial bursa is an extraarticular "potential space" in which the rotator cuff and subacromial arch can be examined. The key to adequate visualization is distension of the bursa. Therefore, this examination is done last, allowing extravasation of fluid from the rest of the examination to distend the bursa. The arthroscope sheath with blunt trocar is advanced through the posterior portal subcutaneously in a superolateral direction toward the readily palpable inferior surface of the acromion. The arthroscope is then introduced and fluid inflow performed through the arthroscope for further distension of the bursa. A lateral portal for instrumentation of the subacromial space is placed at the inferior edge of the lateral tip of the acromion. A metal cannula with blunt trocar is inserted through a stab incision (see Fig 2–25,D).

BIBLIOGRAPHY

Abbott LC, Dec JB, Saunders M, et al: Surgical approaches to the shoulder joint. *J Bone Joint Surg* 1949; 31A:235–255.

Abbott LC, Larsen LJ, Jones EW, et al: Surgical approaches to the joints, in Cole WH (ed): *Operative Technic in Specialty Surgery.* New York, Appleton-Century Crofts, 1956, pp 539–638.

Abbott LC, Lucas DB: The tripartite deltoid and its surgical significance in exposure of the scapulohumeral joint. *Ann Surg* 1952; 136:392–403.

Andrews JR, Carson WG, Ortega K: Arthroscopy of the shoulder: Technique and normal anatomy. *Am J Sports Med* 1984; 12:1–7.

Banks SW, Laufman H: *An Atlas of Surgical Exposures of the Extremities.* Philadelphia, W B Saunders Co, 1953.

Bankhart ASB: The pathology and treatment of recurrent dislocation of the shoulder-joint. *Br J Surg* 1938–39; 26:23–29.

Bateman JE, Welsh RP: *Surgery of the Shoulder.* St. Louis, C V Mosby Co, 1984.

Bayley I, Kessel L (eds): *Shoulder Surgery.* New York, Springer-Verlag New York, 1982.

Bennett GE: Shoulder and elbow lesions of the professional baseball pitcher. *JAMA* 1941; 117:510–514.

Brodsky JW, Tullos HS, Garstman GM: Simplified posterior approach to the shoulder joint. *J Bone Joint Surg* 1987; 69A:773–774.

Consentino R: *Atlas of Anatomy and Surgical Approaches in Orthopedic Surgery.* Springfield, Ill, Charles C Thomas, Publishers, 1960.

Crenshaw AH: *Campbell's Operative Orthopaedics,* ed 7. St. Louis, C V Mosby Co, 1987.

Cubbins WR, Callahan JJ, Scuderi CS: The reduction of old or irreducible dislocations of the shoulder joint. *Surg Gynecol Obstet* 1934; 58:129–135.

Darrach W: Surgical approaches for surgery of the extremities. *Am J Surg* 1945; 67:237–262.

DePalma AF: *Surgery of the Shoulder,* ed 3. Philadelphia, JB Lippincott Co, 1983.

Detrisac DA, Johnson LL: *Arthroscopic Shoulder Anatomy: Pathologic and Surgical Implications.* Thorofare, NJ, Slack, 1986.

Goldstein LA, Dickerson RC: *Atlas of Orthopedic Surgery.* St Louis, The C V Mosby Co, 1974.

Goss CM: *Gray's Anatomy,* ed 29. Philadelphia, Lea & Febiger, 1973.

Grant JC: *An Atlas of Anatomy,* ed 5. Baltimore, Williams & Wilkins Co, 1962.

Guyot J: *Atlas of Human Limb Joints.* New York, Springer-Verlag New York, 1981.

Harty M, Joyce JJ: Surgical approaches to the shoulder. *Orthop Clin North Am* 1975, 6:553–564.

Henry AK: *Extensile exposure.* Baltimore, Williams & Wilkins Co, 1963.

Hollinshead WH: *Anatomy for Surgeons: The Back and Limbs,* ed 3. New York, Harper & Row, 1982.

Hollinshead WH, Jenkins DB: *Functional Anatomy of the Limbs and Back,* ed 5. Philadelphia, WB Saunders Co, 1981.

Johnson LL: Arthroscopy of the shoulder. *Orthop Clin North Am* 1980; 11:197–204.

Johnson LL: *Diagnostic and Surgical Arthroscopy: The Knee and Other Joints,* ed 2. St. Louis, C V Mosby Co, 1981.

Johnson, LL: *Arthroscopic Surgery: Principles and Practice,* ed 3. St Louis, C V Mosby Co, 1986.

Joyce JJ, Harty M: Surgical exposure of the shoulder. *J Bone Joint Surg* 1967; 49A:547–554.

Kessel L: The transacromial approach for rotator cuff rupture, in Bayley I, Kessel LK (eds): *Shoulder Surgery.* New York, Springer-Verlag New York, 1982, pp 39–44.

Leslie JT, Ryan TJ: The anterior axillary incision to approach the shoulder joint. *J Bone Joint Surg* 1962; 44A:1193–1196.

Martini M: The subdeltoid approach to the proximal humerus, in Bayley I, Kessel LK (eds): *Shoulder Surgery,* New York, Springer-Verlag New York, 1982, pp 199–204.

McLaughlin HC: Lesions of the musculotendinous cuff of the shoulder: The exposure and treatment of tears with retraction. *J Bone Joint Surg* 1944; 26:31–51.

Moore, KL: *Clinically Oriented Anatomy,* ed 2. Baltimore, Williams & Wilkins Co, 1985.

Neer CS: Anterior acromioplasty for the chronic impingement syndrome in the shoulder. *J Bone Joint Surg* 1972; 54A:41–50.

Neviaser TJ: Arthroscopy of the shoulder. *Orthop Clin North Am* 1987; 18:361–372.

Post M (ed): *The Shoulder: Surgical and nonsurgical management,* ed 2. Philadelphia, Lea & Febiger, 1988.

Rowe CR, Yee LBK: A posterior approach to the shoulder joint. *J Bone Joint Surg* 1944; 26:581–584.

Slocum DB: *An Atlas of Amputations.* St Louis, C V Mosby Co, 1949.

Toumey JW, Haggart GE: Surgery of the shoulder joint. *Surg Clin North Am* 1942, 22(3):883–897.

Wiley AM, Older MWJ: Shoulder arthroscopy. *Am J Sports Med* 1980; 8:31–38.

Zarins B: Arthroscopy of the shoulder: Technique, in Zarins B, Andrews JR, Carson WG (eds): *Injuries to the Throwing Arm.* Philadelphia, W B Saunders Co, 1985.

Arm

Frederick W. Reckling, M.D.
Melvin P. Mohn, Ph.D.

ANATOMIC FEATURES OF THE ARM

The arrangement of the musculature, nerves, and vessels of the arm is relatively simple. Operations on the arm generally involve open reduction–internal fixation of fractures and/or exploration of neurovascular structures. All approaches to the humerus are potentially dangerous because the major nerves and vessels run much closer to this bone than they do elsewhere in the body (Fig 3–1).

Bony Anatomy

The upper end of the humerus is formed by the head and the greater and lesser tubercles (Fig 3–2). The rounded head, which is covered with articular cartilage, is directed upward medially and posteriorly. The greater tubercle, or tuberosity, is on the lateral side of the upper end of the humerus. The lesser tubercle is on the anterior aspect of the upper end of the humerus. Between the two tubercles lies the intertubercular, or bicipital, groove. The small rim of bone at the edge of the articular surface just proximal to the tubercles is considered the anatomical neck. The narrowest part of the body or shaft of the humerus lies just below the tubercles. This is referred to as the surgical neck because of the relative frequency of fractures that occur there. The shaft of the humerus is cylindrical in shape except for the distal portion, which is flattened in the sagittal plane. In the middle third of the anterolateral surface of the humerus is a prominence, the so-called deltoid tuberosity, on which the deltoid muscle inserts. The posterior surface of the humerus is crossed obliquely by a shallow groove known as the radial or spiral groove that runs downward and laterally from behind the deltoid tuberosity.

The lower end of the humerus has two articular surfaces; a medial trochlea, which articulates with the ulna, and a lateral capitellum, which articulates with the radial head. Just proximal to the trochlea is a cavitation, known as the coronoid fossa, in the anterior surface of the humerus. This cavitation receives the coronoid process of the ulna when the forearm is flexed. On the posterior surface is a larger cavitation, known as the olecranon fossa, which receives the olecranon when the elbow is extended. The flattened lower end of the humerus displays sharp edges known as supracondylar ridges. The medial and lateral intermuscular septa of the arm are attached to these ridges. The lateral supracondylar ridge ends in the lateral epicondyle, and the medial supracondylar ridge ends in the more prominent medial epicondyle.

Muscles

The muscles of the arm consist of the biceps brachii, coracobrachialis, and brachialis muscles, which are found on the anterior, or flexor, surface of the humerus, and the triceps and anconeus, which

ANTERIOR

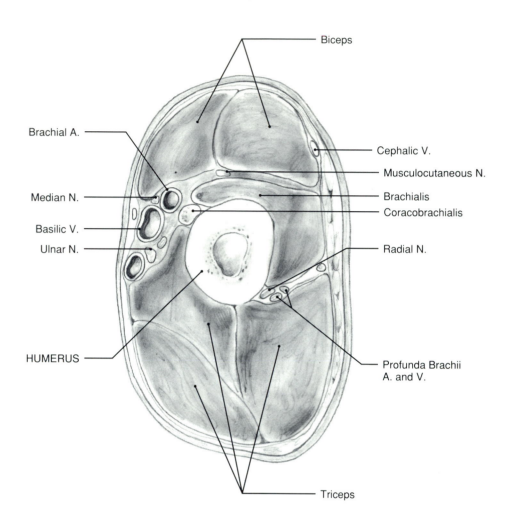

Biceps

Brachial A.

Cephalic V.

Musculocutaneous N.

Median N.

Brachialis

Coracobrachialis

Basilic V.

Ulnar N.

Radial N.

HUMERUS

Profunda Brachii
A. and V.

Triceps

POSTERIOR

FIG 3–1.
Cross-sectional anatomy of the arm at midhumeral-shaft level. Note the close approximation of the neurovascular structures to the humerus.

are found posteriorly (Fig 3–3). Although the brachioradialis and wrist flexors and extensors arise from the distal humerus, they are described in the chapters on the elbow and forearm.

The most superficial muscle of the anterior aspect of the arm is the biceps brachii, which almost entirely covers the underlying brachialis muscle (Fig 3–4). It arises from two heads. The long head arises from the supraglenoid tubercle of the scapula by means of a long tendon that traverses the shoulder joint covered by a reflection of synovial membrane and passes downward between the two humeral tu-

berosities. The weak transverse humeral ligament holds the biceps tendon in the bicipital groove. In this location the tendon is crossed anteriorly by the tendon of the pectoralis major muscle. As the biceps tendon emerges from the capsule of the shoulder joint it forms a muscular belly behind the lower part of the insertion of the pectoralis major. The short head of the biceps arises from the coracoid process. This head of the muscle unites with the long head at a somewhat variable level, commonly about the junction of the middle and lower thirds of the arm. The biceps inserts through two tendinous attach-

FIG 3–2.
Humerus.

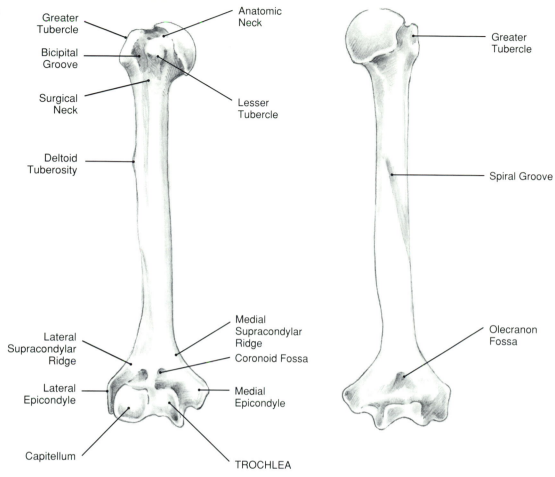

Greater Tubercle
Bicipital Groove
Surgical Neck
Deltoid Tuberosity
Anatomic Neck
Lesser Tubercle
Lateral Supracondylar Ridge
Lateral Epicondyle
Capitellum
Medial Supracondylar Ridge
Coronoid Fossa
Medial Epicondyle
TROCHLEA
Greater Tubercle
Spiral Groove
Olecranon Fossa

ANTERIOR

POSTERIOR

ments, the rounded and strong tendon proper and the rather thin, broad, and flattened bicipital aponeurosis (lacertus fibrosus). The biceps tendon proper passes deeply between the origins of the flexor and extensor forearm muscles into the cubital fossa, where it inserts on the posterior part of the tuberosity of the radius. The medial border of the tendon and the lower medial muscular portion of the muscle give rise to the bicipital aponeurosis. The aponeurosis joins the deep fascia over the upper ends of the flexor muscles of the forearm after passing downward and medially across the cubital fossa. The biceps is an important flexor of the elbow and supinator of the forearm. This is particularly true when the arm is supinated with elbow flexion. The biceps brachii is innervated by the musculocutaneous nerve.

The coracobrachialis muscle arises with the short head of the biceps from the coracoid process and in-serts into the medial border of the midshaft of the humerus. The coracobrachialis is a flexor and adductor of the arm and may help to prevent shoulder subluxation from the powerful downward pull of the adductors, namely the pectoralis major and latissimus dorsi.

The lower one half to two thirds of the anterior surface of the body of the humerus and the adjacent medial and lateral intermuscular septa give rise to the brachialis muscle (Fig 3–5). The body and tendon of the muscle are closely related to the anterior aspect of the elbow joint. The brachialis inserts into the lower part of the coronoid process and the tuberosity of the ulna. Its sole action is elbow flexion. The brachialis is innervated by the musculocutaneous nerve, and it may also receive a branch of the radial nerve. Controversy exists as to whether this is a motor branch or solely a proprioceptive branch to the elbow joint.

FIG 3–3.
Muscles of the arm (lateral view).

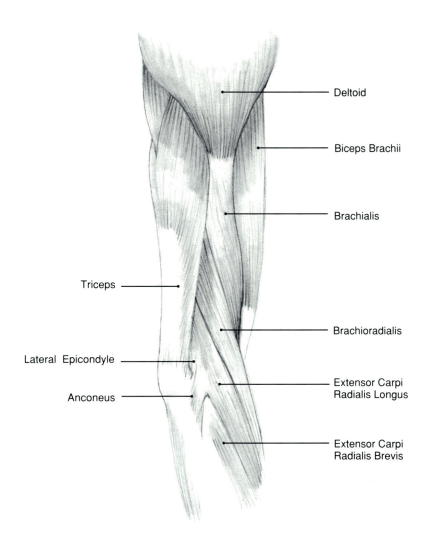

Deltoid

Biceps Brachii

Brachialis

Triceps

Brachioradialis

Lateral Epicondyle

Extensor Carpi
Radialis Longus

Anconeus

Extensor Carpi
Radialis Brevis

FIG 3–4.
Muscles of the front of the arm.

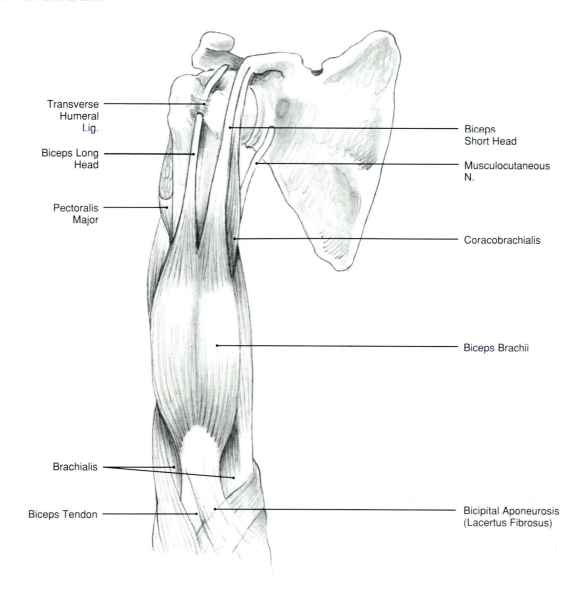

Transverse Humeral Lig.

Biceps Long Head

Pectoralis Major

Biceps Short Head

Musculocutaneous N.

Coracobrachialis

Biceps Brachii

Brachialis

Biceps Tendon

Bicipital Aponeurosis (Lacertus Fibrosus)

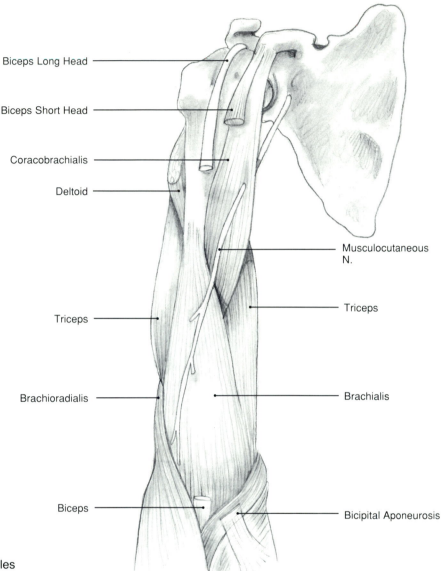

Biceps Long Head

Biceps Short Head

Coracobrachialis

Deltoid

Musculocutaneous N.

Triceps

Triceps

Brachioradialis

Brachialis

Biceps

Bicipital Aponeurosis

FIG 3–5.
Muscles deep to the biceps. Note distribution of the musculocutaneous nerve to the coracobrachialis and brachialis muscles (biceps has been removed).

The triceps occupies almost the whole of the back of the arm (Fig 3–6). As the name implies, it has three heads of origin. The long head originates from the infraglenoid tubercle on the lateral border of the scapula, and as it passes downward it lies in front of the teres minor but behind the teres major. The lateral head of the triceps originates from the posterior surface of the humerus proximal to the radial groove and from the lateral intermuscular septum. The lateral and long heads form the lateral and medial portions of the proximal muscle and unite to form almost the entire portion of the muscle, which is visible superficially. The medial head of the triceps muscle (Fig 3–7), in reality is the deep head. It has an extensive origin from the entire posterior sur-

face of the humerus below the radial groove, from the medial intermuscular septum, and from the lower part of the lateral intermuscular septum, below the point at which the radial nerve passes through this septum. This medial (deep) head of the triceps, present on the medial as well as the lateral side of the arm, attaches to the deep surface of the combined long and lateral triceps heads. The entire muscle crosses the posterior surface of the elbow joint as a broad, powerful tendon and inserts into the olecranon. The muscle is a strong extensor of the elbow and is assisted in this action by the anconeus. The triceps is innervated by the radial nerve.

The anconeus (see Figs 3–3 and 3–6) is a small triangular muscle that originates from the distal end

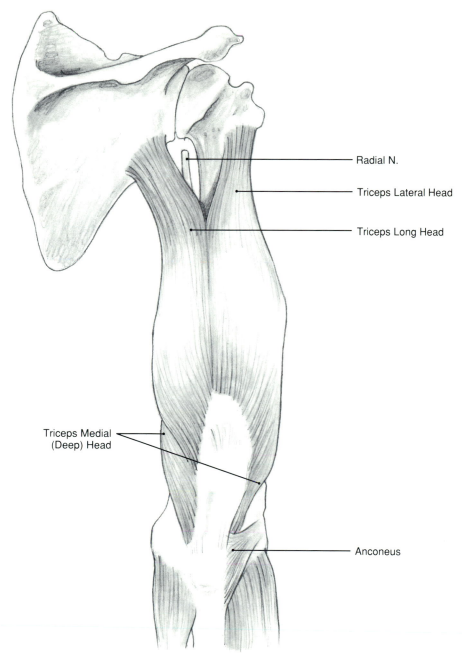

Radial N.

Triceps Lateral Head

Triceps Long Head

Triceps Medial
(Deep) Head

Anconeus

FIG 3–6.
Muscles of the back of the arm. Long and lateral head of the triceps and anconeus.

of the posterior aspect of the lateral epicondyle of the humerus. It spreads out to insert on the lateral side of the olecranon and the proximal posterior surface of the body of the ulna. The anconeus is primarily an elbow extensor, although some investigators have attributed to it an action of abduction of the ulna when the forearm is moved from extreme supination to extreme pronation. The anconeus is innervated by the radial nerve.

Nerves

The muscles on the anterior surface of the arm are innervated by the musculocutaneous nerve, which derives from the lateral cord of the brachial plexus. The muscles on the posterior surface of the arm are innervated by the radial nerve from the posterior cord of the brachial plexus. The median and ulnar nerves traverse the arm on the way to the fore-

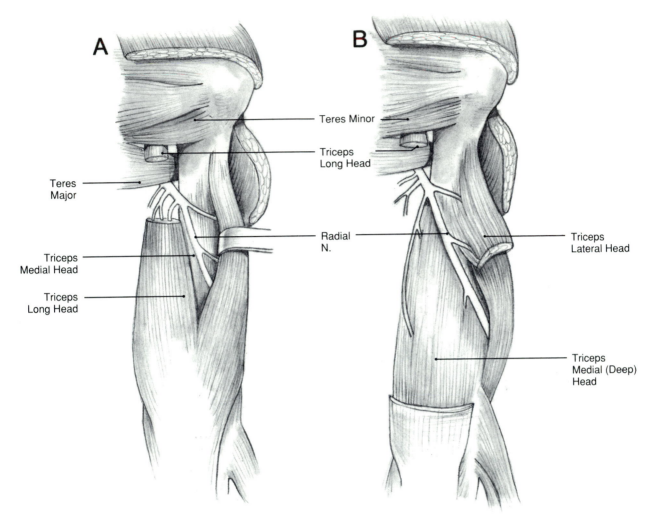

FIG 3–7.
Medial (deep) head of the triceps and distribution of branches of the radial nerve to the triceps. **A,** a portion of the long head of the triceps has been removed. **B,** portions of the long and lateral heads of the triceps have been removed to show the distribution of the radial nerve to the medial (deep) head of the triceps.

arm and hand. These nerves usually give no branches in the arm except perhaps for articular ones to the elbow joint.

The musculocutaneous nerve (Fig 3–8) is one of the terminal branches of the lateral cord. Its fibers arise primarily from the fifth and sixth cervical nerves. As it courses laterally it lies between the co-racobrachialis muscle and axillary artery. It supplies the coracobrachialis muscle via one or more branches, and continues, perforating this muscle. It then lies between the biceps and brachialis muscles and supplies a branch to both heads of the biceps and a branch to the brachialis. From then on it is purely cutaneous and emerges lateral to the tendon of the biceps, becoming the lateral antebrachial cutaneous nerve of the forearm.

The median nerve (Fig 3–9), which has contributions from the lateral and medial cords of the brachial plexus, is formed anterior or anterolateral to the brachial artery. In the middle of the arm it crosses the artery anteriorly. In the antecubital fossa the median nerve lies medial to the artery and deep to the bicipital aponeurosis. In the forearm it disappears between the two heads of the pronator teres muscle.

The ulnar nerve arises from the medial cord where it is situated between the axillary artery and vein. It lies medial or posterior to the brachial artery in the proximal half of the arm but diverges near the middle of the arm to penetrate the medial intermuscular septum. It is joined on the front of the medial head of the triceps muscle by the superior ulnar col-

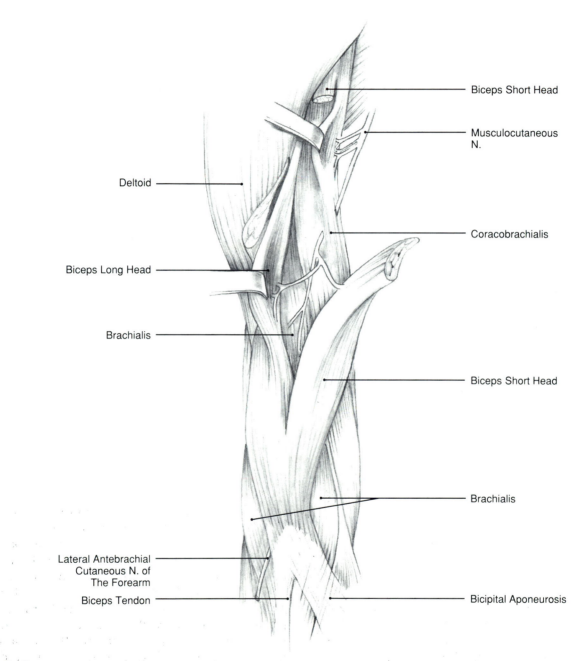

Biceps Short Head

Musculocutaneous N.

Deltoid

Coracobrachialis

Biceps Long Head

Brachialis

Biceps Short Head

Brachialis

Lateral Antebrachial Cutaneous N. of The Forearm

Biceps Tendon

Bicipital Aponeurosis

FIG 3–8.
Relationship of the musculocutaneous nerve to the musculature in the front of the arm.

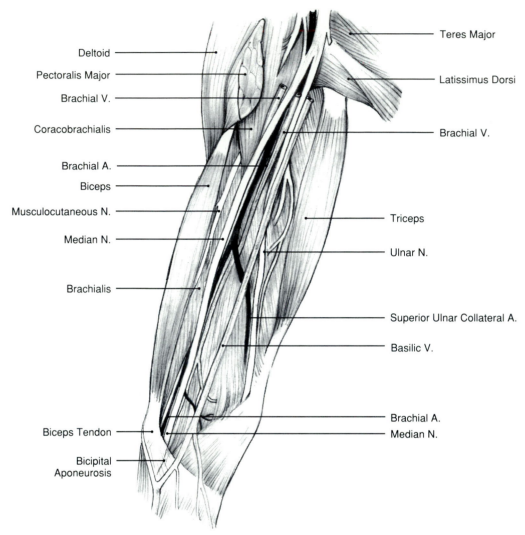

Deltoid

Pectoralis Major

Brachial V.

Coracobrachialis

Brachial A.

Biceps

Musculocutaneous N.

Median N.

Brachialis

Biceps Tendon

Bicipital Aponeurosis

Teres Major

Latissimus Dorsi

Brachial V.

Triceps

Ulnar N.

Superior Ulnar Collateral A.

Basilic V.

Brachial A.

Median N.

FIG 3–9.
Anterior view of right arm: relationship of median and ulnar nerves to the brachial artery.

lateral artery. They descend together on the anterior surface of the triceps muscle and pass behind the medial epicondyle. The nerve enters the forearm between the humeral and ulnar heads of the flexor carpi ulnaris muscle.

The radial nerve (Fig 3–10), the larger of the two terminal branches of the posterior cord, may contain fibers from all the nerves entering the brachial plexus. Most fibers contributing to the nerve are usually from the seventh cervical root. After separating from the other major branch of the posterior cord, the axillary nerve, the radial nerve lies behind the axillary artery. In the axillary area it lies on the surface of the subscapularis, teres major, and latissimus dorsi muscles. As it descends in the proximal arm it lies behind the brachial artery. As the radial nerve passes laterally and posteriorly with the pro-

funda brachii artery, it lies deep to the long head of the triceps muscle. In the posterior aspect of the arm it lies deep to the lateral head and therefore between the lateral and medial (deep) heads of the triceps, close to, but not in, the spiral groove of the humerus. The radial nerve is vulnerable and sometimes injured with humerus fractures in the region. The nerve, along with the radial collateral branch of the profunda brachii artery, pierces the lateral intermuscular septum as it reaches the lateral border of the medial (deep) head of the triceps. As it gains the anterior aspect of the arm it lies between the brachioradialis and brachialis muscle. In this area, where it is intimately associated with the brachialis muscle, the radial nerve is vulnerable to injury. When the distal humerus is exposed anteriorly, careful subperiosteal dissection of the brachialis muscle

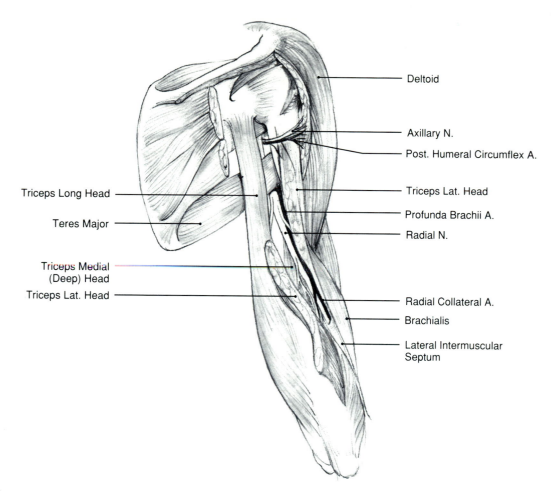

Deltoid

Axillary N.

Post. Humeral Circumflex A.

Triceps Long Head

Teres Major

Triceps Lat. Head

Profunda Brachii A.

Radial N.

Triceps Medial
(Deep) Head

Triceps Lat. Head

Radial Collateral A.

Brachialis

Lateral Intermuscular
Septum

FIG 3–10.
Posterior view: the radial nerve and its relationship to other structures.

must be carried out to prevent injury to the radial nerve.

Arteries

The arterial supply to the arm is via the brachial artery, which is a continuation of the axillary artery (Fig 3–11). There can be considerable anatomical variance of this artery and its branches. The brachial artery begins at the lower border of the teres major muscle. This artery normally undergoes no appreciable diminution in size during its course through the arm, and it ends by dividing into radial and ulnar arteries in the forearm. At first the artery lies on the medial side of the arm in front of the long head of the triceps, and then it lies on the medial head of the triceps. As it descends it courses anteriorly along the medial border of the biceps to the anterior surface of the brachialis muscle. It then passes into the cubital fossa, deep to the aponeurosis of the biceps (lacertus fibrosus). It is usually accompanied by two brachial veins, one medial and one lateral to it, with numerous anastomoses between them. Although there may be considerable variation, the named branches of the brachial artery above its terminal ones are the profunda brachii, the nutrient artery of the humerus, and the superior and inferior ulnar collateral arteries. In addition, the artery gives branches to the muscles of the front and medial side of the arm.

The profunda brachii is the largest branch of the brachial artery in the arm. It arises in the upper part of the arm. It courses downward and laterally behind the brachial artery in conjunction with the radial nerve as they spiral around the posterior surface of the humerus. Just as the profunda reaches the lateral intermuscular septum it divides into two branches. One of these, the middle collateral artery, runs on or in the medial head of the triceps and then takes part in the anastomosis about the elbow. The other branch of the profunda is the radial collateral artery. This artery passes through the lateral intermuscular septum with the radial nerve. It descends

FIG 3–11.
Arteries of the arm (anterior view).

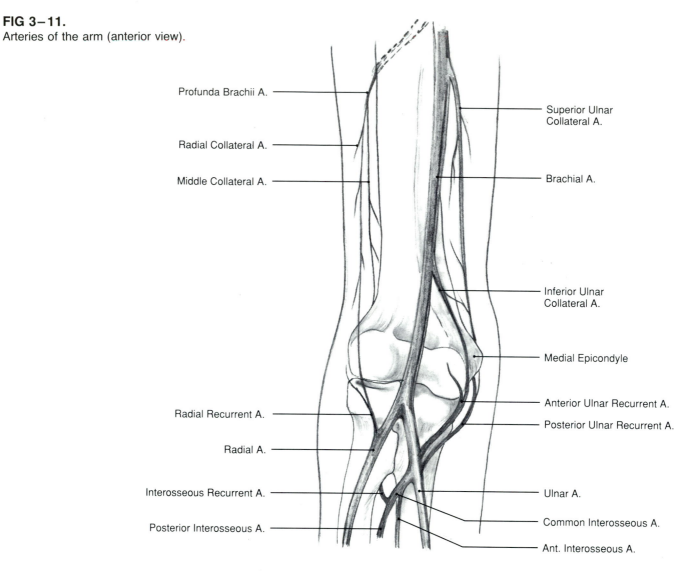

Profunda Brachii A.

Radial Collateral A.

Middle Collateral A.

Superior Ulnar Collateral A.

Brachial A.

Inferior Ulnar Collateral A.

Medial Epicondyle

Radial Recurrent A.

Radial A.

Anterior Ulnar Recurrent A.

Posterior Ulnar Recurrent A.

Interosseous Recurrent A.

Posterior Interosseous A.

Ulnar A.

Common Interosseous A.

Ant. Interosseous A.

with this nerve between the origins of the brachialis muscle and the upper extensor muscles of the forearm. It gives branches to the neighboring muscles and then anastomoses with the radial recurrent artery.

The superior ulnar collateral artery arises from the brachial artery at about the middle of the arm. It passes downward and backward with the ulnar nerve through the medial intermuscular septum to the back of the medial epicondyle, where it anastomoses with the posterior ulnar recurrent artery and at times with the inferior ulnar collateral artery.

The inferior ulnar collateral artery arises from the posteromedial surface of the brachial approximately 4 cm above the medial epicondyle. It runs downward on the brachialis muscle and anastomoses with the posterior ulnar recurrent artery.

SURGICAL APPROACHES TO THE ARM

The humerus may be approached anteriorly, anterolaterally, laterally, or posteriorly to carry out internal fixation of fractures, biopsy or resection of bone tumors, or management of infection. All of these approaches put the neurovascular structures at risk.

Anterior Approach

The anterior approach to the humerus (Fig 3–12) is a distal continuation of the deltopectoral approach to the shoulder. An incision is begun at the coracoid

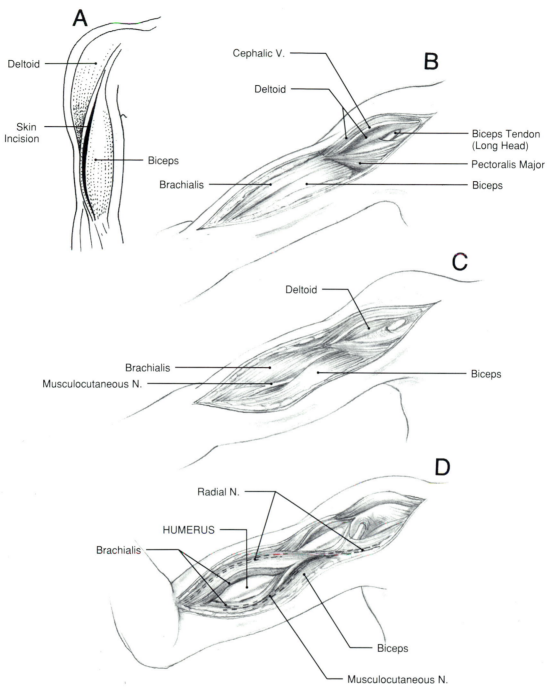

FIG 3–12.
Anterior approach to the arm. **A,** skin incision. **B,** development of the deltopectoral groove proximally. The proximal humerus is exposed by incising the periosteum just lateral to the pectoralis major insertion. Wider exposure may be obtained by reflecting the insertions of the deltoid and pectoralis major. Care must be taken to avoid injury to the axillary nerve when the deltoid is retracted. **C,** distally, the interval between the biceps and brachialis is developed by retracting the biceps medially. The musculocutaneous nerve is identified and gently retracted with the biceps. **D,** note retraction of the musculocutaneous nerve *(dashed line)* with the biceps. The brachialis is split longitudinally and dissected subperiosteally from the humerus. Care is taken to stay in the subperiosteal plane to avoid injury to the radial nerve *(dashed line)* where it lies in the spiral groove on the posterolateral surface of the middle third of the humerus.

(Continued.)

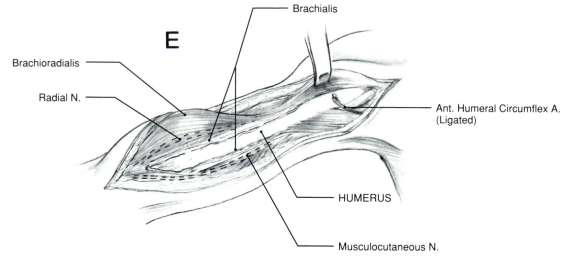

FIG 3–12 (cont.).
E, exposure of entire humerus. Note that proximally the anterior humeral circumflex artery crosses the field from medial to lateral and must be ligated or cauterized.

process and continued distally and laterally over the deltopectoral groove and then distally along the lateral border of the biceps. The incision must end at least 5 cm proximal to the flexion crease of the elbow to prevent injury to the radial nerve as it enters the anterior compartment of the arm between the brachioradialis and brachialis muscles. The deltopectoral interval in the proximal portion of the wound is developed. The proximal portion of the humerus is exposed by an incision into the periosteum just lateral to the pectoralis major. For wider exposure of the humerus the pectoralis major muscle may be reflected off its humeral attachment and the deltoid reflected off its insertion at the deltoid tuberosity. Care must be taken to avoid injury to the axillary nerve when the deltoid is retracted. The anterior humeral circumflex artery, which crosses the field from medial to lateral between the pectoralis major insertion and deltoid, must be ligated or cauterized.

For further exposure of the humeral shaft distally, the deep fascia of the arm is incised in line with the skin incision and the interval between the biceps and brachialis identified. By medial retraction of the biceps, the brachialis muscle, which covers almost the entire anterior portion of the distal humerus, is exposed. The musculocutaneous nerve, which lies between the biceps and brachialis, must be identified and protected. Splitting the fibers of the brachialis longitudinally and incising the periosteum allows exposure of the anterior surface of the humeral shaft. The brachialis muscle is then reflected from its origin. This maneuver is facilitated by flexing the elbow to take tension off the brachialis

while it is stripped from the humerus. Careful reflection of the brachialis muscle in the subperiosteal plane anteriorly will prevent injury to the radial nerve, which lies in the spiral groove in the posterolateral surface of the middle third of the humerus.

Anterolateral Approach to the Shaft of the Humerus

The distal two thirds of the humerus can be exposed from an anterolateral approach to carry out internal fixation of humeral fractures and explore associated radial nerve injuries (Fig 3–13). An incision is made over the lateral border of the biceps, beginning approximately 10 cm above the flexion crease of the elbow and continued distally to the level of the flexion crease. The deep fascia of the arm is incised in line with the skin incision along the lateral border of the biceps. Retraction of the biceps medially reveals the brachialis and brachioradialis muscles. The interval between these muscles is developed. By retraction of the brachialis and biceps medially and the brachioradialis laterally, the radial nerve is located. The nerve can then be traced proximally to where it pierces the lateral intermuscular septum. The radial nerve is retracted laterally with care. The lateral borders of the brachialis muscles are stripped from the humerus and retracted medially. This allows exposure of the distal humeral shaft. During this exposure the lateral antebrachial cutaneous nerve of the forearm (a continuation of the musculocutaneous nerve) should be identified and retracted medially with the biceps and brachialis.

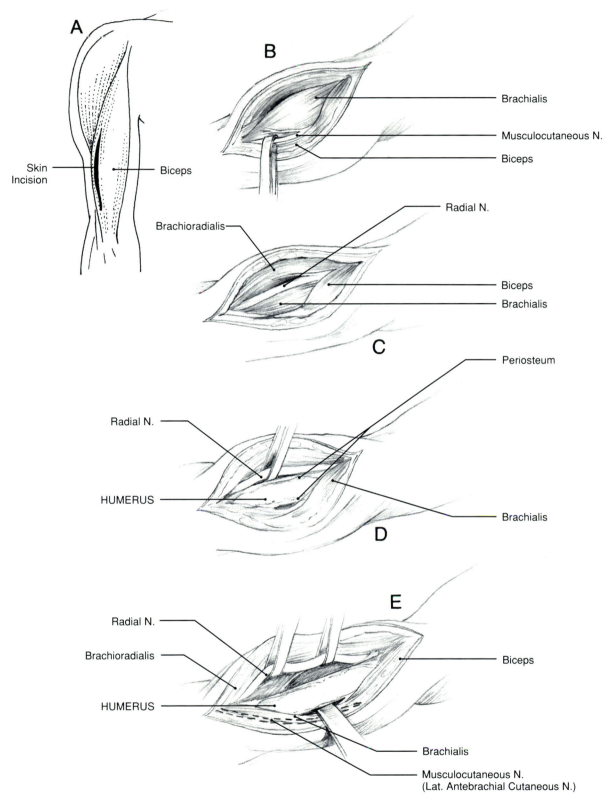

FIG 3–13.
Anterolateral approach to the shaft of the humerus. **A,** skin incision. **B,** fascia incised in line with the skin incision. Retraction of the biceps to reveal the brachialis and brachioradialis and the musculocutaneous nerve. **C,** interval between the brachialis and brachioradialis is developed, exposing the radial nerve. **D,** the radial nerve is carefully retracted laterally and the lateral portion of the brachialis stripped from the humerus. The lateral antebrachial cutaneous nerve of the forearm, which is a continuation of the musculocutaneous nerve, has been identified and retracted with the biceps and brachialis. **E,** wide exposure of the anterolateral shaft of the humerus.

Posterior Approach to the Humerus

The posterior approach to the humerus (Fig 3–14) is most often utilized for exploration of the radial nerve in the spiral groove. This approach also facilitates internal fixation of the humerus when nerve injury is associated with a fracture of the humerus. The posterior approach can also be used in dealing with infections or tumors that involve the distal two thirds of the humerus.

An incision is made in the midline of the posterior arm, beginning about 8 cm below the acromion and continuing down to the olecranon. The fascia is incised in line with the skin incision. The interval between the lateral and long heads of the triceps is developed by blunt dissection, with the lateral head

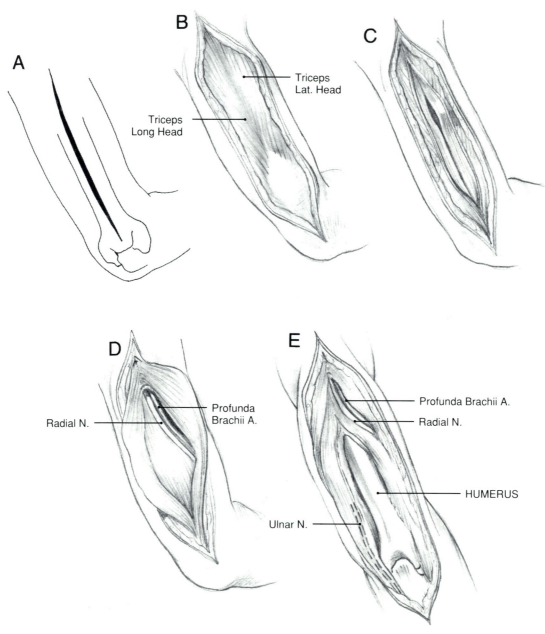

FIG 3–14.

Posterior approach to the humerus. **A,** skin incision. **B,** interval between the lateral and long heads of the triceps is identified. **C,** the interval is developed and the common tendon split distally. **D,** the radial nerve and profunda brachii vessels are identified and exposed. **E,** the medial (deep) head of the triceps is incised in the midline and stripped from the humerus subperiosteally. Care must be taken to keep the dissection subperiosteal to prevent injury to the ulnar nerve, which pierces the medial intermuscular septum as it passes from the anterior to the posterior compartment in the lower third of the arm.

retracted laterally and the medial head medially. As dissection is carried distally the common tendon is split by sharp dissection. The medial (deep) head of the triceps lies below the long and lateral heads. It arises from the posterior humerus, distal to the spiral groove. The radial nerve runs just proximal to the origin of the medial head of the triceps in the spiral groove of the humerus. Care must be taken to identify the radial nerve and the accompanying profunda brachii artery. The medial head of the triceps is incised in the midline, and subperiosteal stripping allows exposure of the distal two thirds of the humerus. Care must also be taken to keep the dissection subperiosteal. This prevents injury to the ulnar

nerve, which pierces the medial intermuscular septum as it passes from the anterior to posterior compartment in the lower third of the arm.

Lateral Approach to the Distal Humerus

The lateral portion of the distal humerus can be approached (Fig 3–15) by developing the plane between the brachioradialis and the triceps. This will allow exposure for open reduction and internal fixation of fractures of the lateral humeral condyle.

A skin incision is made over the supracondylar ridge for a distance of 4 to 6 cm. The interval between the brachioradialis and triceps is identified

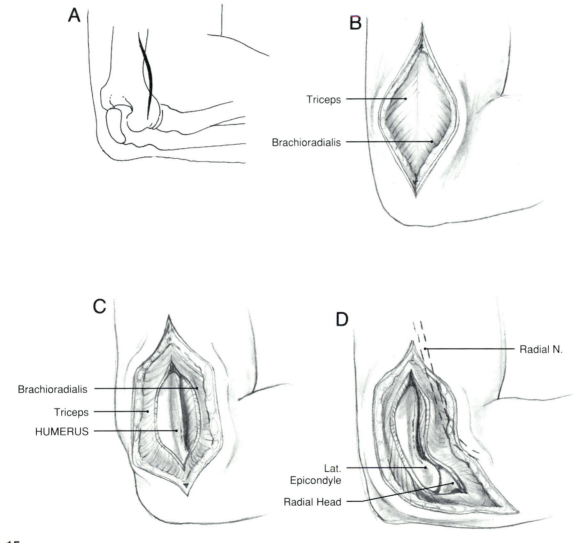

FIG 3–15.
Lateral approach to the distal humerus. **A,** skin incision. **B,** interval between the triceps and brachioradialis is identified. **C,** interval is developed; triceps retraction posteriorly and brachioradialis anteriorly exposes humerus. **D,** distal extension of the dissection exposes the elbow joint. Note: the radial nerve *(dotted lines),* which passes anteriorly between the brachioradialis and brachialis.

and developed. The periosteum is incised, and the triceps is retracted posteriorly and the brachioradialis anteriorly. To avoid injury to the radial nerve, care must be taken not to extend the incision more than 5 to 6 cm proximal to the elbow crease. Extension of this approach distally between the anconeus and extensor carpi ulnaris will allow exposure of the head of the radius.

BIBLIOGRAPHY

Banks SW, Laufman, H.: *An Atlas of Surgical Exposures of the Extremities.* Philadelphia, W B Saunders Co, 1953.

Crenshaw AH: *Operative Orthopaedics,* ed 7. St Louis, C V Mosby Co, 1987.

Grant JC: *Atlas of Anatomy,* ed 8. Baltimore, Williams & Wilkins Co, 1983.

Henry AK: Exposure of the humerus and femoral shaft. *Br J Surg* 1924–25; 12:84–91.

Henry AK: *Extensile Exposure.* Baltimore, Williams & Wilkins Co, 1963.

Hollinshead WH: *Anatomy for Surgeons: The Back and Limbs,* ed 3. Philadelphia, Harper & Row, 1982.

Hoppenfeld S, deBoer P: *Surgical Exposures in Orthopaedics: The Anatomic Approach.* Philadelphia, J B Lippincott Co, 1984.

Moore KL: *Clinically Oriented Anatomy.* Baltimore, Williams & Wilkins Co, 1985.

Thompson JE: Anatomical methods of approach in operations on the long bones of the extremities. *Ann Surg* 1918; 68:309–329.

4

Elbow

Charles E. Rhoades, M.D.

ANATOMIC FEATURES OF THE ELBOW

The elbow is a complex joint that acts as a component link of the lever arm system. Its functions include allowing the hand to be positioned in space, providing power to perform lifting activities, and stabilizing the upper extremity linkage for power and fine work activities.

Bony Anatomy and Articular Surfaces

The osseous structures of the elbow joint include (1) the distal humerus, (2) the proximal radius, and (3) the proximal ulna (Fig 4–1). These bones form three articulations: the ulnohumeral (ulnotrochlear), radiohumeral (radiocapitellar), and proximal radioulnar joints.

The distal humerus consists of two condyles, which provide the two proximal articular surfaces of the elbow, the trochlea and capitellum. A prominent groove separates the capitellum from the trochlea. Just proximal to the articular surfaces are the epicondyles, which serve as sites for muscle and ligament origins. On the anterior surface of the distal humerus are two concavities: a lateral one, known as the radial fossa, which accepts the radial head when the elbow is fully flexed, and a central one, known as the coronoid fossa, which accepts the coronoid process of the ulna when the elbow is fully flexed. On the posterior surface of the distal humerus between the medial and lateral epicondyles is

an indentation known as the olecranon fossa. This fossa accommodates the olecranon when the elbow is extended.

The proximal radius and ulna together form the distal portion of the elbow joint. The cylindrical radial head articulates with the hemispherical capitellum of the humerus and with the radial notch of the proximal ulna. The large cup-shaped proximal end of the ulna, with its coronoid and olecranon processes, articulates with the trochlea of the humerus. The trochlea of the humerus forms the keystone of the elbow. It provides a hinged articulation with the cuplike trochlear notch of the proximal ulna, allowing elbow flexion and extension. The trochlea is pulley-shaped, having ridges medially and laterally with a central groove. The trochlear notch of the ulna (also known as the greater sigmoid or greater semilunar notch), runs from the coronoid to the olecranon process of the ulna. When viewed sagittally, the trochlear notch can be separated into anterior (coronoid) and posterior (olecranon) sections. When seen frontally, the notch is divided in the center by the trochlear ridge, a guiding ridge that articulates with the central trochlear groove of the humerus.

On the anterolateral aspect of the coronoid process of the ulna is a semicircular depression known as the radial notch (lesser sigmoid or lesser semilunar notch), which articulates with the radial head. The cylindrical radial head rotates in this notch during pronation and supination of the forearm. The slightly depressed disclike proximal end of the radial head articulates with the hemispherical capitellum of the humerus to permit forearm rotation and flexion-extension.

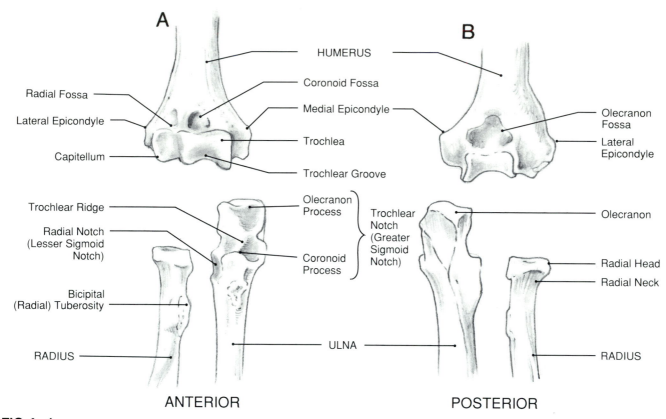

FIG 4–1.
Bony anatomy of elbow. **A,** anterior view. **B,** posterior view.

The articulations of the radius with the capitellum and ulna, combined with bowing of the radial shaft, allow rotation of the radius around the ulna during all degrees of elbow flexion and extension.

Ligamentous Structures

A complex set of ligaments and capsular structures provides stability of the elbow joint (Figs 4–2 and 4–3). On the anterior surface the capsule attaches proximally to the humerus above the coronoid and radial fossae. Distally, the capsule attaches to the coronoid process medially and the annular ligament laterally. Posteriorly, the capsule attaches to the edge of the olecranon fossa of the humerus proximally and the margins of the trochlear notch of the ulna distally. The capsule is relatively thin anteriorly but it is reinforced by the cruciate orientation of its anterior fibers. The anterior capsule is taut in extension and lax in flexion.

The medial collateral ligament is considered the prime stabilizer of the elbow joint. It has three components: the anterior, posterior, and transverse bundles. The anterior bundle is the most important. It originates from the lateral and base portions of the medial epicondyle of the humerus and attaches to the medial side of the coronoid process of the ulna. The posterior bundle is a thickening of the posterior capsule that attaches at the medial humeral epicondyle and the medial portion of the posterior trochlear notch of the ulna. The transverse bundle is inconstant.

The lateral collateral ligament is less well defined than the medial ligament. It originates at the lateral epicondyle of the humerus and inserts diffusely into the annular ligament. The annular ligament is a discrete structure that encircles the radial neck and maintains contact of the radial head with the proximal ulna during pronation and supination. The annular ligament attaches to the anterior and posterior margins of the radial notch (lesser sigmoid notch of the ulna).

According to Morrey there are three defined components of the lateral collateral ligament complex: the radial collateral, accessory collateral, and lateral ulnar collateral ligaments. The radial collateral ligament originates at the lateral humeral epicondyle and inserts into the fibers of the annular ligament. The accessory collateral ligament is a discrete band of the annular ligament that inserts into the supina-

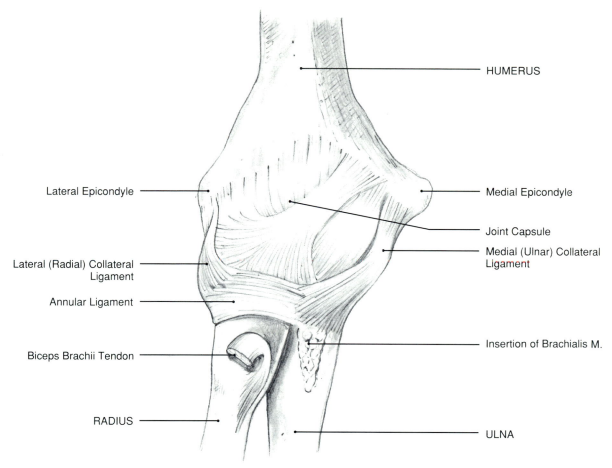

Lateral Epicondyle

Lateral (Radial) Collateral
Ligament

Annular Ligament

Biceps Brachii Tendon

RADIUS

HUMERUS

Medial Epicondyle

Joint Capsule

Medial (Ulnar) Collateral
Ligament

Insertion of Brachialis M.

ULNA

FIG 4–2.
Capsule of elbow joint (anterior view). Note cruciate orientation of fibers. Note medial collateral ligament attachment to the base of the medial epicondyle.

tor tubercle of the ulna. The lateral ulnar collateral ligament originates at the lateral epicondyle of the humerus and likewise inserts at the supinator tubercle of the ulna.

Muscles and Muscle Attachments

The motions of the elbow are flexion, extension, and forearm rotation (pronation and supination).

The most superficial muscle on the anterior aspect of the elbow is the biceps brachii (Fig 4–4). The biceps inserts through two tendinous attachments, the rounded and strong tendon proper and the thin, broad, and flattened bicipital aponeurosis (lacertus fibrosus). The tendon of insertion of the biceps passes deeply between the flexor and extensor muscle origins into the cubital fossa. The tendon attaches to the posterior part of the bicipital tubercle of the radius. The bicipital aponeurosis arises from the medial border of the tendon and from the lower me-

dial muscular portion of the muscle. The aponeurosis passes downward and medially across the front of the cubital fossa to join the deep fascia over the upper ends of the flexor muscles of the forearm. The biceps is a flexor of the elbow and the primary supinator of the forearm. It is innervated by the musculocutaneous nerve.

The brachialis muscle lies beneath the biceps. It overlies the anterior aspect of the distal humerus and inserts into the coronoid process of the ulna. Its sole function is elbow flexion. The brachialis muscle is innervated by the musculocutaneous nerve; according to some authorities it also receives innervation from the radial nerve.

The common flexor tendon arises from the medial epicondyle. This tendon provides origin for the flexor carpi radialis, palmaris longus, and humeral portions of the pronator teres and flexor carpi ulnaris. These muscles are innervated by the median nerve, with the exception of the flexor carpi ulnaris,

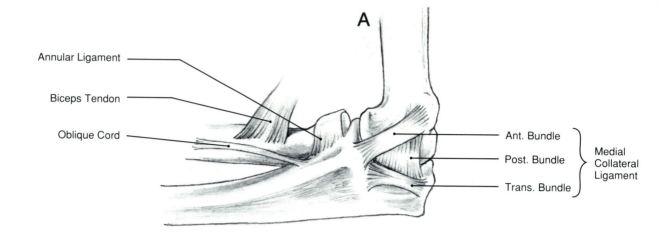

MEDIAL

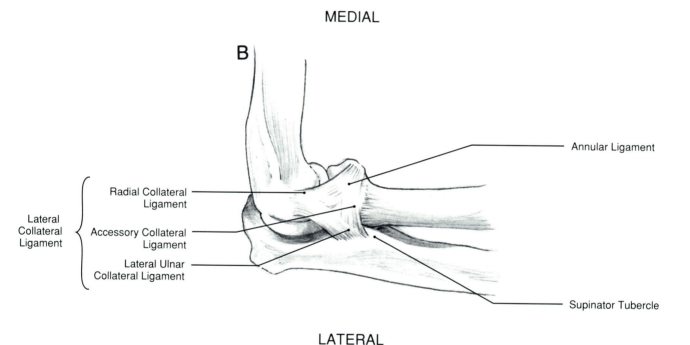

LATERAL

FIG 4-3.
Ligaments of elbow joint. **A,** medial view. Note three components of medial collateral ligament. **B,** lateral view. Note the three somewhat ill-defined components of the lateral collateral ligament.

which is innervated by the ulnar nerve. The pronator teres muscle is primarily a pronator of the forearm and is a weak elbow flexor. The flexor carpi ulnaris and flexor carpi radialis are primary wrist flexors and also weak elbow flexors. The palmaris longus inserts into the palmar fascia of the hand. Although it may be somewhat vestigial, it does aid in wrist flexion. It is commonly used in tendon transfers.

On the lateral aspect of the elbow and forearm,

the "mobile wad of three" (as described by Henry) originates from the lateral supracondylar ridge. This wad consists of the brachioradialis, extensor carpi radialis longus, and extensor carpi radialis brevis. The brachioradialis is a weak secondary elbow flexor, pronator, and supinator. The extensor carpi radialis longus and extensor carpi radialis brevis function as wrist extensors. The brachioradialis and extensor carpi radialis longus are innervated by the radial nerve proper. The extensor carpi radialis

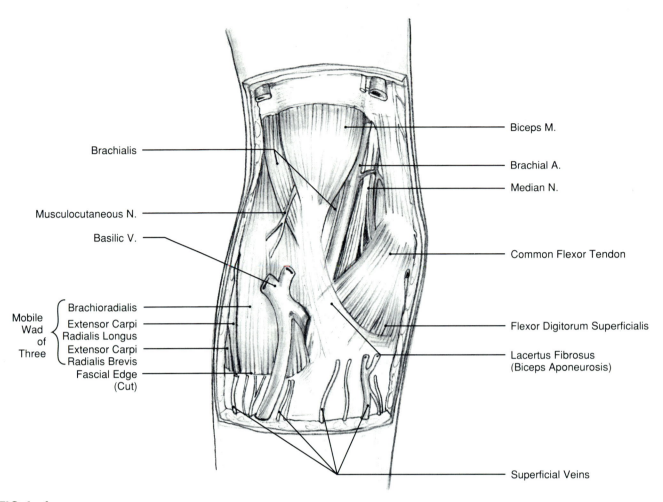

Brachialis

Musculocutaneous N.

Basilic V.

Mobile
Wad
of
Three

- Brachioradialis
- Extensor Carpi
Radialis Longus
- Extensor Carpi
Radialis Brevis
- Fascial Edge
(Cut)

Biceps M.

Brachial A.

Median N.

Common Flexor Tendon

Flexor Digitorum Superficialis

Lacertus Fibrosus
(Biceps Aponeurosis)

Superficial Veins

FIG 4–4.
Anterior elbow (fascia removed). Note brachialis beneath biceps. Note musculocutaneous nerve exiting between biceps and brachialis muscles. Note relationship of biceps muscle tendon, brachial artery, and median nerve: from lateral to medial they spell "man" (*m*uscle, *a*rtery, *n*erve).

brevis is innervated by the posterior interosseous nerve.

The lateral epicondyle of the humerus gives origin to the common extensor tendon, which in turn gives rise to the anconeus, extensor carpi ulnaris, extensor digiti quinti, and extensor digitorum communis. The anconeus is a weak extensor of the elbow that is supplied by the radial nerve. The other muscles (extensor carpi ulnaris, extensor digiti quinti, and extensor digitorum communis) that originate from the common extensor tendon are wrist and finger extensors with little effect on the elbow. These latter three muscles are innervated by the posterior interosseous nerve.

Posteriorly, the triceps brachii inserts into the olecranon process and proximal ulnar shaft. It is the primary extensor of the elbow and is innervated by the radial nerve.

Arteries

The major artery crossing the elbow is the brachial artery (Figs 4–5 and 4–6). It crosses the elbow just superficial to the brachialis muscle belly, lateral to the median nerve, and medial to the biceps tendon. In the cubital fossa it divides into its terminal branches, the radial and ulnar arteries.

There are four collateral circulation systems about the elbow. Laterally, the radial recurrent artery connects proximally and anteriorly to one of the terminal branches of the profunda brachii, the radial collateral artery. The posterior interosseous artery anastomoses, via the interosseous recurrent artery, with the middle collateral artery (the other terminal branch of the profunda brachii). The ulnar artery gives off anterior and posterior recurrent arteries, which anastomose medially with branches of the

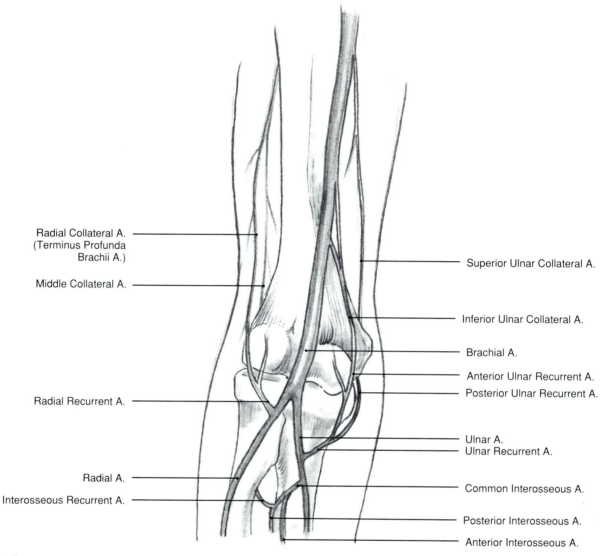

Radial Collateral A.
(Terminus Profunda
Brachii A.)

Middle Collateral A.

Radial Recurrent A.

Radial A.

Interosseous Recurrent A.

Superior Ulnar Collateral A.

Inferior Ulnar Collateral A.

Brachial A.

Anterior Ulnar Recurrent A.
Posterior Ulnar Recurrent A.

Ulnar A.
Ulnar Recurrent A.

Common Interosseous A.

Posterior Interosseous A.

Anterior Interosseous A.

FIG 4–5.
Brachial artery and collateral circulation of the elbow.

brachial artery, the inferior ulnar collateral and superior ulnar collateral arteries, respectively.

Nerves

Three mixed nerves (radial, median, and ulnar) and two sensory nerves (lateral antebrachial cutaneous—a continuation of the musculocutaneous nerve—and medial antebrachial cutaneous) traverse the elbow (see Fig 4–6). Articular branches come from each of the major branches but are inconstant. The median nerve crosses the elbow anteriorly on the medial side of the brachial artery between the biceps and the brachialis. It can usually be found ap-

proximately 3 cm anterior and 3 cm proximal to the medial epicondyle.

The radial nerve enters the area coursing from posterior to anterior in the interval between the origin of the brachioradialis and the muscle belly of the brachialis. It crosses the joint anteriorly and divides to form the superficial radial and posterior interosseous (deep radial) nerves at the level of the radiocapitellar joint.

As the musculocutaneous nerve continues distally beyond the lateral border of the brachialis it is known as the lateral antebrachial cutaneous nerve.

The ulnar nerve passes posterior to the medial epicondyle to enter the cubital tunnel on the medial

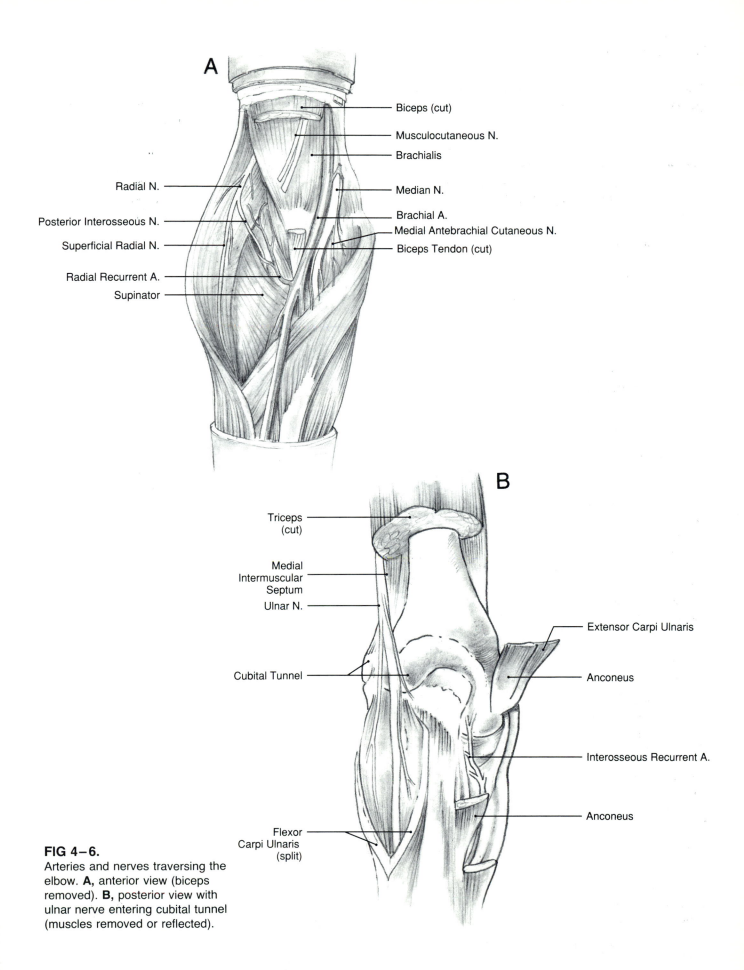

A

Biceps (cut)

Musculocutaneous N.

Brachialis

Radial N.

Posterior Interosseous N.

Superficial Radial N.

Radial Recurrent A.

Supinator

Median N.

Brachial A.

Medial Antebrachial Cutaneous N.

Biceps Tendon (cut)

B

Triceps
(cut)

Medial
Intermuscular
Septum

Ulnar N.

Cubital Tunnel

Flexor
Carpi Ulnaris
(split)

Extensor Carpi Ulnaris

Anconeus

Interosseous Recurrent A.

Anconeus

FIG 4–6.
Arteries and nerves traversing the
elbow. **A,** anterior view (biceps
removed). **B,** posterior view with
ulnar nerve entering cubital tunnel
(muscles removed or reflected).

side of the elbow. It can be palpated subcutaneously against the medial epicondyle in most individuals.

SURGICAL APPROACHES TO THE ELBOW

Selection of an approach to the elbow should be based on the surgery planned and the extensile capability of the exposure. Because of the subcutaneous position of the olecranon and medial and lateral condyles, selection of skin incisions is crucial to avoid problems with skin healing. Straight or gently curved incisions crossing flexor creases are best. Planning incisions to avoid the bony prominences will allow wound healing and ease of subsequent surgical procedures, if required.

Posterior Approaches

Posterior approaches are the most utilitarian of all the approaches to the elbow. They can be used to deal with distal humerus fractures; proximal ulna fractures; tumor excision; loose body retrieval; total joint arthroplasty; and treatment of infections, nonunion, and synovial disorders. Many modifications of the skin incision and the handling of the triceps have been proposed. Most surgeons agree the incision should be longitudinal and avoid the tip of the olecranon. The triceps may be split in the center, opened in a V to Y fashion, elevated with the osteotomized olecranon, or reflected in continuity with the forearm fascia and periosteum.

The landmarks (Fig 4–7) for posterior exposure are the olecranon tip, which may be easily palpated posteriorly, and the medial and lateral epicondyles. The patient should be placed in the supine position with the arm over the chest or in the lateral position with the elbow bent 90 degrees over an appropriate support. The incision is started 5 to 8 cm proximal to the olecranon tip in the midline, carried distally, and curved laterally just above the olecranon tip. It is continued distally over the subcutaneous border of the ulna. Care should be taken to avoid a scar directly over the olecranon tip, which can lead to skin breakdown.

The deep fascia is divided in the midline. The ulnar nerve should be identified at this time. It is freed posterior to the medial epicondyle, tagged with a rubber tape, and carefully protected during all further dissection. If extensive dissection is anticipated, anterior transposition of the ulnar nerve early in the procedure is advisable. The triceps tendon is identified as it inserts onto the olecranon.

If an osteotomy of the olecranon is to be carried out, the olecranon is predrilled and tapped to receive a cancellous screw when reattached to the ulna. The olecranon is osteotomized into the sigmoid notch 2 cm distal to the tip. Sharp medial dissection through the capsule before the osteotomy is made will allow direct visualization of the joint surface and ensure proper placement of the osteotomy. Care must be taken to note the rotation of the olecranon to ensure proper replacement. A small osteotome or electrocautery device may be used to score the osteotomy site before division to aid alignment. With care taken to protect the ulnar nerve, the medial and lateral fascial attachments to the triceps-olecranon complex are released as the triceps is reflected proximally. Hyperflexion of the elbow facilitates a complete view of the joint. Medial and lateral stripping of the humerus may be done subperiosteally to afford more complete exposure. Care must be taken not to strip the posterior humerus proximally farther than one fourth the length of the shaft. The radial nerve may be injured as it spirals around the posterior humerus at this point. Anteriorly the median nerve and brachial artery are at risk with extensive dissection. At the conclusion of the dissection the olecranon is reattached with a cancellous screw. In dealing with fractures of the olecranon, proper alignment is easily noted and maintained because of the irregularity of the fracture surfaces. With an osteotomy, however, correct alignment must be carefully checked and maintained. Though osteotomy of the olecranon is the most common exposure, it does have a drawback: violation of the elbow joint surface by the osteotomy.

Anson and Maddock describe a posterior approach, which they attribute to Campbell (Fig 4–8). It is a triceps-splitting technique that leaves the triceps insertion intact. After the ulnar nerve is identified, the triceps is incised in the midline down to the distal humerus and olecranon. At the olecranon the triceps is carefully kept in continuity with the distal muscular fascial sleeve. This is done by subperiosteally reflecting the split triceps, laterally with the anconeus and distal forearm fascia and medially with the flexor carpi ulnaris and medial forearm fascia. Closure is done with simple sutures proximally and sutures through the tip of the olecranon distally. Early motion after this approach is risky because of the tenuous nature of the closure. Another

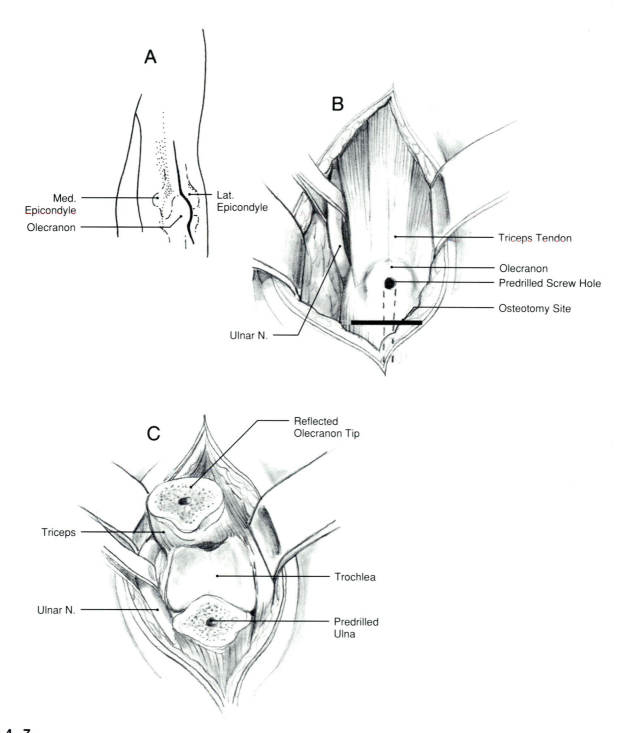

FIG 4–7.
Posterior approach to elbow. **A,** incision and bony anatomy for posterior approach. Note the medial and lateral epicondyles and olecranon are all subcutaneous and palpable; incision deviates around olecranon. **B,** deep dissection of posterior approach. Note olecranon is predrilled prior to osteotomy. Ulnar nerve is identified and protected first. **C,** osteotomized olecranon is reflected with triceps exposing trochlea.

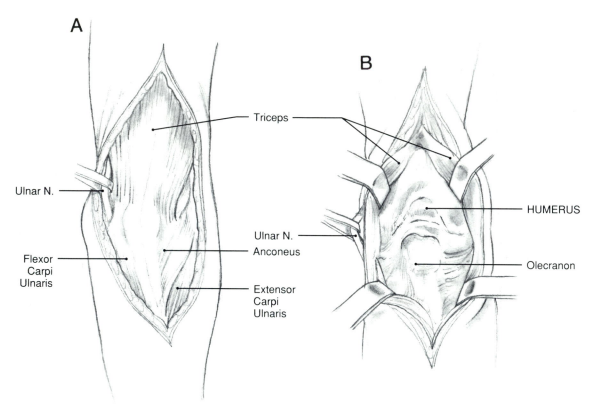

FIG 4–8.
Campbell posterior approach (triceps-splitting). **A,** triceps and olecranon are exposed. **B,** triceps split with exposure of distal humerus, proximal ulna, and joint capsule by subperiosteal dissection along the lateral side of the olecranon and proximal ulnar shaft. (Redrawn from Anson BJ, Maddock WG: *Callendar's Surgical Anatomy,* ed 4. Philadelphia, W B Saunders Co, 1958, p 842.)

drawback is that the intact olecranon limits exposure to the distal humerus and its articular surfaces.

Van Gorder modified Campbell's triceps-splitting approach for exposing the posterior distal humerus (Fig 4–9). In this technique, which is particularly useful in dealing with extension contracture of the elbow, the triceps is divided and either reconnected or lengthened with a V to Y incision. The triceps aponeurosis is incised in the form of an inverted V and reflected from the underlying muscle. A small cuff of aponeurosis must be left proximally to allow reattachment at the resection margins. The tendon is reflected distally to the level of the olecranon. The muscle fibers overlying the distal humerus are divided in the midline and retracted. Subperiosteal stripping of the triceps from the humerus allows extension of the exposure. If triceps lengthening is required to correct elbow extension contracture, the triceps may be lengthened at closure by a V to Y closure of the aponeurosis.

Bryan and Morrey describe a posteromedial ex-

tensile exposure (Fig 4–10) that preserves the continuity of the triceps extensor mechanism with the distal triceps fascia and periosteum. This approach is particularly useful in total elbow arthroplasty. With the shoulder flexed and the arm placed across the chest, a straight posterior incision is made medial to the midline. The incision extends 8 cm above and below the olecranon tip. The medial border of the triceps is identified and dissected free of the intermuscular septum. The ulnar nerve is dissected free and gently retracted medially or transferred anteriorly. The superficial fascia of the proximal forearm is incised directly down to the periosteum along the medial border of the ulna. The entire complex (triceps, forearm fascia, and periosteum) is elevated from the proximal ulna, with continuity maintained, and retracted laterally. Because the junction of the triceps insertion with the periosteum and fascia is very thin, care must be exercised when the structures are dissected free from the proximal ulna. If exposure of the radiocapitellar joint is needed the

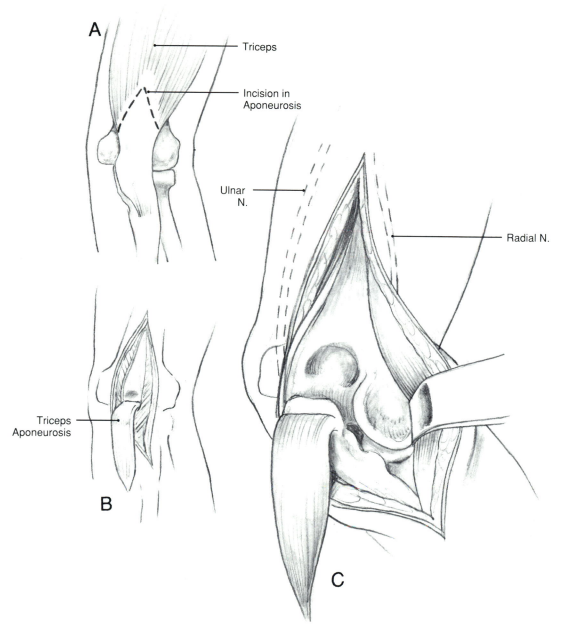

FIG 4–9.
Van Gorder modification of Campbell approach. **A,** tendon incision for V to Y triceps resection approach. Note a small rim of tendon is left attached to muscle to allow reattachment. **B,** reflected tongue of triceps aponeurosis. **C,** proximal extension into triceps muscle. Note location of radial and ulnar nerves. (Modified from Van Gorder GW: Surgical approach in supracondylar "T" fractures of the humerus requiring open reduction. *J Bone Joint Surg* 1940; 22:278–292.)

anconeus is also elevated and reflected laterally. The tip of the olecranon may be excised for additional exposure. Closure is accomplished by suturing the triceps into the bone at the olecranon and carefully attaching the fascia-periosteum complex to the free edge of flexor carpi ulnaris.

There are structures at risk in any of these pos-

terior approaches to the elbow. The ulnar nerve must always be identified and protected by gentle retraction and/or anterior transposition. These approaches may be extended proximally only as far as the radial nerve in the spiral groove, because this nerve may be injured as it spirals around the distal fourth of the humerus. The median nerve and bra-

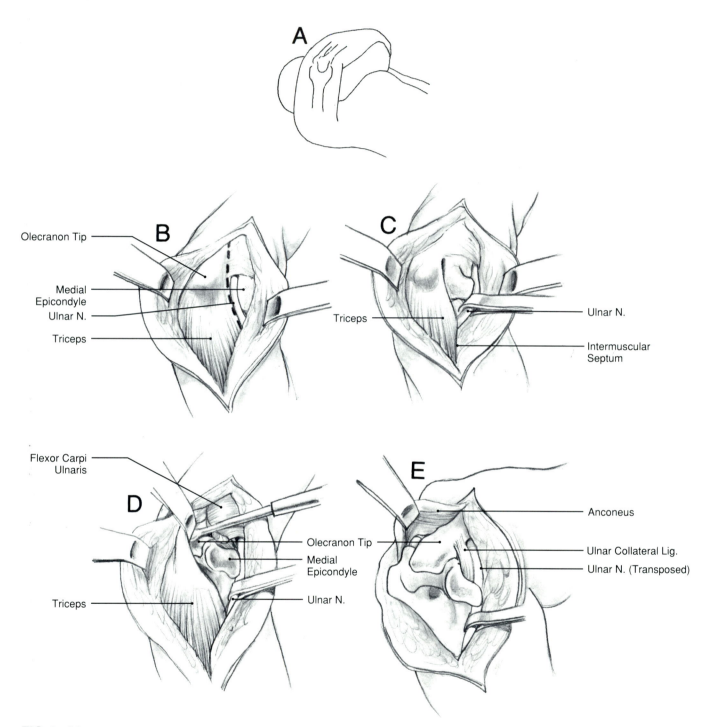

FIG 4–10.
Posteromedial extensile exposure. **A,** patient positioned with shoulder flexed and arm placed over the chest. **B,** incision parallels medial border of triceps, with care taken to avoid ulnar nerve. **C,** deep dissection: ulnar nerve is protected by gentle retraction and triceps freed from intermuscular septum. **D,** elevation of triceps at its distal insertion by subperiosteal dissection. **E,** lateral extension of exposure: anconeus can be subperiosteally raised to gain access to radiocapitellar joint.

(Continued.)

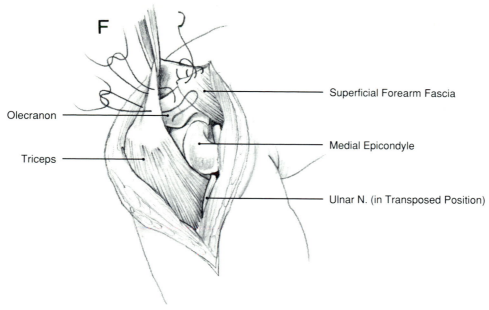

Olecranon

Triceps

Superficial Forearm Fascia

Medial Epicondyle

Ulnar N. (in Transposed Position)

FIG 4–10 (cont.).
F, closure is accomplished by suturing the triceps into the bone at the olecranon and reattaching the fascia-periosteum complex to the free edge of the flexor carpi ulnaris. (Redrawn from Bryan RS, Morrey BF: Extensive posterior exposure of the elbow: a triceps-sparing approach. *Clin Orthop Rel Res* 1982; 166:188–192.)

chial artery can be harmed by overly vigorous anterior dissection along the humerus. Distally, however, the dissection may be extended along the subcutaneous border of the ulna and down the entire length of the forearm.

Posterolateral Approach

The posterolateral (sometimes referred to as lateral) exposure (Fig 4–11) is the most common approach to the elbow joint. It is relatively safe, but it gives access to only the radiocapitellar area. Kaplan and Kocher have described two separate posterolateral approaches. Kaplan's approach uses the interval between the extensor digitorum communis and extensor carpi radialis longus. Kocher advocated use of the interval between the anconeus and extensor carpi ulnaris. Because Kaplan's approach is closer to the posterior interosseous nerve it is used much less commonly and will not be described here. Kocher's approach may be used for all surgery of the radial head including (1) radial head fracture fixation, (2) radial head replacement arthroplasty, (3) tumor resection, and (4) loose body retrieval from the radiocapitellar joint.

The landmarks for Kocher's approach are the lateral epicondyle, the tip and lateral border of the olecranon, and the radial head. The lateral epicondyle and common extensor origin are easily palpable and

guide placement of the incision. The lateral border of the olecranon, which is subcutaneous, is used to identify the insertion of the anconeus. The radial head may be palpated 2 cm distal to the lateral epicondyle. It can be rotated beneath the palpating finger by pronation and supination of the forearm.

The patient is placed in supine or semisupine position with the arm pronated over the chest. A curved incision is made from the lateral epicondyle distal and medial to the lateral border of the olecranon, ending 5 to 6 cm distal to the tip of the olecranon. The deep fascia is identified and entered in line with the incision. The interval between the anconeus and extensor carpi ulnaris is identified *after* the deep fascia is entered. The interval is found distally where both muscles are distinct; proximally, the muscles blend intimately and are difficult to separate. The anconeus is subperiosteally elevated from the ulna and retracted medially. The extensor carpi ulnaris is retracted laterally. The arm should be fully pronated at this point to move the posterior interosseous (deep branch of radial) nerve as far medially as possible. The posterior interosseous nerve, not routinely visualized in this exposure, usually passes around the neck of the radius two fingerbreadths distal to the joint when the arm is pronated. The capsule is entered longitudinally and the joint exposed. To prevent injury to the posterior interosseous nerve, the capsule should not be opened

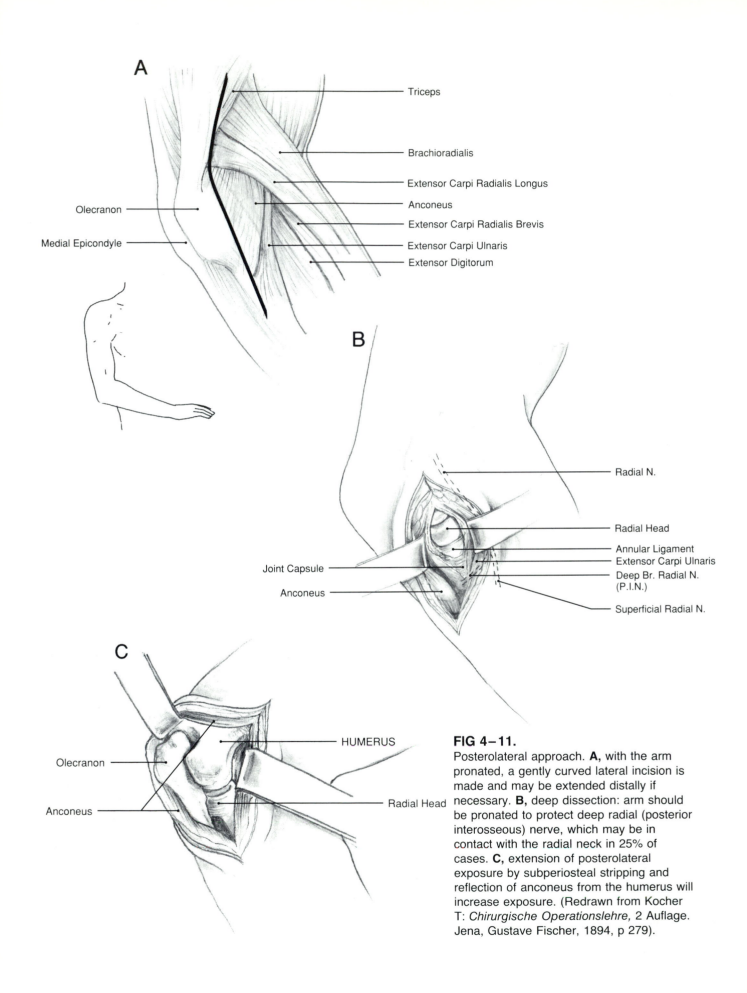

A

Triceps

Brachioradialis

Extensor Carpi Radialis Longus

Anconeus

Extensor Carpi Radialis Brevis

Extensor Carpi Ulnaris

Extensor Digitorum

Olecranon

Medial Epicondyle

B

Radial N.

Radial Head

Annular Ligament

Extensor Carpi Ulnaris

Deep Br. Radial N. (P.I.N.)

Superficial Radial N.

Joint Capsule

Anconeus

C

Olecranon

Anconeus

HUMERUS

Radial Head

FIG 4–11.
Posterolateral approach. **A,** with the arm
pronated, a gently curved lateral incision is
made and may be extended distally if
necessary. **B,** deep dissection: arm should
be pronated to protect deep radial (posterior
interosseous) nerve, which may be in
contact with the radial neck in 25% of
cases. **C,** extension of posterolateral
exposure by subperiosteal stripping and
reflection of anconeus from the humerus will
increase exposure. (Redrawn from Kocher
T: *Chirurgische Operationslehre,* 2 Auflage.
Jena, Gustave Fischer, 1894, p 279).

distal to the annular ligament. Retraction must be very judicious, since the deep radial (posterior interosseous) nerve is closely associated with the bone in the mass of the supinator and commonly (25% of individuals) comes in contact with the radial neck.

Medial Approach

The medial approach gives limited exposure to the entire elbow joint, but it is relatively complex and rarely indicated (Fig 4–12). It is most commonly used to retrieve loose bodies from the ulnotrochlear articulation and to reduce and stabilize fractures of the trochlea, coronoid process, and/or medial epicondyle. This approach requires an osteotomy of the medial epicondyle, during which the ulnar nerve, median nerve, and brachial artery must be protected.

The patient is placed in a supine position with the arm externally rotated and abducted. The medial epicondyle is the solitary landmark for this exposure, and in most individuals the ulnar nerve can be palpated directly posterior to the epicondyle. The incision is centered over the medial epicondyle, starting 6 to 10 cm proximally and extending 6 cm distally. The superficial fascia is carefully incised over the ulnar nerve proximally behind the epicondyle. The ulnar nerve is tagged with a soft rubber tape and retracted posteriorly. The proximal border of the flexor carpi ulnaris may need to be released to facilitate mobilization of the nerve. The deep fascia overlying the pronator teres is retracted laterally and the interval between the pronator teres and the brachialis defined distally. The medial epicondyle is predrilled and tapped for a cortical screw. The epicondyle is then osteotomized *deep* to the common flexor origin but *superficial* to the attachment of the ulnar collateral ligament, the integrity of which should be maintained. The epicondyle with attached wrist flexor origins is gently retracted distally, with care taken not to stretch the branches of the median nerve that supply these muscles. In the proximal portion of the wound the brachialis is retracted anteriorly and the triceps retracted posteriorly. The capsule and collateral ligament are opened longitudinally. The coronoid process and distal humerus may be stripped subperiosteally to afford greater exposure. If need be, the joint can be opened, with care taken not to injure the median nerve. Following capsular closure the epicondyle is reattached anatomically with a small cortical screw.

Extreme care must be taken with this exposure to protect the ulnar nerve during dissection and os-

teotomy of the medial epicondyle. The median nerve must also be protected from excessive traction when the common wrist flexor muscles are reflected. Distal extension of the exposure is limited by the leash of median nerve branches to the common wrist flexors. Proximal extension between the triceps and brachialis is possible along the distal fourth of the humerus.

Anterior Approaches

The anterior approaches are the least commonly used approaches to the elbow. They give limited access to the joint, and the major neurovascular structures are in close proximity to the area of dissection. The anteromedial approach is used only for exploration of the neurovascular structures in the cubital fossa and for exposure of the biceps tendon. The anterolateral approach can be used for limited access to the joint anteriorly. These approaches can be used for (1) repair of lacerations to the brachial artery, (2) repair of lacerations or avulsion of the biceps tendon, (3) repair of median nerve injuries, (4) limited exposure of the proximal radius and capitellum, and (5) release of flexion contractures.

The landmarks for the anterior approaches are the medial and lateral epicondyles, the "mobile wad of three" (Henry) and the biceps tendon. The biceps tendon is easily palpable and serves as the guide to the dissection. The mobile wad is the lateral group of muscles (the brachioradialis, extensor carpi radialis longus, and extensor carpi radialis brevis) that originate from the distal lateral humerus. With the elbow flexed these muscles can be easily palpated and moved as a group. The medial epicondyle can be used as a guide to the median nerve. The nerve can be located 3 cm anterior and 3 cm proximal to the epicondyle in the interval between the biceps and brachialis.

Anteromedial Approach

The incision for the anteromedial approach (Fig 4–13) begins over the biceps-triceps interval 5 to 7 cm proximal to the joint, courses distally and obliquely across the cubital fossa flexor creases, and distally over the interval between the brachioradialis and pronator teres. Care must be taken in the subcutaneous tissues medially and laterally to avoid the medial and lateral cutaneous nerve branches. The superficial veins (basilic, cephalic, cubital, median antecubital, etc.) are ligated. The superficial dissection must be carefully done since the major neurovascular structures are just beneath the fascia.

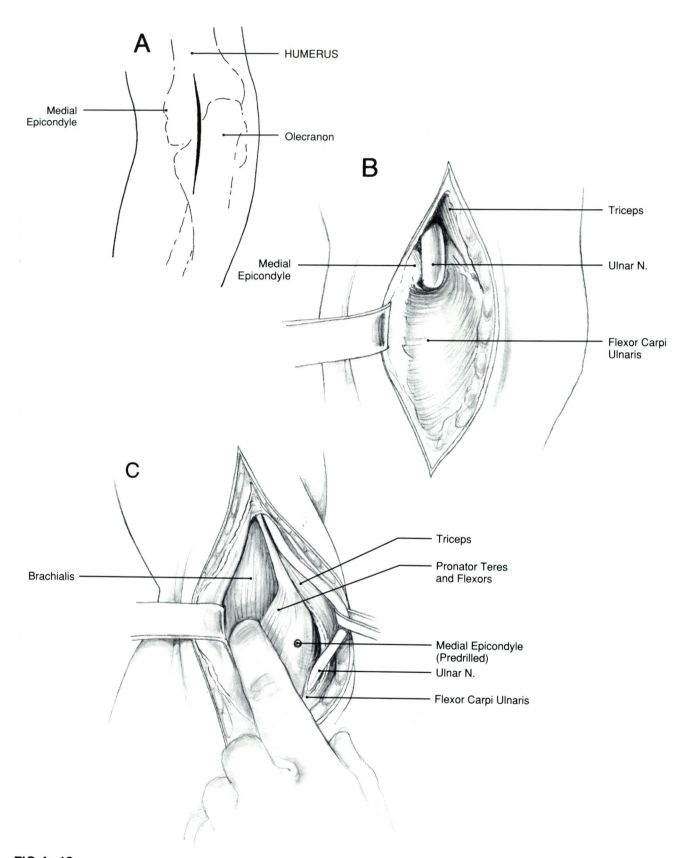

FIG 4–12.
Medial approach to elbow. **A,** bony landmarks and incision. **B,** superficial dissection. Note ulnar nerve is just posterior to epicondyle. **C,** deep dissection; interval between pronator teres and brachialis developed. Medial epicondyle is predrilled.

(Continued.)

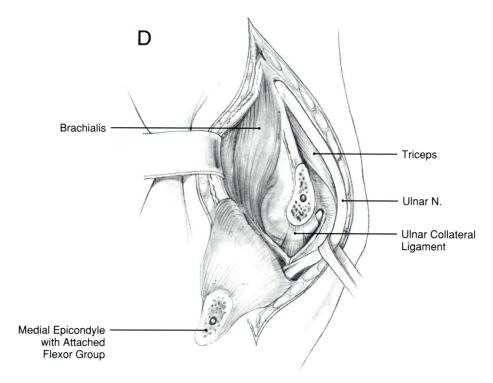

D

Brachialis

Triceps

Ulnar N.

Ulnar Collateral Ligament

Medial Epicondyle with Attached Flexor Group

FIG 4–12 (cont.).
D, after predrilling, medial epicondyle is osteotomized. Ulnar collateral ligament must be left intact. The extent of epicondyle reflection is limited by the neurovascular leash to the muscle flexor group.

The deep fascia is entered proximally, and the median nerve and brachial vessels are identified in the biceps-triceps interval. The median nerve and brachial artery are then mobilized from proximal to distal across the cubital fossa. In order to accomplish this, the lacertus fibrosus (a fascial band originating from the biceps tendon and fascia that sweeps distally and medially to insert into the forearm fascia) must be released carefully, as the median nerve and radial artery pass directly beneath it. The fascia between the pronator teres and brachioradialis is released to allow retraction of the pronator. The median nerve is traced across the joint and between the superficial and deep heads of the pronator teres. The median nerve must be carefully dissected and displaced medially.

The brachial artery branches into the ulnar and radial arteries in the cubital fossa. The ulnar artery courses posterior to the flexor group toward the ulnar border of the arm. The radial artery passes laterally anterior to the biceps tendon to lie between the brachioradialis and pronator teres. Near its origin the radial artery gives off the radial recurrent artery, which courses laterally and proximally. The radial recurrent artery may have to be ligated and released for adequate exposure. In the depths of the dissec-

tion the biceps tendon inserts into the bicipital tuberosity of the proximal radius and may be palpated with the forearm in supination. Access to the joint proper is limited. It can be partially visualized if the brachialis is split or moved to one side or the other. In this way the anterior capsule can be exposed for incision.

In the anteromedial approach to the elbow the very superficial position of the median nerve and brachial artery places these structures at risk. If identified early they can be easily protected, but even so they have limited mobility. The median nerve is tethered medially by the branches to the pronator teres and common flexors. The branching of the brachial artery limits its excursion.

Anterolateral Approach (Modified Henry)

A gently curved incision (Fig 4–14) is made over the anterior aspect of the elbow. The incision begins 5 to 7 cm proximal to the joint between the biceps and brachioradialis muscles and courses distally along the medial border of the brachioradialis muscle. The incision then turns medially over the flexion crease and deviates laterally, continuing distally along the medial border of the brachioradialis into the proximal forearm.

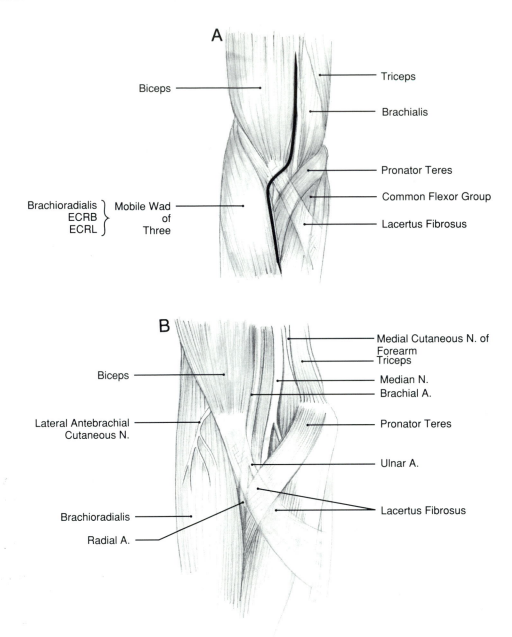

FIG 4–13.
Anteromedial approach. **A,** incision; note oblique crossing of flexor crease. **B,** superficial dissection; note median nerve and brachial artery lie directly under the lacertus fibrosus.   *(Continued.)*

Proximally the interval between the brachioradialis and biceps is bluntly developed. The lateral antebrachial cutaneous nerve is identified in the subcutaneous tissues over the cubital fossa. This is the terminal branch of the musculocutaneous nerve. It enters the distal arm between the biceps and brachialis muscles and is superficial to the fascia of the brachioradialis in the cubital fossa. The lateral antebrachial cutaneous nerve must not be confused with the

radial nerve. The lateral antebrachial cutaneous nerve is gently retracted and preserved.

The radial nerve enters the brachioradialis-brachialis interval at the most proximal origins of the brachioradialis. The radial nerve is traced distally in this interval. It can be protected by early identification and gentle retraction. The deep fascia is developed between the brachioradialis and brachialis proximally and the brachioradialis and pronator dis-

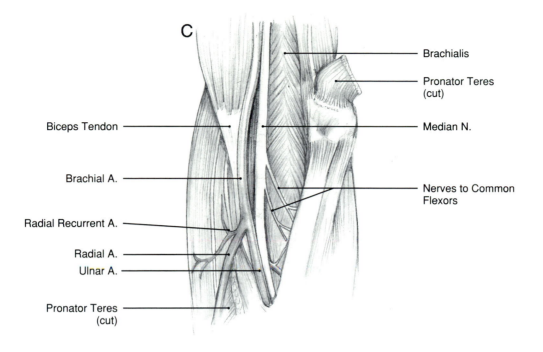

C

Brachialis

Pronator Teres (cut)

Biceps Tendon

Median N.

Brachial A.

Radial Recurrent A.

Nerves to Common Flexors

Radial A.

Ulnar A.

Pronator Teres (cut)

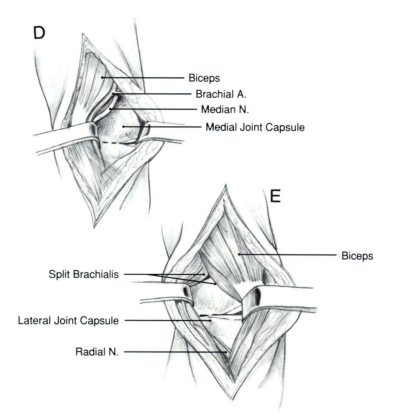

D

Biceps

Brachial A.

Median N.

Medial Joint Capsule

E

Biceps

Split Brachialis

Lateral Joint Capsule

Radial N.

FIG 4–13 (cont.).
C, deep dissection; note branches of median nerve medially and radial recurrent artery laterally. Biceps tendon is prominent palpable landmark which can guide dissection distally. Medial **(D)** and lateral **(E)** access to joint capsule can be obtained with retraction of biceps tendon and brachialis muscle. Anterior capsule can be entered transversely from either side.

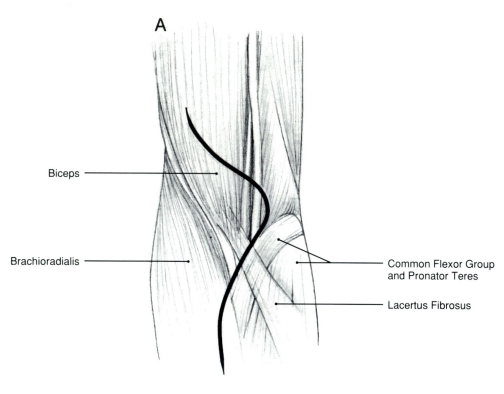

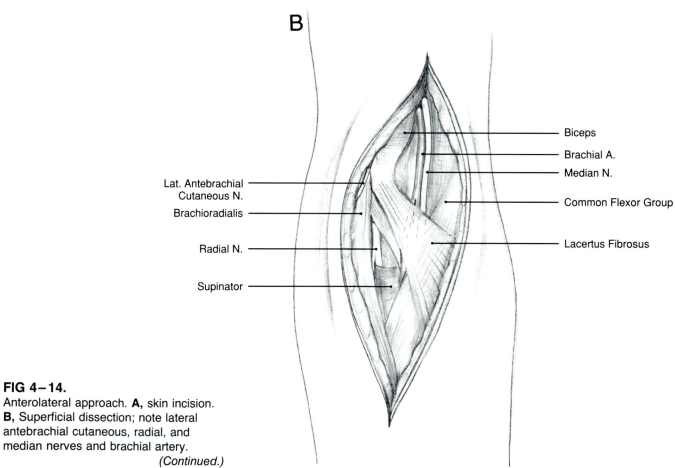

FIG 4–14.
Anterolateral approach. **A,** skin incision.
B, Superficial dissection; note lateral
antebrachial cutaneous, radial, and
median nerves and brachial artery.

(Continued.)

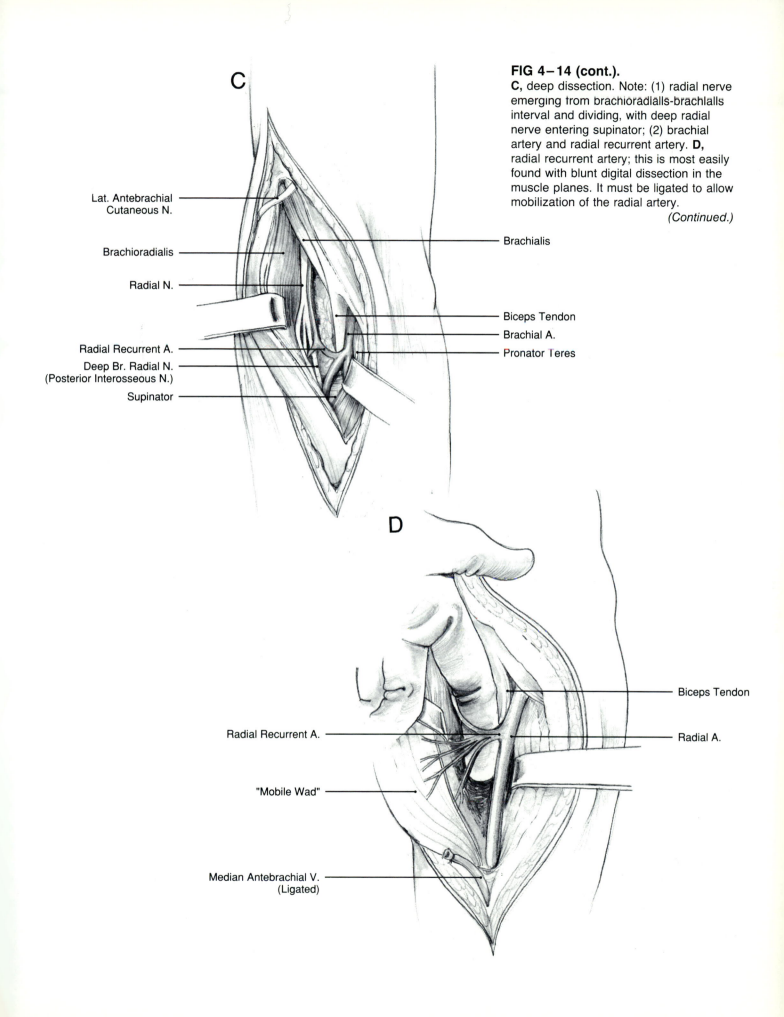

C

Lat. Antebrachial Cutaneous N.

Brachioradialis

Radial N.

Radial Recurrent A.

Deep Br. Radial N. (Posterior Interosseous N.)

Supinator

Brachialis

Biceps Tendon

Brachial A.

Pronator Teres

FIG 4–14 (cont.).
C, deep dissection. Note: (1) radial nerve emerging from brachioradialis-brachialis interval and dividing, with deep radial nerve entering supinator; (2) brachial artery and radial recurrent artery. **D,** radial recurrent artery; this is most easily found with blunt digital dissection in the muscle planes. It must be ligated to allow mobilization of the radial artery.

(Continued.)

D

Biceps Tendon

Radial Recurrent A.

Radial A.

"Mobile Wad"

Median Antebrachial V. (Ligated)

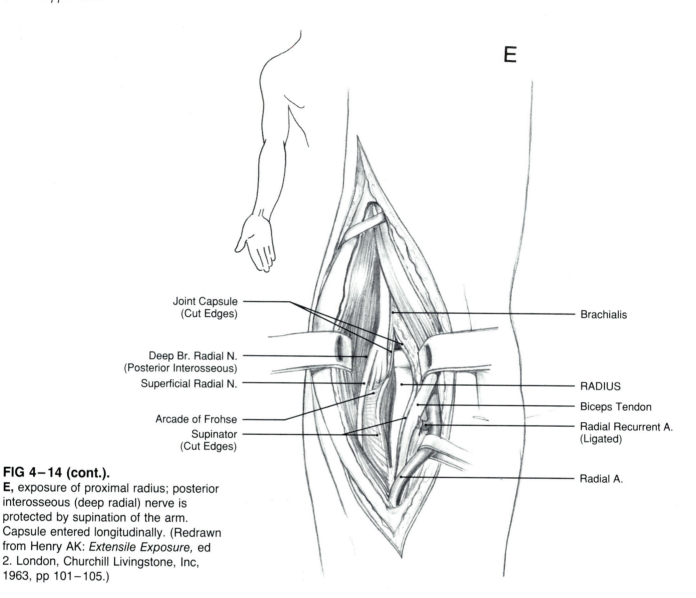

Joint Capsule (Cut Edges)

Deep Br. Radial N. (Posterior Interosseous)

Superficial Radial N.

Arcade of Frohse

Supinator (Cut Edges)

Brachialis

RADIUS

Biceps Tendon

Radial Recurrent A. (Ligated)

Radial A.

E

FIG 4–14 (cont.).
E, exposure of proximal radius; posterior interosseous (deep radial) nerve is protected by supination of the arm. Capsule entered longitudinally. (Redrawn from Henry AK: *Extensile Exposure,* ed 2. London, Churchill Livingstone, Inc, 1963, pp 101–105.)

tally. The radial nerve is freed distally to its three terminal branches: the posterior interosseous nerve, superficial radial nerve, and nerve to the extensor carpi radialis brevis. These branches are all lateral and allow limited lateral retraction of the nerve. The posterior interosseous nerve dives into the substance of the supinator muscle, the superficial radial nerve continues distally beneath the brachioradialis, and the nerve to the extensor carpi radialis brevis enters the muscle immediately.

The radial artery is identified as it passes anterior to the biceps tendon. The recurrent branch of the radial artery is identified and, if necessary for additional exposure, ligated and released. If torn, this vessel may be difficult to find, and postoperative hematoma with possible compartment syndrome may occur.

The biceps tendon is retracted medially, and the muscle fibers of the brachialis that cover the joint capsule can be bluntly elevated and retracted medially.

If greater exposure is needed the dissection may be extended to the proximal radius. To do so an incision is made through the supinator attachment to the radius. When the supinator is released the deep branch of the radial (posterior interosseous) nerve can be protected by full supination of the forearm. This maneuver rolls the nerve laterally approximately 1 cm. The supinator is subperiosteally elevated off the radius and retracted laterally. The posterior interosseous nerve is protected by the muscle fibers of the supinator, but retraction must be gentle to avoid traction injury to the nerve. If necessary the capsule is opened longitudinally for joint access.

This will expose the proximal radius, capitellum, and distal humerus. Care should be taken not to divide the annular ligament. The exposure may be extended proximally into an anterolateral exposure of the humeral shaft. In doing so, the radial nerve, which has already been identified, can be protected. Distal exposure into the forearm can also be done.

ANATOMICAL CONSIDERATIONS IN ELBOW ARTHROSCOPY

George A. Richardson, M.D.

Elbow arthroscopy has been found to be a safe and effective procedure when performed in a systematic and reproducible manner with proper indications. Attention to detail, particularly when arthroscopic portals are established, is essential to avoid injury to neurovascular structures. The most common indication for diagnostic arthroscopy is disparity between the objective findings and the patient's subjective complaint. Removal of loose bodies and resection of olecranon osteophytes are the most common arthroscopic operative procedures.

Because of the high degree of articular congruence in the elbow, arthroscopy of this joint is a technically demanding procedure. In addition, the diagnostic and treatment options in elbow arthroscopy are limited when compared to other joints. However, almost the entire elbow joint can be visualized through the arthroscope; thus the main indication for elbow arthroscopy is intraarticular pathologic conditions that cannot be identified by noninvasive means. In addition to removal of loose bodies and olecranon osteophytes, elbow arthroscopy may be useful in the treatment of synovitis, adhesions, osteochondritis dissecans of the capitellum, and chondromalacia of the radial head. It may also be used for evaluation of subtle fractures of the capitellum and radial head.

Elbow arthroscopy is performed with a 2.7 to 4 mm 30-degree arthroscope. The patient is placed in the supine position on a standard operating table under general anesthesia (Fig 4–15). A tourniquet is applied, the arm placed in an arthroscopic shoulder holder and suspended with about 6 pounds of overhead skin traction, and the elbow flexed 90 degrees. With this technique the elbow can be assessed medi-

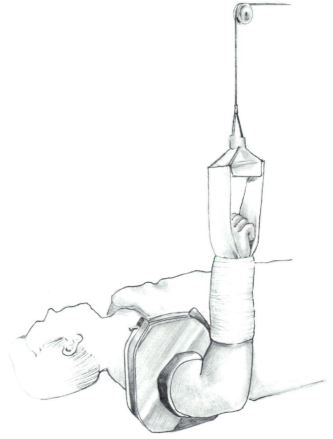

FIG 4–15.
Positioning technique for elbow arthroscopy.

ally, laterally, and posteriorly. Pronation and supination of the forearm can be done to help identify bony landmarks.

Bony Landmarks

With the patient appropriately positioned, the palpable bony landmarks should be outlined with a pen before the procedure is started, as they will quickly become obscured by fluid extravasation during the procedure (Fig 4–16). The lateral landmarks so identified are the radial head and the lateral epicondyle. Medially, the medial epicondyle and, posteriorly, the tip of the olecranon are similarly outlined.

Portal Placement

The five portals most commonly used are direct lateral, anterolateral, anteromedial, posterolateral, and straight posterior.

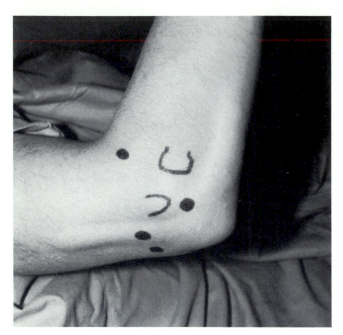

FIG 4–16.
Bony landmarks (radial head and lateral epicondyle). Portal locations are indicated by dark circles.

Direct Lateral Portal

The direct lateral portal is used for initial distension of the elbow joint (Fig 4–17). An 18-gauge needle is placed in the soft spot, proximal and posterior to the radial head. This can be palpated between the lateral epicondyle, olecranon tip, and radial head (this is the same portal routinely used for aspiration of the elbow joint). Once the joint is maximally distended, the other portals may be established. Particular attention to bony landmarks and instrument placement is important because of the proximity of the neurovascular structures.

Anterolateral Portal

To establish the anterolateral portal, an 18-gauge needle is placed 3 cm distal and 2 cm anterior to the lateral epicondyle with the elbow flexed 90 degrees (Fig 4–18). The needle is aimed directly toward the center of the joint just anterior to the radial head, which can be identified by pronation and supination of the forearm. Once the joint has been further distended to displace the antecubital structures anteriorly, the arthroscope or other instruments may be introduced. This portal passes through the extensor carpi radialis brevis and may come within 7 mm of the radial nerve. The anterolateral portal allows visualization of the distal humerus, trochlear ridges, and coronoid process.

Anteromedial Portal

The anteromedial portal (Fig 4–19) is established under direct visualization with the arthroscope already in the anterolateral portal. An 18-gauge spinal needle is passed 2 cm anterior and 2 cm distal to the

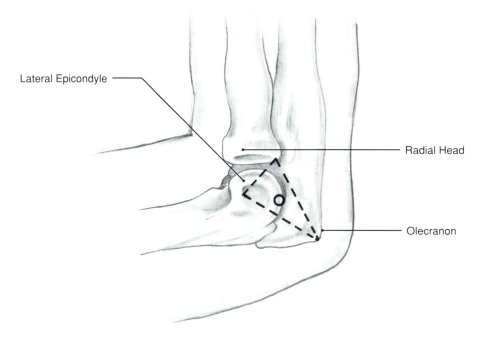

Lateral Epicondyle

Radial Head

Olecranon

FIG 4–17.
Direct lateral portal is used for initial elbow joint distension. This can also be used as an arthroscopic portal. It is located at the "soft spot," centered in the middle of a triangle formed by lines connecting the lateral epicondyle, olecranon tip, and posterior rim of the radial head.

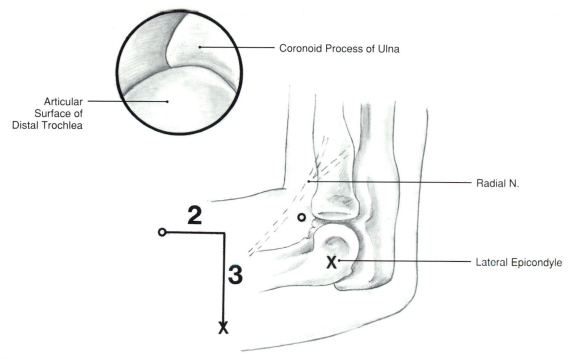

FIG 4–18.
The anterolateral portal is placed 3 cm distal and 2 cm anterior to the lateral epicondyle. The radial nerve *(dashed line)* must be avoided when this portal is established.

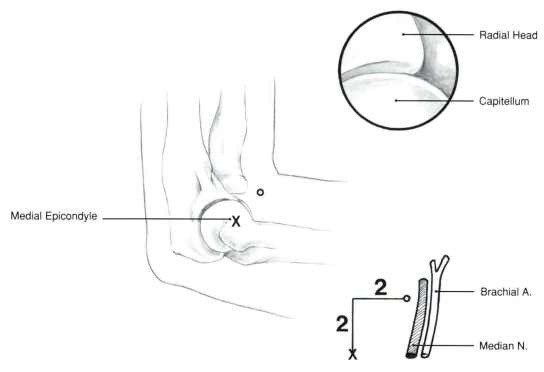

FIG 4–19.
Anteromedial portal is established 2 cm distal and 2 cm anterior to the medial epicondyle. The median nerve and brachial artery *(inset)* must be avoided when this portal is established.

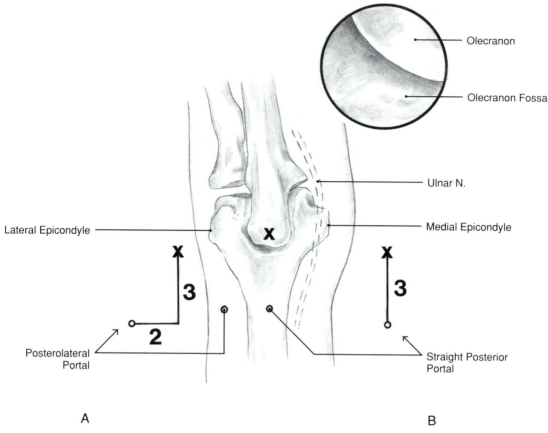

Olecranon

Olecranon Fossa

Ulnar N.

Medial Epicondyle

Lateral Epicondyle

X

3

2

Posterolateral
Portal

X

3

Straight Posterior
Portal

A

B

FIG 4–20.
A, posterolateral portal is located 3 cm proximal and 2 cm lateral to the olecranon tip at the lateral margin of the triceps tendon. **B,** straight posterior portal is placed 3 cm proximal to the olecranon tip. The ulnar nerve *(dashed line)* is close to the portal and must be avoided.

medial epicondyle and directed toward the center of the elbow joint. With the arthroscope in the anterolateral portal the needle will be seen to pass just anterior to the medial epicondyle and inferior to the antecubital structures. After the needle is properly placed, it is withdrawn and the arthroscope inserted.

This portal passes through the pronator teres, just medial to the median nerve and brachial artery. The anteromedial portal provides excellent visualization of the lateral elbow, where most pathologic processes are located.

The direct lateral portal, which was used initially to distend the joint, allows a third working portal anteriorly and permits better visualization of the radial head and capitellum.

Posterolateral Portal

The posterolateral portal (Fig 4-20,A) allows visualization of the olecranon fossa. This portal is established 3 cm proximal and 2 cm lateral to the ole-

cranon tip, just superior and posterior to the lateral epicondyle at the lateral margin of the triceps. The elbow should be flexed only 20 to 30 degrees, with the arthroscope directed toward the olecranon fossa.

Straight Posterior Portal

The straight posterior portal (Fig 4–20,B) is established as a working operative portal for removal of loose bodies and resection of osteophytes of the posteromedial olecranon. This portal is established under direct visualization 3 cm proximal to the olecranon tip, directly through the triceps, with the elbow flexed 20 to 30 degrees. This portal passes very close to the ulnar nerve.

BIBLIOGRAPHY

Albee FH: Arthoplasty of the elbow. *J Bone Joint Surg* 1933; 15:979–985.
Andrews JR, St Pierre RK, Carson WG Jr: Arthroscopy of the elbow. *Clin Sports Med* 1986; 5:653–662.

Anson BJ, Maddock WG: *Callendar's Surgical Anatomy*, ed 4. Philadelphia, W B Saunders Co, 1958.

Armistad RB, Linscheid RL, Dobyns JH, et al: Ulnar lengthening in the treatment of Kienbock's disease. *J Bone Joint Surg* 1982; 64A:170–178.

Banks S, Laufman H: *An Atlas of Surgical Exposures of the Extremities*. Philadelphia, W B Saunders Co, 1953.

Boast FC, et al: Surgical approaches to the elbow joint. *Am Acad Orthop Surg Instr Course Lectures* 1953; 10:180–189.

Boyd HB: Surgical approaches to the elbow joint. *Am Acad Orthop Surg Instr Course Lectures* 1947; 4:147.

Bryan RS, Morrey BF: Extensive posterior exposure of the elbow: A triceps-sparing approach. *Clin Orthop Rel Res* 1982; 166:188–192.

Campbell WC: Incision for exposure of the elbow joint. *Am J Surg* 1932; 15:65–67.

Carson WG Jr, Andrews JR: Arthroscopy of the elbow, in Zarins B, Andrews JR, Carson WG (eds): *Injuries to the Throwing Arm*. Philadelphia, W B Saunders Co, 1985.

Cassebaum WH: Operative treatment of T & Y fractures of the lower end of the humerus. *Am J Surg* 1952; 83:265–270.

Crenshaw AH: *Campbell's Operative Orthopaedics*, ed 7. St Louis, C V Mosby Co, 1987.

Durig M, Muller W, Ruedi TP, et al: The operative treatment of elbow dislocation in the adult. *J Bone Joint Surg* 1979; 61A:239–244.

Grant JCB: *An Atlas of Anatomy*, ed 6. Baltimore, Williams & Wilkins Co, 1972.

Gray H: *The Anatomy of the Human Body*, ed 29. Philadelphia, Lea & Febiger, 1975.

Hall RM: Recurrent posterior dislocation of the elbow joint in a boy. *J Bone Joint Surg* 1953; 35B:56.

Hasmann GC, Neer CS: Recurrent dislocation of the elbow. *J Bone Joint Surg* 1975; 57A:1080–1084.

Henry AK: *Extensile Exposure*, ed 2. New York, Churchill Livingston, Inc, 1963.

Hollinshead WH: *Anatomy for Surgeons: The Back and Limbs*, ed 3. New York, Harper & Row, 1982.

Hoppenfeld S: *Surgical Exposures in Orthopaedics: The Anatomical Approach*, ed 1. Philadelphia, J B Lippincott Co, 1984.

Inglis AE, Ranawat CS, Straub LR: Synovectomy and debridement of the elbow in rheumatoid arthritis. *J Bone Joint Surg* 1971; 53A:652–662.

Johansson H, Olerud S: Operative treatment of inter-condylar fractures of the humerus. *J Trauma* 1971; 11:836–843.

Kaplan EB: Surgical approach to the proximal end of the radius and its use in fractures of the head and neck of the radius. *J Bone Joint Surg* 1941; 23:86–92.

Kelly RP, Griffin TW: Open reduction of T-condylar fractures of the humerus through an anterior approach. *J Trauma* 1969; 9:901–914.

King T: Recurrent dislocations of the elbow. *J Bone Joint Surg* 1953; 35B:50–54.

Kocher T: *Chirurgische Operationslehre*. 2 Auflage. Jena, Gustave Fischer, 1894.

Kocher T: *Textbook of Operative Surgery* (Translated from 4th German edition by HJ Stiles). London, Adam & Charles Black, 1903.

Molesworth HWL: Operation for the complete exposure of the elbow joint. *Br J Surg* 1930; 18:303–307.

Morrey BF, Chao EY, Hui FC: Biomechanical study of the elbow following excision of the radial head. *J Bone Joint Surg* 1979; 61A:63–68.

Morrey BF, Kainan AN: Articular and ligamentous contributions to the stability of the elbow joint. *Am J Sports Med* 1983; 11:315–319.

Morrey BF: *The Elbow and Its Disorders*, ed 1. Philadelphia, W B Saunders Co, 1985.

Osborn G, Cotterill P: Recurrent dislocation of the elbow. *J Bone Joint Surg* 1966; 48B:340–346.

Swanson AB, Jaeger SH, LaRochelle D, et al: Comminuted fractures of the radial head. *J Bone Joint Surg* 1981; 63A:1039–1049.

Symeonides PP, Paschaloglou C, Stavrou Z, et al: Recurrent dislocation of the elbow. *J Bone Joint Surg* 1975; 57A:1084–1086.

Taylor TK, Scham SM: A posterior medial approach to the proximal end of the ulna for the internal fixation of olecranon fractures. *J Trauma* 1969; 9:594–602.

Tullos HS, Schwab G, Bennett JB, et al: Factors influencing elbow stability. *Am Acad Orthop Surg Instr Course Lectures* 1981; 30:185–199.

Urbaniak JR, et al: Correction of post-traumatic flexion contracture of the elbow by anterior capsulotomy. *J Bone Joint Surg* 1985; 67A:1160–1164.

Van Gorder GW: Surgical approach in old posterior dislocation of the elbow. *J Bone Joint Surg* 1932; 14:127–143.

Van Gorder GW: Surgical approach in supracondylar "T" fractures of the humerus requiring open reduction. *J Bone Joint Surg* 1940; 22:278–292.

5

Forearm

Charles E. Rhoades, M.D.

ANATOMIC FEATURES OF THE FOREARM

Rotation (pronation and supination) of the forearm allows placement of the hand in the most appropriate position for a specific task. The forearm muscles apply or resist forces to accomplish such tasks.

Bony Anatomy and Ligamentous Structures

The two bones of the forearm (Fig 5–1), the radius and the ulna, articulate with each other, the distal humerus, and the carpal bones of the wrist. The five articulations—the ulnohumeral (ulnotrochlear), radiohumeral (radiocapitellar), the proximal radioulnar, distal radioulnar, and radiocarpal—allow flexion and extension of the elbow and wrist, as well as rotation of the radius (in relation to the fixed ulna) for supination and pronation.

The proximal ulna consists of the olecranon and coronoid processes with the broad ulnotrochlear articular surface (trochlear, or greater sigmoid, notch) between them. The bone extends distally in a triangular shape with posterior, radial (interosseous), and anterior borders. Its distal half tapers to a round shaft, ending in the ulnar head and styloid process. The coronoid process and tuberosity of the ulna, situated just below the elbow joint, are the site of insertion of the brachialis muscle. The proximal ulna has a radial (lesser sigmoid) notch that provides a concavity for articulation with the radial head. The ulnar head articulates with the ulnar notch, a con-

cavity in the ulnar side of the distal radius. The distal end of the ulna is covered by the triangular fibrocartilage complex, which arises from the ulnar side of the distal radius just proximal to the articular surface and attaches to the base of the ulnar styloid process.

The radius is the converse of the ulna in that it is round proximally and provides the major articulation for the wrist joint distally. The radial head is completely covered with cartilage and rotates in the radial notch of the ulna. It also articulates with the capitellum of the humerus. The annular ligament firmly anchors the slender radial neck to the proximal ulna. The biceps tendon inserts on the radial (bicipital) tuberosity just distal to the annular ligament. Below the tuberosity the radius assumes a roughly triangular shape with anterior, posterior, and medial borders. It expands at its distal end to provide the radiocarpal articulation. The lower volar surface of the radius is relatively flat. The lower dorsal surface has a bony prominence, known as Lister's tubercle, around which courses the tendon of the extensor pollicis longus.

The interosseous membrane is a broad, strong, fibrous connection that runs in an oblique direction from the proximal radius to the distal ulna. This membrane coordinates rotation and prevents proximal migration of the radius. It begins just below the radial tuberosity and ends at the distal radioulnar joint. There is a gap of approximately 1.9 cm proximal to the distal radioulnar joint where the anterior interosseous artery dives posteriorly to join the posterior interosseous artery.

Proximally there is a narrow fibrous cord, known as the oblique cord. This cord courses dis-

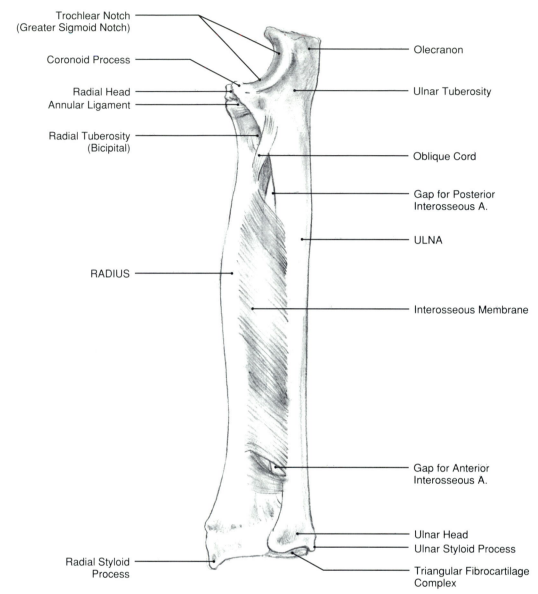

Trochlear Notch
(Greater Sigmoid Notch)

Coronoid Process

Radial Head
Annular Ligament

Radial Tuberosity
(Bicipital)

RADIUS

Radial Styloid
Process

Olecranon

Ulnar Tuberosity

Oblique Cord

Gap for Posterior
Interosseous A.

ULNA

Interosseous Membrane

Gap for Anterior
Interosseous A.

Ulnar Head
Ulnar Styloid Process

Triangular Fibrocartilage
Complex

FIG 5–1.
Bony and ligamentous configuration of the right forearm (side view, volar aspect).

tally from its ulnar origin just below the coronoid process to insert on the radius below the radial tuberosity. The posterior interosseous (or deep radial) nerve gains access to the extensor compartment as it passes through the gap between the oblique cord and interosseous membrane.

Muscles and Muscle Attachments

Anterior Forearm

The muscles of the anterior forearm consist of three radially grouped muscles known as the "mobile wad of three" (the brachioradialis, extensor carpi radialis longus, and extensor carpi radialis brevis), and three additional muscular layers: superficial, intermediate, and deep (Fig 5–2). The superficial layer consists of the pronator teres, flexor carpi radialis, palmaris longus, and flexor carpi ulnaris. The intermediate layer is composed entirely of the flexor digitorum superficialis. The deep layer consists of the supinator, flexor digitorum profundus, flexor pollicis longus, and pronator quadratus.

Mobile Wad of Three.—The mobile wad of three is a mobile muscle mass bordering the radial side of the forearm. It is an easily palpable landmark

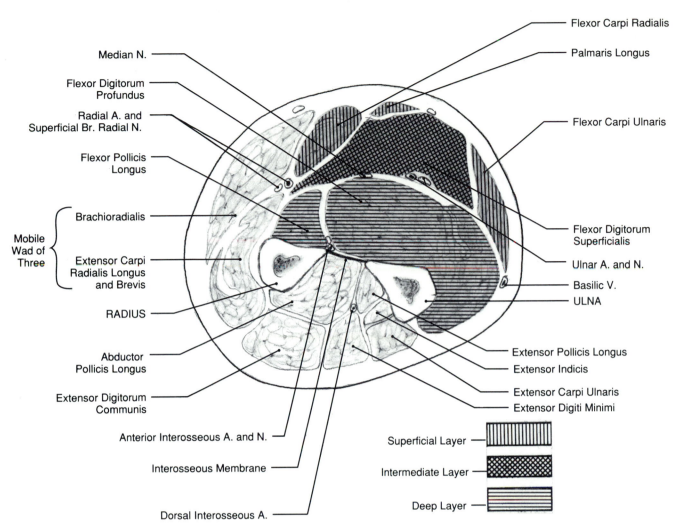

Median N.

Flexor Digitorum Profundus

Radial A. and Superficial Br. Radial N.

Flexor Pollicis Longus

Brachioradialis

Mobile Wad of Three

Extensor Carpi Radialis Longus and Brevis

RADIUS

Abductor Pollicis Longus

Extensor Digitorum Communis

Anterior Interosseous A. and N.

Interosseous Membrane

Dorsal Interosseous A.

Flexor Carpi Radialis

Palmaris Longus

Flexor Carpi Ulnaris

Flexor Digitorum Superficialis

Ulnar A. and N.

Basilic V.

ULNA

Extensor Pollicis Longus

Extensor Indicis

Extensor Carpi Ulnaris

Extensor Digiti Minimi

Superficial Layer

Intermediate Layer

Deep Layer

FIG 5–2.
Cross section through middle of supinated right forearm (as seen from a distal position, looking proximally), depicting superficial, intermediate, and deep layers of flexor muscles. Note supinator, pronator teres, and pronator quadratus muscles are not located in the midforearm.

that separates the flexor group on the volar aspect of the forearm from the common extensor muscles on the dorsal aspect of the forearm. It consists of one elbow flexor and two wrist extensor muscles. All three muscles of the mobile wad (brachioradialis, extensor carpi radialis longus and extensor carpi radialis brevis) originate from the lateral supracondylar ridge of the humerus. The brachioradialis inserts into the base of the radial styloid process. The extensor carpi radialis longus inserts into the dorsal surface of the base of the second (index) metacarpal and the extensor radialis brevis into the dorsal surface of the base of the third metacarpal. All three muscles are innervated by direct branches of the radial nerve and serve as borders for dissection anteriorly and posteriorly. The major function of the brachioradialis is el-

bow flexion, while the extensor carpi radialis longus and brevis are primarily wrist extensors.

Superficial Layer of Anterior Forearm.—Henry (Fig 5–3) describes a useful method of remembering the relationship of the four superficial muscles of the anterior forearm (pronator teres, flexor carpi radialis longus, palmaris longus, and flexor carpi ulnaris). When the heel of the opposite hand is placed on the medial epicondyle with the fingers extended distally, the thumb parallels the pronator teres, the index finger indicates the flexor carpi radialis, the long finger is on the palmaris longus, and the ring finger locates the flexor carpi ulnaris.

These four muscles share a common origin from the medial humeral epicondyle. Two of the muscles

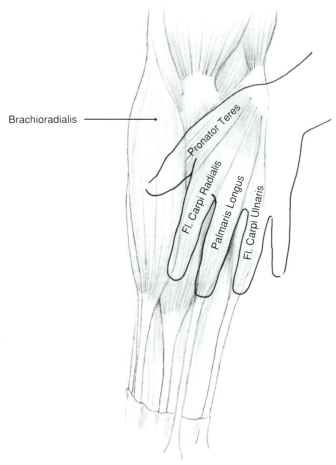

Brachioradialis

Pronator Teres

Fl. Carpi Radialis

Palmaris Longus

Fl. Carpi Ulnaris

FIG 5–3.
Superficial (common flexor) muscles of the anterior palmar forearm. Henry's mnemonic. (Redrawn from Henry AK: *Extensile Exposure*, 1963, Baltimore, Williams & Wilkins Co, p 95.)

Intermediate Layer of Anterior Forearm.—The flexor digitorum superficialis forms the intermediate muscle layer (Fig 5–4). Its origin is trigastric (humeral head, ulnar head, and a head from the proximal radius). It has superficial and deep planes. The superficial plane forms a slender sheet of muscle from the ulna to the radius and divides into the tendons to the long and ring fingers. The deep plane gives rise to the tendons to the index and little finger. The proximal border of the flexor digitorum superficialis forms a muscular arcade beneath which the median nerve passes in the proximal forearm. In the midforearm the thick tendinous portion of the muscle can be mistaken for the median nerve. The median nerve innervates this muscle, and its action is flexion of the proximal interphalangeal joints of the index through fifth fingers.

Deep Layer of Anterior Forearm.—The supinator is the most proximal deep muscle of the forearm (Fig 5–5). It originates from the radial side of the ulna and wraps around the radius from posterior to anterior to insert along the anterior shaft of the proximal radius. It is important to note that the deep branch of the radial nerve (the posterior interosseous nerve) passes through the body of the muscle into the extensor compartment. The supinator is innervated by a muscular branch of the radial nerve; as its name suggests, its function is supination of the forearm.

The flexor digitorum profundus originates from the ulna and forms a common motor tendon unit with all four tendons abreast. These flexor tendons insert into the distal phalanx of the index through fifth fingers. Innervation derives jointly from the anterior interosseous nerve (a branch of the median nerve) in its radial half (tendons to index and long finger) and the ulnar nerve in its ulnar half (tendons to ring and little finger). The flexor pollicis longus originates from the midshaft of the radius and inserts into the volar aspect of the distal phalanx of the thumb. It is innervated by the anterior interosseous nerve. The pronator quadratus originates from the distal ulna and inserts directly into the distal radius. It is innervated by the anterior interosseous nerve, and its function is pronation of the forearm.

Posterior Forearm

The muscles of the extensor (posterior) surface of the forearm (Fig 5–6) include the mobile wad of three, the common extensor group, and the deep group. The mobile wad of three was discussed in the section on the anterior forearm, since it overlies

have additional origins: the flexor carpi ulnaris originates partially from the olecranon and the pronator teres partially from the anterior ulna. The pronator teres inserts at the junction of the proximal and middle portions of the radius. It functions as a strong pronator of the forearm as well as a weak flexor of the elbow. The flexor carpi radialis inserts into the base of the index and sometimes the third (long) metacarpal, and its major function is wrist flexion. The palmaris longus inserts into and becomes continuous with the palmar aponeurosis and is a weak wrist flexor. The flexor carpi ulnaris inserts into a carpal bone (the pisiform), and its major functions are flexion and ulnar deviation of the wrist.

The pronator teres, flexor carpi radialis longus, and palmaris longus are innervated by the median nerve, while the flexor carpi ulnaris is supplied by the ulnar nerve.

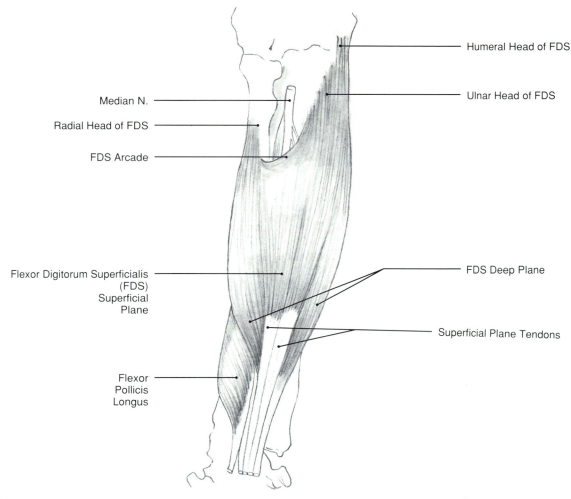

Humeral Head of FDS

Ulnar Head of FDS

Median N.

Radial Head of FDS

FDS Arcade

Flexor Digitorum Superficialis
(FDS)
Superficial
Plane

FDS Deep Plane

Superficial Plane Tendons

Flexor
Pollicis
Longus

FIG 5–4.
Intermediate muscle layer of anterior forearm: flexor digitorum superficialis muscle. (Superficial muscle layer has been removed.) Note heads of origin and arrangement of muscle tendons. Note median nerve passing beneath flexor digitorum superficialis arcade.

part of the anterior as well as the posterior forearm and contains one elbow flexor and two wrist extensor muscles.

Common Extensor Group of the Posterior Forearm.—The common extensor group includes the anconeus, extensor digitorum communis, extensor digiti minimi (quinti), and extensor carpi ulnaris. The anconeus originates from the lateral humeral epicondyle and inserts into the proximal ulna. Its function is a subject of debate. Suggestions have included elbow extension, ulnar abduction during pronation, and elbow joint stabilization. The anconeus is an important landmark in various surgical exposures of the elbow. The extensor digitorum communis originates from the lateral humeral epicondyle and divides into three or four extensor tendons,

which participate in the complex extensor function of the index through fifth fingers. The extensor digiti minimi (quinti) arises from the common extensor tendon and proceeds to the dorsum of the first phalanx of the fifth finger. The extensor carpi ulnaris has humeral and ulnar origins and inserts on the dorsal base of the fifth metacarpal. It is a wrist extensor and adductor (ulnar deviation).

All the muscles except the anconeus are innervated by the deep radial (posterior interosseous) nerve. The anconeus receives separate innervation from posterior muscular branches of the radial nerve.

Deep Muscles of the Posterior Forearm.—The deep muscles are the abductor pollicis longus, extensor pollicis brevis, extensor pollicis longus, and ex-

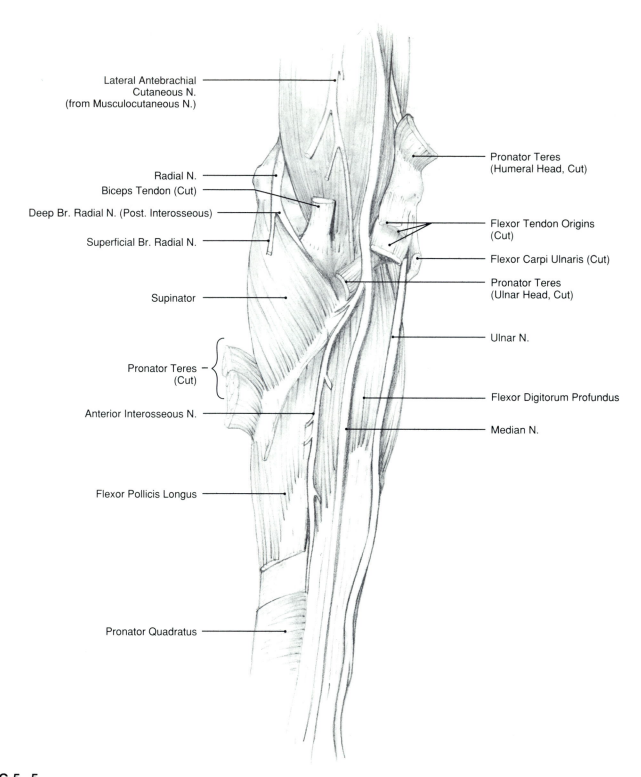

Lateral Antebrachial
Cutaneous N.
(from Musculocutaneous N.)

Radial N.

Biceps Tendon (Cut)

Deep Br. Radial N. (Post. Interosseous)

Superficial Br. Radial N.

Supinator

Pronator Teres
(Cut)

Anterior Interosseous N.

Flexor Pollicis Longus

Pronator Quadratus

Pronator Teres
(Humeral Head, Cut)

Flexor Tendon Origins
(Cut)

Flexor Carpi Ulnaris (Cut)

Pronator Teres
(Ulnar Head, Cut)

Ulnar N.

Flexor Digitorum Profundus

Median N.

FIG 5–5.
Deep flexors of anterior forearm (superficial and intermediate muscle layers have been removed) and their relationship to the nerves of the forearm.

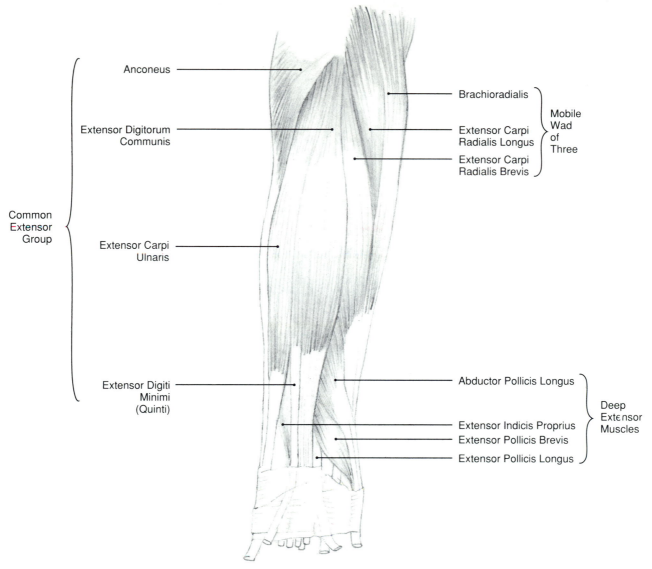

Anconeus

Extensor Digitorum
Communis

Brachioradialis

Extensor Carpi
Radialis Longus

Extensor Carpi
Radialis Brevis

Mobile
Wad
of
Three

Common
Extensor
Group

Extensor Carpi
Ulnaris

Extensor Digiti
Minimi
(Quinti)

Abductor Pollicis Longus

Extensor Indicis Proprius

Extensor Pollicis Brevis

Extensor Pollicis Longus

Deep
Extensor
Muscles

FIG 5–6.
Muscles on extensor (posterior) surface of the right forearm and mobile wad of three. Note common extensor tendon is separate from mobile wad of three; common extensor tendon originates from the lateral epicondyle, whereas mobile wad of three originates from the lateral supracondylar ridge.

tensor indicis proprius. The abductor pollicis longus originates from the proximal radius and intermuscular septum. It wraps around the radius radially, lying next to the extensor pollicis brevis. The extensor pollicis brevis originates from the middistal radius. It parallels the abductor pollicis longus into the first dorsal compartment of the wrist. The extensor pollicis longus originates from the intermuscular septum and radial border of the ulna. The extensor indicis proprius originates distal to the extensor pollicis longus from the intermuscular septum and ulna. All of the deep extensors are innervated by the muscular

branches of the posterior interosseous nerve. Their function includes wrist and hand abduction, as well as extension of the digits upon which they insert. Further details can be found in the chapter on the wrist and hand.

Arteries

The two major arteries in the forearm are the radial and ulnar arteries (Figs 5–7 and 5–8). They arise from the brachial artery as it exits the antecubital fossa. At the elbow the brachial artery passes

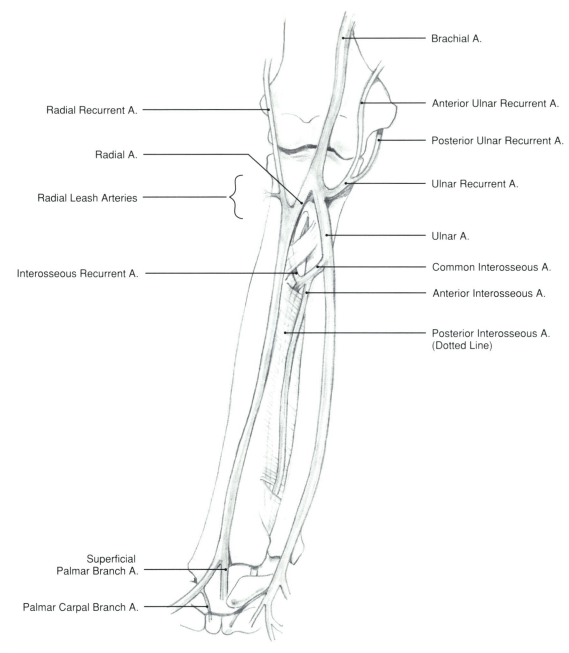

Brachial A.

Radial Recurrent A.

Anterior Ulnar Recurrent A.

Posterior Ulnar Recurrent A.

Radial A.

Ulnar Recurrent A.

Radial Leash Arteries

Ulnar A.

Common Interosseous A.

Interosseous Recurrent A.

Anterior Interosseous A.

Posterior Interosseous A.
(Dotted Line)

Superficial
Palmar Branch A.

Palmar Carpal Branch A.

FIG 5–7.
Arteries of right forearm, anterior view.

medial to the biceps tendon, a constant relationship that aids dissection. It divides into radial and ulnar branches at the level of the biceps insertion on the radial tuberosity.

Radial Artery and Branches

The radial artery courses laterally and distally just beneath the lacertus fibrosus (see Chapter 4), intimately following the proximal belly of the pronator

teres. As the pronator teres descends to insert on the radius, the radial artery passes superficial to the pronator teres and flexor digitorum superficialis to lie next to the superficial radial nerve under cover of the brachioradialis.

A constant branch, the radial recurrent artery, exits laterally approximately 2 cm distal to the biceps tendon insertion. It then ascends, giving off a leash of small muscular perforators that supply flexors

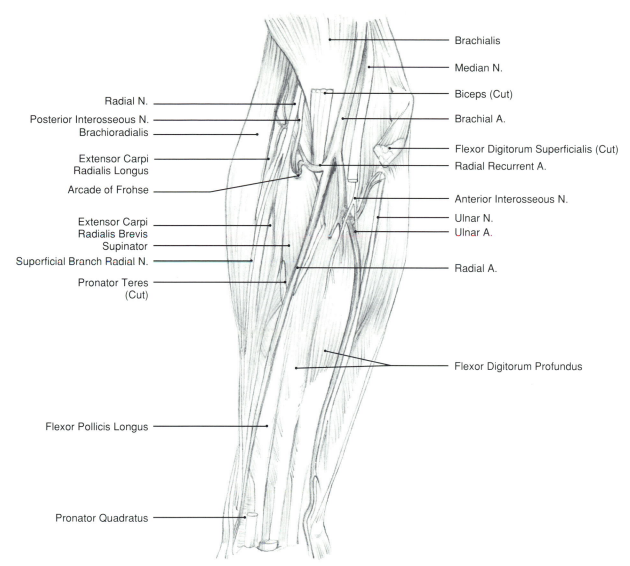

Brachialis
Median N.
Biceps (Cut)
Brachial A.
Flexor Digitorum Superficialis (Cut)
Radial Recurrent A.
Anterior Interosseous N.
Ulnar N.
Ulnar A.
Radial A.

Radial N.
Posterior Interosseous N.
Brachioradialis
Extensor Carpi Radialis Longus
Arcade of Frohse
Extensor Carpi Radialis Brevis
Supinator
Superficial Branch Radial N.
Pronator Teres (Cut)

Flexor Digitorum Profundus

Flexor Pollicis Longus

Pronator Quadratus

FIG 5–8.
Relationship of nerves, arteries, and deep flexor muscles in the anterior aspect of the forearm. (Superficial and intermediate muscle layers have been removed.)

and extensors on the radial side of the forearm. The radial recurrent artery turns back in a proximal direction (lying adjacent to the radial nerve) and anastomoses with the radial collateral artery, a branch of the deep radial (profunda) artery. It must be divided and carefully ligated to allow mobilization of the mobile wad of three.

As the radial artery descends in the forearm it maintains its position between the flexor carpi radialis and brachioradialis to the end of the forearm, where it gives off the superficial palmar branch to the thenar muscles and the palmar carpal branch. The radial artery then passes dorsally beneath the tendons of the abductor pollicis longus and extensor pollicis brevis to enter the anatomic snuff-box in the dorsoradial aspect of the wrist.

Ulnar Artery and Branches

The ulnar artery arises from the bifurcation of the brachial artery and passes deep to the median nerve and ulnar head of the pronator teres. It travels with the ulnar nerve down the forearm. It traverses from the midline to the ulnar border of the forearm in the plane between the flexor digitorum superficialis and flexor digitorum profundus. It maintains a position radial to the ulnar nerve into the wrist. Two branches, the ulnar recurrent and common interosseous, are given off proximally. The ulnar recurrent artery divides into anterior and posterior ulnar recurrent branches. These ascend around the medial epicondyle of the humerus and then anastomose with the inferior ulnar collateral and superior ulnar collateral arteries, respectively.

The common interosseous artery separates from the ulnar artery approximately 2.5 cm distal to the bifurcation of the brachial artery. It is almost equal in size to the distal ulnar artery (which represents the continuation of the ulnar artery). The common interosseous artery divides into the anterior and posterior interosseous arteries. The anterior interosseous artery lies on the palmar surface of the interosseous membrane until it passes dorsally through the gap in the membrane to join the poste-

rior interosseous artery, approximately 1.9 cm proximal to the distal radioulnar joint. The posterior interosseous artery runs dorsal to the interosseous membrane with the posterior interosseous nerve to terminate in the distal forearm and wrist. An interosseous recurrent branch arises from the posterior interosseous artery to anastomose about the elbow in an arborization known as the rete articulare cubiti.

Nerves

The three major nerves of the forearm are the median, ulnar, and radial nerves (Figs 5–5, 5–8, and 5–9). The lateral antebrachial cutaneous nerve (which is a continuation of the musculocutaneous nerve) and medial antebrachial cutaneous nerve provide terminal sensory branches to the forearm.

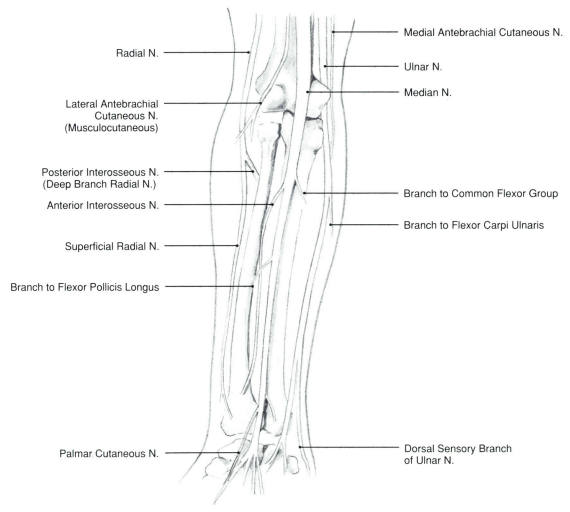

FIG 5–9.
Major nerves of forearm, anterior view.

Median Nerve and Branches

The median nerve is the largest and most important nerve in the forearm and hand. It provides the "eyes of the hand" via its large sensory distribution. It enters the antebrachial fossa medial to the biceps tendon and brachial artery. Branches are given to the common flexor group. The median nerve passes through the two heads of the pronator teres (or deep to the humeral head only). It courses between the two heads of the flexor digitorum superficialis to travel along the dorsal fascia of the flexor digitorum superficialis to the wrist.

The largest branch of the median nerve, the anterior interosseous nerve, arises dorsally distal to the pronator teres. This branch lies on the palmar surface of the flexor digitorum profundus. It innervates the radial half of the flexor digitorum profundus, then travels distally between the flexor digitorum profundus and flexor pollicis longus to lie on the volar aspect of the interosseous membrane. It innervates the flexor pollicis longus and pronator quadratus. Near the wrist the median nerve emerges to lie superficial to the tendons of the flexor digitorum superficialis. It enters the carpal tunnel on the radial

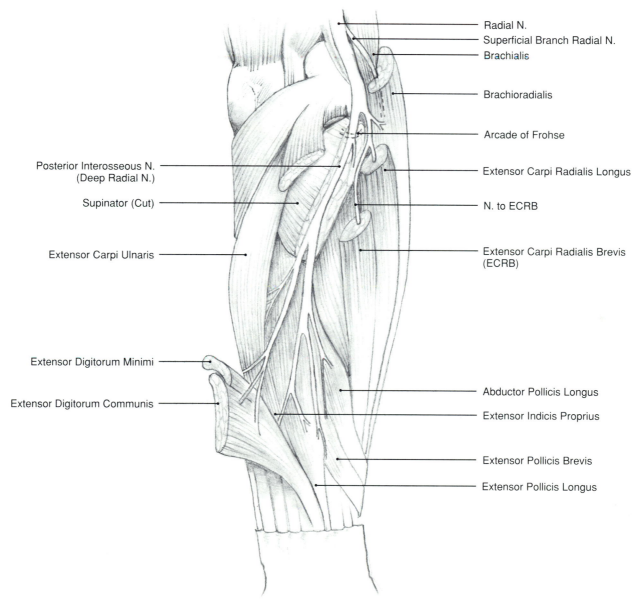

Radial N.

Superficial Branch Radial N.

Brachialis

Brachioradialis

Arcade of Frohse

Posterior Interosseous N.
(Deep Radial N.)

Extensor Carpi Radialis Longus

Supinator (Cut)

N. to ECRB

Extensor Carpi Ulnaris

Extensor Carpi Radialis Brevis
(ECRB)

Extensor Digitorum Minimi

Extensor Digitorum Communis

Abductor Pollicis Longus

Extensor Indicis Proprius

Extensor Pollicis Brevis

Extensor Pollicis Longus

FIG 5–10.
Path of radial nerve through supinator muscle to extensor (posterior) surface of forearm.

side of the palmaris longus tendon, but this relationship is somewhat inconstant.

The palmar cutaneous branch arises from the median nerve approximately 5 cm proximal to the wrist crease. It runs distally, radial to the median nerve and outside the carpal canal, to supply sensation to the thenar eminence.

Ulnar Nerve and Branches

The ulnar nerve enters the forearm from behind the medial epicondyle of the humerus through the two heads of the flexor carpi ulnaris. It gives off a few articular branches as it passes the elbow joint. Its first muscular branch is to the flexor carpi ulnaris. It then travels between the flexor carpi ulnaris and the flexor digitorum profundus to the wrist. It gives branches to the ulnar half of the flexor digitorum profundus. The ulnar artery joins the ulnar nerve midway down the forearm and lies radial to the nerve throughout. A dorsal sensory branch exits the main nerve approximately 7 cm proximal to the wrist crease. It passes deep to the tendon of the flexor carpi ulnaris and enters the extensor surface between the flexor carpi ulnaris and extensor carpi ulnaris.

Radial Nerve and Branches

The radial nerve (Fig 5–10) is the nerve to the mobile wad of three and the extensor compartment. It emerges from posterior to anterior between the brachialis and brachioradialis muscles just above the elbow. The branches to the brachioradialis and extensor carpi radialis longus are given off above the elbow. At the level of the lateral epicondyle the main trunk divides into two main terminal branches: the posterior interosseous and superficial radial nerves. A separate twig to the extensor carpi radialis brevis is either a separate branch or comes from one of the terminal branches. The superficial radial nerve courses distally beneath the brachioradialis tendon to reach the dorsum of the wrist and hand.

Posterior Interosseous Nerve

The posterior interosseous (deep radial) nerve is of great surgical significance. Its position, wrapped around the radial neck, puts it in jeopardy with forearm fractures and surgical procedures in this area. After dividing from the superficial branch, the deep radial nerve enters the supinator muscle. In approximately 25% of limbs, the nerve comes into contact with the radial neck (a point of clinical importance). It runs obliquely through the supinator, dividing the

muscle into deep and superficial layers, and around the radial neck to emerge on the extensor surface. The proximal edge of the supinator muscle has a fibrous arcade (the arcade of Frohse), which can be a point of posterior interosseous nerve compression.

As the posterior interosseous nerve emerges from the supinator, it gives off a leash of nerves to the extensor digitorum communis, extensor digitorum minimi, and extensor carpi ulnaris. The length of this leash can be the limiting structural feature in mobilizing the extensor digitorum communis from the mobile wad of three (extensor carpi radialis brevis, extensor carpi radialis longus, and brachioradialis). The posterior interosseous nerve continues distally along the interosseous membrane to innervate the abductor pollicis longus, the extensor pollicis brevis, the extensor pollicis longus, and finally the extensor indicis proprius. A sensory contribution is given terminally to the dorsal wrist capsule.

SURGICAL APPROACHES TO THE FOREARM

Anterior Approach to Radius

The anterior approach, attributed to Henry, is an extensile approach that can give full visualization of the radial shaft, radial artery, radial nerve, and superficial branch of the radial nerve. It can be expanded to visualize all muscles of the anterior forearm as well as the median and ulnar nerves (Fig 5–11).

The procedure is carried out with the patient supine. The proximal dissection is performed with the forearm supinated. During the procedure the forearm is slightly pronated to obtain access to muscle attachments on the middle and distal portions of the radius, then returned to a supinated position to carry out extensive procedures on the radius. In the supinated position, stretch injuries to the deep radial nerve are less likely.

A straight, or preferably curvilinear, skin incision begins proximally at the interval between the brachioradialis and pronator teres, extends down the forearm, and ends proximal to the wrist crease. It can be lengthened distally or proximally for extensile exposure. The skin can be generously undermined and retracted for wide access.

The superficial fascia is opened in line with the radius, with the prominent veins ligated and retracted as needed. The interval between the brachioradialis and flexor carpi radialis is most easily identified distally and developed proximally. The tendon of the flexor carpi radialis is a characteristically broad, flat tendon that is easily recognized. The superficial radial nerve is retracted radially with the brachioradialis. The radial artery is identified as it lies along the flexor carpi radialis.

As the interval is developed proximally, the pronator teres becomes the medial border of the wound. Care must be taken when the fascia is entered proximally between the brachioradialis and pronator teres, as the radial artery can lie very superficially beneath the lacertus fibrosus. Blunt scissor dissection is recommended. The belly of the brachioradialis may wrap around the radius and lie farther medially than expected. Blunt finger dissection effectively separates the brachioradialis and pronator

teres. This exposes the radial nerve and artery in the depths of the wound, as well as the lateral antebrachial cutaneous nerve (a continuation of the musculocutaneous nerve) coming from under the biceps. The lateral antebrachial cutaneous nerve must not be mistaken for the radial nerve.

The biceps tendon is the key to proximal dissection. It is easily tensed and palpated. The radial artery passes medial to the tendon, then crosses to the radial side of the forearm. Blunt dissection along the radial side of the artery will encounter resistance in the perivascular fat approximately 2 cm distal to the biceps tendon. This identifies the site of the radial recurrent artery and radial leash vessels. The vessels of the leash may form anterior and posterior bundles around the superficial radial nerve. These radial leash vessels, as well as the radial recurrent artery,

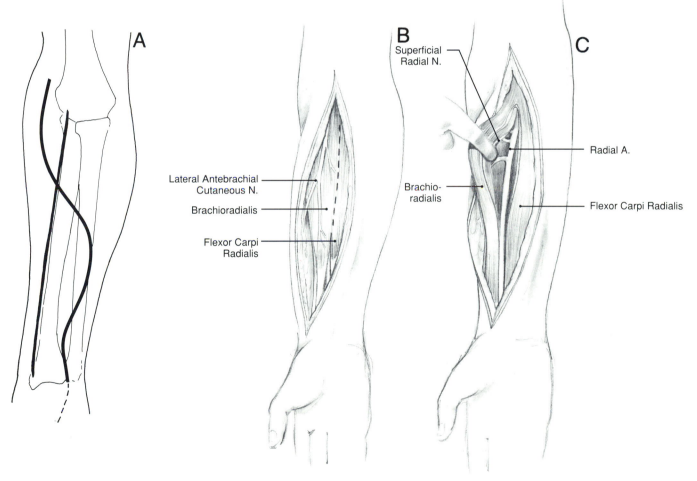

FIG 5–11.
Anterior approach to radius. **A,** skin incisions for an extensile anterior approach to forearm. Curved incision is preferred. The incision can be extended into the volar aspect of the wrist, if necessary *(dashed lines)*. **B,** superficial fascial incision *(dashed line)*. **C,** interval developed between brachioradialis and flexor carpi radialis. Note radial artery's relationship to flexor carpi radialis. Superficial radial nerve lies beneath the brachioradialis muscle and tendon. *(Continued.)*

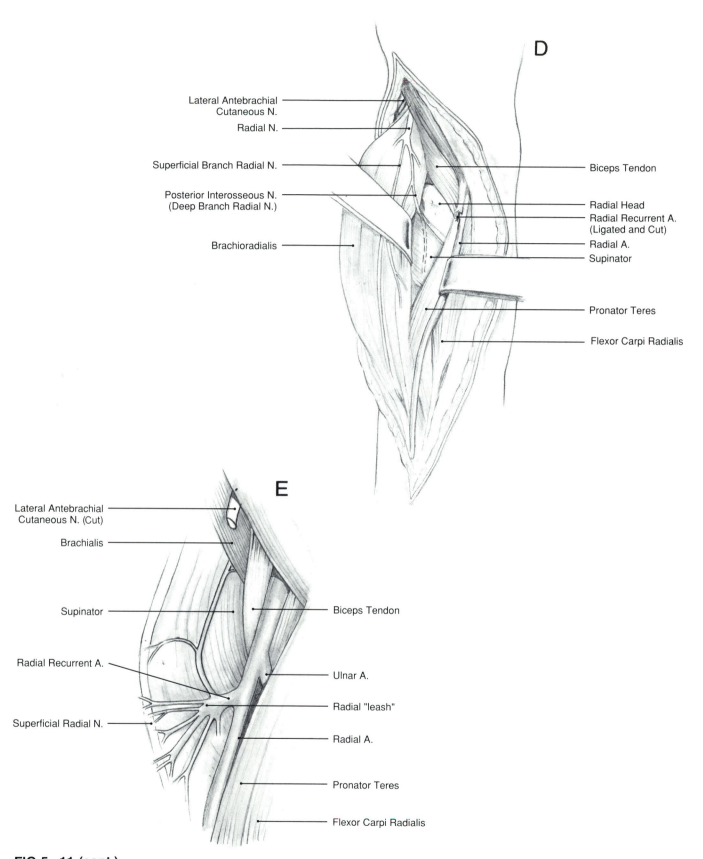

Lateral Antebrachial Cutaneous N.

Radial N.

Superficial Branch Radial N.

Posterior Interosseous N. (Deep Branch Radial N.)

Brachioradialis

D

Biceps Tendon

Radial Head

Radial Recurrent A. (Ligated and Cut)

Radial A.

Supinator

Pronator Teres

Flexor Carpi Radialis

Lateral Antebrachial Cutaneous N. (Cut)

Brachialis

Supinator

Radial Recurrent A.

Superficial Radial N.

E

Biceps Tendon

Ulnar A.

Radial "leash"

Radial A.

Pronator Teres

Flexor Carpi Radialis

FIG 5–11 (cont.).
D, deep dissection: radial recurrent artery has been ligated and mobile wad of three retracted laterally with superficial radial nerve. Pronator teres is limiting structure for visualization. Supinator muscle fibers cross field almost transversely. Note relationship of posterior interosseous nerve and supinator muscle. **E,** relationship of radial leash to surrounding structures.

(Continued.)

must be identified and ligated to allow adequate mobilization of the mobile wad of three.

The plane between the brachioradialis and pronator teres can now be fully developed. The fibers of the supinator muscle can be seen wrapping around the radius. There is a bursa between the lateral edge of the biceps tendon and the medial edge of the supinator that serves as a guide for release of the supinator. With the arm in full supination, which moves the posterior interosseous nerve laterally, dissection through the supinator directly lateral to the biceps provides access to the proximal one third of the radius. The posterior interosseous nerve is protected by lifting the supinator subperiosteally, which car-ries the nerve safely in the muscle substance. Care must be taken to avoid overzealous retraction of the supinator due to the limited excursion of the posterior interosseous nerve. The retractor must also be placed carefully to avoid injury to the posterior interosseous nerve, particularly in limbs (25%) in which this nerve is in direct contact with the neck of the radius.

If exposure to the middle and distal portions of the radius is needed, further dissection can be carried out.

Exposure to the middle one third of the radius is developed by pronating the arm to roll the insertion of the pronator teres into view. The muscle is

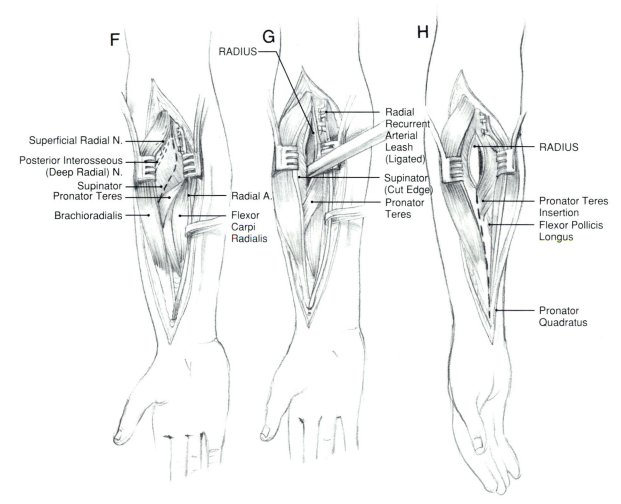

FIG 5–11 (cont.).
F, incision *(heavy dashed line)* through supinator for deep exposure of the proximal radius. Note location of underlying posterior interosseous nerve *(light double-dashed line)*. **G,** subperiosteal dissection of supinator with forearm supinated to move deep branch of radial (posterior interosseous) nerve as far laterally as possible. With this maneuver, proximal radius is exposed. **H,** pronation of the forearm allows visualization of the attachment of the pronator teres, flexor pollicis longus, and pronator quadratus, which can be detached from the radius to allow exposure of middle and distal shaft *(dashed lines)*.

(Continued.)

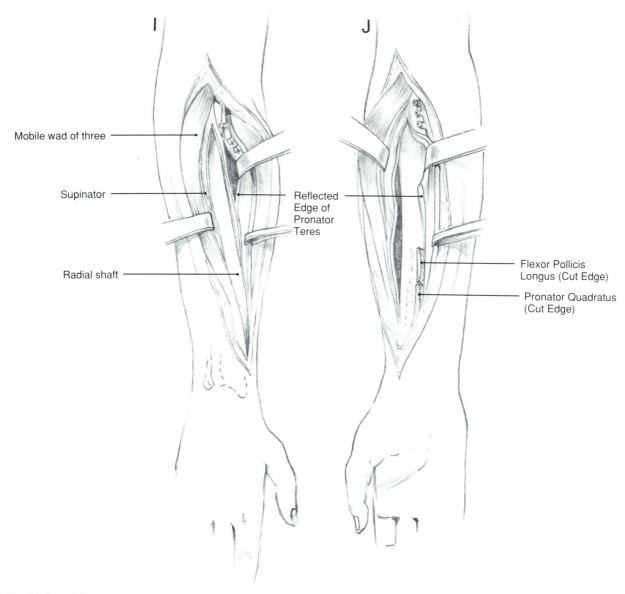

FIG 5–11 (cont.).

I, complete exposure of the radial shaft. **J,** forearm is returned to supinated position. Sharp periosteal elevation of all attachments to radial shaft. Note hand supinated to maintain safe position of superficial and deep radial nerves. (Modified from Henry AK: *Extensile Exposure,* 1963, Baltimore, Williams & Wilkins Co.)

sharply incised at its distal margin and subperiosteally elevated medially. With medial retraction of these elevated structures and rotation of the bone, the entire midshaft of the radius is exposed.

The distal one third of the radius is covered anteriorly by the flexor pollicis longus and pronator quadratus. Their attachments can be sharply reflected from the radius and raised subperiosteally to expose the distal radius.

The forearm is then returned to a supinated position in which the superficial and deep radial nerves are less prone to stretch injuries while operative procedures are carried out.

Direct Approach to the Ulnar Shaft

The ulna, being subcutaneous in its entire length, can be easily approached. The arm is slightly pronated to expose the dorsal ulnar border. An incision of desired length (Fig 5–12) follows the palpable bone from the tip of the olecranon to the ulnar styloid. Sharp dissection is carried down to the

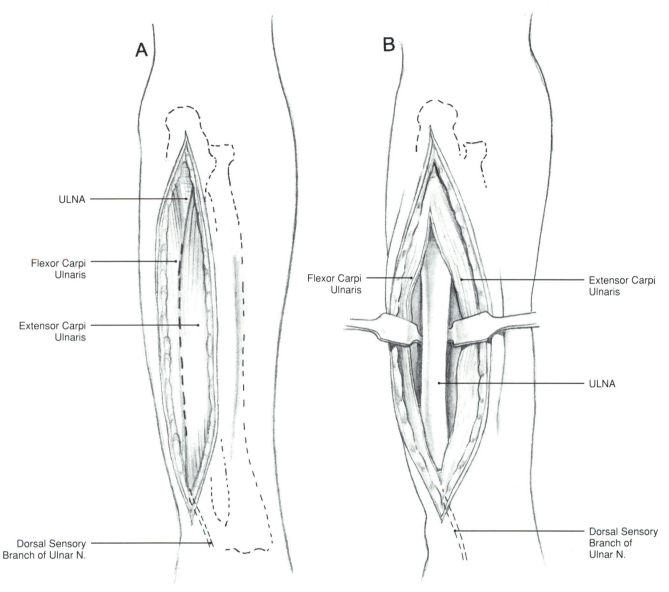

FIG 5–12.
Direct approach to ulnar shaft. **A,** skin incision has been made directly over the shaft of the ulna. Deep fascial incision *(dashed line)* is made in line with the skin incision in the internervous plane between the flexor carpi ulnaris (innervated by the ulnar nerve) and extensor carpi ulnaris (innervated by the posterior interosseous nerve). **B,** safe subperiosteal plane of dissection and retraction showing almost entire circumference of the ulna. Note dorsal sensory branch of the ulnar nerve *(double dashed line).*

bone. The interval between the extensor carpi ulnaris (innervated by the posterior interosseous [deep radial] nerve) and the flexor carpi ulnaris (innervated by the ulnar nerve) forms a safe internervous dissection plane. Subperiosteal reflection of these muscles exposes almost the entire circumference of the ulna. The only structure at risk is the dorsal sensory branch of the ulnar nerve, which crosses the ulna in the distal one fourth of the forearm. All other structures are safe if a subperiosteal dissection

plane is maintained. If the body of the flexor carpi ulnaris is violated, the ulnar artery and ulnar nerve can be encountered; however, reasonable care should prevent this.

Posterior Approach to Radius (Thompson)

The posterior approach as originally described by Thompson for the proximal posterior radius can easily be expanded to expose the entire radius (Fig 5–13).

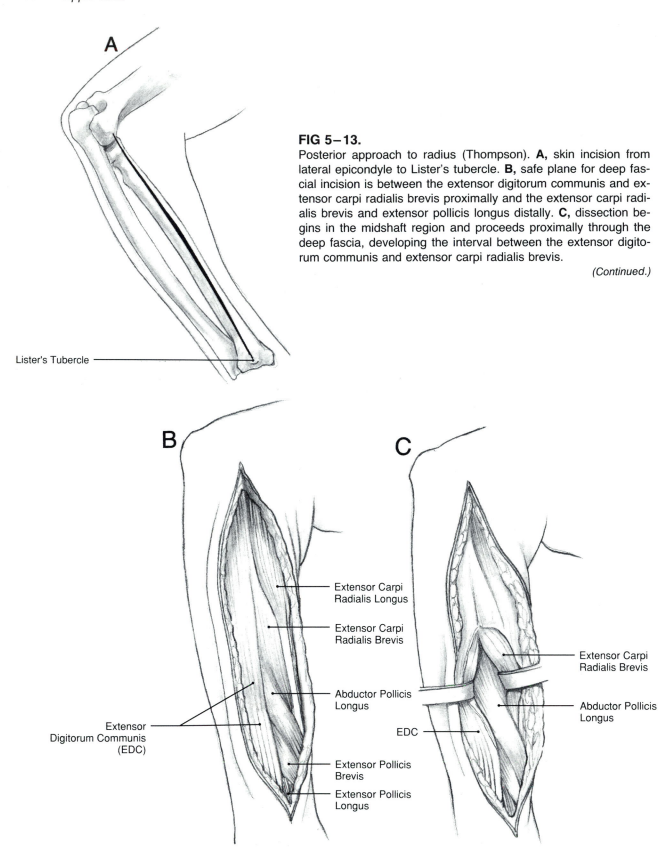

Lister's Tubercle

FIG 5–13.
Posterior approach to radius (Thompson). **A,** skin incision from lateral epicondyle to Lister's tubercle. **B,** safe plane for deep fascial incision is between the extensor digitorum communis and extensor carpi radialis brevis proximally and the extensor carpi radialis brevis and extensor pollicis longus distally. **C,** dissection begins in the midshaft region and proceeds proximally through the deep fascia, developing the interval between the extensor digitorum communis and extensor carpi radialis brevis.

(Continued.)

Extensor Carpi
Radialis Longus

Extensor Carpi
Radialis Brevis

Abductor Pollicis
Longus

Extensor
Digitorum Communis
(EDC)

Extensor Pollicis
Brevis

Extensor Pollicis
Longus

Extensor Carpi
Radialis Brevis

Abductor Pollicis
Longus

EDC

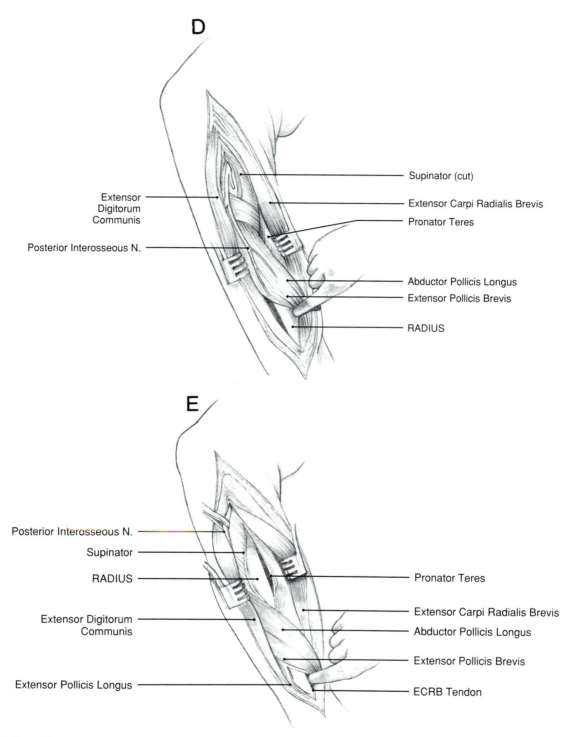

D

Supinator (cut)

Extensor Carpi Radialis Brevis

Pronator Teres

Extensor Digitorum Communis

Posterior Interosseous N.

Abductor Pollicis Longus

Extensor Pollicis Brevis

RADIUS

E

Posterior Interosseous N.

Supinator

RADIUS

Pronator Teres

Extensor Carpi Radialis Brevis

Abductor Pollicis Longus

Extensor Digitorum Communis

Extensor Pollicis Brevis

Extensor Pollicis Longus

ECRB Tendon

FIG 5–13 (cont.).
D, dissection deep to the extensor digitorum communis. The vigor of retraction of the extensor digitorum communis must be limited to prevent stretch injury to the posterior interosseous nerve. Extensor carpi radialis brevis is retracted radially. Abductor pollicis longus and extensor pollicis brevis are usually left attached with their origins undisturbed; dissection is carried out under this bridge of muscle. **E,** complete exposure of the radius is accomplished by retraction of the cut edges of the supinator and pronator teres in the proximal wound; mobilization of the muscle bridge composed of the abductor pollicis longus and extensor pollicis brevis; and, in the distal portion of the wound, retraction of the extensor pollicis longus ulnarly and the extensor carpi radialis brevis tendon radially.

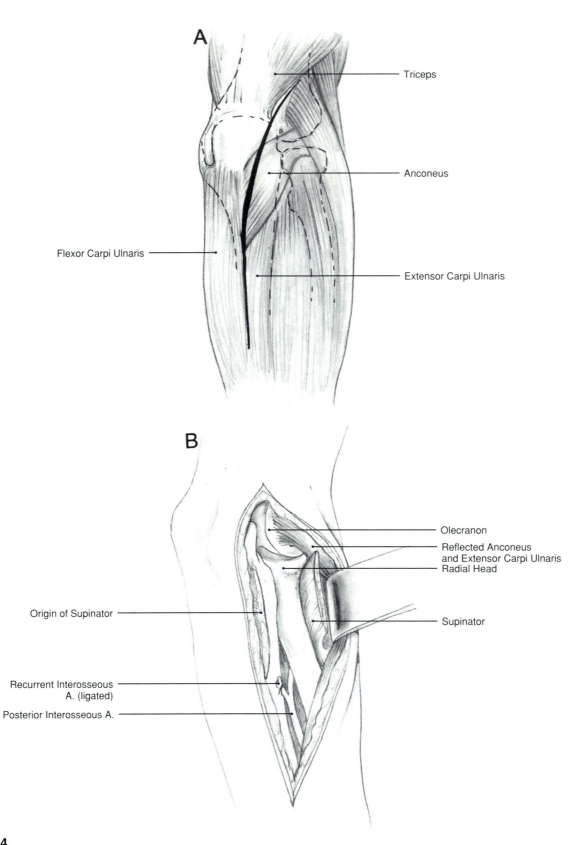

FIG 5–14.
Posterior approach to proximal radius and ulna (Boyd approach). **A,** incision through the origins of the anconeus and extensor carpi ulnaris. **B,** anconeus and extensor carpi ulnaris reflected off the ulna. Origin of supinator dissected from the ulna and reflected medially with the posterior interosseous nerve to allow limited exposure of the proximal radius. The nerve is in the body of the supinator and will not be visualized. (Redrawn from Boyd HB: Surgical exposure of the ulna and proximal third of the radius through one incision. *Surg Gynecol Obstet* 1940; 71:87–88.)

The patient is placed in a supine position and the arm pronated or laid over the chest. The skin is incised from the lateral epicondyle to Lister's tubercle in a slightly curved fashion. The deep fascial incision is located in the interval between the extensor digitorum communis and extensor carpi radialis brevis proximally and the extensor carpi radialis brevis and extensor pollicis longus distally. This interval represents a safe plane between the muscles innervated by the radial nerve itself (extensor carpi radialis brevis) and its posterior interosseous (or deep radial) branch (extensor digitorum communis and extensor pollicis longus). The plane between the extensor carpi radialis brevis and extensor digitorum communis is distinct. It is identified in the midforearm and developed proximally to the common aponeurosis.

Splitting the common aponeurosis and retracting the mobile wad radially and the extensor digitorum communis ulnarly expose the supinator muscle. Emerging from the supinator, approximately 1 cm proximal to the distal edge, is the posterior interosseous (deep radial) nerve. It gives a leash of nerves to the extensor digitorum communis, extensor digitorum minimi, and extensor carpi ulnaris. The leash is the limiting structure to retraction of these muscles and must not be overdistracted. The supinator can be split in line with the posterior interosseous nerve to allow complete visualization of the nerve. Note that the fibers of the supinator run around the radius circumferentially, while the posterior interosseous nerve passes at 90 degrees to these fibers. After the radial nerve is exposed proximally, the arm can be supinated to bring the anterior shaft of the radius and the insertion of the supinator into view. The supinator can be released at its insertion and retracted. The pronator teres insertion can be stripped subperiosteally from the proximal portion of the middle one third of the radius to complete circumferential exposure.

The middle one third is covered by the bellies of the abductor pollicis longus and extensor pollicis brevis. The proximal and distal margins of contact between these two muscles and the radius can be incised and the muscles lifted with the periosteum. Retraction of the two muscle bellies proximally or distally exposes the middle one third of the radius.

The distal one third can be easily exposed by developing the interval between the extensor carpi radialis brevis tendon and the extensor pollicis longus. There are no underlying structures here and the radius is readily accessible.

Posterior Approach to Proximal Radius and Ulna (Boyd)

Boyd described a dorsal ulnar approach to both bones of the proximal forearm (Fig 5–14). The patient is placed in a supine position with the arm pronated or laid over the chest. A slightly curved incision is made on the radial side of the triceps tendon, starting from a point 2.5 cm proximal to the olecranon tip. The incision extends to the subcutaneous border of the ulna along the proximal one fourth of the ulna. The anconeus and extensor carpi ulnaris are reflected off the ulna. The insertion of the anconeus is sharply elevated from the olecranon. Deeper dissection exposes the origin of the supinator, which is elevated subperiosteally from the ulna. The entire muscle flap is retracted radially to expose the radial side of the olecranon and the proximal one fourth of the radius. The exposure can be increased by ligating the interosseous recurrent artery (but preserving the posterior interosseous artery) to allow further retraction. The posterior interosseous nerve is protected within the muscle belly of the supinator.

BIBLIOGRAPHY

Alonso-Llames M: Bilaterotricipital approach to the elbow. *Acta Orthop Scand* 1972; 43:479–490.

Banks S, Laufman H: *An Atlas of Surgical Exposures of the Extremities.* Philadelphia, W B Saunders Co, 1953.

Boyd HB: Surgical exposure of the ulna and proximal third of the radius through one incision. *Surg Gynecol Obstet* 1940; 71:87–88.

Darrach W: Surgical approaches for surgery of the extremities. *Am J Surg* 1945; 67:237–262.

Davies F, Laird M: The supinator muscle and the deep radial (posterior interosseous) nerve. *Anat Rec* 1948; 101:243–250.

Fearn CBd'A, Goodfellow JW: Anterior interosseous nerve palsy. *J Bone Joint Surg* 1965; 47B:91–93.

Gordon ML: Monteggia fracture: A combined surgical approach employing a single lateral incision. *Clin Orthop Rel Res* 1967; 50:87–93.

Grant JCB: *An Atlas of Anatomy,* ed 6. Baltimore, Williams & Wilkins Co, 1972.

Henry AK: *Extensile Exposure,* ed 2. New York, Churchill-Livingstone, Inc, 1963.

Hollinshead WH: *Anatomy for Surgeons: The Back and Limbs,* ed 3. New York, Harper & Row, 1982.

Hoppenfeld S: *Surgical Exposures in Orthopaedics: The Anatomical Approach,* ed 1. Philadelphia, J B Lippincott Co, 1984.

Kaplan EB: Surgical approach to the proximal end of the radius and its use in fractures of the head and neck of the radius. *J Bone Joint Surg* 1941; 23:86–92.

Kiloh LG, Nevin S: Isolated neuritis of the anterior interosseous nerve. *Br Med J* 1952; 1:850–851.

Kopell HP, Thompson WAL: Pronator syndrome: A confirmed case and its diagnosis. *N Engl J Med* 1958; 259:713–715.

Pankovich AM: Anconeus approach to the elbow joint and the proximal part of the radius and ulna. *J Bone Joint Surg* 1977; 59A:124–126.

Roles NC, Maudsley RH: Radial tunnel syndrome: Resistant tennis elbow as a nerve entrapment. *J Bone Joint Surg* 1972; 54B:499–508.

Salsbury CR: The nerve to the extensor carpi radialis brevis. *Br J Surg* 26:95–97.

Sharrard WJW: Posterior interosseous neuritis. *J Bone Joint Surg* 1966; 48B:777–780.

Solnitzky O: Pronator syndrome: Compression neuropathy of the median nerve at level of pronator teres muscle. *Georgetown Med Bull* 1960; 13:232.

Spinner M: The anterior interosseous-nerve syndrome: With special attention to its variations. *J Bone Joint Surg* 1970; 54A:84–94.

Spinner M: The arcade of Frohse and its relationship to posterior interosseous nerve paralysis. *J Bone Joint Surg* 1968; 50B:809–812.

Strachan JCH, Ellis BW: Vulnerability of the posterior interosseous nerve during radial head resection. *J Bone Joint Surg* 1971; 53B:320–323.

Straub LR: Congenital absence of the ulna. *Am J Surg* 1965, 109:300–305.

Thompson JE: Anatomical methods of approach in operations on the long bones of the extremities. *Ann Surg* 1918; 68:309–329.

Travill AA: Electromyographic study of the extensor apparatus of the forearm. *Anat Rec* 1962; 144:373–376.

Vanderpool DW, Chalmers J, Lamb DW, et al: Peripheral compression lesions of the ulnar nerve. *J Bone Joint Surg* 1968, 50B:792–803.

Weinberger LM: Non-traumatic paralysis of the dorsal interosseous nerve. *Surg Gynecol Obstet* 1939; 69:358–363.

Yong-Hing K, Tchang SPK: Traumatic radio-ulnar synostosis treated by excision and a free fat transplant. *J Bone Joint Surg* 1983, 65B:433–435.

6

Wrist and Hand

George A. Richardson, M.D.
James H. Whitaker, M.D.

ANATOMIC FEATURES OF THE WRIST AND HAND

The hand functions to grasp, release, and transport objects. Like the eye and ear, it is also a sensory organ, serving as a tactile extension of the brain. The wrist is a link between the forearm and the hand. The purpose of the entire upper extremity is to position the hand in space so that it can perform its functions.

Bony Anatomy and Ligamentous Structures

The boundaries of the wrist lie between the distal edge of the pronator quadratus and the carpometacarpal joints. Its bony structures include the distal ends of the radius and ulna, as well as the eight carpal bones (Fig 6–1). The carpal bones are held in tight proximity by intracapsular ligaments, which are both interosseous and intraosseous. The wrist as a whole is concave anteriorly and convex posteriorly.

The proximal carpal row consists of the scaphoid, lunate, and triquetrum. These three bones articulate with the radius proximally, with one another, and with the distal carpal row distally. The pisiform, which articulates with the volar surface of the triquetrum, is a type of sesamoid bone. It serves as part of the attachment of the flexor carpi ulnaris. The scaphoid has a large convex surface proximally, which articulates with the scaphoid fossa of the radius. The scaphoid bridges the proximal and distal carpal rows and serves as an intercalated link between them. This bone bridge helps prevent the two carpal rows from collapsing on one another in a zigzag fashion during wrist movements. The lunate is convex proximally where it articulates with the lunate fossa of the radius and concave distally for its articulation with the capitate. The triquetrum does not articulate directly with the ulna but rather through its attachments to the triangular fibrocartilage ligaments.

The distal carpal row consists of the trapezium, trapezoid, capitate, and hamate. These bones articulate distally with the metacarpals and proximally with the proximal carpal row. There is very little motion between the bones of the distal carpal row; they function as a unit. The trapezium has a large saddle-shaped surface distally for articulation with the thumb metacarpal, thus allowing the thumb its important rotational component during opposition. The trapezoid is the smallest carpal bone, except for the pisiform. The capitate is the largest carpal bone. The capitate has two facets proximally for articulation with the scaphoid and lunate. Distally it articulates with the second, third, and fourth metacarpals. The hamate is a triangular bone with a distal saddle-shaped articular surface. There is minimal motion between the trapezoid and capitate and the second and third metacarpals. In contrast, there is significant motion between the fourth and fifth metacarpals and the hamate, which contributes to grip strength during finger flexion. On its volar side the hook of the hamate serves as an attachment for the transverse carpal ligament (flexor retinaculum of the wrist). The pisiform serves as the other attachment for this ligament on the ulnar side of the wrist. Both

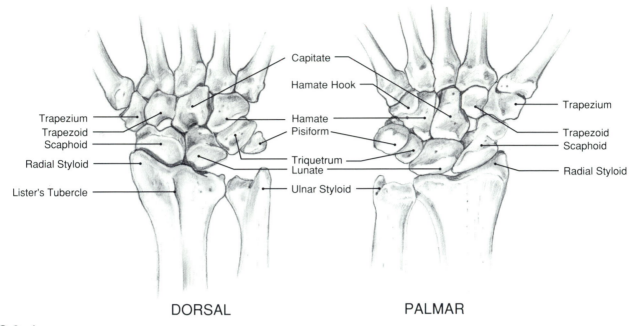

FIG 6–1.
Dorsal and palmar view of the wrist showing skeletal anatomy.

of these structures can be palpated, with the pisi-form being the more proximal and superficial of the two. The hook of the hamate is palpable just distal and radial to the pisiform. The radial attachments of the flexor retinaculum are the ridge of the trape-zium, which can be palpated at the base of the thumb, and the tubercle of the scaphoid. The scaph-oid tubercle is barely palpable just distal to the end of the radius; it is more prominent with the wrist in radial deviation.

The strongest and most important ligaments of the wrist are on the volar side (Fig 6–2). They are in-tracapsular and thus not well visualized unless the capsule is taken down. The general configuration of these ligaments is a double V, with the apices point-ing distally and proximally over the midcapitate and radial styloid regions. The space of Poirier is an area of potential weakness between the two V configura-tions in the vicinity of the volar lunate capitate artic-ulation. Traumatic carpal dislocations most com-monly occur through this space. The primary stabi-lizer of the proximal pole of the scaphoid is the volar radioscapholunate ligament. This ligament must rupture before rotary subluxation of the scaphoid can occur. In addition to these volar ligaments there are interosseous ligaments between the carpal bones and dorsal ligaments, but their contribution to wrist stability is less significant. The so-called ulnar and radial collateral ligaments probably do not exist as distinct ligaments but as part of the wrist capsule.

They do not contribute significantly to wrist stabil-ity.

The distal radioulnar joint consists of the articu-lating surfaces of the ulnar head, the sigmoid notch of the radius and the stabilizing ligaments, which are collectively referred to as the triangular fibrocar-tilage complex (Fig 6–3). During forearm rotation, the sigmoid notch of the radius rotates around the ulnar head; both are semicylindrical surfaces. The triangular fibrocartilage complex consists of the tri-angular fibrocartilage and ulnar carpal ligaments. The base of the triangular fibrocartilage attaches to the edge of the sigmoid notch on the radius. The apex attaches to the concavity of the ulnar head ad-jacent to the styloid process. The ulnocarpal liga-ment also has its apex adjacent to the ulnar styloid. It fans out from there to insert across the lunate and triquetrum. Functionally, this ligamentous complex absorbs some of the compressive loading across the ulnar side of the wrist and suspends the ulnar car-pus from the dorsal ulnar margin of the radius.

The second, third, fourth, and fifth digits of the hand are referred to as the index, middle, ring, and little fingers, respectively (Fig 6–4). Each finger con-sists of three phalanges and is associated with one metacarpal. The phalanges are named proximal, middle, and distal, and each has a shaft with a prox-imal base and distal head. The second, third, fourth, and fifth metacarpals function as intermediaries be-tween the fingers and carpus. The second metacar-

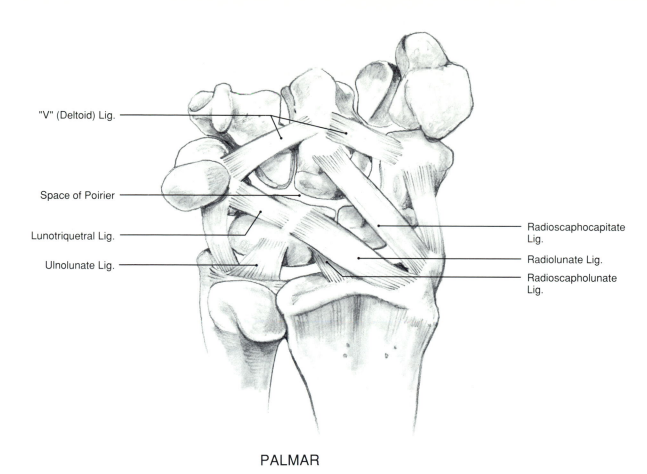

"V" (Deltoid) Lig.

Space of Poirier

Lunotriquetral Lig.

Ulnolunate Lig.

Radioscaphocapitate Lig.

Radiolunate Lig.

Radioscapholunate Lig.

PALMAR

FIG 6–2.
Palmar view of the wrist, showing the volar ligaments. The radioscapholunate ligament is thought to be the most important stabilizer of the proximal pole of the scaphoid. Note the space of Poirier, a weak area over the capitolunate articulation.

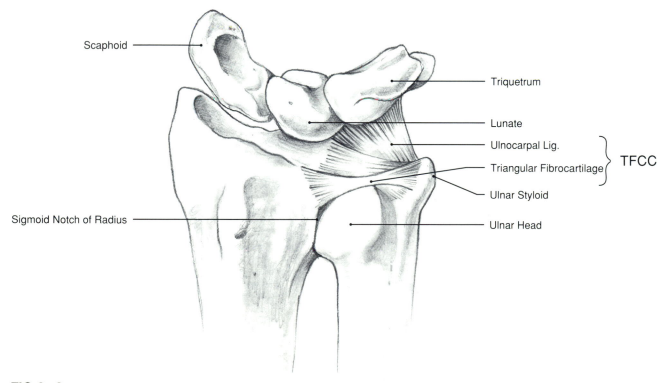

Scaphoid

Triquetrum

Lunate

Ulnocarpal Lig.

Triangular Fibrocartilage

Ulnar Styloid

} TFCC

Sigmoid Notch of Radius

Ulnar Head

FIG 6–3.
Dorsal view of wrist showing triangular fibrocartilage complex (TFCC)—triangular fibrocartilage and ulnocarpal ligament.

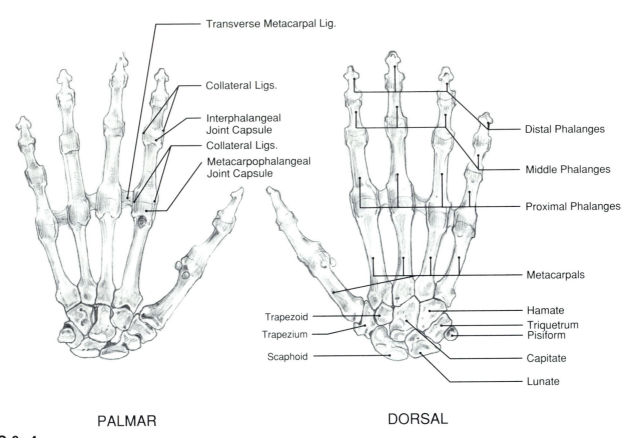

FIG 6−4.
Palmar and dorsal views of the carpal, metacarpal, and phalangeal bones.

pal has a fork-shaped base and articulates with the trapezium and trapezoid. The dorsoradial side of this fork is the area of insertion of the extensor carpi radialis longus tendon. The third metacarpal articulates with the second and fourth metacarpals on either side and with the capitate proximally. The fourth metacarpal has radial and ulnar sides at its base. This metacarpal articulates with the capitate and third metacarpal on the radial side and with the hamate and fifth metacarpal on the ulnar side. The fifth metacarpal articulates at its base with the ulnar side of the hamate.

The metacarpophalangeal (MP) joints consist of the irregularly spheroidal metacarpal heads, which articulate with the broad concave bases of the proximal phalanges (Figs 6–4 and 6–5). Unlike the interphalangeal (IP) joints, the MP joints are not hinge joints. Rather, they constitute a multiaxial condyloid joint, which permits lateral motion and a small amount of circumduction, as well as flexion and extension. The MP joints to the fingers all have the same basic anatomic form, which biomechanically favors palmar flexion with limited extension. Each joint has a capsule and a pair of strong collateral lig-

aments that extend volarly into the palmar, or volar, plate. This volar plate is divided into a tough fibrous portion volar to the joint surface and a membranous portion that extends proximally onto the metacarpal neck. The MP joints provide mobility in the radioulnar and dorsopalmar planes. This is possible because of the eccentric arc of radius of the metacarpal head and the position of the collateral ligaments. The ligaments are slack in extension, thereby allowing lateral movement. As the joint flexes, the ligaments become maximally tight at about 70 degrees of flexion because of their eccentric insertion on the metacarpal head and the camlike action produced by the shape of the palmar portion of the metacarpal head. This has important clinical significance when the hand is immobilized after an injury or surgery and when testing is done for ligamentous stability in this area. The MP joints should be flexed at least 70 degrees in order to correctly test their stability or prevent contractures of the capsular collateral ligaments when the fingers are immobilized. Although the collateral ligaments provide inherent static stability of the MP joints, dynamic stability is provided by balanced interaction of the intrinsic muscles and the

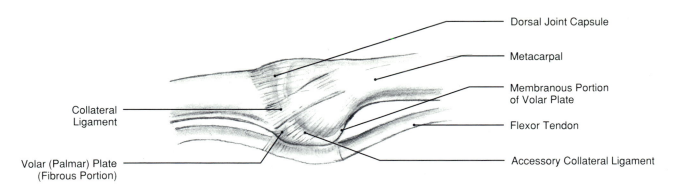

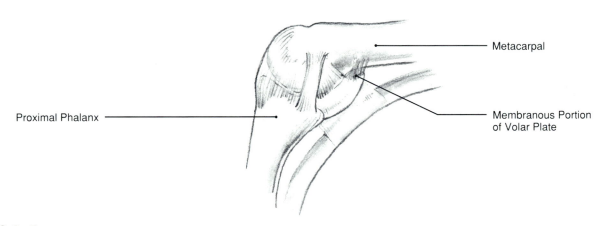

FIG 6–5.
Metacarpophalangeal (MP) joint. Note the relationship of the dorsal capsule, collateral ligament and volar (palmar) plate in extension and flexion, and the eccentric arc of radius of the metacarpal head.

flexor and extensor mechanisms. The volar plate, with its two accessory collateral ligaments (one on each side), extends proximally to the level of the metacarpal neck and thus enlarges the cavity of the MP joint. This allows the metacarpal head to remain in the joint cavity when the proximal phalanx is in full flexion. The volar plates of all four fingers are connected by the deep transverse metacarpal ligament. The interosseous muscles pass dorsal to the transverse metacarpal ligaments but palmar to the axis of rotation of the MP joints (see Fig 6–13). The lumbrical muscles, along with the flexor tendons and neurovascular bundles, lie volar to the ligaments. The tendons of the interossei are located in a depression on each side of the metacarpal neck and head, adjacent to the collateral ligaments.

Unlike the ball and socket configuration of the MP joints, the proximal IP joint is a hinge joint with little movement other than flexion and extension

(Fig 6–6). Stability is derived from the articular contours and ligamentous structures of the joint. Secondary reinforcement is provided by the flexor and extensor tendons and the retinacular system. The proximal side of the joint consists of a pair of symmetric condyles separated by an intercondylar notch. The condyles articulate with two corresponding depressions in the base of the middle phalanx, which in turn are separated by a median ridge. This tongue and groove configuration contributes to lateral and rotatory stability.

The joint capsule of the proximal IP joint consists of the paired collateral ligaments on either side, the volar plate palmarly, and the extensor mechanism dorsally. The collateral ligaments are 2 to 3 mm thick and arise from a depression just dorsal and proximal to each condyle. They pass in a volar oblique direction to insert along the volar third of the middle phalanx and the lateral margin of the volar

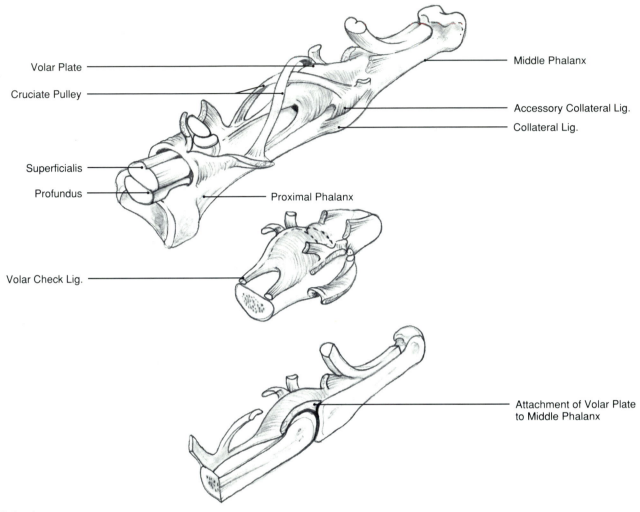

Volar Plate

Cruciate Pulley

Superficialis

Profundus

Volar Check Lig.

Middle Phalanx

Accessory Collateral Lig.

Collateral Lig.

Proximal Phalanx

Attachment of Volar Plate to Middle Phalanx

FIG 6–6.
Proximal interphalangeal (IP) joint (palmar view). Note relationship between flexor tendons (superficialis and profundus), collateral ligaments, and volar plate.

plate. The thick volar plate, which forms the floor of the joint, is attached to the collateral ligaments by accessory ligaments. Together with them, it inserts into the lateral margins of the middle phalanx. The central portion of the volar plate tapers proximally into a thin sheet but has a thick attachment laterally on either side. These attachments are confluent with the attachments of the pulley system. Together they form paired cordlike structures called volar check ligaments. These ligamentous structures prevent hyperextension but allow a full range of flexion. In addition, the paired collateral ligaments and volar plate form a ligamentous boxlike configuration. This configuration strongly resists any proximal IP joint displacement unless disrupted in at least two planes.

The distal IP joint is similar to the proximal IP joint. It has a bicondylar convex surface proximally,

which articulates with the double concave articular surface of the distal phalanx. The flexor and extensor tendons insert at the level of this joint, and injury to the joint or either tendon produces characteristic deformities that can seriously impair digital function. Like the proximal IP joint, the distal IP joint has substantial collateral ligaments, which blend palmarly with a thick volar plate. Unlike in the proximal IP joint, no "checkrein" ligaments are involved in the attachment to the middle phalanx. This allows some hyperextension of the distal IP joint.

Skin and Aponeurosis

There are significant differences between the dorsal and palmar skin of the hand. The dorsal skin is thin, mobile, and loosely attached to its underlying structures, except over the proximal and distal IP joints. Simple defects in the dorsal skin can be easily closed by shifting the skin around without a flap or a graft. The volar skin, by contrast, is much thicker and more firmly attached to the underlying structures.

The palmar aponeurosis (Fig 6–7) is a specialized thickening in the deep fascia underlying the palmar skin. This aponeurosis extends from the distal edge of the flexor retinaculum, where it is continuous with the tendon of the palmaris longus, to the level of the metacarpal heads. As the aponeurosis approaches the fingers its longitudinally directed fibers form four slips, one to each finger. These slips blend into the flexor tendon sheath and the underlying metacarpals. As the four slips reach the level of the web spaces they are reunited by transverse fibers, which constitute the superficial transverse metacarpal ligaments. These are the natatory ligaments (from the Latin *natatorius,* meaning adapted for swimming). The neurovascular bundles pass between each of these longitudinal slips and deep to the natatory ligaments. Both the natatory ligaments and the longitudinal slips of the palmar aponeurosis are of particular importance in Dupuytren's contracture, which involves the palmar fascia.

The palmar aponeurosis and longitudinal fibers, which continue into the fingers, give off superficial attachments to the skin. These are most prominent at the palmar and digital creases. These fibers are important in anchoring the skin to the skeleton of the hand, and they provide stability of the skin for prehension.

The palmar aponeurosis continues deep to form the thenar and hypothenar septa, which delineate the three deep compartments of the hand (Fig 6–7,B). The thenar compartment contains the short muscles of the thumb, except for the adductor pollicis. The hypothenar compartment contains the short muscles of the little finger. Between these two compartments lies the central compartment, which contains the flexor tendons to the fingers, the palmar arterial arches, and most of the digital neurovascular structures. Also located here are the thenar and palmar spaces, which in reality are only potential spaces. (Note that "compartment" is not synonymous with "space"—see Fig 6–53.)

Muscles and Tendons

There are three direct motors for wrist flexion and three for wrist extension. The flexors are the flexor carpi radialis, flexor carpi ulnaris, and palmaris longus (Fig 6–8). The flexor carpi radialis is the most superficial forearm muscle and lies just anterior to the flexor digitorum superficialis. It crosses the wrist just ulnar to the radial artery and superficial to the carpal canal. It passes adjacent to the trapezium in a separate compartment of its own and inserts onto the base of the second metacarpal. The flexor carpi ulnaris lies on the ulnar border of the wrist and has an extensive insertion into the pisiform. It also sends expansions out onto the hook of the hamate and the ulnar side of the volar carpal ligament, which in turn forms the roof for the ulnar nerve and artery as they pass between the transverse carpal and volar carpal ligaments (Guyon's canal—see Fig 6–16). The palmaris longus is a slender, flat muscle that descends to the wrist in the midline and blends into the midpalmar fascia. This muscle is absent unilaterally or bilaterally in about 12% of the population. When present, it serves as a useful landmark, because the median nerve is found directly dorsal and ulnar to the tendon in the proximal wrist. The palmaris longus is useful for tendon grafting because it is readily accessible and expendable.

The extensors of the wrist consist of the extensor carpi radialis longus, extensor carpi radialis brevis, and extensor carpi ulnaris (Fig 6–9). The extensor carpi radialis longus and brevis are located within the second of six dorsal wrist compartments, which contain the wrist and finger extensors. The two tendons run deep to the abductor pollicis longus and extensor pollicis brevis, which cross them in the lower third of the forearm. Upon emerging from under the dorsal retinaculum, which covers the compartment, the longus and brevis insert into the bases of the second and third metacarpals, respectively. The extensor carpi ulnaris courses within the sixth dorsal wrist compartment and crosses the ulnar side of the wrist to insert into the base of the fifth metacarpal. Radial deviation of the wrist is accomplished primarily by the abductor pollicis longus and extensor pollicis brevis, with assistance from the primary wrist flexors and extensors. Ulnar deviation of the wrist is a combined action of the flexor carpi ulnaris and extensor carpi ulnaris.

At the wrist level, the deep forearm fascia thickens, forming a band 2 to 3 cm wide that extends from the distal part of the radius, around the dorsum of the wrist, to the ulnar styloid and ulnar carpal bones. This extensor retinaculum keeps the extensor tendons close to the bones as they cross the wrist. It differs from the flexor retinaculum in that it

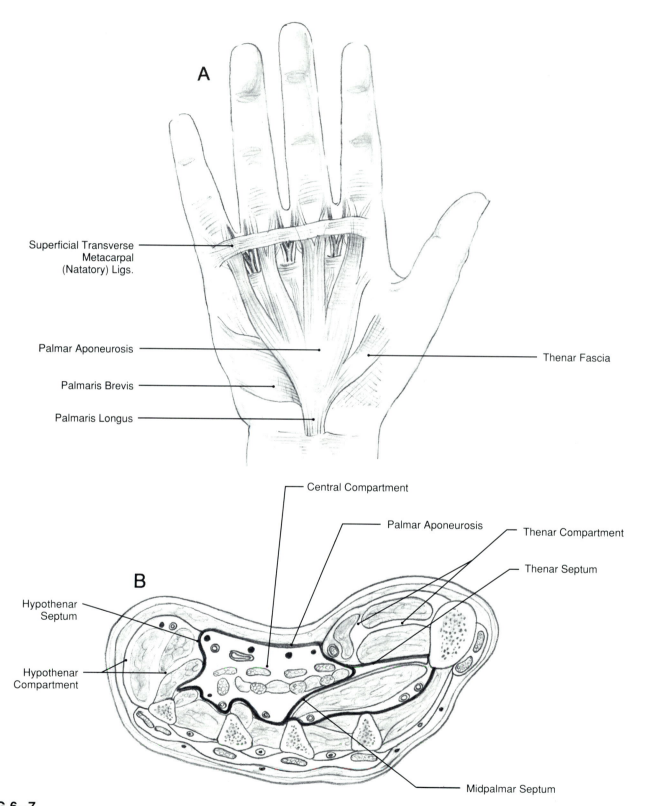

FIG 6–7.
A, palmar aponeurosis and superficial transverse metacarpal ligaments. **B,** cross section (viewed from proximal to distal) showing septa and deep compartments.

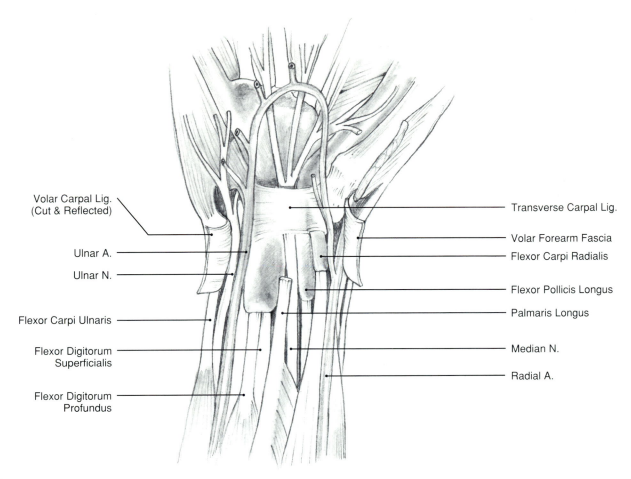

Volar Carpal Lig.
(Cut & Reflected)

Ulnar A.

Ulnar N.

Flexor Carpi Ulnaris

Flexor Digitorum
Superficialis

Flexor Digitorum
Profundus

Transverse Carpal Lig.

Volar Forearm Fascia

Flexor Carpi Radialis

Flexor Pollicis Longus

Palmaris Longus

Median N.

Radial A.

FIG 6–8.
Wrist and finger flexor tendons.

is divided by septa into compartments, which contain tendons or groups of tendons. There are usually six compartments (Fig 6–10). Starting from the radial side, they contain (1) the abductor pollicis longus and extensor pollicis brevis, (2) the extensor carpi radialis longus and brevis, (3) the extensor pollicis longus, (4) the extensor digitorum and extensor indicis proprius, (5) the extensor digiti minimi, and (6) the extensor carpi ulnaris. Each tendon or group of tendons is surrounded by a synovial sheath, which begins just proximal to the extensor retinaculum and continues a short distance onto the dorsum of the hand distal to the retinaculum. None of the sheaths continues into the fingers. A good way to remember the compartments and the numbers of tendons within them is the mnemonic 22-12-11. The first two compartments each have two tendons; the third compartment has one tendon; and the fourth compartment has two tendons, if you think of the common extensors as a group of one and the exten-

sor indicis proprius as the other. The fifth and sixth compartments each contain one tendon.

The abductor pollicis longus and extensor pollicis brevis cross superficial to the two wrist extensors. Together they form the radial, or lateral, boundary of the anatomic snuff-box, which is a depression in the radial side of the wrist seen when the thumb is extended (Fig 6–11). The dorsal, or medial, boundary is formed by the extensor pollicis longus, which passes obliquely across the forearm deep to the common extensors. It then passes under the retinaculum and courses around Lister's tubercle, over the two radial wrist extensors, and onto the thumb, where it inserts into the base of the distal phalanx.

The long extensors of the fingers are the four common extensors, the extensor indicis to the index finger and the extensor digiti minimi to the little finger (see Fig 6–9). The extensor indicis passes over the wrist deep to the common extensors and inserts

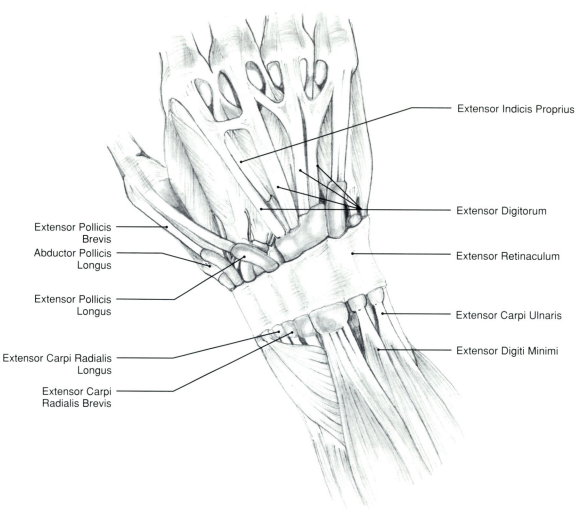

FIG 6–9.
Wrist and finger extensors.

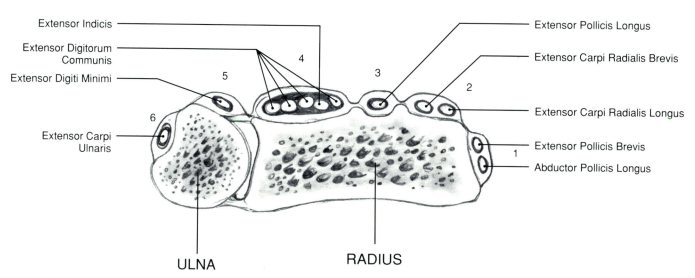

FIG 6–10.
The six dorsal compartments of the wrist. (Cross section of pronated right wrist viewed from distal to proximal.)

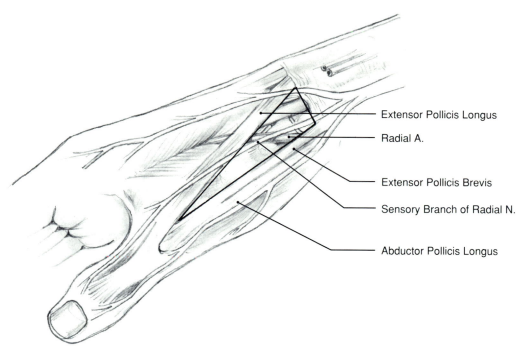

Extensor Pollicis Longus

Radial A.

Extensor Pollicis Brevis

Sensory Branch of Radial N.

Abductor Pollicis Longus

FIG 6–11.
Anatomic snuff-box (triangle-bordered dorsally by the extensor pollicis longus and radially by the abductor pollicis longus). Note that the radial artery and sensory branches of the radial nerve cross through this area.

into the extensor hood on the ulnar side of the index finger. Because of the consistent presence of the common extensor to the index finger, the extensor indicis is expendable and can be used for tendon transfers. The extensor digiti minimi arises in common with the extensor digitorum and inserts on the ulnar side of the extensor hood of the little finger. It is frequently the only extensor to the little finger, since the common extensor to this digit is absent or significantly deficient in up to 75% of people. The tendons of the extensor digitorum are usually joined together just proximal to the MP joints by intertendinous connections called junctura. These typically arise from the ring finger common extensor tendon and pass obliquely and distally to the other fingers. Extensor tendon lacerations proximal to the junctura may not be appreciated on clinical examination, because the finger can be extended by the other tendons through the junctura.

On the fingers the extensor tendons are joined by the lumbricals and interossei to form a complex structure referred to as the extensor aponeurosis (expansion) (Fig 6–12). As the extensor tendons approach the metacarpal head, they expand to form a "hood." This hood completely covers the dorsum of the MP joints and extends around on either side to connect with the volar plate and transverse metacarpal ligaments. Through this hood the long extensors

extend the proximal phalanx. At this level the extensor mechanism is joined by the interosseous and lumbrical tendons. Dorsally, the extensor tendon continues as the central slip but also forms two lateral bands on either side of the finger, to which the lumbricals and interossei contribute. The central slip inserts into the base of the middle phalanx and serves to extend this joint in conjunction with the lateral bands. The lateral bands then come together dorsally just proximal to the distal IP joint to form a conjoined tendon, which inserts at the base of the distal phalanx to provide distal IP joint extension. Over the dorsum of the middle phalanx the triangular ligament helps stabilize the lateral bands against volar subluxation. Each lateral band is also attached to a retinacular ligament laterally that allows proximal and distal migration but limits dorsal displacement. This transverse retinacular ligament is anchored volarly to the edge of the flexor tendon sheath at the proximal IP joint. A "swan-neck deformity" can result if the transverse retinacular ligaments are injured and the lateral bands are allowed to ride up dorsally to cause hyperextension of the proximal IP joint. A "boutonniére deformity" may occur with rupture of the central slip into the middle phalanx, resulting in a flexion deformity at the proximal IP joint. In this situation the transverse retinacular ligaments become contracted. The lateral bands,

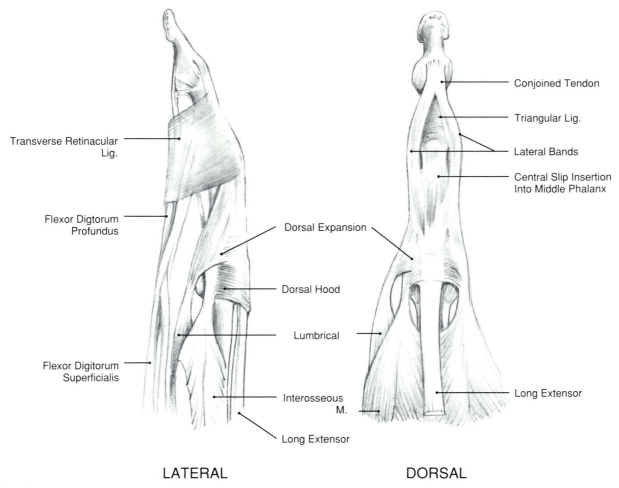

Transverse Retinacular Lig.

Flexor Digtorum Profundus

Flexor Digitorum Superficialis

Conjoined Tendon

Triangular Lig.

Lateral Bands

Central Slip Insertion Into Middle Phalanx

Dorsal Expansion

Dorsal Hood

Lumbrical

Interosseous M.

Long Extensor

Long Extensor

LATERAL   DORSAL

FIG 6–12.
The extensor mechanism is an intricate complex composed of the long extensor, the interossei, and the lumbricals and their expansions.

which continue to function, will cause a concomitant hyperextension of the distal IP joint.

The interossei are the deepest muscle layer in the hand (Figs 6–13 and 6–14). They lie between and take their origins from the metacarpals. There are four dorsal and three palmar interossei. The dorsal interossei take their origin from adjacent sides of contiguous metacarpals. They cross the MP joints dorsal to the deep transverse metacarpal ligament but volar to the axis of rotation. The first, second, and fourth dorsal interossei have two heads, one of which inserts at the base of the proximal phalanx and the other into the extensor aponeurosis. The dorsal interossei abduct (relative to the long finger) the index, ring, and little fingers. In addition, by virtue of their insertion into the extensor aponeurosis, they are primary flexors of the MP joints and aid in proximal and distal IP extension.

Three palmar interossei arise from the shafts of

the second, fourth, and fifth metacarpals. They insert into the extensor aponeurosis on the ulnar side of the index finger and the radial sides of the ring and little fingers. They adduct the index, ring, and little fingers, relative to the long finger. All of the interossei are innervated by the deep branch of the ulnar nerve, which courses around the palm with the deep palmar arterial arch on the volar surface of the interossei.

The lumbrical muscles are four in number and take their origin from the four flexor profundi tendons in the palm (Fig 6–15). They cross the MP joints volar to the deep transverse metacarpal ligament and insert into the radial lateral bands at the midportion of each proximal phalanx. The two most radial lumbrical muscles are innervated by the median nerve and the most lateral two (third and fourth) by the ulnar nerve. They aid in MP joint flexion and interphalangeal joint extension.

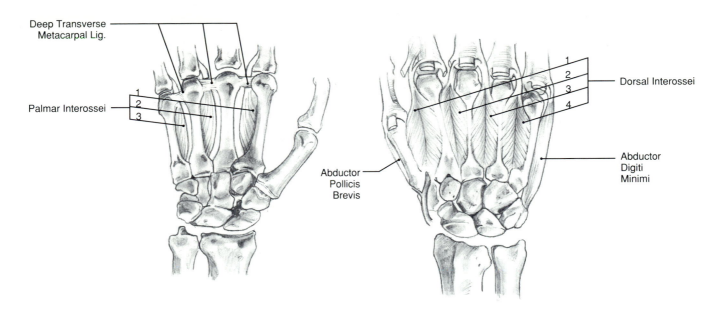

PALMAR
DORSAL

FIG 6–13.
Deepest muscle layer in the hand: four dorsal and three palmar interossei.

VOLAR

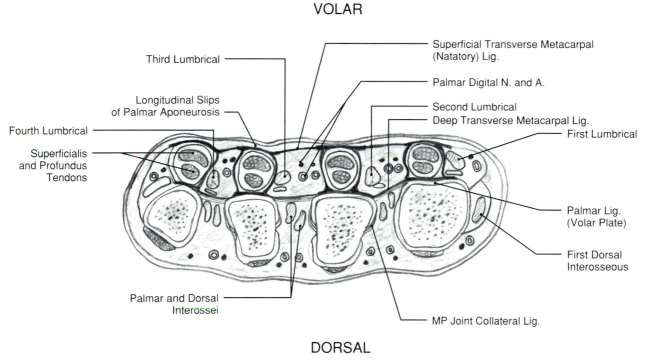

DORSAL

FIG 6–14.
Cross section of supinated right hand viewed from proximal to distal at the level of the MP joints. Note relationship of the deep transverse metacarpal ligaments to the intrinsic (interosseous and lumbrical) muscles and neurovascular bundles. The interossei lie dorsal to the deep transverse metacarpal ligaments. Lumbricals and neurovascular structures are palmar to these ligaments.

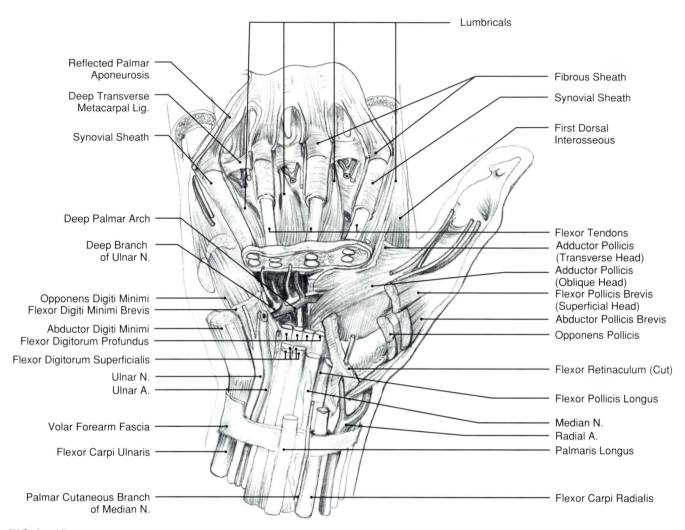

FIG 6-15.
Thenar (abductor pollicis brevis, flexor pollicis brevis, opponens pollicis, and adductor pollicis) and hypothenar (palmaris brevis, abductor digiti minimi, flexor digiti minimi brevis, and opponens digiti minimi) muscles and portions of flexor tendons and intrinsics have been cut away to reveal their relationship to one another and to the nerve branches and the two palmar arches.

The intrinsic muscles of the thumb (thenar muscles) consist of the abductor pollicis brevis, flexor pollicis brevis, opponens pollicis, and adductor pollicis. The abductor pollicis brevis, flexor pollicis brevis (superficial head), and opponens pollicis are innervated by the motor branch of the median nerve and take their origin largely from the flexor retinaculum. The abductor pollicis brevis inserts into the radial side of the base of the proximal phalanx of the thumb. This muscle serves to abduct the thumb from the palm. The flexor pollicis brevis has two heads, which are separated by the flexor pollicis longus tendon as it passes to its insertion on the base of the distal thumb phalanx. The deep head of the flexor pollicis brevis is innervated by the ulnar

nerve. This muscle inserts into the radial base of the proximal phalanx, flexes the thumb at the MP joints, and pronates the thumb in opposition. The opponens pollicis lies deep to the short abductor and flexor pollicis. This muscle inserts on the radial anterior surface of the first metacarpal, where it provides opposition. The adductor pollicis arises by two heads: the oblique head arises from the second and third metacarpals and the transverse head from the third metacarpal. The two heads converge as they pass superficial to the interossei radial to the third metacarpal. This muscle inserts into the ulnar side of the base of the proximal phalanx of the thumb and the ulnar sesamoid. The adductor pollicis adducts the first metacarpal and aids in flexion of the MP joints. It is innervated by the ulnar nerve, and some authorities consider it a palmar interosseous muscle.

The hypothenar muscles consist of the palmaris brevis, abductor digiti minimi, flexor digiti minimi brevis, and opponens digiti minimi. The palmaris brevis is quite superficial. It arises from the palmar aponeurosis and extends into the skin along the ulnar border of the palm. It is supplied by the superficial branch of the ulnar nerve and serves to deepen the hollow of the palm by drawing in the skin on the ulnar border of the hand. The three deeper muscles take their origin from the pisiform, hamate, and flexor retinaculum. The more superficial abductor digiti minimi inserts into the base of the proximal phalanx of the little finger and serves to abduct the little finger. The flexor digiti minimi brevis joins the insertion of the abductor digiti minimi but has a more palmar course. This muscle serves to flex the proximal phalanx at the proximal MP joint. The opponens digiti minimi inserts along the ulnar border of the fifth metacarpal and draws it forward, thus contributing to power grip along the ulnar border of the palm and to opposition between the thumb and

the little finger. These three muscles (abductor, flexor, and opponens of the little finger) are innervated by the deep branch of the ulnar nerve.

Nine flexor tendons pass through the carpal canal (Fig 6–16) along with the median nerve: two flexors for each of the four fingers and the long flexor for the thumb. The flexor digitorum superficialis (sublimis) tendons lie anterior to the profundus tendons and are grouped in two layers at the level of the carpal canal. The tendons to the middle and ring fingers lie volar to those of the index and little fingers. In the palm all four superficialis tendons lie in the same plane, volar to the profundi. As the profundus tendons enter the carpal canal there are often only two tendons, one for the index finger and a large, flat tendon for the other three fingers. These become more distinct in the palm. This has clinical significance, since any situation that limits the excursion of one of these three fingers may limit profundus motion of the other two fingers as well. This is known as the quadrigia effect. (A quadrigia is a two-wheeled chariot drawn by a team of four.) The flexor pollicis longus is the most radial tendon pass-

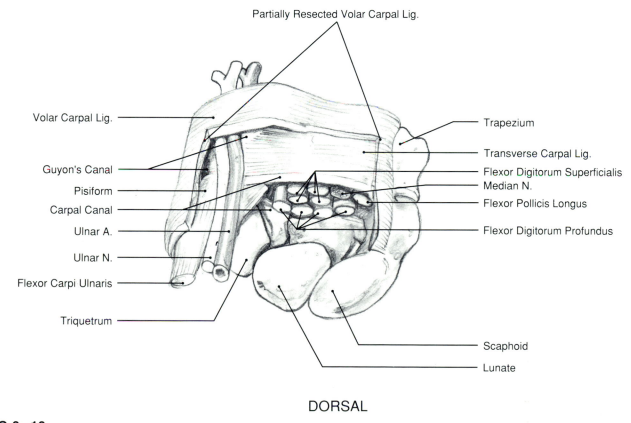

Partially Resected Volar Carpal Lig.

Volar Carpal Lig.

Guyon's Canal

Pisiform

Carpal Canal

Ulnar A.

Ulnar N.

Flexor Carpi Ulnaris

Triquetrum

Trapezium

Transverse Carpal Lig.

Flexor Digitorum Superficialis

Median N.

Flexor Pollicis Longus

Flexor Digitorum Profundus

Scaphoid

Lunate

DORSAL

FIG 6–16.
Guyon's canal and carpal canal and contents. (Cross section of supinated right wrist, viewed from proximal to distal). Note the relationship between the transverse carpal ligament and volar carpal ligament (partially resected).

ing through the carpal canal as it courses around the scaphoid toward the thumb. The flexor pollicis longus has a synovial tendon sheath that starts just proximal to the carpal canal and is continuous with the digital tendon sheath in the thumb. The little finger has a similar synovial sheath that runs out into the finger. This synovial sheath also surrounds the other flexor tendons in the palm and carpal canal. These synovial sheaths usually connect each other in the carpal canal.

As each paired superficialis (sublimis) and profundus tendon approaches its finger, it enters a well-defined digital fibro-osseous tunnel which starts just proximal to the MP joint of each finger (Fig 6–17). This digital fibrous sheath consists of thick fibrous bands, known as pulleys, which keep the tendons firmly adherent to the phalanges and prevent bowstringing during flexion of the finger.

There are four annular (A) pulleys and three cruciate (C) pulleys. The two pulleys critical for proper tendon excursion are the A-2 and A-4 pulleys, which are located over the proximal phalanx and middle phalanx, respectively. The A-1 pulley is over the MP joint and the A-3 pulley over the proximal IP joint. The C-1 pulley is over the middle of the proximal phalanx, the C-2 pulley over the proximal end of the middle phalanx, and the C-3 pulley over the distal end of the middle phalanx.

As the flexor tendons enter their digital sheaths the superficialis tendon is volar to the profundus. However, over the proximal phalanx it splits to allow the profundus tendon to pass through it and continue on to insert onto the base of the distal phalanx (Fig 6–18). The two slips of the superficialis tendon split and rotate away from the midline so that the most medial fibers become the most volar

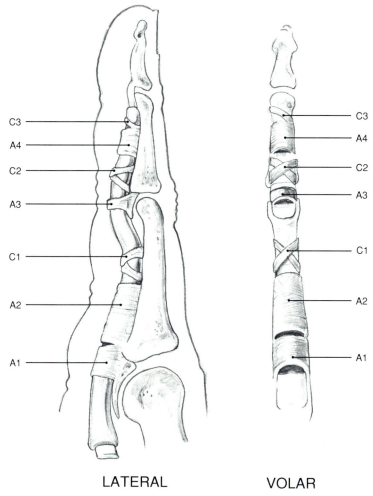

LATERAL   VOLAR

FIG 6–17.
The digital bursa has been stripped away to show individual pulleys and their relationship to joints and phalanges. (A = annular. C = cruciate.)

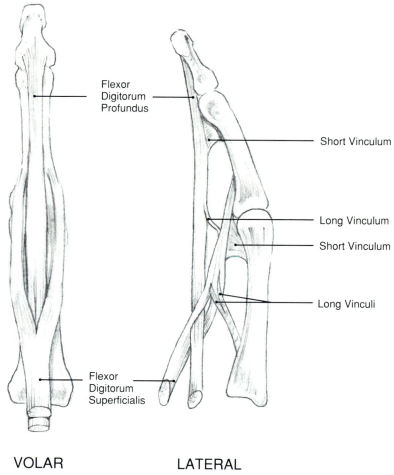

Flexor
Digitorum
Profundus

Short Vinculum

Long Vinculum

Short Vinculum

Long Vinculi

Flexor
Digitorum
Superficialis

VOLAR   LATERAL

FIG 6–18.
Long and short vinculae carry blood supply to finger flexors.

ones and the most lateral fibers become the most dorsal as the tendon inserts onto the base of the middle phalanx.

Nutrition to the flexor tendons within the digital sheath comes from two sources: diffusion of nutrients from the synovial fluid surrounding the tendons and vascular perfusion from the vincular system (see Fig 6–18). Each tendon has a long and a short vinculum, which are folds of the mesotenon running from the dorsal portion of the dorsal wall of the tendon sheath to the superficial and deep flexor tendons. The short vinculae, which are located over the ends of the proximal and middle phalanges, are the more important ones. They carry blood vessels to the tendons from the branches of the digital vessels that are given off to the proximal and distal IP joints.

The flexor pollicis longus also has a fibrous tendon sheath as it emerges from between the two heads of the flexor digitorum brevis. There is an an-

nular pulley over the thumb MP joint, another one over the IP joint, and an oblique (cruciate) pulley in between.

Arteries and Veins

The blood supply to the hand comes primarily from the radial and ulnar arteries, both located on the volar side of the wrist and hand.

The ulnar artery, accompanied by the ulnar nerve on its medial side, descends into the distal forearm and wrist deep to the flexor carpi ulnaris. The nerve and artery then pass through Guyon's canal between the pisiform and the more distal hook of the hamate. The transverse carpal ligament, which covers the median nerve and the finger and thumb flexors, forms the floor of Guyon's canal, and the volar carpal ligament forms its roof. Distal to Guyon's canal, lying between the palmaris brevis and the flexor retinaculum, the ulnar artery continues as the superficial palmar arch (Fig 6–19). Distal to the retinaculum, the arch turns radially and courses across the palm, lying between the palmar aponeurosis and the branches of the median nerve. The arch is concave proximally and lies approximately at the level of the proximal transverse palmar crease. The main branches of the superficial palmar arch are the four digital arteries. While the ulnar artery is under cover of the palmaris brevis, the proper digital artery to the ulnar side of the little finger is given off. As it courses across the palm on top of the median nerve branches, the arch gives off three common digital arteries to the adjacent side of the four fingers. The common digital arteries are accompanied by corresponding common digital nerves. At the point where each common digital nerve branches into its proper digital nerve, each common digital artery assumes a more dorsal position and branches more distally at about the base of the proximal phalanx. At the level of the interdigital cleft the nerves and arteries are superficial and can be easily transected. Beyond the origin of the most radial

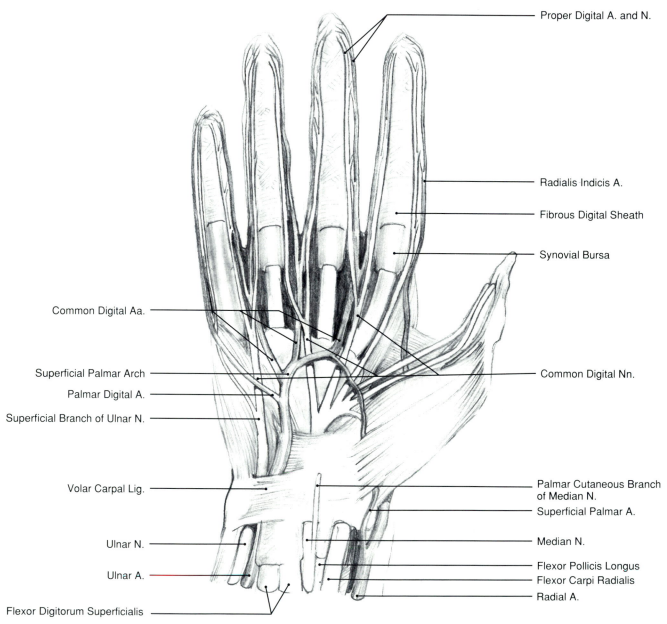

FIG 6–19.
Superficial palmar arch. Note relationship to digital nerves in hand.

common digital artery the superficial palmar arch usually curves into the thumb muscles. It may end here or anastomose with the superficial palmar branch of the radial artery.

The radial artery crosses the volar aspect of the wrist between the flexor carpi radialis and the brachioradialis. At this point, where it overlies the pronator quadratus, the artery is readily palpable by compression against the radius (Fig 6–20). Just proximal to the wrist the artery gives off a superficial palmar branch. It then courses radially and dorsally deep to the abductor pollicis longus and extensor pollicis brevis, under the extensor pollicis longus, and into the anatomic snuff-box (see Fig 6–11) on the dorsolateral aspect of the wrist. Here it gives off branches to form the dorsal intercarpal arch and a

longer first dorsal metacarpal branch to the dorsum of the thumb and the radial side of the index finger (Fig 6–21). This branch may be encountered during dorsal exposure of the first metacarpal trapezial joint or scaphoid (see Fig 6–40,B). As the radial artery leaves the dorsum of the hand it passes between the two heads of the first dorsal interosseous muscle and branches to form the deep palmar arch and the princeps pollicis arteries. The deep palmar arch turns ulnarly and courses between the first dorsal interosseous and adductor pollicis across the metacarpals and interossei (see Fig 6–20). The deep arch is usually completed on the ulnar side by anastomosing with the deep branch of the ulnar artery, which arises just distal to the pisiform and passes with the deep branch of the ulnar nerve between the

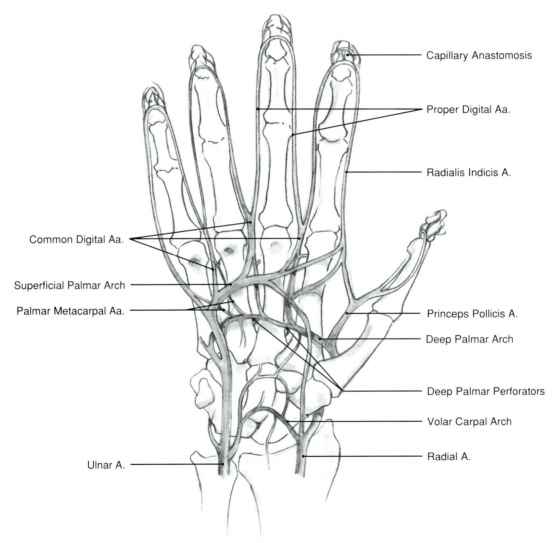

Capillary Anastomosis

Proper Digital Aa.

Radialis Indicis A.

Common Digital Aa.

Superficial Palmar Arch

Palmar Metacarpal Aa.

Princeps Pollicis A.

Deep Palmar Arch

Deep Palmar Perforators

Volar Carpal Arch

Ulnar A.

Radial A.

FIG 6–20.
Most common pattern of arterial supply to hand. Note radial artery and deep palmar arch.

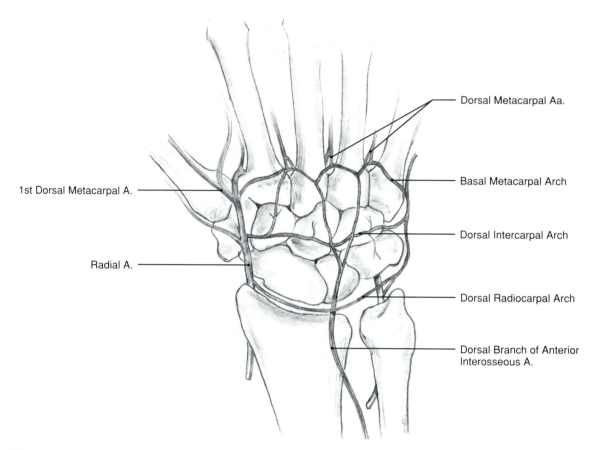

FIG 6–21.
Dorsal arterial supply of wrist.

origins of the short abductor and short flexor of the little finger. The princeps pollicis artery runs between the first dorsal interosseous and adductor pollicis, at the distal edge of which it divides into two branches to either side of the thumb. The radialis indicis artery is usually a branch of the deep arch to the radial side of the index finger, but it may also arise from the superficial arch. The deep palmar arch gives off perforating branches between the heads of the second, third, and fourth dorsal interossei, which join the dorsal metacarpal arteries. In addition, the arch gives off a variable number of palmar metacarpal arteries, which join the common digital artery of each interspace. Distally, between the metacarpal heads, the dorsal metacarpal arteries are connected to the volar digital arteries by perforators. It is the presence of these branches, as well as the often-present direct radial branch into the superficial arch, that allows the hand to usually survive so well following division of the radial or ulnar artery. It should be noted however, that incomplete arches exist in up to 20% of hands. The collateral circulation

cannot always be relied upon when one of the arteries is severed.

The carpal bones receive their blood supply from a network of dorsal and volar carpal arches (see Figs 6–20 and 6–21). The blood supply to the scaphoid is particularly significant, because the scaphoid is second only to the femoral head in its frequency of posttraumatic avascular necrosis (Fig 6–22). Thirty percent of middle one-third fractures and nearly 100% of proximal one-fifth fractures of the scaphoid are associated with avascular necrosis of the proximal pole. This is because the majority of the blood supply to the scaphoid enters in its distal portion. There are dorsal and volar branches to the distal two thirds of the scaphoid, but the proximal pole is intraarticular and has essentially no independent blood supply.

The main arterial supply to the fingers comes from the previously mentioned digital arteries, which run along either side of the four fingers and thumb next to the flexor tendon sheath. The two arteries anastomose to form an arch across the distal

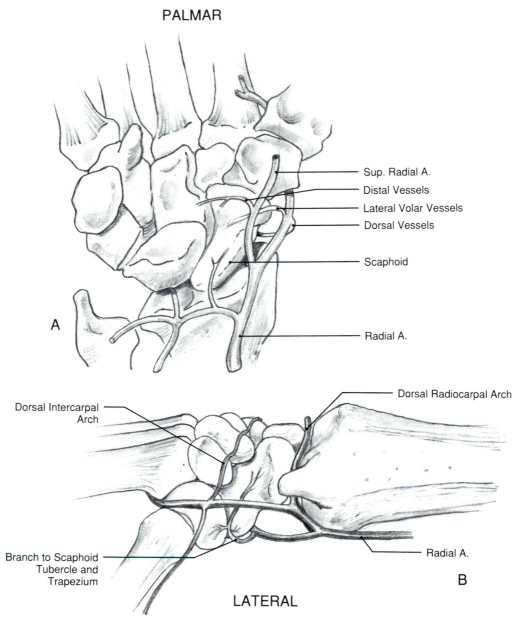

PALMAR

A

— Sup. Radial A.
— Distal Vessels
— Lateral Volar Vessels
— Dorsal Vessels

— Scaphoid

— Radial A.

Dorsal Intercarpal Arch —

Dorsal Radiocarpal Arch —

Branch to Scaphoid Tubercle and Trapezium —

— Radial A.

B

LATERAL

FIG 6–22.
Arterial supply of scaphoid. Note that the majority of scaphoid blood supply enters distally. **A,** palmar view. **B,** lateral view.

phalanx, from which a fine network of vessels extends into the pulp of the distal phalanx. The dorsal metacarpal arteries extend into the phalanges but cannot be counted on to perfuse more than the proximal phalanx of each finger.

The venous drainage of the hand consists of deep and superficial systems (Fig 6–23). The deep veins accompany the palmar and dorsal arterial arches and are usually of much smaller caliber than the arteries. This deep system of veins usually extends into the fingers as well. The superficial veins

of the dorsum of the fingers run in a pattern of several trunks parallel with the long axis of the finger. This larger system collects the veins from the volar and lateral sides of the fingers. They also collect most of the subungual and terminal volar plexuses and finally are directed toward the interdigital spaces to form a venous network over the dorsum of the hand. There is great variability in the dorsal veins of the hand, but they eventually connect with cephalic and basilic veins in the forearm and arm.

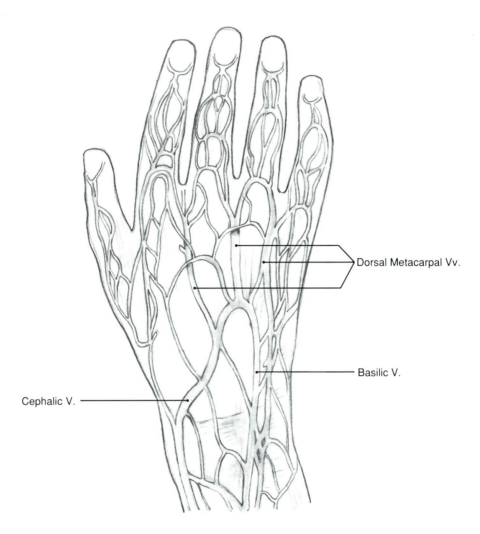

Dorsal Metacarpal Vv.

Basilic V.

Cephalic V.

FIG 6–23.
Venous drainage of the hand.

Nerves

Sensation of the wrist and hand is provided by the musculocutaneous, radial, median, and ulnar nerves (Fig 6–24). The lateral antebrachial cutaneous nerve, a continuation of the musculocutaneous nerve, is purely sensory at this level. It supplies the skin and joints over the radial side of the forearm, wrist, and proximal thumb. Sensation of the remainder of the wrist and hand is supplied by the other three nerves.

The superficial branch of the radial nerve is purely sensory and emerges from under the tendon of the brachioradialis 8 cm proximal to the tip of the radial styloid, perforates the fascia, and divides into a lateral and medial branch (Fig 6–25). Three fourths of individuals have complete or incomplete overlap of the innervation of the radial and lateral antebrachial cutaneous nerves on the radial side of the wrist and hand.

After giving off all of its motor branches, the posterior interosseous branch of the radial nerve (now known as the dorsal interosseous nerve) runs on the posterior surface of the interosseous membrane and divides into numerous branches to supply the ligaments of the radiocarpal, carpal, and carpometacarpal joints (Fig 6–26). This nerve has been implicated as a source of wrist pain in patients with symptomatic dorsal wrist ganglia.

The median nerve approaches the carpal canal superficial to the flexor superficialis of the index and middle fingers and just radial and deep to the palmaris longus tendon (Fig 6–27). The median nerve, in addition to supplying most of the extrinsic flexors of the wrist and fingers and a portion of the intrinsic thumb and lumbrical muscles, also provides sensory innervation for most of the finger joints. In addition, it provides sensation (see Fig 6–24) to more than half of the palmar skin, a portion of the dorsal skin of the fingers, and the subungual portion of the thumb. The anterior interosseous branch of the median nerve, after giving off its motor branches more

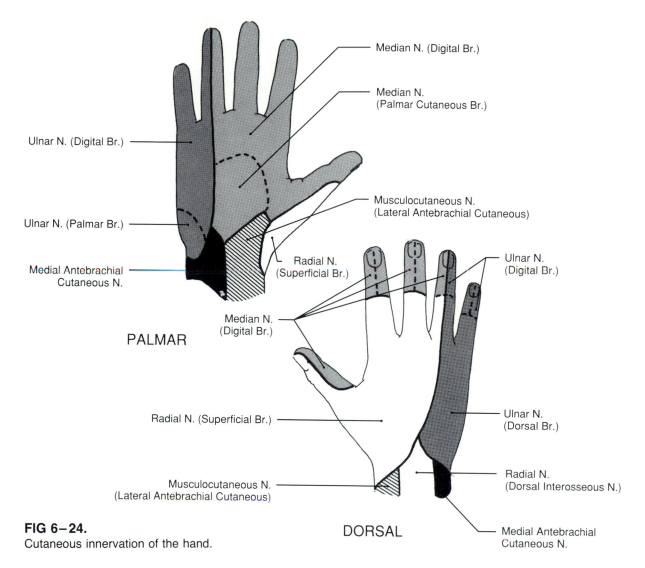

Median N. (Digital Br.)

Median N.
(Palmar Cutaneous Br.)

Ulnar N. (Digital Br.)

Musculocutaneous N.
(Lateral Antebrachial Cutaneous)

Ulnar N. (Palmar Br.)

Ulnar N.
(Digital Br.)

Medial Antebrachial
Cutaneous N.

Radial N.
(Superficial Br.)

Median N.
(Digital Br.)

PALMAR

Radial N. (Superficial Br.)

Ulnar N.
(Dorsal Br.)

Musculocutaneous N.
(Lateral Antebrachial Cutaneous)

Radial N.
(Dorsal Interosseous N.)

FIG 6–24.
Cutaneous innervation of the hand.

DORSAL

Medial Antebrachial
Cutaneous N.

proximally in the forearm, gives a branch to the pronator quadratus and then innervates the anterior portion of the radiocarpal joint. The palmar cutaneous branch of the median nerve (see Fig 6–15) consistently originates from the radial side of the median nerve 5 to 7 cm proximal to the wrist crease and parallels the parent nerve, crossing the base of the thenar eminence over the prominence of the tubercle of the scaphoid. It is particularly vulnerable to transection at this point. Here, the nerve divides into a radial branch, which supplies the skin to the base of the thenar area and radial palm, and several ulnar branches, which perforate the transverse carpal ligament.

At the distal border of the carpal canal the median nerve divides into muscular and digital branches. The motor or recurrent branch of the median nerve arises from the anterior or radial aspect

of the median nerve and courses anteriorly and laterally into the muscles of the thenar eminence. The motor branch usually courses distal to and behind the flexor retinaculum, but may also pierce the retinaculum itself before entering the thenar musculature. After penetrating the septum between the central palmar compartment and thenar muscles, the motor branch supplies the superficial head of the flexor pollicis brevis, which is the larger portion of this muscle. It then supplies the abductor pollicis brevis and terminates in the opponens pollicis.

The median nerve commonly gives off its digital branches at about the same level as the motor branch. At this level it lies just deep to the superficial palmar arch. The digital branches then pass slightly ventral so that they or their proper digital branches come to lie volar to the arteries before reaching the digits. There are two common digital

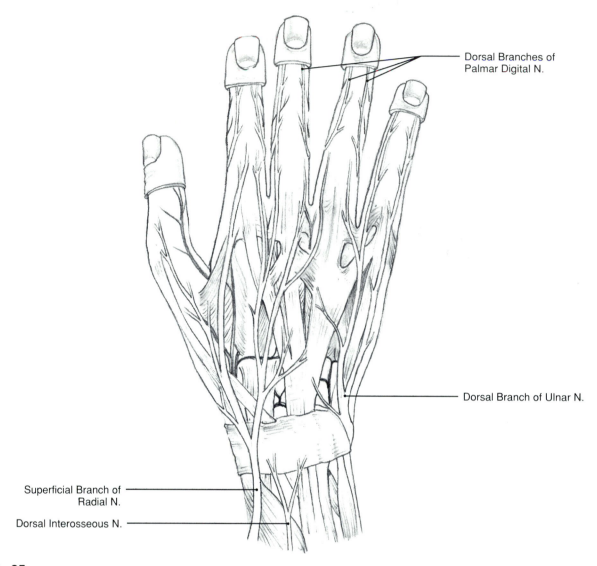

Dorsal Branches of
Palmar Digital N.

Dorsal Branch of Ulnar N.

Superficial Branch of
Radial N.

Dorsal Interosseous N.

FIG 6–25.
Dorsal cutaneous nerve branches of the hand. Note the relatively nerve-free interval between the dorsal branch of the ulnar nerve and superficial branch of the radial nerve.

nerves, one for the adjacent sides of the index and middle fingers and one for the adjacent sides of the middle and ring fingers. There is a proper digital nerve for the radial side of the index finger. The digital nerves to the thumb may arise separately or by a short common stem. The digital arteries typically divide into their proper digital branches distal to the corresponding nerve division. Prior to reaching the bases of the digits, the nerves and vessels lie between the long flexor tendons with their associated lumbrical muscles. The proper digital nerve to the radial side of the index finger gives off a motor branch to the first lumbrical. The common digital nerve to the adjacent sides of the index and middle fingers gives off a branch to the second lumbrical.

As the proper digital nerve proceeds into the digit just volar to the artery, both the nerve and artery lie at the sides of the flexor tendons at about the level of the palmar surface of the phalanges (Fig 6–28). They are thus protected from being squeezed between the flexor tendons and skin during grasp. The nerve and artery pass between the palmar and dorsal cutaneous ligaments of the fingers (known respectively as Grayson's and Cleland's ligaments). During its course along the digits, the digital nerve gives off numerous branches, which end in large lamellated structures known as pacinian corpuscles. During surgical dissection, recognition of these corpuscles usually heralds the proximity of the nerve and vessel. The digital nerves in the index, middle,

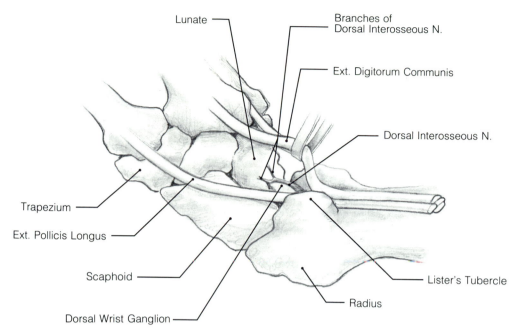

FIG 6–26.
Relationship of the posterior interosseous nerve to dorsal wrist ganglion.

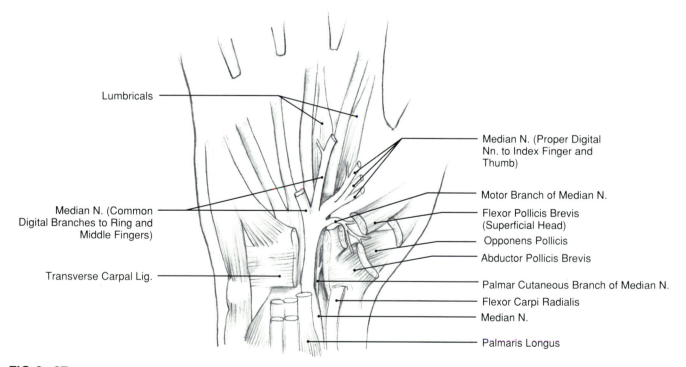

FIG 6–27.
Sensory and motor branches of the median nerve. The palmaris brevis and the palmar cutaneous branch of the median nerve have been removed to show the course of the deep branch. Note: in the proximal wrist the median nerve lies just under and slightly radial to the palmaris longus.

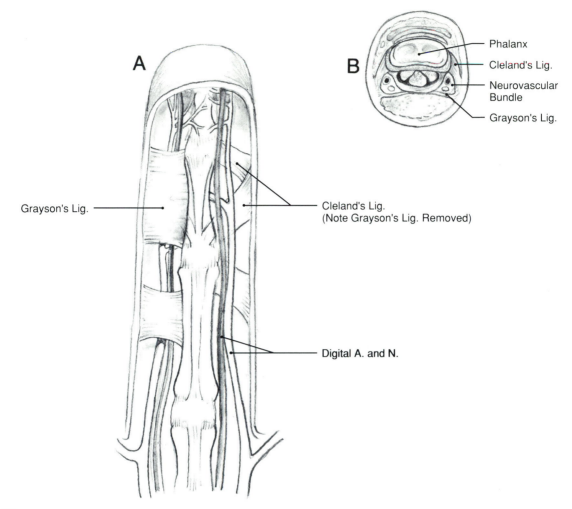

FIG 6–28.
A, Cleland's and Grayson's ligaments. Note that Cleland's ligament is dorsal to the neurovascular bundle while Grayson's is volar. **B,** cross-section.

and ring fingers give off dorsal branches proximal to the proximal IP joint. These branches supply the dorsum of the index and middle fingers and the radial side of the ring finger distal to the midportion of the middle phalanx (Fig 6–29). In addition, the digital nerves give off articular branches to the MP and proximal IP joints. Branches of the radial nerve innervate the dorsum of the thumb, except for the subungual region of the tip of the thumb, which is innervated by the median nerve.

At the wrist, the ulnar nerve travels through Guyon's canal, with the ulnar artery located just radial to the nerve (see Fig 6–16). The canal is bounded on either side by the pisiform and the hook of the hamate and covered volarly by the volar carpal ligament, which is an expansion of the flexor carpi ulnaris. The dorsal cutaneous branch of the ulnar nerve arises approximately 6 cm proximal to the styloid process of the ulna and perforates the fascia to lie on the dorsum of the wrist. It supplies the ulnar side of the dorsal hand, the dorsum of the little finger, and the dorsum of the radial side of the ring finger. It is useful to remember that there is a nerve-free interval between the branches of the dorsal ulnar nerve and the superficial radial nerve (see Fig 6–25). Dissecting between the extensor pollicis longus and extensor carpi ulnaris reduces the possibility of injuring a dorsal nerve.

Unlike the median nerve, the ulnar nerve does not have a consistent palmar cutaneous branch. Usually, multiple small branches from the superficial and/or dorsal branch of the ulnar nerve supply sensory fibers to the hypothenar region. The ulnar nerve divides within Guyon's canal, and the superfi-

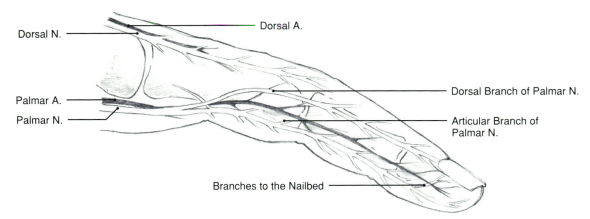

Dorsal N.

Dorsal A.

Palmar A.

Palmar N.

Dorsal Branch of Palmar N.

Articular Branch of Palmar N.

Branches to the Nailbed

FIG 6–29.
Distribution of digital nerves.

cial branch continues into the palm under the palmaris brevis muscle, giving off a small branch to this muscle (Fig 6–30). The nerve then gives off a proper digital branch to the ulnar side of the little finger and a common digital branch to the radial side of the little finger and ulnar side of the ring finger (see Fig 6–19). Like their median counterparts, these nerves have branches that supply their respective MP joints and dorsal branches for the dorsum of the fingers starting at the middle of the middle phalanx. The

deep, or motor, branch of the ulnar nerve divides in Guyon's canal and curves around the hook of the hamate, coursing in the interval between the abductor and flexor digiti minimi brevis while innervating these two muscles. It then passes through the opponens of the little finger, giving branches to this muscle, and enters the midpalmar space dorsal to the flexor tendons. As it courses across the palm it gives off branches to the ulnar two lumbricals and the interossei. It then penetrates through the open-

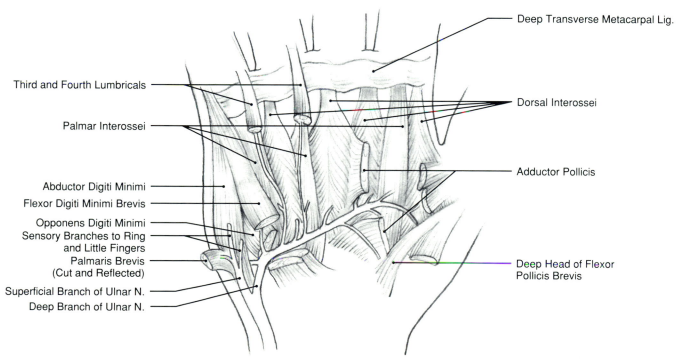

Third and Fourth Lumbricals

Palmar Interossei

Abductor Digiti Minimi

Flexor Digiti Minimi Brevis

Opponens Digiti Minimi

Sensory Branches to Ring and Little Fingers

Palmaris Brevis (Cut and Reflected)

Superficial Branch of Ulnar N.

Deep Branch of Ulnar N.

Deep Transverse Metacarpal Lig.

Dorsal Interossei

Adductor Pollicis

Deep Head of Flexor Pollicis Brevis

FIG 6–30.
Motor branches from the ulnar nerve supply most of the hand intrinsics.

ing (interval between transverse and oblique heads) of the adductor pollicis to supply this muscle, the first dorsal interosseous, and the deep head of the flexor pollicis brevis.

SURGICAL APPROACHES TO THE WRIST

Volar Incisions

The incision to expose the carpal tunnel contents should be kept just at the ulnar side of the thenar skin crease. It can be extended proximally quite satisfactorily by oblique extension at the level of the wrist flexor crease (Fig 6–31). The dissection is kept in line with the ring finger metacarpal to avoid the palmar cutaneous branches of the median and ulnar nerves. The dissection is carried down through the palmar fascia, palmaris brevis muscle, and transverse carpal ligament. To protect the nerve a spatula-type instrument can be placed under the ligament prior to its actual sectioning, or the nerve can be identified proximally and the ligament incised with the nerve under direct vision (Fig 6–32). Within the carpal tunnel deeper dissection should be kept to the ulnar side of the median nerve. This will avoid damage to the motor branch of the median nerve, which arises on the radial aspect of the nerve at the intersection of Kaplan's cardinal line with the thenar skin crease (Fig 6–33). However, the surgeon must also be aware of the ulnar artery and nerve, which lie in Guyon's canal just ulnar to this line of dissection. Inspection of the carpal tunnel floor should be done routinely, as bony spurs can cause tendon attrition and subsequent rupture. In cases of carpal bone trauma and/or distal radial fractures, this exposure can be extended proximally by curvilinear extension and reflection of the pronator quadratus muscle off the radius and toward the distal ulna (Fig 6–34). This allows complete exposure of the entire distal radius and carpal bones while simultaneously decompressing the carpal tunnel. Care must be taken in retraction of the radial artery and median nerve.

The Russe or Herbert approach can be used for scaphoid exposure or for exposure of the flexor pollicis longus and radial digital flexors (Fig 6–35). It is carried out with a longitudinal incision, which runs between the flexor carpi radialis tendon and radial artery. With the wrist in full radial deviation the scaphoid tubercle can be palpated. The incision is curved distally beyond the wrist flexor crease to ex-

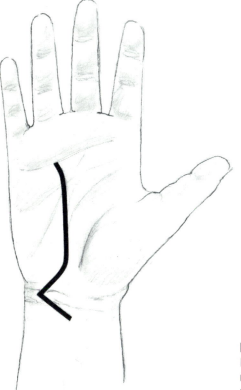

FIG 6–31.
Incision to decompress the carpal tunnel. Note incision is kept in line with the ring digit to avoid the palmar cutaneous branches of the median nerve and the ulnar nerve.

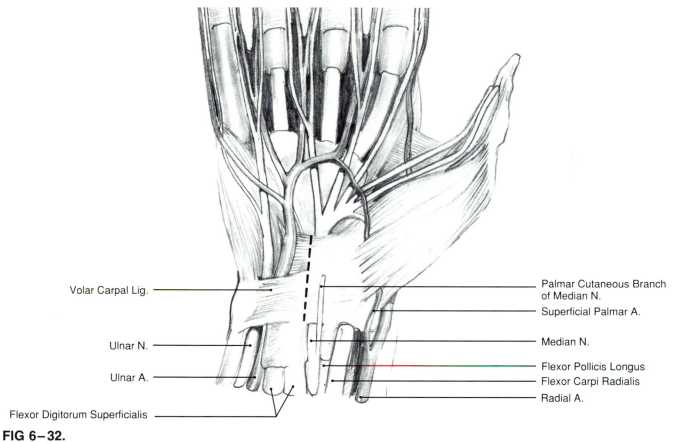

Volar Carpal Lig.

Ulnar N.

Ulnar A.

Flexor Digitorum Superficialis

Palmar Cutaneous Branch
of Median N.

Superficial Palmar A.

Median N.

Flexor Pollicis Longus

Flexor Carpi Radialis

Radial A.

FIG 6–32.
Relationship of the optimum incision through the transverse carpal ligament to the median nerve, its branches, and the ulnar neurovascular complex at the wrist.

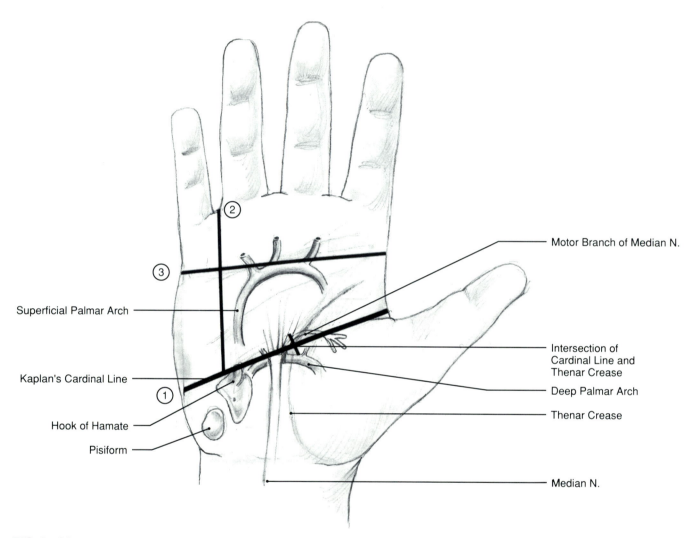

Motor Branch of Median N.

Superficial Palmar Arch

Kaplan's Cardinal Line

Hook of Hamate

Pisiform

Intersection of
Cardinal Line and
Thenar Crease

Deep Palmar Arch

Thenar Crease

Median N.

FIG 6–33.
Kaplan's cardinal line *(1)* is a line drawn from the apex of the interdigital fold between the thumb and index finger toward the ulnar side of the hand parallel with the proximal palmar crease. A second line *(2)* parallels the ulnar side of the ring finger and intersects the cardinal line. The point of intersection defines the ulnar artery, sensory branch of the ulnar nerve (not shown), and hook of the hamate. The intersection of the thenar crease with the cardinal line (Note small line marking intersection) corresponds to the emergence of the motor branch of the median nerve. A line drawn from the radial side of the proximal palmar flexion crease to the ulnar side of the distal palmar flexion crease *(3)* corresponds to the level of the superficial palmar arterial arch.

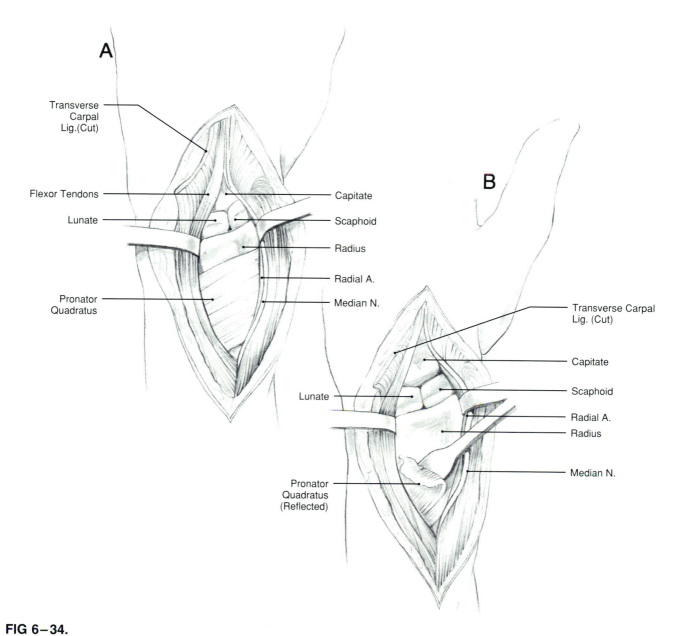

FIG 6–34.
A, proximal extension of the carpal tunnel incision. **B,** the pronator quadratus muscle is resected off the radius, then reflected in an ulnar direction. Care must be taken in retracting the radial artery and median nerve.

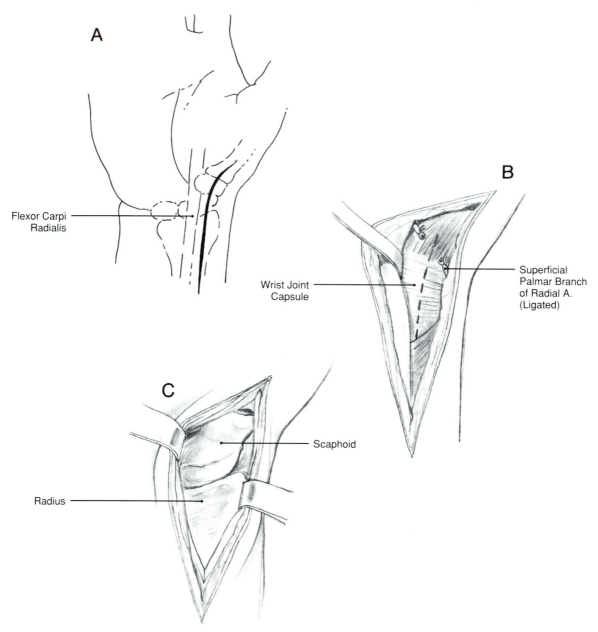

FIG 6–35.
The Russe or Herbert approach enters the wrist just radial to the flexor carpi radialis and extends into the thumb carpometa-carpal area. **A,** skin incision. **B,** site of capsule incision *(dashed line);* ligated superficial palmar branch of radial artery. **C,** exposure of scaphoid and distal radius.

pose the distal scaphoid. The superficial palmar branch of the radial artery is encountered as it passes ulnarly to join the superficial palmar arch. This branch should be ligated rather than electroco-agulated. The surgeon must also be aware of the lateral antebrachial cutaneous nerve (Fig 6–36), which lies radial to the palmar cutaneous branch of the median nerve and volar to the superficial branch of the radial nerve. It represents the most distal end of the

musculocutaneous nerve and if injured can be the source of symptomatic neuroma formation.

The approach to Guyon's canal follows the hy-pothenar skin crease in the palm at the base of the ring finger. It crosses the wrist flexor crease obliquely, staying radial to the flexor carpi ulnaris and extending proximally in a zigzag or curvilinear fashion (Fig 6–37). The nerve is identified proximally first where it lies deep to the artery and veins above

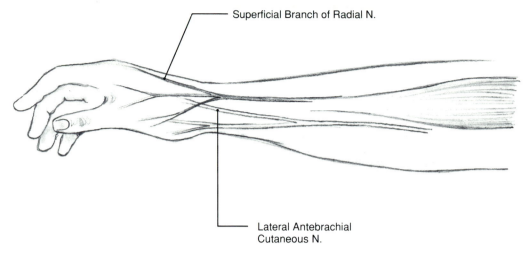

FIG 6–36.
Relationship between the lateral antebrachial cutaneous nerve and the superficial branch of the radial nerve.

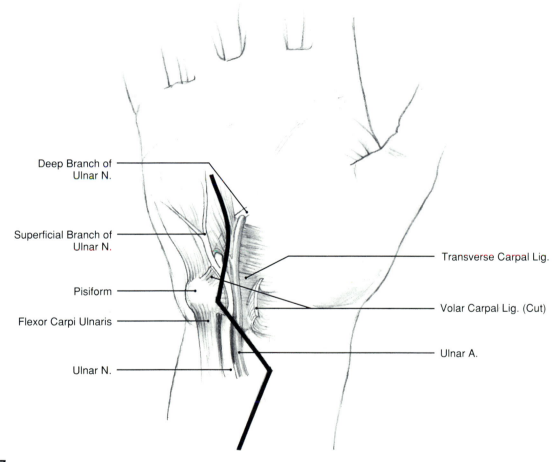

FIG 6–37.
Guyon's canal exposure with the volar carpal ligament transected and reflected radially and the ulnar nerve and artery running on top of the transverse carpal ligament.

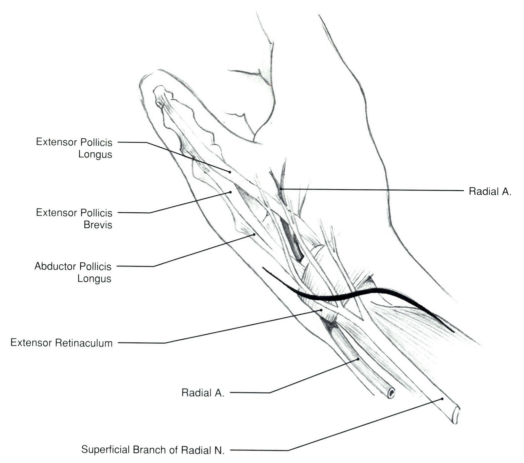

FIG 6–38.
Incision *(solid line)* for exposure to the first dorsal compartment showing the location of the superficial branch of the radial nerve on top of the extensor retinaculum.

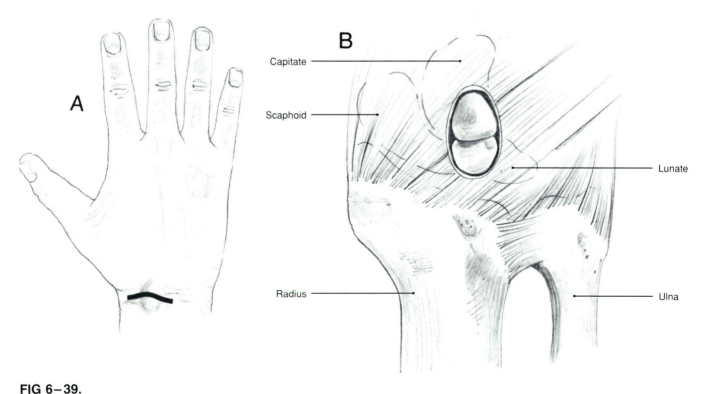

FIG 6–39.
A, transverse incision used to excise a typical ganglion cyst from the dorsal radiocarpal area. **B,** completed excision of dorsal ganglion cyst along with a small segment of capsule.

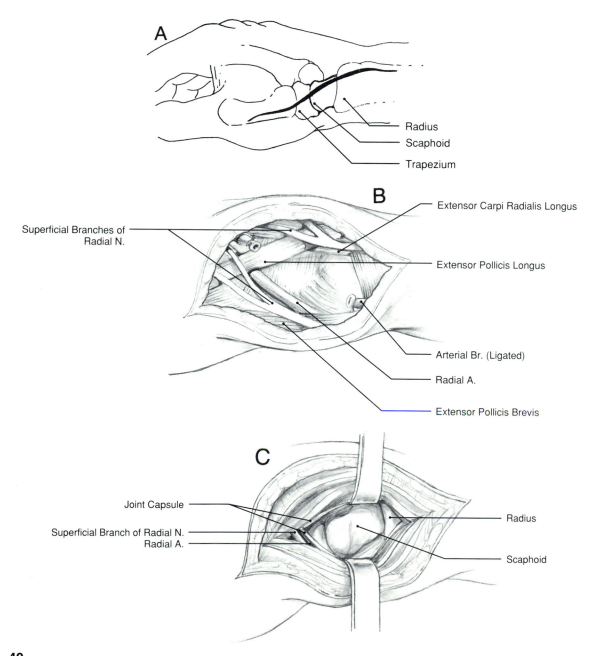

FIG 6–40.
Exposure of the radioscaphoid joint from the dorsal approach. **A,** skin incision. **B,** exposure of radial artery and branches and superficial radial nerve. **C,** capsular incision exposing scaphoid.

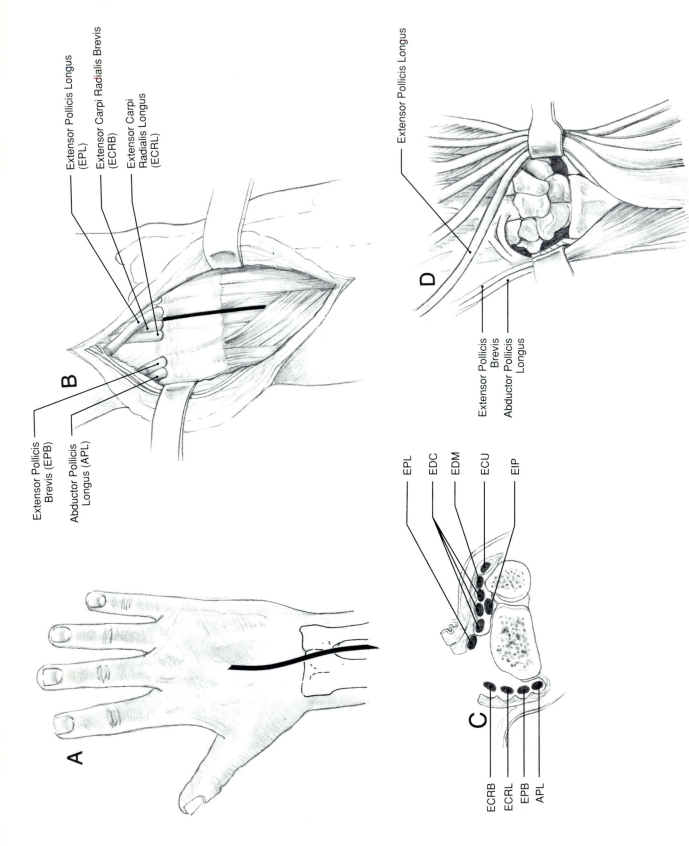

Extensor Pollicis Longus (EPL)

Extensor Carpi Radialis Brevis (ECRB)

Extensor Carpi Radialis Longus (ECRL)

Extensor Pollicis Brevis (EPB)

Abductor Pollicis Longus (APL)

B

A

Extensor Pollicis Longus

D

Extensor Pollicis Brevis

Abductor Pollicis Longus

EPL

EDC

EDM

ECU

EIP

ECRB

ECRL

EPB

APL

C

FIG 6–41.
A, dorsal midline wrist incision. **B**, dissection between the second and third compartments allows the extensor tendons to be elevated. **C**, cross-section of wrist with elevation of extensor tendons. **D**, complete carpal bone and distal radius exposure.

the wrist. At the wrist, the nerve is located on the ulnar side of the artery. These two structures run on top of the transverse carpal ligament and below the volar carpal ligament. The ulnar nerve has a palmar cutaneous branch similar to the median nerve, but it need not be exposed during the approach just described. The anatomic location is inconsistent. Symptomatic neuromas of this branch of the nerve are rare.

Dorsal Incisions

Dorsal wrist incisions may be either longitudinal or transverse. Great care must be taken to neither traumatize (cut) directly nor vigorously retract the sensory nerves in this area. The superficial branches of the radial nerve, as well as the dorsal sensory branches of the ulnar nerve, are located in the tissue planes between the skin and extensor retinaculum. These nerves are prone to neuroma formation with minimal insult.

Stenosing tenosynovitis of the tendons (abductor pollicis longus and extensor pollicis brevis) of the first dorsal compartment is a common clinical problem that requires surgical decompression at times. A safe approach to use in decompression of the first dorsal compartment is through a longitudinal curved incision over the radial styloid (Fig 6–38). The superficial radial nerve and its branches are retracted from the surface of the extensor retinaculum, and the first dorsal compartment is identified and released.

Ganglion cysts over the dorsum of the wrist can be exposed through a transverse incision. The skin creases in this area are transverse, making for an ideal cosmetic approach (Fig 6–39). The retinaculum is incised longitudinally over the mass and the extensor tendons retracted. The cyst and a small segment of underlying capsule are excised (see Fig 6–39), along with any segments of posterior interosseous nerve in the area (see Fig 6–26). This procedure partially denervates the wrist and may help decrease pain associated with ganglion cysts.

A dorsal radial incision allows satisfactory visualization of the radial styloid and the entire scaphoid (Fig 6–40). This dorsoradial curvilinear incision allows entry to the wrist joint between the first and third dorsal compartments. The extensor pollicis longus and extensor carpi radialis longus are retracted dorsally, and the radial artery and branches and the superficial radial nerve are retracted volarly. Small radial artery branches may require ligation and transection. Capsular incision allows exposure

of the radioscaphoid area. Radial and ulnar deviation of the wrist will allow more extensive visualization of the carpal bones.

Longitudinal dorsal wrist incisions are generally employed for more extensive wrist exposure. Procedures such as wrist arthrodesis, treatment of fracture-dislocations, or wrist arthroplasty can be approached via either a straight longitudinal or a curvilinear incision (Fig 6–41). The extensor retinaculum is divided between the second and third compartments, and the tendons are retracted to allow visualization of the entire distal radial metaphysis and carpal bony architecture.

Some surgeons prefer transverse wrist incisions for more limited arthroplasty or arthrodesis procedures (Fig 6–42). When limited wrist arthrodeses are performed, the distal radius can be approached through a second transverse incision to obtain donor bone for grafting. These incisions heal with a less conspicuous scar than longitudinal incisions, but the superficial cutaneous nerves are more vulnerable to injury. Longitudinal retinacular incisions are employed with these transverse skin incisions.

Another dorsal wrist approach is that to the distal radioulnar joint (Fig 6–43). A longitudinal, serpentine skin incision between the fourth and fifth extensor compartments is made. The dorsal sensory

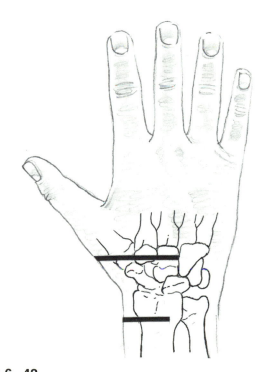

FIG 6–42.
Transverse incisions may be utilized to carry out limited arthrodeses and to obtain bone graft from the distal radius.

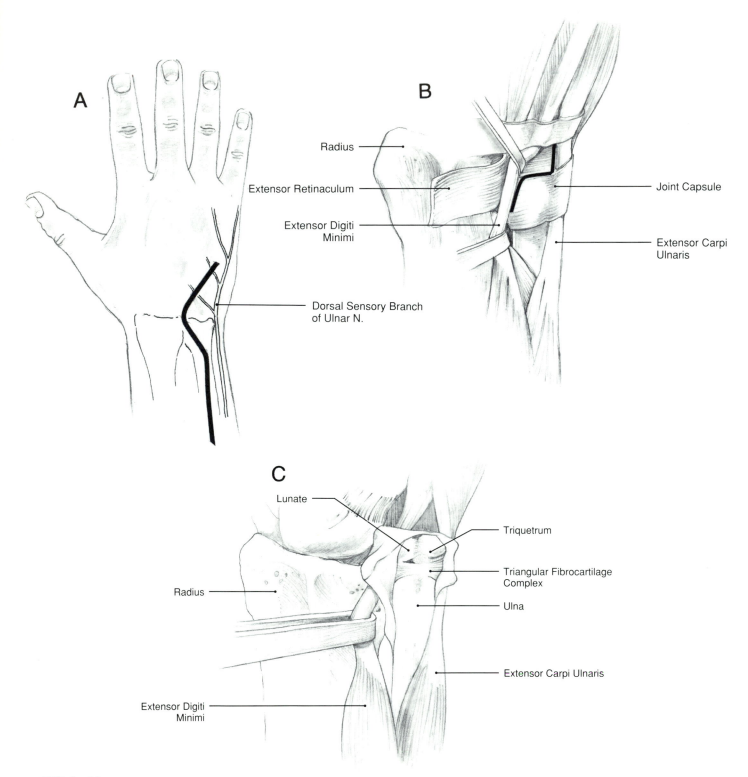

FIG 6–43.
A, skin incision for exposure of the distal radioulnar joint. Note the location of the dorsal sensory branch of the ulnar nerve. **B,** deeper dissection *(solid line)* through the retinaculum with the forearm in pronation exposes the capsule of the distal radioulnar joint. The extensor digiti minimi is reflected radially, and the extensor carpi ulnaris remains on the ulnar border of the ulna. **C,** the capsule is reflected and the distal radioulnar joint exposed. The triangular fibrocartilage complex (TFCC) and the lunotriquetral surfaces can be seen as well.

branch of the ulnar nerve is identified and protected. With the forearm fully pronated, the skin flaps are developed and the retinaculum exposed. The proximal and ulnar half of the extensor retinaculum is incised and reflected radially, uncovering the extensor digiti minimi and extensor carpi ulnaris. The extensor digiti minimi is retracted radially to expose the capsule of the distal radioulnar joint. A bayonet capsular incision allows exposure of the distal end of the ulna, the distal radioulnar joint, and the lunotriquetral articular surfaces.

SURGICAL APPROACHES TO THE HAND

The MP joints of the fingers are best approached, either singly or multiply, through a transverse incision. The incision is made dorsally along the apex of the flexed MP joints and can be curved between the metacarpal heads to give a scalloped appearance (Fig 6–44). This exposure is particularly useful for work on multiple joints in the rheumatoid hand. The transverse incision is made only down to the extensor tendons. Care is taken to preserve the dorsal veins and sensory nerves, which are branches of the radial and ulnar nerves. Incisions into the joints are made longitudinally through the dorsal hood, preferably on the ulnar side of the extensor tendon.

Alternatively, any of the MP joints may be approached through a longitudinal incision. The MP joint of the index finger can be accessed through a curved incision over the radial side of the joint. The MP joint of the middle or ring finger can be approached through a straight longitudinal incision between these two joints. A similar incision can be made between the ring and little fingers to gain access to either of their joints.

Fractures of the metacarpal shafts may be exposed through straight longitudinal incisions made just to one side of the extensor tendon of the involved bone (Fig 6–45). If all four metacarpals are involved, they may be exposed through an incision

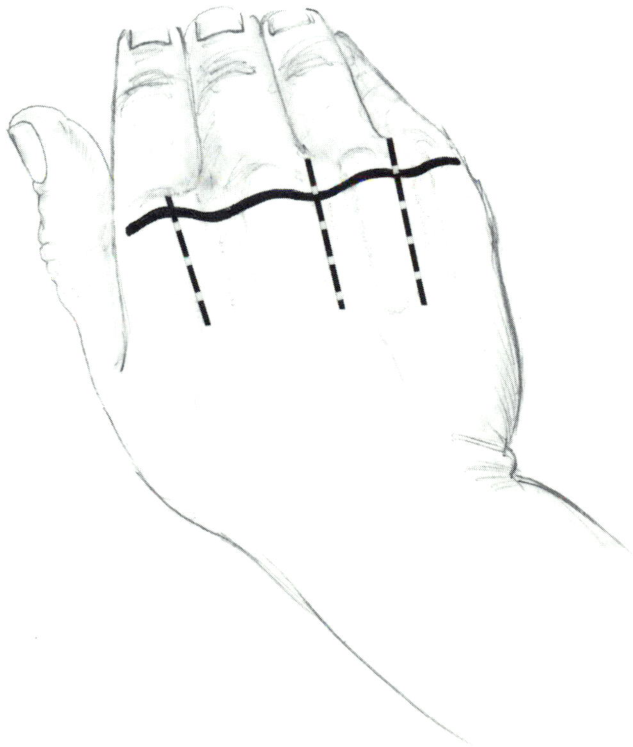

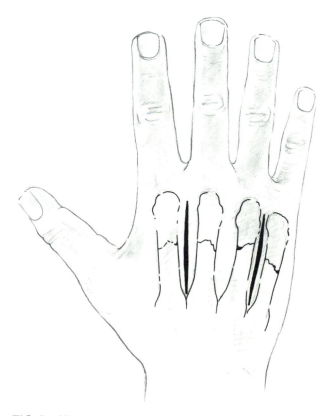

FIG 6–44.
Incisions for approaching metacarpophalangeal joints. Part or all of transverse incision may be used, depending upon the exposure required. Alternatively, longitudinal incisions *(dashed lines)* may be preferred.

FIG 6–45.
Dorsal approaches to fractured metacarpals. Note that metacarpals 2 through 5 can be reached through two incisions.

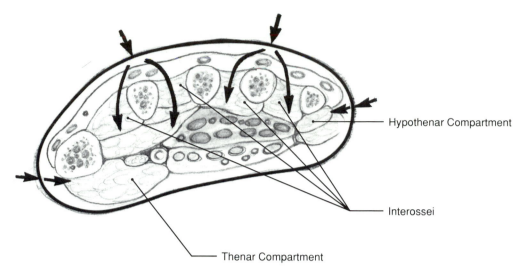

FIG 6–46.
Cross-section of pronated right hand (viewed from proximal to distal) showing incisions used for decompressing compartments of the hand.

between the second and third metacarpals and a second incision between the fourth and fifth metacarpals.

In a compartment syndrome of the hand, the deep muscle compartments (containing the dorsal and volar interossei and the thumb adductor) can be exposed through two dorsal longitudinal incisions

centered over the second and fourth metacarpals (Fig 6–46). After the fascia is incised over the dorsal interossei, the volar interossei and the adductor compartment can be decompressed by blunt dissection with a hemostat. The thenar and hypothenar compartments are exposed through incisions over the radial side of the first metacarpal and the ulnar

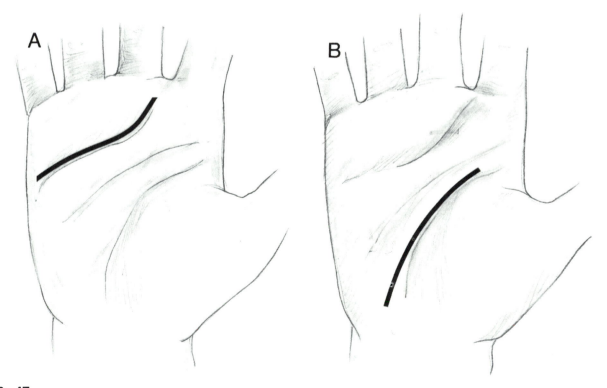

FIG 6–47.
A, transverse incision, in region of distal palmar crease, to decompress palm. **B,** curved incision following the volar thenar crease to decompress proximal palm.

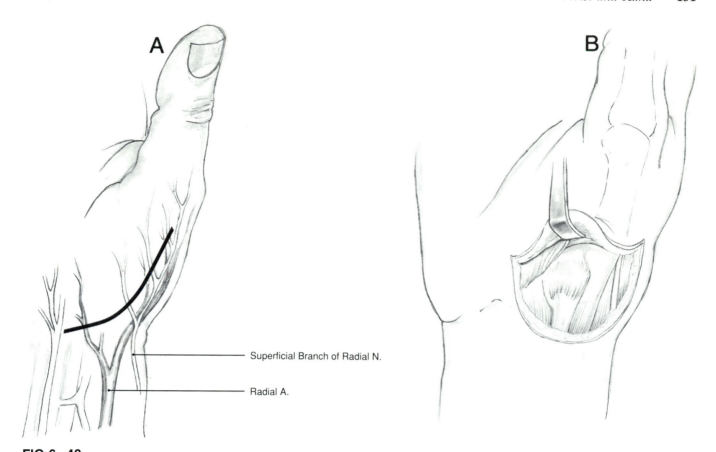

Superficial Branch of Radial N.

Radial A.

FIG 6–48.
A, hockey-stick incision for approach to the basal thumb joint. Note superficial radial nerve and branch of radial artery. **B,** alternate (transverse) approach to basal thumb joint.

side of the fifth metacarpal, respectively. The fingers are decompressed by fasciotomies through midlateral incisions.

Palmar incisions may be needed for exposure of the flexor tendons or the volar nerves and vessels (Fig 6–47). In the distal palm, incisions should be made transversely, following the proximal or distal palmar crease. In the proximal palm, incisions are more longitudinal, with the distal end curving parallel to the nearest major skin crease. Most of the vital structures lie just deep to the palmar fascia, except in the distal palm, where the structures between the metacarpal heads are not protected by the palmar fascia. In the very distal palm the neurovascular structures and tendons are all oriented longitudinally. More proximally, the thenar motor branch of the median nerve and the palmar arches curve transversely, and are at risk during palmar dissections. These structures can be identified topographically if Kaplan's cardinal line and a few landmarks are remembered (see Fig 6–33).

Exposure of the basal thumb joint is often needed for fracture repair or for arthrodesis or ar-

throplasty in patients with carpometacarpal joint arthritis. A curved transverse incision, or alternatively a hockey-stick incision, centered over the carpometacarpal joint provides excellent exposure (Fig 6–48). The sensory branch of the radial nerve should be identified in the subcutaneous tissues and protected. The dorsal continuation of the radial artery should also be identified as it courses around the radial side of the wrist under the abductor pollicis longus. Finally, the palmar cutaneous branch of the median nerve and the branches of the lateral antebrachial cutaneous nerves should be located and protected.

SURGICAL APPROACHES TO THE DIGITS

Midlateral Incision

The midlateral incision is useful for digital nerve exploration, flexor tendon exploration for repair or tendolysis, and incision and drainage of purulent tenosynovitis. The midaxial line has no variation of length with flexion and extension so contraction of the scar and restriction of joint motion are avoided (Fig 6–49). This incision allows good exposure of the flexor tendons and their sheath and one or both neurovascular bundles. The incision should be made along the dorsal margin of the flexor creases at the distal and proximal IP joints. This can be determined by flexing the finger and noting the dorsal extent of the flexor crease. Distally, the incision can be started at the lateral nail margin. Proximally, it is difficult to extend this incision into the palm, particularly in the middle and ring fingers, where the web spaces and natatory (superficial transverse metacarpal) ligaments should be preserved to prevent scar contractures.

After the skin incision, Cleland's ligament is cut and the neurovascular bundle carried with the volar flap. The flexor tendon sheath and, if necessary, the opposite neurovascular bundle can then be exposed. Alternatively, the artery and nerve can be identified and the tendon sheath approached anterior to the neurovascular bundle. This alternative approach avoids injury to the dorsal digital nerve branches, which supply the skin.

The midlateral incision is also useful for approaching fractures involving the distal one third of the proximal or middle phalanx. The transverse retinacular ligament is released to allow dorsal retraction of the lateral band and exposure of the fracture by lifting the extensor mechanism off the fracture site. To facilitate exposure, part or all of the collateral ligament may need to be released. If possible, this incision should be avoided on the ulnar side of the little finger and the radial side of the index finger, because these are contact surfaces for touching and pinching. The radial side of the middle and ring fingers are also contact areas for tip-to-side thumb pinching, and care should be taken to protect the dorsal nerve branches to the skin when these areas are explored.

Volar Incisions

The volar zigzag (Bruner) incisions provide a direct approach to the flexor tendons and digital neurovascular bundles for repair (Fig 6–50). They are particularly useful if extension into the palm is required, since the neurovascular bundles are not mobilized in the flaps. The three-flap incision, with the apices at the three volar skin creases of the digit is preferred. The digital nerves and vessels lie just under the point of each flap, and the dissection should only be skin deep at these points.

In children it is important to carry the apex of the flap to the dorsal limit of the flexor skin creases. This is because the scars tend to straighten as the child matures, resulting in a contracture. In adults this is usually not a problem, but necrosis of the flap tip can occur if the apex is placed too far dorsally. In the thumb, it may be preferable to extend the incision across the IP joint along the midlateral line on the radial side so as to avoid a scar in the pulp tip. This incision is also useful for excision of cysts and tumors. The main disadvantage of this incision is that the loss of volar skin continuity can interfere with early finger mobilization postoperatively.

An alternative to the classic Bruner incision is the running W design, which utilizes smaller flaps but still provides excellent exposure. An additional advantage to this incision is that it may be converted to a W-Y at any level to provide more horizontal exposure. This approach is also useful in a contracted finger, where the volar skin can be lengthened by converting the W-Y to a W-Y-V.

Explorations of structures underlying lacerations can be facilitated by proximal and distal extension of the wound. The lacerations can usually be incorporated into the basic zigzag incision, taking care to keep all angles at 90 degrees or greater.

Dorsal Incisions

The proximal IP joint and extensor mechanism may be approached through a gently curved incision (Fig 6–51). On the index, long, and ring fingers the apex of the curve should be on the ulnar side. In the little finger, the apex should be on the radial side. The base of the flap should not extend past the midlateral line. This incision protects most of the dorsal nerve supply and avoids the highly specialized skin over the joint. The dorsal incision is very useful for exposing fractures of the proximal two thirds of the proximal phalanx if the extensor mechanism is split after the skin incision is made. Alternatively, one may incise alongside the extensor tendon and retract it laterally.

An S-shaped incision may be used to approach the proximal IP joint and is especially suited for extending transverse wounds over the fingers. On the index, long, and ring fingers, the incision is begun on the ulnar side of the proximal phalanx in the midlateral line. The incision is extended transversely across the midjoint skin crease to the midaxis of the

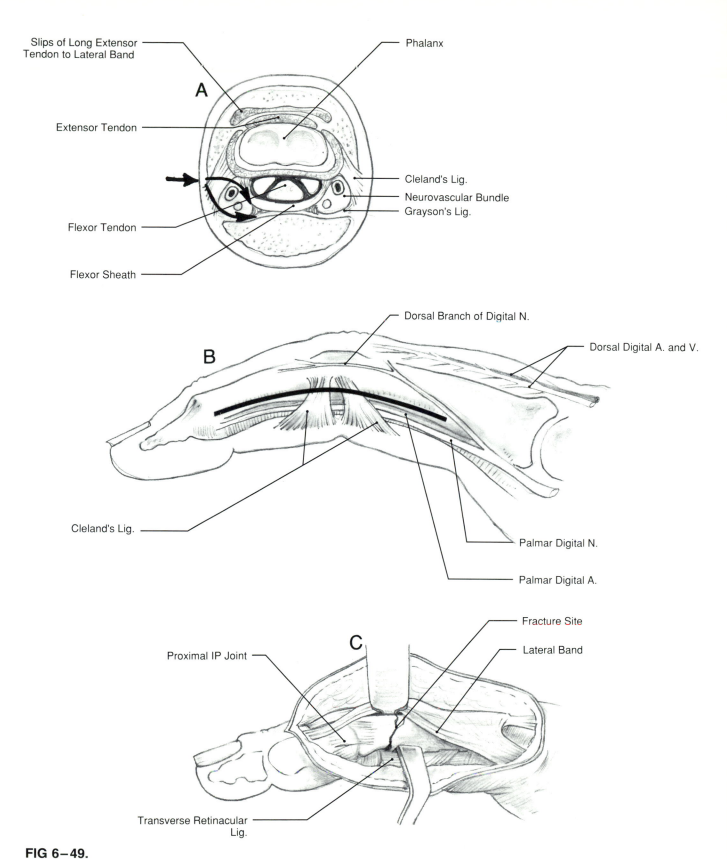

FIG 6–49.

A, cross-section shows midlateral approach through Cleland's ligament with the option of dissecting dorsal or volar to the neurovascular bundle. **B,** note that the incision lies between the palmar digital nerve and its dorsal branch. **C,** midlateral approach for fractures of the distal third of the proximal phalanx. The transverse retinacular ligament has been released to allow dorsal retraction of the lateral bands.

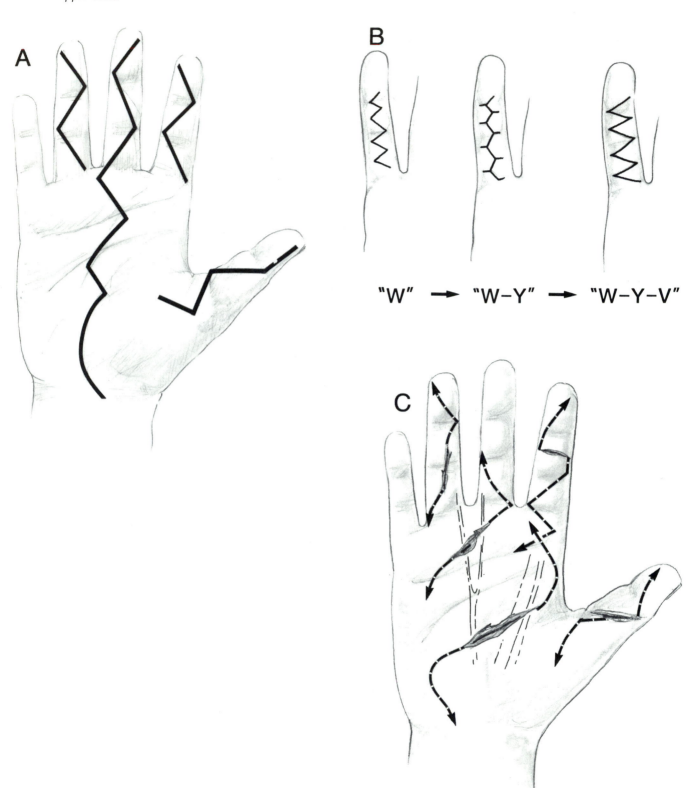

FIG 6–50.
A, zigzag (Bruner) incisions with flap apices at each digital flexion crease. **B,** when the running Y incision is connected to a W-Y in the contracted finger, it will open up into a series of Vs as the finger is straightened out. **C,** extension of wounds for primary repair of underlying structures. Note that transverse finger lacerations are extended in a bayonet fashion at the edges so as not to compromise the skin flaps.

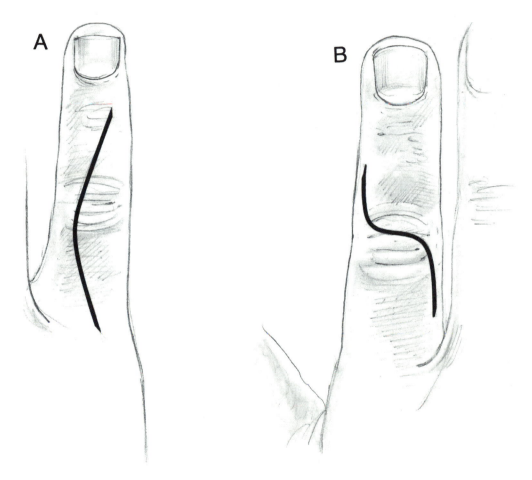

FIG 6–51.
Proximal interphalangeal joint approaches. **A,** gently curved dorsal approach to the proximal IP joint of the little finger. (The apex of the curve is on the radial side in the little finger and on the ulnar side in the index, long, and ring fingers.) **B,** S-shaped approach to index, long, and ring fingers. (The limbs of the incision are reversed on the little finger.)

radial side. The limbs should be reversed in the little finger.

Exposure of the distal IP joint for arthrodesis or correction of a mallet deformity may be accomplished through an S-shaped incision as described above (Fig 6–52). On the index, long, and ring fingers, the incision is begun on the ulnar side of the middle phalanx in the midlateral line and extended transversely across the midjoint skin crease to the midaxis of the radial side. This approach protects the dorsal sensory branch of the radial digital nerve. The limbs should be reversed in the little finger. The dissection is best done with a knife and a skin hook, taking the flap all the way down to the extensor ten-

don. The dorsal veins at this level may be sacrificed, but care should be taken to avoid injury to the nail matrix. Placing the proximal limb of the incision on the ulnar side avoids the dorsal sensory branch of the radial digital nerve. The juncture of the limbs of this incision should be gently curved to protect the flap tips.

An incision that provides wide exposure of the distal IP joint for arthroplasty or arthrodesis is the distally based Y or "Mercedes" incision. The limbs of the Y fan out on either side of the nail, thus avoiding the matrix. To expose the joint, the extensor mechanism may be cut either transversely or in a step-cut fashion. Midline dorsal incisions at this

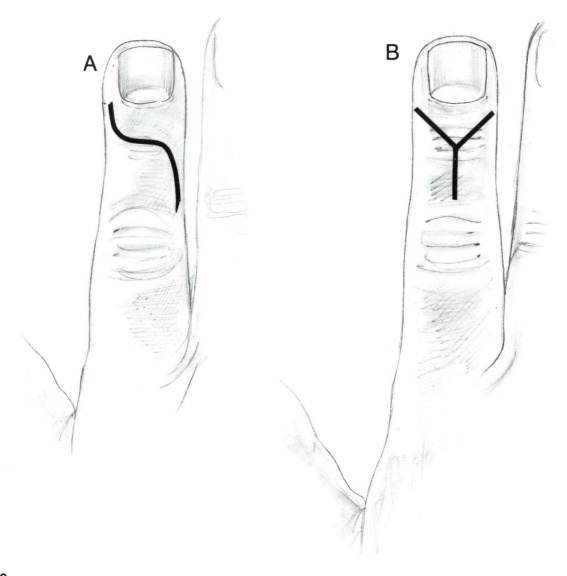

FIG 6–52.
Approaches to the distal interphalangeal joint. **A,** S-shaped incision to the distal IP joint of the index, long, and ring fingers (limbs of incision are reversed on the little finger). **B,** "Mercedes" incision. Note that both incisions avoid the proximal nail bed.

level should be avoided, as they can cause a scar contracture across the IP joint and/or damage the nail bed.

SURGICAL DRAINAGE OF INFECTIONS OF THE HAND AND DIGITS

All surgical approaches to the infected hand should permit easy extension in any direction and avoid crossing any flexion creases at a right angle. In general, surgically drained infections should be left open, or they may be closed over irrigation catheters.

Hand Infections

Midpalmar space (Fig 6–53) infections can occur from penetrating trauma, extension of a distal palmar abscess through the lumbrical canal, or rupture of an infected flexor tendon sheath in the ulnar three fingers. The midpalmar space, which lies over the ulnar three metacarpals between the flexor tendons and interossei, may be approached through a transverse or longitudinal incision (see Fig 6–47). The transverse incision parallels the distal palmar crease; the nerves and vessels are protected and the flexor tendons to the ring finger retracted to expose the abscess. The longitudinal approach provides more ex-

posure and is centered over the third metacarpal, between the distal palmar and thenar creases. This approach will expose the superficial palmar arch, which must be carefully protected.

A web space or collar button abscess usually involves the volar side. It may be subepidermal or involve the superficial transverse metacarpal ligament. As in most hand infections, there is usually more dorsal swelling, regardless of which side the abscess is on. The web space should be opened through two incisions (Fig 6–54). A volar zigzag incision will expose the neurovascular bundles and the superficial transverse metacarpal ligament. A straight longitudinal dorsal incision is then made and a generous communication established between the two incisions.

Thenar space infections (see Fig 6–53), which also result from penetrating trauma or extensions of infections in adjacent areas, present with marked pain and swelling of the thenar eminence and abduction of the thumb. This space lies just anterior to the adductor pollicis, but clinically the infection can extend to the subcutaneous region of the first web space. Like web space infections, thenar space infections are best drained through a combined dorsal and volar approach (Fig 6–55). The volar approach follows the thenar crease, placing both the palmar cutaneous and motor branch of the median nerve at risk. The palmar cutaneous nerve lies subcutaneously, under the proximal part of the incision. The motor branch of the median nerve lies deeper, near the juncture of the proximal and middle thirds of the incision. Once the skin incision is made, the deeper

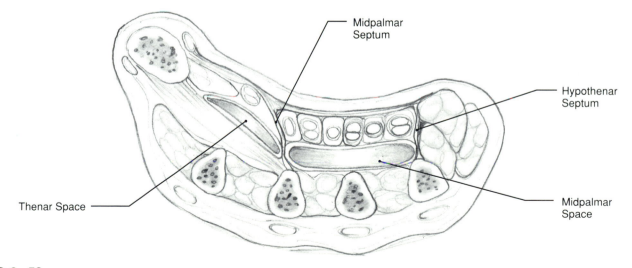

FIG 6–53.
Cross-section of supinated right midhand, viewed from distal to proximal. The midpalmar and thenar spaces are only potential spaces that do not become apparent unless an infection develops in them.

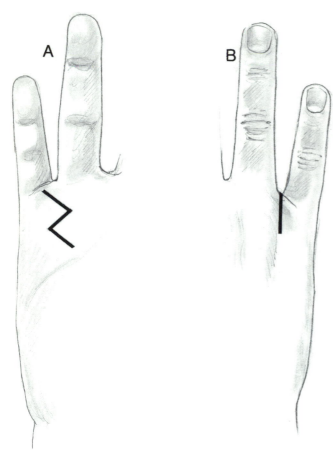

FIG 6–54.
Two separate incisions are preferred for web space drainage. **A,** volar. **B,** dorsal.

dissection should be done bluntly towards the adductor pollicis, until pus is encountered.

Finger Infections

The most common hand infection is the acute paronychia, or "runaround." It occurs between the base of the nail and the eponychium and, like most hand infections, is usually caused by *Staphylococcus aureus.* If the infection fails to respond to warm saline soaks and oral antibiotics, it may be approached surgically in one of two ways (Fig 6–56). One fourth of the nail on the involved side may be excised after it is separated from the underlying nailbed. If this does not adequately decompress the infection, the paronychial fold may be incised, with care taken to direct the blade away from the nailbed and matrix.

A felon is an infection of the distal pulp of a finger with involvement of the fibrous trabeculae, which divide the pulp into several small compartments. If the abscess has "pointed," it may be relieved by an incision directly over it (Fig 6–57,A and B). If it has not pointed, a lateral incision is preferred

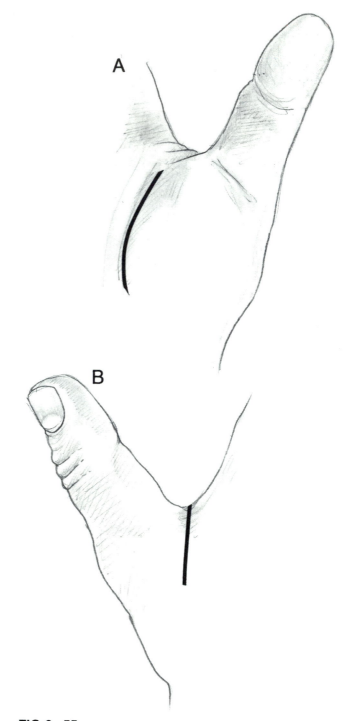

FIG 6–55.
Thenar space infections are deeper than other web space infections. They should also be drained through two incisions. **A,** volar. **B,** dorsal.

(Fig 6–57,C and D). In the index, middle, and ring fingers, a lateral incision is made on the ulnar side. In the thumb and little finger, the incision is made on the radial side. Fishmouth or bilateral incisions should be avoided.

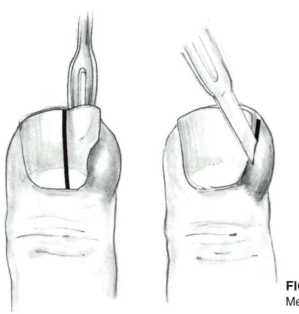

FIG 6–56.
Methods for drainage of acute paronychia.

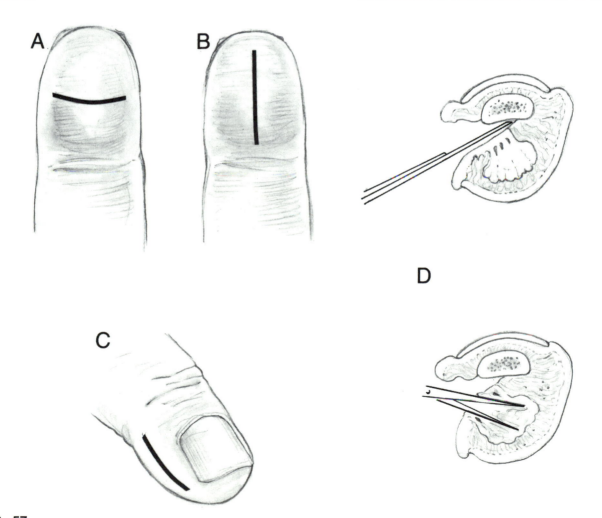

A

B

C

D

FIG 6–57.
Drainage of a felon. **A** and **B,** accepted incisions for localized areas of purulence that have "pointed." **C** and **D,** standard approach. Note that the incision is dorsal to the midline and does not extend around the tip of the finger.

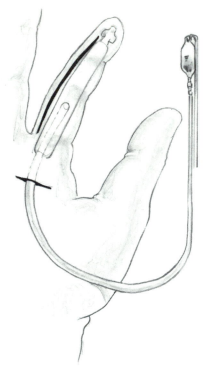

FIG 6–58.
Midlateral finger incision and palmar incision for drainage of infected flexor tendon sheaths. Closed irrigation may be added after surgical drainage has been established.

Pyogenic flexor tenosynovitis is the most dreaded hand infection, as it can result in loss of the tendon-gliding mechanism and destruction of the blood supply to the digit. Kanavel's four classic signs of this infection are (1) flexed position of the involved finger, (2) symmetric swelling of the finger, (3) tenderness over the tendon sheath only, and (4) pain with passive finger extension. Flexor sheath infections should be drained through either a midlateral or volar oblique incision in the finger and a second incision in the palm, at the level of the proximal margin of the A1 pulley (Fig 6–58). The midlateral incision is extended into the distal phalanx, the neurovascular bundle is reflected volarly, and the sheath distal to the A4 pulley is resected. This allows placement of a continuous irrigation catheter in the sheath between the two incisions. A similar approach is used with a volar oblique incision.

WRIST ARTHROSCOPY

Wrist arthroscopy is a promising new tool for diagnosis and management of difficult intraarticular wrist problems. It allows detailed examination of the capsular and ligamentous structures and articular surfaces of the wrist joint. Currently, wrist arthroscopy appears to be useful in three situations. In ligamentous tears, particularly of the triangular fibrocartilage complex (TFCC), arthroscopy is useful for debridement of unstable flaps or assessment of the extent of injury if a stabilization procedure is being considered. Second, arthroscopy is useful for reduction of intraarticular fractures and dislocations about the wrist. Finally, wrist arthroscopy can be helpful in patients with persistent symptoms who have had a negative conventional workup. However, although wrist arthroscopy may facilitate the diagnosis and treatment of certain intraarticular wrist problems, it should not replace conservative management or traditional radiographic diagnostic techniques.

All of the arthroscopic portals are located on the dorsal aspect of the wrist, avoiding most of the neurovascular structures (Fig 6–59). There are seven portals for visualizing the radiocarpal, ulnocarpal, distal radioulnar, and midcarpal joints. The five portals involving the radiocarpal and ulnocarpal interval are named after the six extensor compartments. They are the 1-2 portal, between the first and second compartments; the 3-4 portal, between the third and fourth compartments; the 4-5 portal, between the fourth and fifth compartments; and the 6R and 6U portals, radial and ulnar to the sixth dorsal compartment. The midcarpal portal is located radial to the third ray, just distal to the proximal carpal row at the level of the scaphocapite interval. The seventh portal visualizes the distal radioulnar joint and the proximal surface of the TFCC. This joint is entered by supinating the wrist and palpating the radial side of the ulnar head with the scope between the TFCC and the fovea on the head of the ulna.

Arthroscopy is performed with a 2 to 3 mm small-joint arthroscope with or without a sheath. The patient is placed in the supine position on the operating table with the upper extremity suspended from fingertraps with 5 pounds of countertraction over the tourniquet on the upper arm. This provides adequate distraction of the joint for visualizing intraarticular structures (Fig 6–60).

The radiocarpal joint is distended with saline using an 18-gauge needle through either the 6R or 4-5 portal. The 3-4 portal is best for looking at the scapholunate interval and the radial aspect of the wrist and is preferable for general examination of the entire radiocarpal interval. A 4 mm longitudinal incision is made 1 cm distal and just ulnar to Lister's tubercle. Subcutaneous tissues are spread with a he-

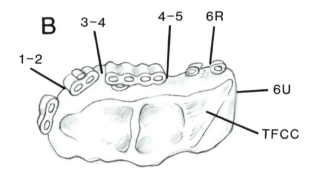

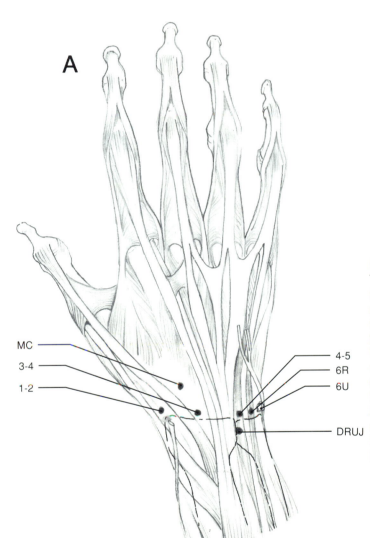

FIG 6–59.
The seven preferred arthroscopic portals of the wrist (1-2 portal, 3-4 portal, MC portal, DRUJ portal, 4-5 portal, 6R portal, and 6U portal). Portals involving the radiocarpal and ulnocarpal interval are named after the six extensor compartments: the 1-2 portal is located between the first and second compartments, etc.; 6R and 6U are radial and ulnar to the sixth dorsal compartment. (MC = midcarpal portal. DRUJ = distal radioulnar joint portal.) **A,** dorsal view. **B,** cross-section of midwrist, viewed from proximal to distal. Note extensor pollicis longus tendon at this level lies almost directly dorsal to the ECRL and ECRB. TFCC = triangular fibrocartilage complex.

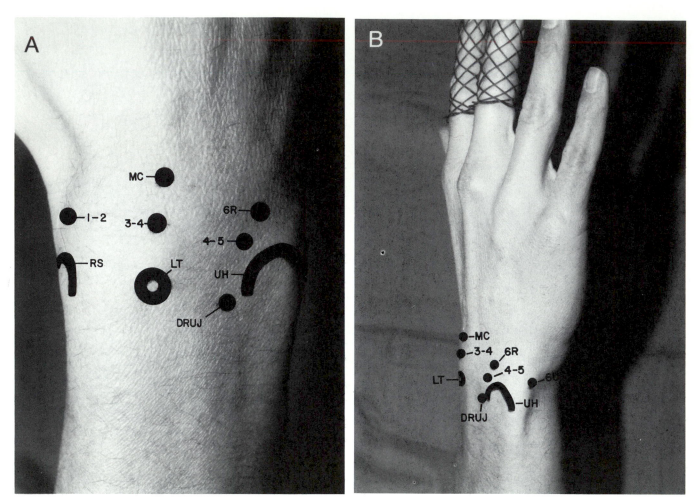

FIG 6–60.
With the wrist distracted in fingertrap traction, the seven arthroscopic portals are accessed from the dorsal side. The radial styloid *(RS)*, Lister's tubercle *(LT)* and the ulnar head *(UH)* are useful landmarks to help identify entry points. **A,** dorsoradial view. **B,** dorsoulnar view.

mostat to avoid dorsal veins and nerves. The arthroscope is then inserted using a blunt trocar. The 1-2 portal gives good visualization of the scaphoid fossa and proximal pole of the scaphoid. It is also useful for placement of probes or other instruments. When the 1-2 portal is used, it is important to remember that the dorsal continuation of the radial artery passes under the first dorsal compartment as it enters the anatomic snuff-box. The 4-5 portal enters the joint directly adjacent to the midportion of the TFCC and is most useful for exploration of this ligament. The 6R and 6U portals are ideal for placement of instruments to assess the TFCC. The midcarpal portal is used to visualize the entire midcarpal joint. Its site is palpable as a small depression on the dorsum of the wrist radial to the extensor digitorum communis tendon of the index finger.

BIBLIOGRAPHY

Adamson JE, Fluery AF Jr: Incisions in the hand and wrist, in Green DP (ed): *Operative Hand Surgery,* ed 2. New York, Churchill Livingstone, Inc, 1988, pp 1785–1804.

Andrews JR, Pierre RK, Carson WG: Arthroscopy of the elbow. *Clin Sports Med* 1986; 5:653–662.

Ashbell TS: The scalloped dorsal metacarpophalangeal skin incision. *J Bone Joint Surg* 1969; 51A:787–788.

Bingham DIC: Acute infections of the hand. *Surg Clin North Am* 1960; 40:1285–1298.

Bruner JM: The zig-zag volar-digital incision for flexor-tendon surgery. *J Plast Reconstr Surg* 1967; 40:571–574.

Carroll RE, Green DP: Significance of the palmar cutaneous nerve at the wrist. *Clin Orthop Rel Res* 1972; 83:24–29.

Carroll RE, Hill NA: Arthrodesis of the carpometacarpal joint of the thumb. *J Bone Joint Surg* 1973; 55B:292–294.

Dellon AL: Partial dorsal wrist denervation: Resection of

the distal posterior interosseous nerve. *J Hand Surg* 1985; 10A:527–533.

Dray GJ, Eaton RG: Dislocations and ligament injuries in the digits, in Green DP (ed): *Operative Hand Surgery*, ed 2. New York, Churchill Livingstone, Inc, 1988, pp 777–811.

Eaton RE, Littler JW: Ligament reconstruction for the painful thumb carpometacarpal joint. *J Bone Joint Surg* 1973; 55A:1655–1666.

Engber WD, Cameiner JG: Palmar cutaneous branch of the ulnar nerve. *J Hand Surg* 1980; 5:26–39.

Ertel AN, Millender LH, Nalebuff E, et al: Flexor tendon ruptures in patients with rheumatoid arthritis. *J Hand Surg* 1988; 12A:860–866.

Flynn JE: The grave infections, in Flynn JE (ed): *Hand Surgery*. Baltimore, Williams & Wilkins Co, 1966, pp 815–832.

Gelberman RH, et al: Vascularity of the scaphoid. *J Hand Surg* 1980; 5:508–513.

Grant JCB: *Grant's Atlas of Anatomy*, ed 5. Baltimore, Williams & Wilkins Co, 1962.

Gray H: *Anatomy of the Human Body*, ed 30. Philadelphia, Lea & Febiger, 1973.

Hollinshead WH: *The Back and Limbs*. New York, Harper & Row, 1982.

Hoppenfeld S, deBoer P: *Surgical Exposures in Orthopaedics: The Anatomic Approach*. Philadelphia, J B Lippincott Co, 1984.

Johnson RK, Shrewsbury MM: The anatomical course of the thenar branch of the median nerve: Usually in a separate tunnel through the transverse carpal ligament. *J Bone Joint Surg* 1970; 52A:269.

Kanavel AB: *Infections of the Hand: A Guide to the Surgical Treatment of Acute and Chronic Suppurative Processes in the Fingers, Hand and Forearm*. Philadelphia, Lea & Febiger, 1965.

Kaplan EB, Spinner M: The hand as an organ, in Spinner M (ed): *Kaplan's Functional and Surgical Anatomy of the Hand* (ed 3). Philadelphia, J B Lippincott Co, 1984, pp 1–19.

MacKinnon SE, Dellon AL: The overlap patterns of the lateral antebrachial cutaneous nerve and the superficial branch of the radial nerve. *J Hand Surg* 1985; 10A:522–526.

Mannerfelt N, Norman O: Attritional ruptures of flexor tendons in rheumatoid arthritis caused by bony spurs in the carpal tunnel. *J Bone Joint Surg* 1988, 51B:270–277.

Milford L: Surgical technique and aftercare, in Crenshaw AH (ed): *Campbell's Operative Orthopaedics*, ed 7. St Louis, C V Mosby Co, 1987, pp 119–122.

Moore KL: *Clinically Oriented Anatomy*, ed 2. Baltimore, Williams & Wilkins Co, 1985.

Morrey BF: Arthroscopy of the elbow, in Morrey BF (ed): *The elbow and its disorders*. Philadelphia, W B Saunders Co, pp 114–121.

Morrey BF: Elbow arthroscopy: A critical assessment. Presented at American Academy of Orthopaedic Surgery Course, Denver, Colorado, September, 1986, p 25.

Murray GM: Bone-graft for non-union of the carpal scaphoid. *Br J Surg* 1934–1935, 22:63–68.

Netter FH: *The Ciba Collection of Medical Illustrations: Musculoskeletal System*, vol 8. Summit, NJ, Ciba-Geigy Corp, 1987.

Neviaser RJ: Infections, in Green DP (ed): *Operative Hand Surgery*, ed 2. New York, Churchill Livingstone, Inc, 1988, pp 1027–1047.

O'Brian ET: Fractures of the metacarpals and phalanges, in Green DP (ed): *Operative Hand Surgery*, ed 2. New York, Churchill Livingstone, Inc, 1988, pp 709–775.

Posner MA, Kaplan EB: The fingers: Osseus and ligamentous structures, in Spinner M (ed): *Kaplan's functional anatomy of the hand*, ed 3. Philadelphia, J B Lippincott Co, 1984, pp 23–50.

Pratt ER: Exposing fractures of the proximal phalanx of the finger longitudinally through the dorsal extensor apparatus. *Clin Orthop Rel Res* 1959; 15:22–26.

Rowland SA: Fasciotomy: The treatment of compartment syndrome, in Green DP (ed): *Operative Hand Surgery*, ed 2. New York, Churchill Livingstone, Inc, 1988, pp 678–679.

Schultz RJ, Kaplan EB: Nerve supply to the muscles and skin of the hand, in Spinner, M (ed): *Kaplan's functional anatomy of the hand*, ed 3. Philadelphia, J B Lippincott Co, 1984, pp 222–243.

Taleisnik J: Fractures of the carpal bones, in Green DP (ed): *Operative Hand Surgery*, ed 2. New York, Churchill Livingstone, Inc, 1988, pp 835–837.

Taleisnic J: The palmar cutaneous branch of the median nerve in the approach to the carpal canal. *J Bone Joint Surg* 1973; 55A:1212–1217.

Watson HK, Hempton RF: Limited wrist arthrodesis. I: The triscaphoid joint. *J Hand Surg* 1980; 5:320–327.

Watson HK, Ryw J: Degenerative disorders of the carpus. *Orthop Clin North Am* 1984; 15:337–353.

Whipple TL, et al: Techniques of wrist arthroscopy. *Arthroscopy* 1986; 2:244–252.

PART III

Spine

Overview

Marc A. Asher, M.D.
Gopal Jayaraman, Ph.D.

The spinal column serves as the axial support for the trunk, head, and extremities and provides a protected conduit for the communication system linking them. It is organized as a segmented column of alternating stiff (vertebrae) and flexible (discs and connecting joints and ligaments) elements allowing motions in space that involve rotation and translations of the stiff segments (Fig III–1).

Superficially, the spine's design seems a monotonous repetition of the stiff and flexible segments. All are covered by sheets of muscles characterized by indistinct planes and confusing, seemingly overlapping names. However, it is readily apparent that there are major anatomical and mechanical differences among the major regions of the spine (cervical, thoracic, lumbar, and sacral). One result is the modification of the spine from a nonuniform, segmented, elastic rod to one with transitions from relatively mobile to relatively (or absolutely) immobile portions at the occipitocervical, cervicothoracic, thoracolumbar, and lumbosacral junctions. Most mechanical problems of the spine occur at these junctions.

Although not part of the spinal column, the rib cage plays an important role in spinal stability. Lacking the ventral support of the rib cage, the cervical and lumbar regions gain added stability by assuming a lordotic posture. This shifts more intervertebral compression force dorsally. By the same token, being unrestricted by the rib cage, the cervical and lumbar spine have greater mobility (Fig III–2). This places greater mechanical demand on the intrinsic stabilizing factors (joints and ligaments), no doubt making degenerative disease more likely in these regions.

In addition to the apparent regional differences, there are segmental differences; some are striking, such as those between C1, C2, and C3. Others are less obvious. For instance, the spinous process orientation varies in the thoracic spine, with the upper and lower four segments being relatively perpendicular and the middle four segments being relatively parallel to the long axis of the body. These positions have a marked effect on the accessibility of the ligamentum flavum and interlaminar openings. The pedicles likewise are quite variable in their size and orientation. These differences have important implications for surgical approaches to the spine.

Impressive as it is, the spine's design is only marginally capable of meeting the mechanical demands placed upon it. This is particularly true at the lumbosacral junction, where the forces and moments experienced are particularly large. For instance, when lifting a 224 newton (50 lbf) object 0.45 meters (18 in) from the body (L5 to hand horizontal distance), a person weighing 762 newtons (170 lb) develops a compressive force on the L5-S1 disc that may reach 4,200 newtons (900 lbf). This leaves little margin of safety, considering that 10,000 newtons (2,500 lbf) of compressive force is likely to cause vertebral rupture and 5,600 newtons (1,250 lbf) of compressive force may rupture the normal intervertebral disc. The compression load tolerated when the intervertebral disc is degenerated is as low as approximately 1,800 newtons (400 lbf).

The structure of the lumbosacral junction, with its large concave facet joints, extensive lumbosacral ligaments, and strong musculature, is adequate in most instances to handle the loads presented. However, congenital, developmental, traumatic, and de-

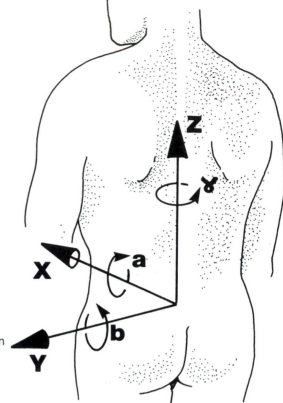

FIG III–1.
The three planes of and six motion possibilities with a right-hand orthogonal (90-degree angle) coordinate axis system. Shown is an anatomic axis system for the conventional anatomic planes of the human body with the origin at the center of the superior endplate of S1 and a gravity line Z axis (ISO axis convention). The planes are coronal *(YZ)*, sagittal *(XZ)*, and transverse or axial *(XY)*. Translation and rotation may occur in each plane.

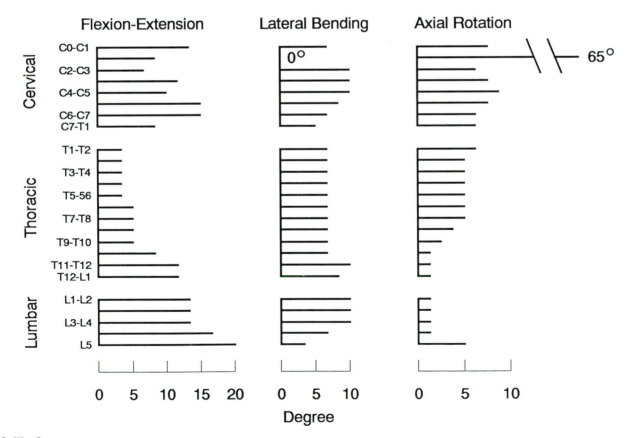

FIG III–2.
Composite of rotation in the traditional modalities and traditional planes of movement for the different regions of the spine. (Redrawn from White AA III, Panjabi MM: *Clinical Biomechanics of the Spine,* ed 2. Philadelphia, J B Lippincott Co, 1990.)

generative variances regularly test these adaptations. As a result, back pain is the leading cause of disability in workers aged 18 to 44 years, and second only to the common cold in its frequency as the cause of time loss from work.

The complexity and inaccessibility of the spine has limited our understanding of its pathophysiology and our capacity to deal with it surgically. This is quickly changing. The rapid accumulation of knowledge about spinal physiology and pathology has made it necessary to approach the spine surgically from every conceivable angle and lent a special urgency to the study of spinal anatomy.

REFERENCES

Borenstein BG, Wiesel SW: *Low Back Pain: Medical Diagnosis and Comprehensive Management.* Philadelphia, W B Saunders Co, 1989.

Brown T, Hansen RJ, Yorra AJ: Some mechanical tests on the lumbosacral spine with particular reference to the intervertebral disk: A preliminary report. *J Bone Joint Surg* 1957; 39A:1135–1164.

Chaffin DB, Anderson GBJ: *Occupational Biomechanics.* New York, John Wiley & Sons, 1984.

Jayson MIV, Herbert CM, Barks JF: Intervertebral disk: Nuclear morphology and bursting pressures. *Ann Rheum Dis* 1973: 32:308–315.

Limitation of Activity Due to Chronic Conditions. Rockville, MD, US Department of Health and Human Services, DHHS Publication No 80-10.

Nordin M, Frankel VH: *Basic Biomechanics of the Musculoskeletal System*, ed 2. Lea & Febiger, Philadelphia, 1989.

White AA III, Panjabi MM: *Clinical Biomechanics of the Spine,* ed 2. Philadelphia, J B Lippincott Co, 1990.

7

Cervical Spine

Pasquale X. Montesano, M.D.
Frederick W. Reckling, M.D.
Melvin P. Mohn, Ph.D.

ANATOMIC FEATURES OF THE NECK

The cervical spine has at least three fundamental biological functions. First, it transfers the weight and bending moments of the head to the trunk. Second, it allows sufficient physiological motion. Finally, and most importantly, it protects the delicate spinal cord from potentially damaging forces or motions produced by trauma. These functions are accomplished through the highly specialized mechanical properties of the normal cervical spine anatomy.

Bony Anatomy

There are seven cervical vertebrae. Because of specific anatomical features the first, second, and seventh cervical vertebrae will be discussed individually. The anatomical features of the third through sixth cervical vertebrae are quite similar and will be discussed collectively.

The atlas (C1) obtains its name from the fact that it supports the "globe" of the head. It consists of two lateral masses, which are connected by anterior and posterior arches (Fig 7–1). The atlas has no body or spinous process. In many ways the atlas functions as an ossified meniscus between the occiput and axis (C2). The superior surface of the atlas has two concave facets for articulation with the

condyles of the occiput. This allows flexion and extension of the head. The inferior facets of the atlas are concave and oval, which allows rotation of the atlas on the axis. Each transverse process of the atlas contains a bony transverse foramen through which a vertebral artery passes. Both the anterior and posterior arches have medially flared tubercles on which ligaments attach. The medial aspect of each lateral mass also has a small tubercle for attachment of the transverse ligament. Occasionally (12% of the time) the posterior arch of C1 forms a deep groove or canal (the ponticulus posticus), which contains the vertebral artery.

The axis, or C2, is distinguished by a vertical process connected to its body, the odontoid process (dens) (Fig 7–2). The odontoid process actually represents the body of the atlas that has been embryologically separated from the atlas and united with the axis. The odontoid process provides a pivot around which the axis rotates. Anteriorly this process has a small convex facet that articulates with a concave facet on the posterior aspect of the anterior arch of the atlas. Posteriorly, the odontoid is grooved by the transverse ligament. A small bursa is usually interposed between the transverse ligament and posterior odontoid. The superior surfaces of the lateral masses of the axis have two large oval convex facets facing posteriorly and superiorly. Anteriorly the body of the axis is concave on each side of the

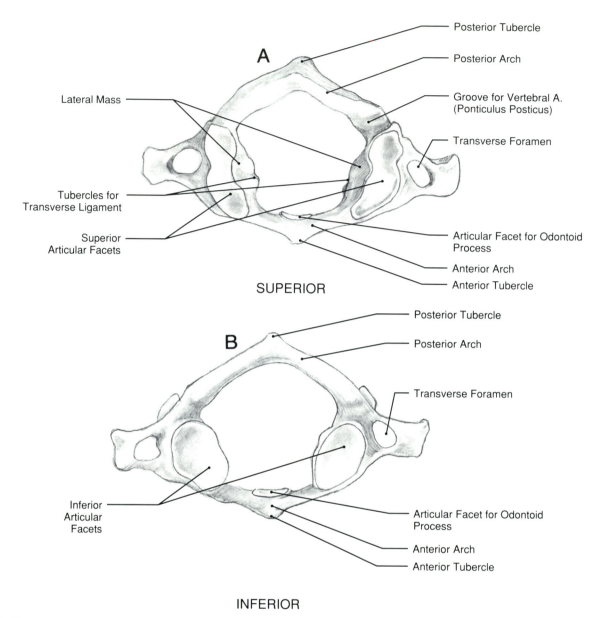

FIG 7–1.
Atlas (C1). **A,** superior view. **B,** inferior view.

midline. This is where the longus colli muscles attach. The pedicles of the axis are quite large. On their inferior surfaces, at the junction of the pedicles and laminae, are the inferior facets that articulate with the superior facets of C3. The inferior axial facets are oriented forward and lateral and, when viewed laterally, are located posterior to the superior axial facets. The laminae of the axis are thick, providing a broad attachment for ligaments, and fused posteriorly to form a stout bifid spinous process.

The third through sixth cervical vertebrae have similar features (Fig 7–3). Typically they have a small vertebral body. Their pedicles project posteriorly and laterally from the midpoint of the vertebral body, while their laminae are directed medially and posteriorly. Their spinous processes are short and bifid. The superior and inferior facets are in the same vertical plane, creating an articular pillar. When viewed laterally, the intervertebral facet joints are oriented approximately 45 degrees from anterosuperior to posteroinferior (Fig 7–4). Laterally, each vertebra displays a transverse process. This process contains the transverse foramen (foramen transversarium), through which the vertebral artery passes.

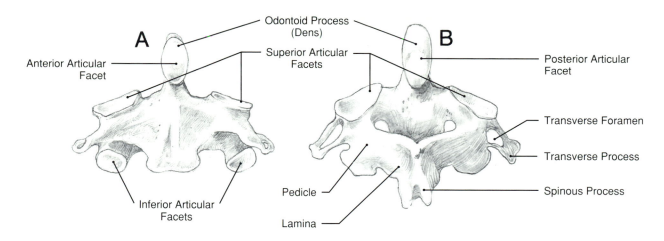

ANTERIOR   POSTERIOR

FIG 7–2.
Axis (C2). **A,** anterior view. **B,** posterior view.

Projections or ridges located on the superolateral margins of the vertebral bodies create the so-called joints of Luschka (Figs 7–3 and 7–5).

The seventh cervical vertebra, like the atlas and unlike the second through sixth vertebrae, does not have a bifid spinous process (Fig 7–6). Instead it has a long and prominent spinous process on which a variety of muscles and ligaments attach. Sometimes the seventh cervical vertebra lacks a transverse foramen on one or both sides. If present, the foramina

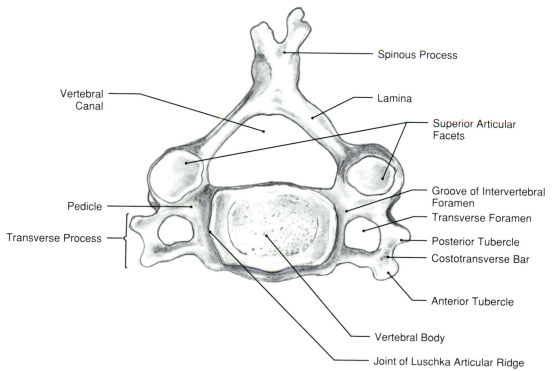

FIG 7–3.
Superior view of fifth cervical vertebra (C5).

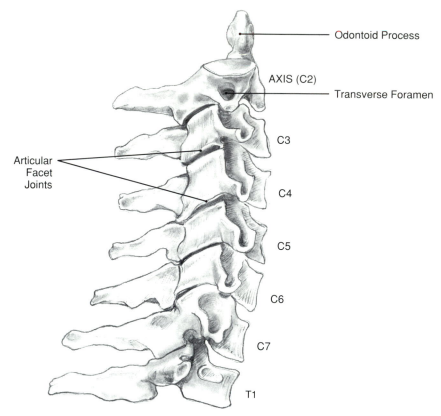

FIG 7–4.
Lateral view of cervical vertebrae (C2-C7) and first thoracic vertebra (T1).

contain only small accessory vertebral veins. The vertebral artery does not pass through the transverse foramen of the seventh cervical vertebra.

Ligaments

A number of ligaments connect the occiput, atlas, and axis. These ligaments provide support and security, yet allow normal movement of the head.

They can be broadly classified as external craniocervical ligaments, which lie outside the vertebral canal, and internal craniocervical ligaments, which lie within the vertebral canal.

External Craniocervical Ligaments

The ligamentum nuchae extends from the external occipital protuberance to the posterior tubercle of the atlas and all other spinous processes of the cervi-

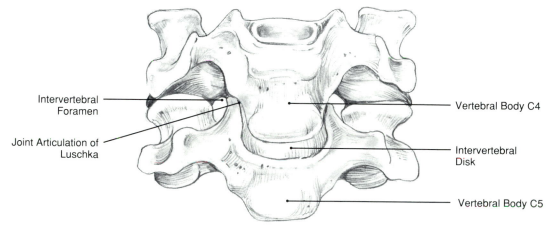

FIG 7–5.
Anterior view of C4-C5 articulation. Note intervertebral foramina and their relationship to the joints of Luschka.

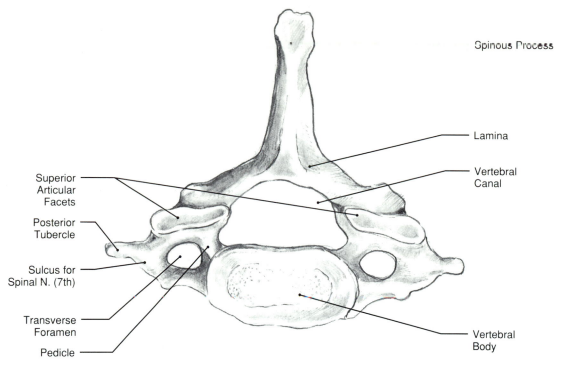

Spinous Process

Lamina

Vertebral Canal

Superior Articular Facets

Posterior Tubercle

Sulcus for Spinal N. (7th)

Transverse Foramen

Pedicle

Vertebral Body

FIG 7–6.
Superior view of seventh cervical vertebra (C7).

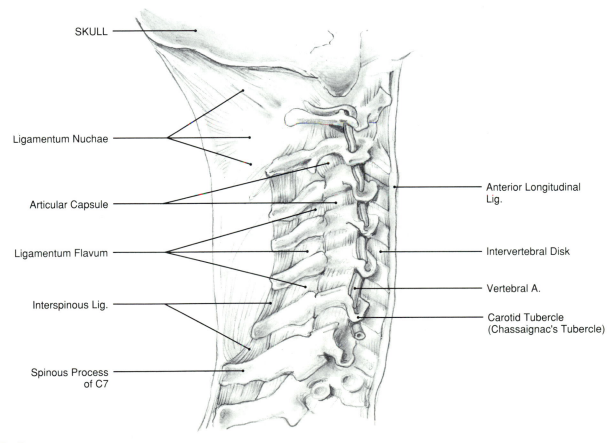

SKULL

Ligamentum Nuchae

Articular Capsule

Ligamentum Flavum

Interspinous Lig.

Spinous Process of C7

Anterior Longitudinal Lig.

Intervertebral Disk

Vertebral A.

Carotid Tubercle (Chassaignac's Tubercle)

FIG 7–7.
Lateral view of cervical spine. Note the vertebral artery entering the transverse foramen of C6 and exiting transverse foramen of C1. Note carotid (Chassaignac's) tubercle.

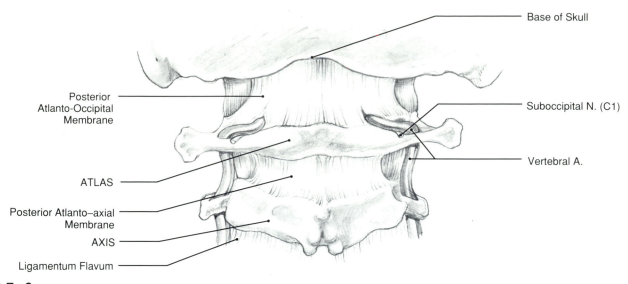

FIG 7–8.
Posterior view of ligaments from base of skull to the axis. Note relationship of the first spinal nerve (suboccipital nerve) to the vertebral artery.

cal vertebrae (Fig 7–7). It is not nearly as well developed in humans as in quadrupeds.

The yellow elastic fibers that connect the laminae of adjacent vertebrae are referred to as ligamentum flavum. Such fibers are not found between the atlas and skull but are present between the arch of the atlas and the lamina of the axis. There are no intervertebral disks between the occiput and atlas or between the atlas and axis.

Wide, dense fibroelastic bands referred to as the anterior atlanto-occipital and posterior atlanto-occipital membranes stretch between the anterior margin of the foramen magnum and the upper border of the anterior arch of the atlas, and the posterior margin of the foramen magnum and the upper border of the posterior arch of the atlas, respectively (Fig 7–8). Although the membrane stretching between the posterior arch of the atlas and the lamina of the axis re-

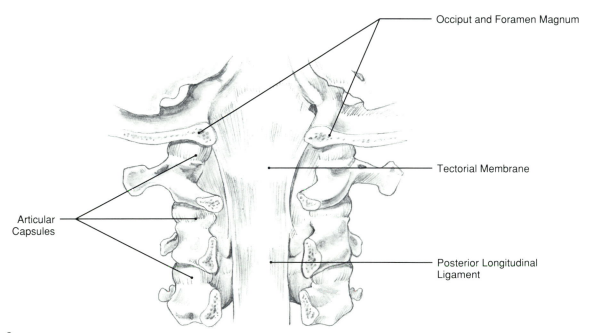

FIG 7–9.
Ligaments on posterior aspect of upper cervical vertebral bodies. The spinous processes, portions of the vertebral arches, and contents of the vertebral canal have been removed.

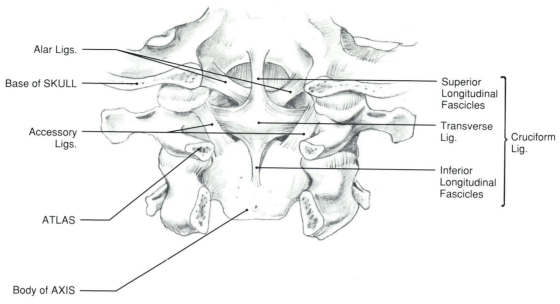

Alar Ligs.

Base of SKULL

Accessory Ligs.

ATLAS

Body of AXIS

Superior Longitudinal Fascicles

Transverse Lig.

Inferior Longitudinal Fascicles

Cruciform Lig.

FIG 7–10.
Deeper, cruciform ligament exposed after removal of the tectorial membrane.

sembles the ligamentum flavum, it is usually referred to as the atlantoaxial membrane. In addition, capsular ligaments surround the joints between the occipital condyles of the skull and the superior atlantal facets, as well as around the atlantoaxial facet articulations.

Internal Craniocervical Ligaments

Several ligaments on the posterior aspects of the vertebral bodies are arranged to prevent excessive movement and provide strength to the articulations. A strong, broad band called the tectorial membrane is a cranial prolongation of the posterior longitudinal ligament. It extends from the posterior surface of the

body of the axis to the anterior edge of the foramen magnum and blends with the cranial dura mater (Fig 7–9). The tectorial membrane lies posterior to and covers the odontoid process and its associated ligaments, providing added protection to the junction between the medulla oblongata and spinal cord.

The important transverse ligament of the atlas passes posterior to the odontoid process and attaches to the tubercles located on the inner side of each lateral mass of the atlas (Figs 7–10 and 7–12). It prevents the odontoid process from moving posteriorly and threatening the spinal cord. From the midpoint of the transverse ligament, fibrous projections extend vertically upward and downward to at-

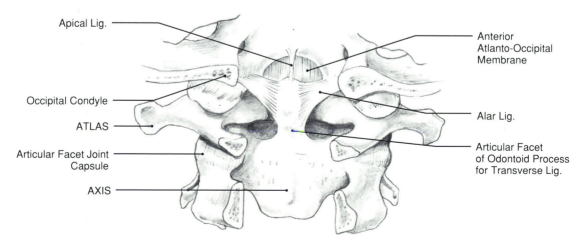

Apical Lig.

Occipital Condyle

ATLAS

Articular Facet Joint Capsule

AXIS

Anterior Atlanto-Occipital Membrane

Alar Lig.

Articular Facet of Odontoid Process for Transverse Lig.

FIG 7–11.
Deepest (alar and apical) ligaments exposed by removal of cruciform ligaments.

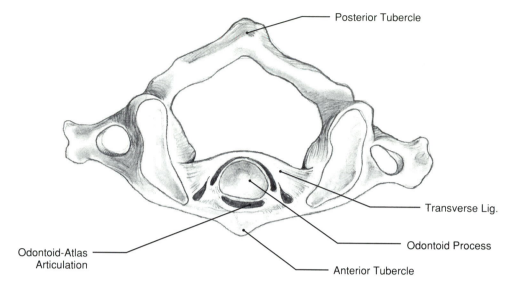

FIG 7–12.
Superior view of the atlas articulating with odontoid process (dens) of the axis. Note transverse ligament.

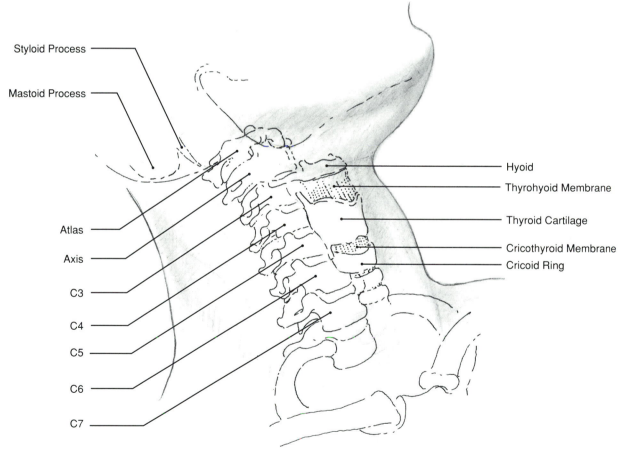

FIG 7–13.
Topographic landmarks of the neck.

tach to the basilar part of the occipital bone and to the posterior surface of the body of the axis, respectively. Together these transverse and vertical bands form the so-called cruciform ligament (see Fig 7–10).

A slender band referred to as the apical ligament connects the very apex of the odontoid to the anterior midpoint of the foramen magnum (Fig 7–11). The alar ligaments are two strong bands that stretch obliquely upward and outward from the superolateral aspect of the odontoid process to the inner sides of the occipital condyles. These ligaments act to check rotation of the occiput-C1 complex on C2. In addition, extensions of the anterior longitudinal ligament, the so-called accessory ligaments, may run from the base of the odontoid to the lateral mass of the atlas.

There are synovial joints composed of the articular facets of the lateral masses of the atlas and the axis. These joints have thin, loose articular capsules.

Topographic Landmarks

The important topographic landmarks of the anterior aspect of the neck include the hyoid bone, thyroid cartilage, and cricoid cartilage (Fig 7–13). These structures lie roughly at the level of the third,

fourth, and sixth cervical vertebrae, respectively. The carotid tubercle (Chassaignac's carotid tubercle) is an enlargement of the anterior tubercle of the transverse process of C6 (see Fig 7–7). It is larger than all the other vertebral tubercles and may be palpable. The carotid artery lies just anterior to this tubercle and can be compressed against it. The important landmarks of the posterior aspect of the neck are the prominent spinous processes of the axis (C2) and the seventh cervical vertebra.

Another important landmark is the sternocleidomastoid muscle, which is prominent and easily identifiable. This muscle has its origin on the mastoid bone of the skull and a dual insertion on the clavicle and manubrium (Fig 7–14). The anterior border of the sternocleidomastoid muscle forms the posterior limb of the anterior cervical triangle, whereas the posterior border of the sternocleidomastoid muscle forms the anterior limb of the posterior cervical triangle.

Muscles and Fascia
Anterior
The key to dissection in the anterior aspect of the neck is the relationship of the fascial layers to

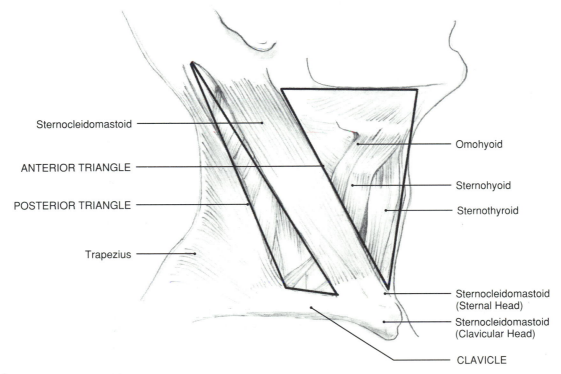

FIG 7–14.
Lateral view of neck. Note prominent sternocleidomastoid muscle. The anterior cervical triangle is bounded by the anteromedian line of the neck, inferior border of the mandible, and anterior border of the sternocleidomastoid muscle. The posterior cervical triangle is bounded anteriorly by the sternocleidomastoid muscle, posteriorly by the anterior border of the trapezius muscle, and inferiorly by the middle third of the clavicle.

the neurovascular structures, trachea, and esophagus (Fig 7–15). The most superficial muscle in the anterior aspect of the neck is the platysma. It extends from the mandible to the thorax and is encased in the superficial fascia of the neck.

Directly beneath the platysma is the so-called investing layer of deep fascia. This fascial layer surrounds the entire neck, ensheathes the sternocleidomastoid and trapezius muscles and external jugular vein, and forms the so-called "roof" of the posterior triangle of the neck. Posteriorly the fascia joins the ligamentum nuchae. The transverse cervical, supraclavicular, lesser occipital, and greater auricular nerves pierce this fascial layer in the posterior triangle of the neck.

The middle cervical and pretracheal fascia lie directly below the deep (investing) fascia. The middle cervical fascia extends from the hyoid bone to the anterior chest wall and ensheathes the strap muscles (sternohyoid, sternothyroid, omohyoid, and thyrohyoid). The pretracheal fascia surrounds the pharynx, larynx, trachea, esophagus, and thyroid gland. At its lateral margin the pretracheal fascia is continuous with the carotid sheath, which contains the common carotid artery, internal jugular vein, deep cervical lymph trunk, and vagus nerve. The superior laryngeal nerve and the superior and inferior thyroid vessels penetrate the pretracheal fascia as they course from the carotid sheath towards the midline. These structures are at risk when the cervical vertebrae are approached anteriorly.

The deepest layer of fascia is referred to as the prevertebral fascia. It is a strong fibrous membrane that covers the prevertebral muscles (longus capitis

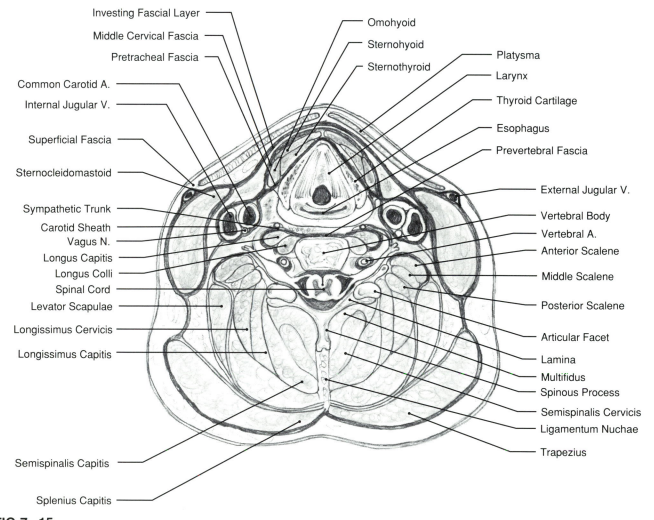

FIG 7–15.
Cross-section of the neck at the level of the thyroid cartilage (C4). Note pretracheal and prevertebral fascia and their relationship to contents of the carotid sheath, trachea, esophagus, and vertebral body.

and longus colli) and the scalene muscles (anterior, middle, and posterior). The vertebral bodies and disks lie beneath these muscles. The cervical sympathetic trunk lies on the surface of the prevertebral fascia. The upper cervical nerves (C1-C4) pierce this fascia to form the cervical plexus, and the lower spinal nerves (C5-T1) emerge between the anterior and middle scalene muscles to form the brachial plexus.

Posterior

The musculature associated with the posterior cervical vertebrae consists of three layers, superficial, intermediate, and deep. In addition to these three layers is a fourth layer associated with the suboccipital region.

The superficial muscle layer (Fig 7–16) is represented by the upper portion of the trapezius muscle, which is encased by the investing layer of deep cervical fascia. The trapezius arises from the superior nuchal line, external occipital protuberance, ligamentum nuchae, spine of the seventh cervical vertebra, and all the thoracic vertebrae and interspinous ligaments. The trapezius inserts on the lateral third of the posterior surface of the clavicle, the medial border of the acromion, and the spine of the scapula.

The second, or intermediate, layer consists of the splenius capitis and cervicis, which are large flat muscles that arise from the midline structures (the caudal half of the ligamentum nuchae, the spine of the seventh cervical vertebra, and the upper three thoracic vertebral spinous processes). They insert

into the lateral aspect of the occipital bone and mastoid process and the transverse processes of vertebrae C1, C2, and C3.

The third, or deep, layer is in turn subdivided into three parts: superficial, middle, and deep (Fig 7–17). The superficial portion is the semispinalis capitis, which lies immediately beneath the splenius capitis. It is a relatively large muscle that takes its origin from the transverse processes of the cervical vertebrae and inserts into the occipital bone. The middle layer is the semispinalis cervicis, which arises from the transverse processes of the upper five or six thoracic vertebrae and inserts into the midline spinous processes four to six segments higher than its origins. The deep component of the deep layer consists of the multifidi and the long and short rotators (transversospinal muscles), which arise from the transverse processes and insert on the spinous processes of the next higher vertebrae.

Suboccipital Triangle and Related Structures.— The cervical region just distal to the occiput is referred to as the suboccipital area (Fig 7–18). There are several vital structures in this region that should be avoided when the area is approached surgically. The muscles found here are the rectus capitis posterior minor, the rectus capitis posterior major, and the superior and inferior oblique muscles of the head. All of these lie directly deep to the semispinalis capitis muscle. The rectus capitis posterior major muscle arises from the spinous process of the axis and the rectus capitis posterior minor from the tu-

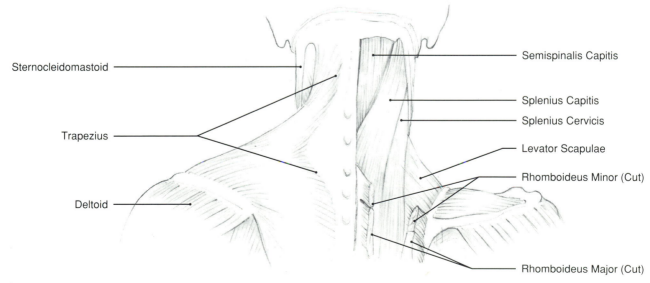

FIG 7–16.
Superficial and intermediate muscle layers of posterior neck and suboccipital region.

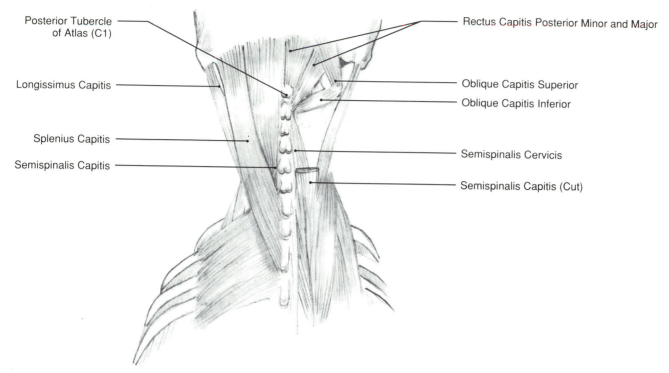

Posterior Tubercle of Atlas (C1)

Longissimus Capitis

Splenius Capitis

Semispinalis Capitis

Rectus Capitis Posterior Minor and Major

Oblique Capitis Superior

Oblique Capitis Inferior

Semispinalis Cervicis

Semispinalis Capitis (Cut)

FIG 7–17.
Deep muscular layer of the posterior neck.

bercles of the posterior arch of the atlas. Both muscles insert into the inferior nuchal line of the occipital bone. The inferior oblique muscle of the head arises from the spinous process of the axis, travels laterally, and ends in the transverse process of the atlas. The superior oblique muscle of the head arises from the transverse process of the atlas and passes cephalad and medial to insert on the occipital bone. All of these suboccipital muscles extend the head and rotate it with the atlas toward the same side.

The suboccipital triangle is an area bounded by the two oblique muscles and the rectus capitis major muscle. The floor of this triangle is formed by the posterior atlanto-occipital membrane. Just deep to this membrane lies the vertebral artery, which passes through a groove on the upper surface of the posterior arch of the atlas and courses medially toward the foramen magnum. The first cervical nerve, the so-called suboccipital nerve (dorsal ramus C1), penetrates the atlanto-occipital membrane between the vertebral artery and the posterior arch of the atlas to innervate the suboccipital muscles. The second cervical nerve, the so-called greater occipital nerve (medial branch of the dorsal ramus of C2), exits below the inferior oblique muscle of the head, turns cranially to cross the suboccipital triangle, and pierces the semispinalis capitis and trapezius to reach the scalp. There it supplies sensation as high as the vertex of the scalp.

Arteries

The arteries of concern when the cervical spine is approached from the anterior aspect are the common carotids and their branches. From the posterior aspect, the vertebral arteries are of concern (Fig 7–19). The right common carotid artery begins at the bifurcation of the brachiocephalic trunk, just craniad to the sternoclavicular joint. The left common carotid begins at the highest part of the arch of the aorta. In the neck the common carotid arteries travel in the carotid sheath along with the internal jugular vein, deep cervical lymph trunk, and vagus nerve. At the upper border of the thyroid cartilage they divide into internal and external carotid arteries. The internal carotid artery has no branches in the neck and ascends to the base of the skull to enter the carotid canal of the temporal bone. The external carotid begins at about the level of the C3-C4 disk space and travels cranially to a point midway between the mastoid process and the angle of the jaw. There it divides into superficial temporal and maxillary arteries. Caudad to the level of the greater cornu of the hyoid bone, the superior thyroid, occip-

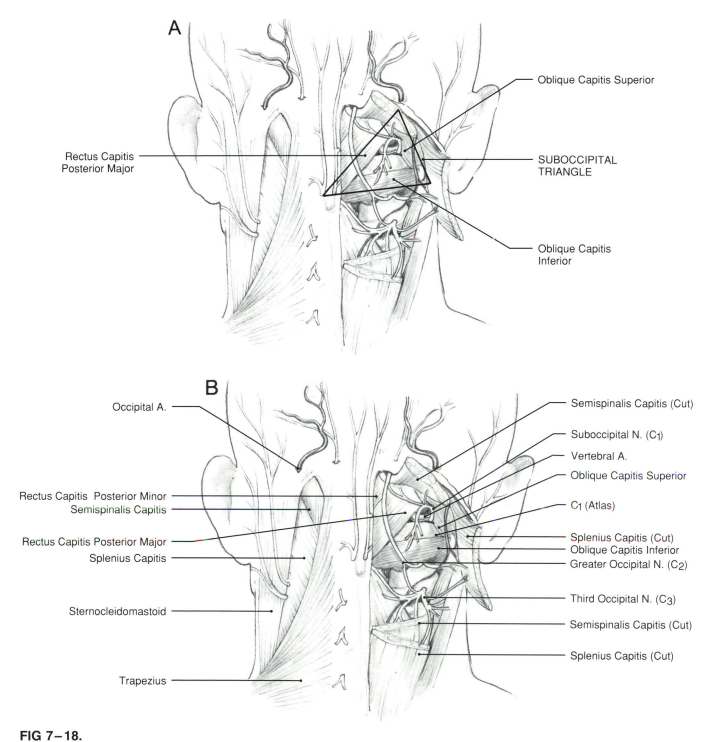

A

Oblique Capitis Superior

Rectus Capitis
Posterior Major

SUBOCCIPITAL
TRIANGLE

Oblique Capitis
Inferior

B

Occipital A.

Semispinalis Capitis (Cut)

Suboccipital N. (C$_1$)

Vertebral A.

Oblique Capitis Superior

Rectus Capitis Posterior Minor
Semispinalis Capitis

C$_1$ (Atlas)

Rectus Capitis Posterior Major
Splenius Capitis

Splenius Capitis (Cut)
Oblique Capitis Inferior
Greater Occipital N. (C$_2$)

Sternocleidomastoid

Third Occipital N. (C$_3$)

Semispinalis Capitis (Cut)

Splenius Capitis (Cut)

Trapezius

FIG 7–18.
A, suboccipital triangle and related structures. **B,** note the relations of the vertebral artery and suboccipital and greater occipital nerves to the triangle.

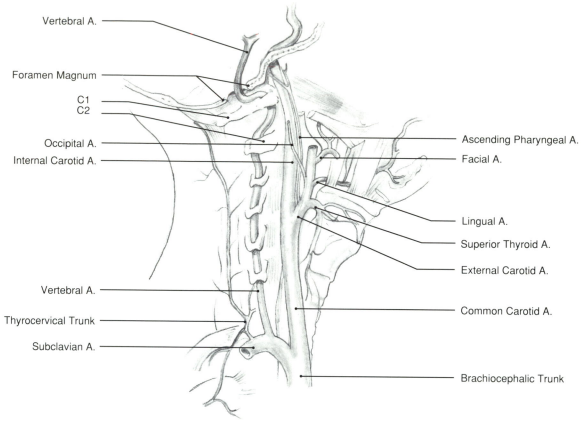

FIG 7–19.
The common, internal, and external carotid and vertebral arteries.

ital, and ascending pharyngeal arteries take origin from the external carotid artery. The lingual artery arises from the external carotid at the level of the greater cornu and the facial artery from just above this level.

Another major artery encountered in the anterior aspect of the neck is the inferior thyroid artery (Fig 7–20). The inferior thyroid artery arises from the subclavian artery close to the medial border of the scalenus anticus muscle as part of the thyrocervical trunk, which also has ascending cervical, transverse cervical, and suprascapular branches. The inferior thyroid artery courses cranially and medially to the lower border of the inferior lobe of the thyroid.

The vertebral arteries are paired arteries that are the first branches of each of the subclavian arteries (see Fig 7–19). They ascend through the transverse foramina of the C1-C6 vertebrae and enter the skull through the foramen magnum. Their relation to the atlas (C1) should be noted: they exit from its transverse foramen and then course posteriorly and medially, lying in the groove of the posterior arch of

the atlas. They enter the foramen magnum by passing forward past the lateral edge of the posterior atlantooccipital membrane and piercing the dura mater. Each vertebral artery forms a loop between the atlas and the base of the skull.

Posteriorly the terminal portion of the occipital artery courses deep to the sternocleidomastoid muscle and travels across the suboccipital triangle to the scalp (see Fig 7–18).

Veins

The external jugular vein commences at the level of the angle of the mandible from the retromandibular and posterior auricular veins. It courses caudally toward the middle of the clavicle (Fig 7–21,A). It crosses the middle of the sternocleidomastoid muscle obliquely and penetrates the deep fascia to drain into the subclavian vein.

The internal jugular vein begins at the base of the skull in the jugular foramen (Fig 7–21,B). It is a direct continuation of the sigmoid sinus. In the neck it travels in the carotid sheath with the carotid artery

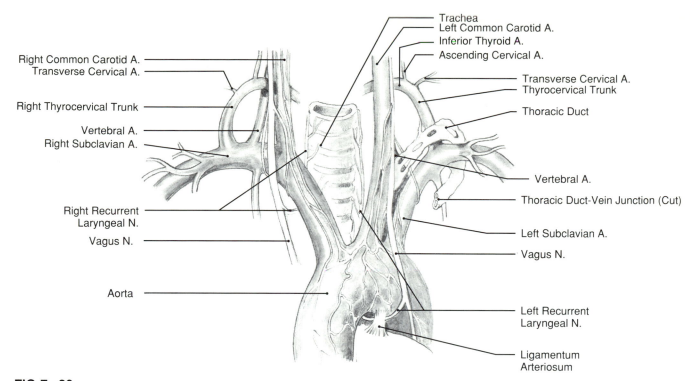

Right Common Carotid A.
Transverse Cervical A.

Right Thyrocervical Trunk

Vertebral A.
Right Subclavian A.

Right Recurrent
Laryngeal N.

Vagus N.

Aorta

Trachea
Left Common Carotid A.
Inferior Thyroid A.
Ascending Cervical A.

Transverse Cervical A.
Thyrocervical Trunk

Thoracic Duct

Vertebral A.

Thoracic Duct-Vein Junction (Cut)

Left Subclavian A.

Vagus N.

Left Recurrent
Laryngeal N.

Ligamentum
Arteriosum

FIG 7–20.
Relationship of arteries, nerves, and the thoracic duct in the anterior inferior neck. Note point at which thoracic duct empties into venous system (veins not shown).

and vagus nerve. It unites with the subclavian vein to form the brachiocephalic vein at the root of the neck. The superior and middle thyroid veins cross the anterior triangle of the neck to join the internal jugular vein. The middle thyroid vein has no arterial counterpart. The inferior thyroid vein arises in the thyroid gland and runs in a caudal direction to join the brachiocephalic vein.

Important vessels of the posterior neck include the occipital veins, deep cervical veins, and the vertebral plexus of veins (Fig 7–21,C).

Thoracic Duct

The thoracic duct is vulnerable to injury when dissection is carried out in the region of the left lower cervical spine. The thoracic duct forms an arch as it passes into the root of the left side of the neck about 3 to 4 cm above the clavicle (see Figs 7–20 and 7–22). As it ascends it passes ventral to the subclavian artery, vertebral artery, and thyrocervical trunk and its branches and dorsal to the common carotid artery, vagus nerve, and internal jugular vein. It ends by curving around the subclavian artery and opening into the venous system at the angle formed

by the junction of the left subclavian and left internal jugular veins.

Nerves

There are eight cervical spinal nerves, each emerging through its respective intervertebral foramen. The first exits the spinal canal between the occiput and atlas (see Fig 7–18). Each cervical nerve exits above the pedicle of its respective vertebral body, with the exception of C8, which exits between C7 and T1. The anterior or ventral rami of the cervical nerves forms the so-called cervical and brachial plexuses. The dorsal rami innervate the deep back muscles and skin. The dorsal ramus of C1 is called the suboccipital nerve. The medial branch of the dorsal ramus of C2 is called the greater occipital nerve. The dorsal ramus of C3 is called the third occipital nerve.

The vagus nerve takes its origin from the medulla oblongata, passes caudally through the jugular foramen, and then travels within the carotid sheath (see Fig 7–20). It enters the thorax posterior to the brachiocephalic vein. It is composed of motor and sensory fibers.

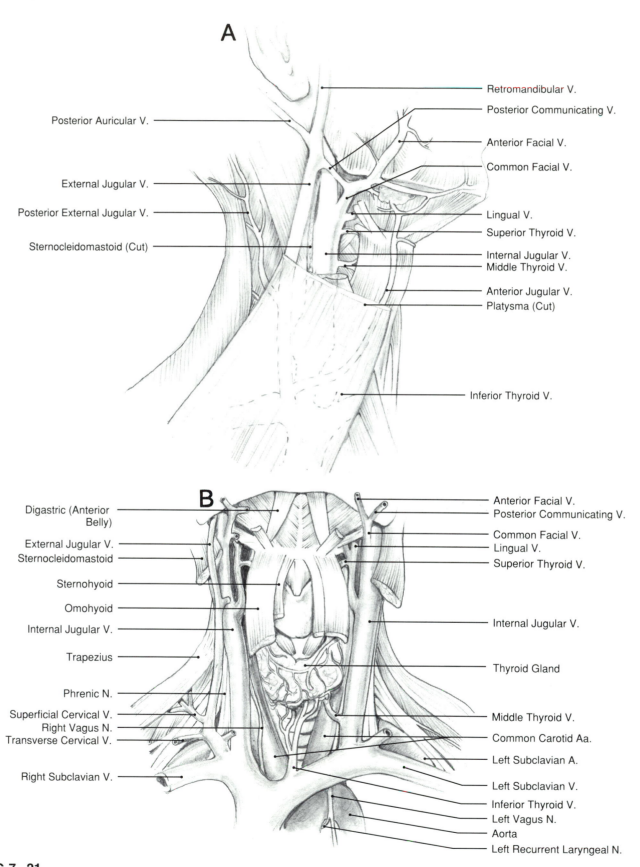

A

Posterior Auricular V.

External Jugular V.

Posterior External Jugular V.

Sternocleidomastoid (Cut)

Retromandibular V.

Posterior Communicating V.

Anterior Facial V.

Common Facial V.

Lingual V.

Superior Thyroid V.

Internal Jugular V.

Middle Thyroid V.

Anterior Jugular V.

Platysma (Cut)

Inferior Thyroid V.

B

Digastric (Anterior Belly)

External Jugular V.

Sternocleidomastoid

Sternohyoid

Omohyoid

Internal Jugular V.

Trapezius

Phrenic N.

Superficial Cervical V.

Right Vagus N.

Transverse Cervical V.

Right Subclavian V.

Anterior Facial V.

Posterior Communicating V.

Common Facial V.

Lingual V.

Superior Thyroid V.

Internal Jugular V.

Thyroid Gland

Middle Thyroid V.

Common Carotid Aa.

Left Subclavian A.

Left Subclavian V.

Inferior Thyroid V.

Left Vagus N.

Aorta

Left Recurrent Laryngeal N.

FIG 7–21.
Veins of the neck. **A,** anterolateral aspect. **B,** root.

(Continued.)

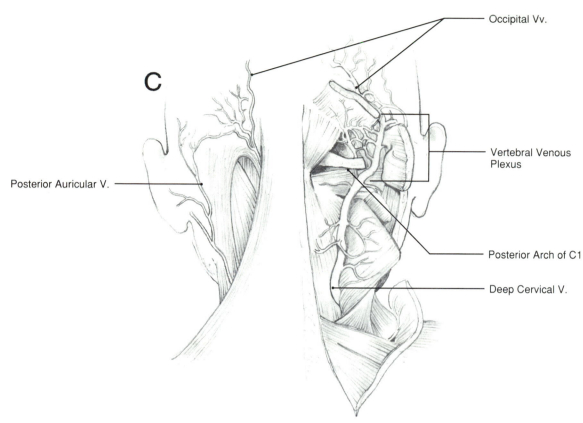

C

Occipital Vv.

Posterior Auricular V.

Vertebral Venous Plexus

Posterior Arch of C1

Deep Cervical V.

FIG 7–21 (cont.).
C, posterior aspect.

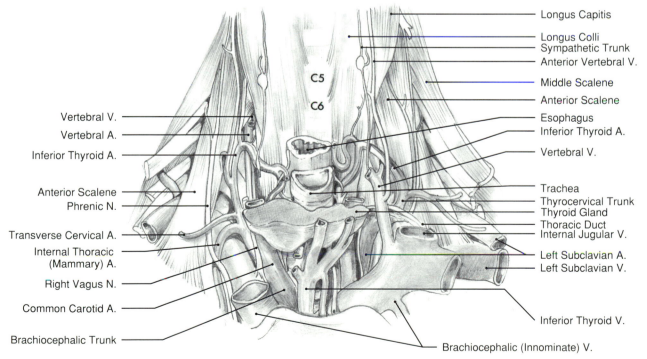

Longus Capitis

Longus Colli
Sympathetic Trunk
Anterior Vertebral V.

Middle Scalene

Anterior Scalene

C5

C6

Esophagus
Inferior Thyroid A.

Vertebral V.
Vertebral A.
Inferior Thyroid A.

Vertebral V.

Trachea
Thyrocervical Trunk
Thyroid Gland
Thoracic Duct
Internal Jugular V.

Anterior Scalene
Phrenic N.

Transverse Cervical A.

Left Subclavian A.
Left Subclavian V.

Internal Thoracic
(Mammary) A.

Right Vagus N.

Common Carotid A.

Inferior Thyroid V.

Brachiocephalic Trunk

Brachiocephalic (Innominate) V.

FIG 7–22.
Anatomical structures in the root of the neck.

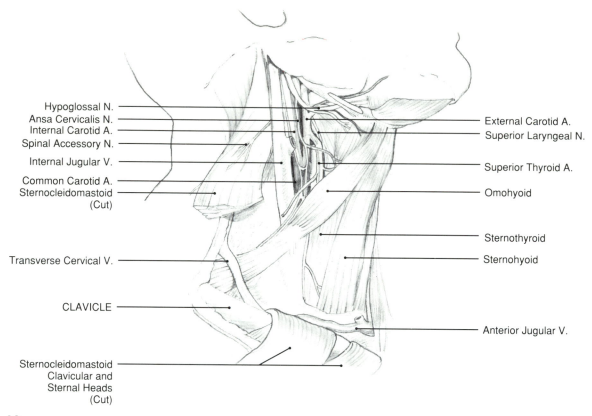

Hypoglossal N.	External Carotid A.
Ansa Cervicalis N.	Superior Laryngeal N.
Internal Carotid A.	
Spinal Accessory N.	
Internal Jugular V.	Superior Thyroid A.
Common Carotid A.	Omohyoid
Sternocleidomastoid (Cut)	
	Sternothyroid
Transverse Cervical V.	Sternohyoid
CLAVICLE	
	Anterior Jugular V.
Sternocleidomastoid Clavicular and Sternal Heads (Cut)	

FIG 7–23.
Superior laryngeal, spinal accessory, and hypoglossal nerves in the anterior triangle.

The superior laryngeal nerve (Fig 7–23) arises from the vagus nerve. It passes obliquely, downward and medially behind and medial to both the internal and external carotid arteries, toward the larynx. The nerve is accompanied in this course by the superior thyroid artery.

The right and left recurrent laryngeal nerves (see Fig 7–20) differ in their origin and anatomic course. On the right, the recurrent laryngeal nerve takes its origin from the vagus anterior to the subclavian artery, then winds beneath and posterior to it. It then ascends obliquely and travels with the inferior thyroid artery. The left recurrent laryngeal nerve takes its origin from the left vagus anterior to the arch of the aorta. It then loops under the aorta just lateral to the ligamentum arteriosum and enters the plane between the trachea and esophagus.

In the anterior triangle of the neck the spinal accessory and hypoglossal nerves may be encountered (see Fig 7–23). The spinal accessory nerve is composed of cranial and spinal portions. Actually the cranial roots travel with it for only a short distance before they join the vagus nerve. The spinal roots originate as far caudal as the fifth cervical vertebra.

The spinal portion of the accessory nerve ascends cranially behind the dorsal roots of the spinal nerves and enters the foramen magnum with the vertebral artery. It then travels laterally within the cranium to the jugular foramen, where it exits the skull and passes caudally and laterally to enter the sternocleidomastoid muscle. It then emerges at the posterior margin of the sternocleidomastoid muscle and traverses the posterior triangle of the neck to reach the deep surface of the trapezius muscle.

The hypoglossal nerve is the motor nerve to the tongue. It travels through the hypoglossal canal in the occipital bone and descends between the internal jugular vein and internal carotid artery until it reaches the angle of the jaw, where it courses anteriorly to enter the tongue.

The ansa cervicalis is a nerve loop from the cervical plexus in the anterolateral aspect of the neck. It is attached anteriorly and superiorly to the hypoglossal nerve and originates from the anterior ramus of the first cervical spinal nerve. Posteriorly the nerve loop arises from the second and third cervical nerves and innervates the strap muscles.

SURGICAL APPROACHES
TO THE CERVICAL SPINE

Transoral Approach

Fang and Ong have advocated a direct transoral approach to C1 and C2 as well as the inferior portion of the clivus (the bony surface of the cranial fossa that slopes upward from the foramen magnum to the dorsum sellae). Because of the association of postoperative infections with the transoral approach, it should be reserved for anterior decompression and/or biopsy of the region of the occipital-cervical junction.

The patient is positioned supine on the operating table with the head slightly extended (Fig 7–24). After endotracheal anesthesia is established a tracheostomy is performed. The endotracheal tube is removed and anesthesia continued through a short cuffed tube inserted through the tracheostomy. A three-ring retractor is then inserted. This will allow for retraction of the uvula and tongue while the mouth is held open. The uvula may be further retracted superiorly by placement of a rubber catheter through the nostrils and out the mouth. Alternatively, the soft palate may be folded back on itself and temporarily sutured to its junction with the hard palate. Radiographic confirmation of the level of dissection is then obtained. The oral pharynx is cultured and prepared with antiseptic. The posterior pharyngeal tissue area is injected with lidocaine and epinephrine to aid hemostasis. After palpation and radiographic confirmation of the ring of C1, a vertical incision is made from approximately 1 cm cephalad to the tip of the odontoid to 2 cm distal to the anterior tubercle of the ring of C1. The four layers (posterior pharyngeal mucosa, superior constrictor muscles of the pharynx, prevertebral fascia, and anterior longitudinal ligament) are incised directly down to bone. The soft tissues are dissected off the odontoid and off the ring of C1. These soft tissues may be stripped and retracted as far laterally as the lateral masses of C1 and C2 and anchored with stay sutures. Biopsy or decompression can then be carried out. The wound is closed in layers with absorbable suture material.

Anterolateral Approach

The anterolateral approach can be used for exposure of the first and second cervical vertebrae; biopsy; tumor, infection, or odontoid resection; and fusion of the first through third cervical vertebrae.

Henry originally described this approach as a means of access to the vertebral arteries. Whitesides and Kelly have advocated its use for treatment of patients with instability, particularly in the C1-C2 area. This approach allows access without sacrificing the branches of the external carotid artery or injuring the hypoglossal and/or laryngeal nerves. The plane of dissection is anterior and medial to the sternocleidomastoid muscle but lateral and posterior to the carotid sheath.

Before the procedure is begun, spinal stability is considered and the need for skeletal traction determined. Nasotracheal intubation or tracheostomy is preferred to orotracheal intubation, because the latter may limit exposure by the position of the jaw. A bolster is placed between the scapulae to create slight cervical extension. Skin preparation should include the entire outer surface of the ear. The earlobe is then sutured to the cheek (Fig 7–25). A hockey-stick incision is begun under the mastoid process. It proceeds in a transverse direction and turns caudally along the anterior margin of the sternocleidomastoid muscle. The sternocleidomastoid and the posterior belly of the digastric muscle are divided near their origins on the mastoid, with fascial remnants left for reattachment. The spinal accessory nerve is identified as it enters the sternocleidomastoid muscle. It should be remembered that the spinal accessory nerve exits the skull through the jugular foramen, medial to the jugular bulb, and courses laterally to reach the deep surface of the sternocleidomastoid muscle approximately 3 cm caudal to the muscle's origin. Dissection of this nerve from the internal jugular vein will allow its mobilization; however, the relationship of the nerve and vein is variable. In two thirds of individuals the nerve descends superficial to the internal jugular vein and in one third it courses deep to the vein.

The middle layer of the deep cervical fascia is now encountered. This fascia is incised lateral to and parallel with the carotid sheath. This allows medial retraction of the carotid sheath and its enclosed structures. The vagus nerve enters the carotid sheath cranial to C2 and can usually be retracted medially with the sheath. If it appears to be a direct tether to medial retraction, it can be dissected distally from the sheath. The hypoglossal nerve may be exposed and is easily retracted medially. The transected sternocleidomastoid muscle with the accompanying accessory nerve is then retracted laterally to allow palpation of the upper cervical vertebrae. The retropharyngeal space is developed by blunt finger dissection. The prevertebral layer of cer-

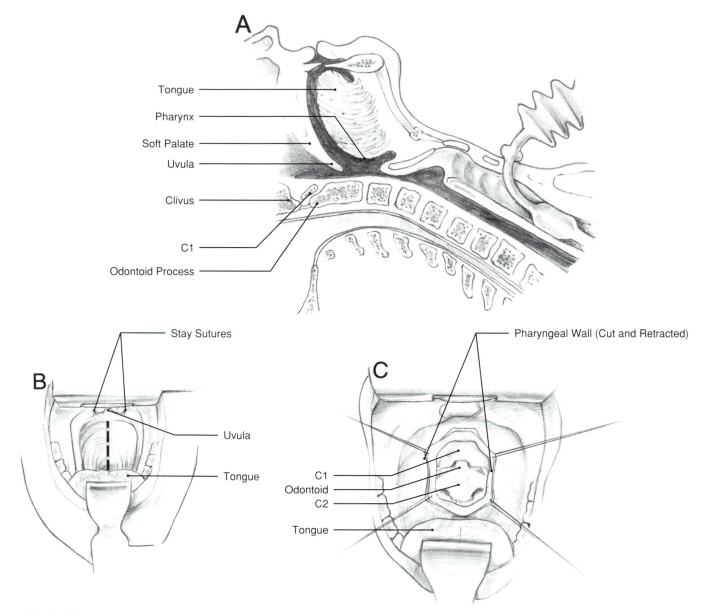

FIG 7–24.
Transoral approach. **A,** relationship of the posterior pharynx and bony structures of the craniocervical junction. Note anesthetic is administered via tracheostomy. **B,** incision on posterior pharyngeal wall *(dashed line)*. The soft palate has been folded on itself and secured with two stay sutures. **C,** cut edge of the posterior pharyngeal wall retracted, to expose C1, odontoid, and body of C2. (Drawn after Fang HSY, Ong GB: Direct anterior approach to the upper cervical spine. *J Bone Joint Surg* 1962; 44A:1588–1604.)

vical fascia is encountered and incised in a longitudinal direction. The longus colli and longus capitis muscles with the overlying sympathetic chain are visualized. With care taken to avoid injury to the sympathetic chain, the longus colli and longus capitis muscles are dissected off the cervical vertebra. The anterior longitudinal ligament is then incised and subperiosteally dissected off the underlying vertebral body. Radiographic confirmation of the level of

exposure is necessary before the desired surgical procedure is carried out. Closed suction drainage is established before wound closure.

Anterior Approach

The anterior vertebral bodies of C3-T1 can best be exposed through an anteromedial approach to carry out procedures such as biopsy of the vertebral

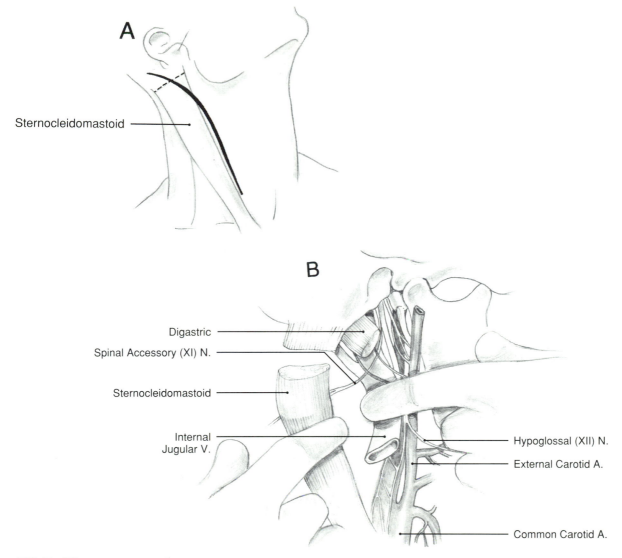

Sternocleidomastoid

Digastric
Spinal Accessory (XI) N.

Sternocleidomastoid

Internal
Jugular V.

Hypoglossal (XII) N.

External Carotid A.

Common Carotid A.

FIG 7–25.
Anterolateral approach to right side of neck. **A,** hockey-stick skin incision along anterior border of sternocleidomastoid muscle. *Dashed line* indicates resection site of sternocleidomastoid. (Note earlobe retracted by suturing to cheek.) **B,** blunt finger dissection of the craniocervical junction region. Note that the sectioned sternocleidomastoid muscle and the spinal accessory nerve are retracted laterally and the internal jugular vein, carotid artery and branches, and hypoglossal and vagus nerves are retracted medially.
(Continued.)

bodies or disk spaces, removal of herniated disks, drainage of abscesses, foraminal decompression, excision of tumor, and interbody fusion. The underlying principle is that dissection can be safely carried out by retraction of the vital structures in the carotid sheath (carotid artery, internal jugular vein, and vagus nerve) laterally and the esophagus and trachea medially.

The patient is placed supine on the operating table with a bolster between the scapulae. If neck stability is in question, cervical tongs or halo traction can be maintained. If there is no stability problem,

the head is placed in slight extension and rotated to the side opposite to that being exposed. Exposure can be made from either side, but the right recurrent laryngeal nerve is more vulnerable to injury than the left. This is because the right recurrent laryngeal nerve arises from the vagus in the root of the neck and runs cranially toward the larynx, crossing over from lateral to medial in the lower part of the neck to reach the midline of the trachea. The left recurrent laryngeal nerve arises from the vagus in the thorax, loops under the aortic arch, and ascends in the neck between the trachea and esophagus. Be-

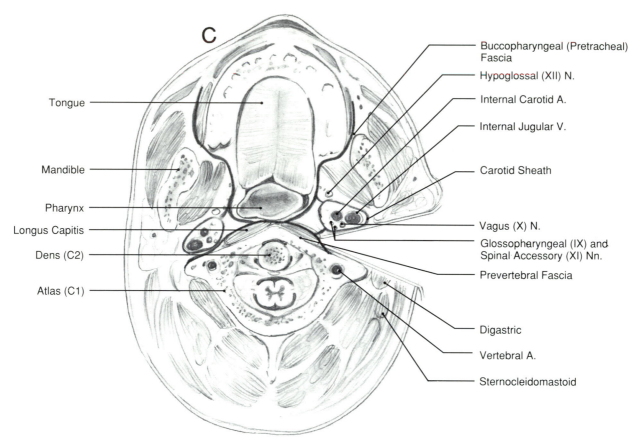

FIG 7–25 (cont.).
C, cross section (viewed from proximal to distal) at C1-C2 level showing plane of dissection anterior and medial to the sternocleidomastoid muscle but lateral and posterior to the carotid sheath. (Modified and adapted from Henry AK: *Extensile Exposure*, ed 2. Edinburgh, E & S Livingston, 1957; Watkins RG: *Surgical Approaches to the Spine.* New York, Springer-Verlag, 1983; and Whitesides TE Jr, Kelly RP: Lateral approach to the upper cervical spine for anterior fusion. *South Med J* 1966; 59:879–883.)

cause of this anatomic arrangement of the recurrent laryngeal nerves, some surgeons always approach this portion of the cervical spine from the left. Other surgeons approach from either side, depending on the location of the pathologic process.

The topographical landmark is the medial border of the sternocleidomastoid muscle. The skin incision is placed transversely, centered over the medial border of the sternocleidomastoid muscle (Fig 7–26). Depending upon the intended level of exposure, the incision is placed at the level of the hyoid bone, thyroid cartilage, or cricoid cartilage, which correspond to the C3, C4, and C6 cervical vertebrae, respectively. Alternatively, the distance from the clavicle to the intended level can be measured on an anteroposterior radiograph of the cervical spine and the incision made that same distance on the patient. If several vertebral bodies are to be exposed, an ob-

lique incision in line with the anteromedial edge of the sternocleidomastoid may be preferable.

Once the skin incision has been made, the platysma muscle is identified and divided in line with its muscle fibers or the skin incision. The platysma is dissected off the investing layer of deep cervical fascia. The investing and middle layers of cervical fascia are incised parallel to the medial edge of the sternocleidomastoid muscle. This usually requires sectioning of transversely crossing cervical veins and superficial transverse cervical nerves. The sternocleidomastoid muscle is retracted laterally and the strap muscles medially. The pretracheal layer of the deep cervical fascia is identified. The omohyoid muscle passes proximal and medial to posterolateral at the level of C6-C7. It may be retracted or require resection and subsequent repair. The pretracheal layer of the deep cervical fascia, which fuses with the carotid sheath, is incised just medial to the carotid sheath. With finger dissection, the exposure is expanded and spread. The middle thyroid vein, which is inconstant but sometimes encountered at the C5 level, must be ligated and divided. Dissection above C4 will be limited by the superior thyroid, lingual, and facial arteries, which may be ligated to increase exposure. Also limiting cranial dissection are the superior laryngeal and hypoglossal nerves, which must be protected.

The sternocleidomastoid muscle and carotid sheath, with its contents, are retracted laterally. The strap muscles, trachea, and esophagus are retracted medially. Prior placement of a nasogastric tube will help identify the esophagus. The recurrent laryngeal nerves lie between the esophagus and trachea. To prevent injury to the laryngeal nerves, care must be taken in retracting these structures not to insert the retractor tip in the interval between them. The prevertebral layer of cervical fascia is now encountered. The prevertebral fascia is incised in a longitudinal direction in the midline. With a periosteal elevator, the longus colli muscle is dissected off the vertebral body and anterior longitudinal ligament, which lie just beneath it. There is a rich vascular bed intimately related to the longus colli muscle. Electrocauterization may be required to obtain hemostasis. The sympathetic chain lies on the longus colli, just lateral

to the vertebral bodies. Injury to the sympathetic chain may result in a Horner's syndrome. If dissection is carried out laterally as far as the transverse processes, the vertebral artery will be in jeopardy.

During wound closure the omohyoid muscle and platysma muscle are repaired. Closed suction drainage is established.

Anterior Approach to the Cervical-Thoracic Junction

The cervical-thoracic junction is a difficult anatomical region to approach surgically because it represents the apex of two physiological curvatures of the spine, and the thoracic inlet is crowded with important vascular structures that can be easily injured. However, it can be approached anteriorly to carry out biopsies; excisions of tumors or infections; decompression of the spinal cord for neoplastic, infectious, or traumatic lesions; decompression of herniated nucleus pulposus from C7 to T2; or for fusion procedures of the cervical-thoracic junction. An anterior approach will also allow for internal fixation by either cervical plating or insertion of methylmethacrylate with wire mesh for vertebral body replacement.

Few authors have described methods of approaching this region. We prefer a transsternal ap-

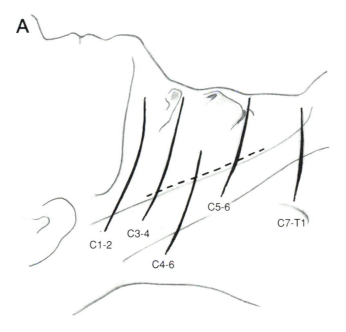

FIG 7–26.
Anterior approach. **A,** skin incision is placed in a slightly oblique transverse direction, in line with the skin folds and centered over the medial border of the sternocleidomastoid at the level of the intended exposure *(solid lines)*. Alternatively, a longitudinal oblique incision can be made along the anteromedial edge of the sternocleidomastoid muscle *(dashed line)*.

(Continued.)

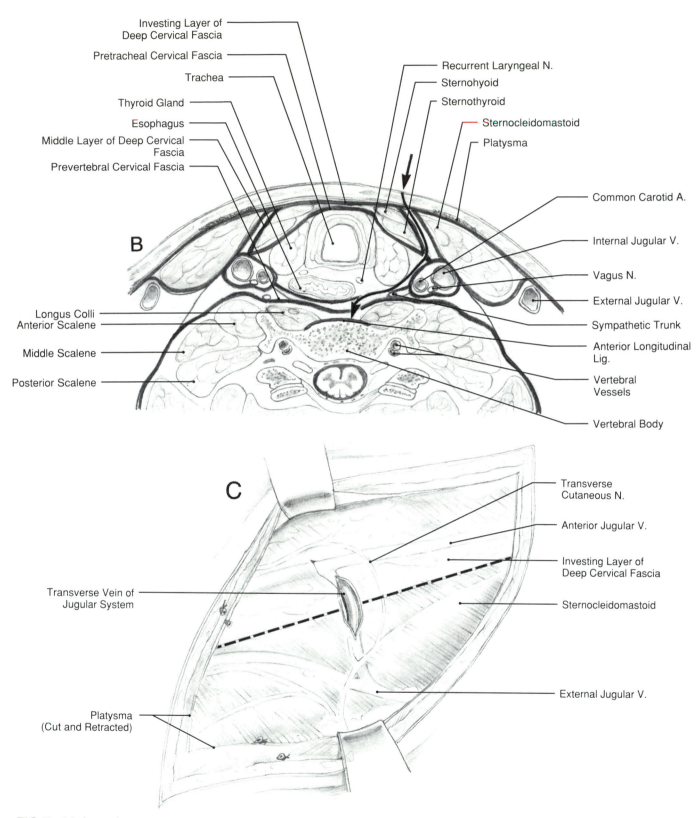

Investing Layer of
Deep Cervical Fascia

Pretracheal Cervical Fascia

Trachea

Thyroid Gland

Esophagus

Middle Layer of Deep Cervical
Fascia

Prevertebral Cervical Fascia

Recurrent Laryngeal N.

Sternohyoid

Sternothyroid

Sternocleidomastoid

Platysma

Common Carotid A.

Internal Jugular V.

Vagus N.

External Jugular V.

Sympathetic Trunk

Anterior Longitudinal
Lig.

Vertebral
Vessels

Vertebral Body

B

Longus Colli
Anterior Scalene

Middle Scalene

Posterior Scalene

C

Transverse
Cutaneous N.

Anterior Jugular V.

Investing Layer of
Deep Cervical Fascia

Sternocleidomastoid

Transverse Vein of
Jugular System

External Jugular V.

Platysma
(Cut and Retracted)

FIG 7–26 (cont.).
B, cross section of midcervical area. Dissection plane *(arrows)* between the sternocleidomastoid laterally and strap muscles medially with retraction of the structures of the carotid sheath laterally and the trachea and esophagus medially allows safe exposure to the bodies of the cervical vertebrae and disks. **C,** platysma has been incised and reflected. Transverse veins exposed for ligation as necessary. *Dashed line* indicates transection of the outer investing layer of deep cervical fascia parallel to the anterior border of the sternocleidomastoid.

(Continued.)

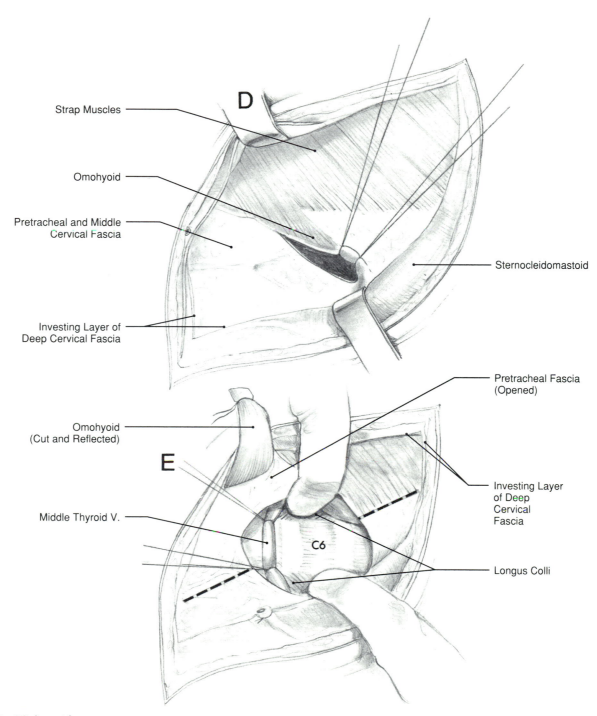

Strap Muscles

Omohyoid

Pretracheal and Middle
Cervical Fascia

Investing Layer of
Deep Cervical Fascia

Sternocleidomastoid

Omohyoid
(Cut and Reflected)

Middle Thyroid V.

C6

Pretracheal Fascia
(Opened)

Investing Layer
of Deep
Cervical
Fascia

Longus Colli

FIG 7–26 (cont.).
D, in the lower portion of the neck in the region of C6-C7 the omohyoid muscle crosses the operative field. Retraction and/or division may be required. **E,** the exposure is expanded and spread by finger dissection. The middle thyroid vein, which is inconstant but sometimes encountered at the level of C5, must be ligated and divided. *(Continued.)*

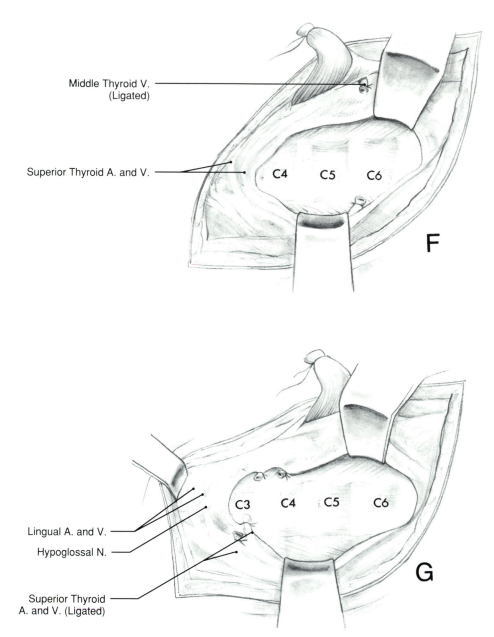

Middle Thyroid V.
(Ligated)

Superior Thyroid A. and V.

C4　C5　C6

F

Lingual A. and V.

Hypoglossal N.

Superior Thyroid
A. and V. (Ligated)

C3　C4　C5　C6

G

FIG 7–26 (cont.).
F, exposure of C4 to C6. Note superior thyroid vessels underlying fascia in cranial portion of wound. **G,** if more cranial exposure is desired with this approach, transection and ligation of the superior thyroid, lingual, and facial arteries may be required. The superior laryngeal and hypoglossal nerves will be encountered in this region and must be preserved.

(Continued.)

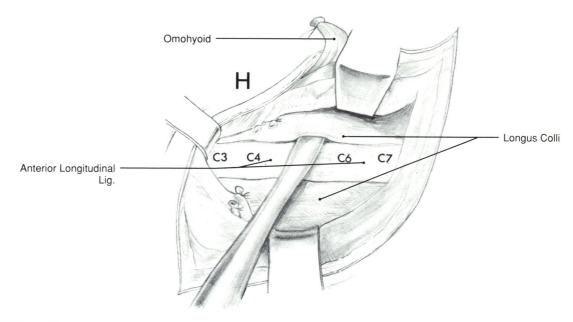

Omohyoid

H

Anterior Longitudinal
Lig.

C3 C4 C6 C7

Longus Colli

FIG 7–26 (cont.).
H, prevertebral cervical fascia has been divided, exposing longus colli and anterior longitudinal ligament. Subperiosteal dissection of the ligament and muscle exposes the vertebral bodies and disk spaces. (Modified from Bauer R, Kerschbaumer F, Poisel S: *Operative Approaches in Orthopedic Surgery and Traumatology.* New York, Thieme Medical Publishers Inc, 1987.)

proach as described by Sundaresan, Shah, and Feghall. Spinal stability must be evaluated and instability managed as previously described. A bolster is placed between the scapulae to facilitate exposure. The skin preparation includes the neck and proximal thorax. A T-shaped incision is used (Fig 7–27). The transverse part of the T is placed 1 cm above the sternoclavicular joint. It extends from the lateral border of the sternocleidomastoid muscle on one side to the lateral border of the sternocleidomastoid muscle on the other side. The longitudinal part of the incision is centered over the sternum. The sternocleidomastoid muscle insertion and pectoralis major muscle origins are detached subperiosteally from the medial one third of the clavicle and from the manubrium on the preferred side. In a similar fashion the insertions of the sternohyoid and sternothyroid muscles are subperiosteally dissected off the deep surface of the manubrium. Now free of muscular attachments, the medial one third of the clavicle is removed. A rectangular section of the superficial cortex and medulla of the manubrium is removed with a high-speed burr and rongeurs. Forty-five-degree-angle Kerrison rongeurs can then be used to remove the deep cortex of the manubrium subperiosteally, leaving the underlying periosteum to protect the mediastinal structures until careful separation and removal of the periosteum can be carried out. An avascular plane medial to the carotid sheath and lat-

eral to the trachea and esophagus is developed. The inferior thyroid vein is doubly ligated and sectioned. The thymus and surrounding fat are bluntly dissected free as necessary. If dissection is done on the left side of the neck, the left recurrent laryngeal nerve should be identified and gently retracted with the esophagus and trachea. As dissection is carried into the mediastinum, the subclavian arteries and veins and aortic arch can be retracted gently in a caudal direction. The prevertebral layer of fascia is then incised in a longitudinal direction. Gentle dissection removes the longus colli muscle from the underlying anterior longitudinal ligament and vertebral bodies. The anterior longitudinal ligament is incised longitudinally and the vertebral bodies and disk spaces exposed by subperiosteal dissection. This exposure can be used to deal with lesions from C7 to T2. If more distal exposure is desired, the manubrium and body of the sternum can be bisected and retracted, allowing visualization to T3-T4.

During wound closure, the sternocleidomastoid muscle insertion and pectoralis major origins are attached to the remaining periosteum of the clavicle and manubrium with nonabsorbable suture. The wound is drained by closed suction.

Along with those problems which may occur with the anterior approach to the midcervical spine, approaches to the cervical-thoracic junction may precipitate additional complications. Care must be

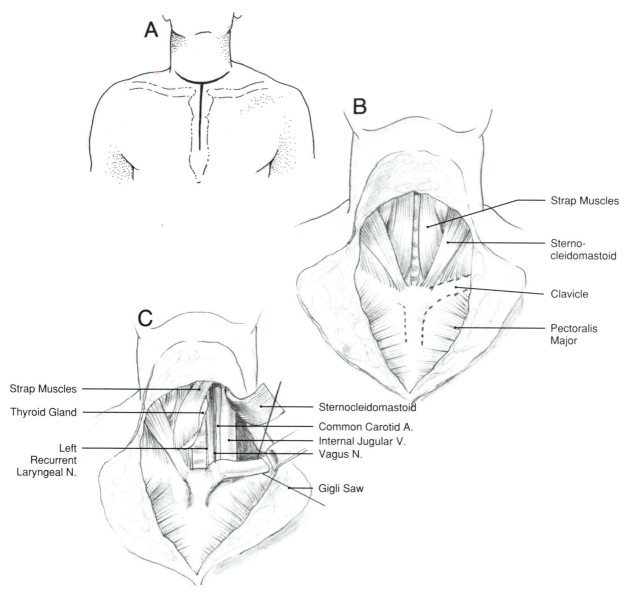

FIG 7–27.
Anterior approach to the cervical-thoracic junction. **A,** skin incision. **B,** skin flaps are developed, and strap muscles, sternoclei-domastoid, and pectoralis muscles are exposed. *Dashed lines* indicate where muscles are resected from clavicle and manu-brium. **C,** the carotid sheath, trachea and esophagus, manubrium, and medial clavicle are exposed by retraction of the strap muscles, sternocleidomastoid, and pectoralis major. Note Gigli saw positioned to resect clavicle.   *(Continued.)*

taken to avoid injury to the aorta and subclavian or carotid artery; subclavian, jugular, or innominate vein and superior vena cava; or inferior portion of the brachial plexus. Pneumothorax and hemothorax must also be avoided.

Posterior Approach

The posterior approach to the cervical spine is commonly used to provide safe access for excision of herniated disks, nerve root exploration, treatment of

facet joint dislocations, and posterior cervical spine fusions. Through this approach spinal stability can be achieved easily and safely. However, the approach is a poor choice for removing lesions that compress the spinal cord from an anterior direction, such as may occur with vertebral body fractures, certain neoplasms, and infectious processes.

The patient is intubated with great care, especially if the spine is unstable due to trauma or rheumatoid arthritis. Nasotracheal intubation or tracheostomy should be considered if the cervical spine is

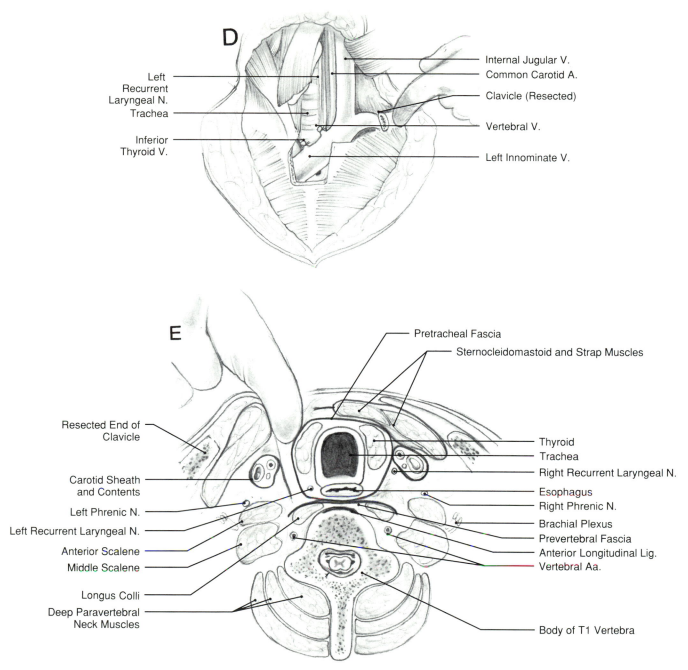

FIG 7–27 (cont.).
D, the medial third of the left clavicle and a portion of the manubrium are removed. Branches of the innominate artery and vein are ligated. **E,** cross section at level of cervical-thoracic junction, viewed from cranial to caudal. *(Continued.)*

markedly unstable. Once the patient is intubated, anesthesia is induced. The patient is then logrolled to the proper position on either the operating table or a Stryker frame. The head must be controlled at all times to prevent unwanted motion. If the head holder is to be used it is attached to the operating table. Lateral cervical spine radiographs are then ob-

tained to check for cervical alignment. The length and location of the midline posterior approach are determined, keeping in mind that the posterior processes of C2 and C7 are most prominent. Infiltration of the skin with 1:200,000 to 1:500,000 epinephrine will aid in hemostasis.

A skin incision of the desired length is placed in

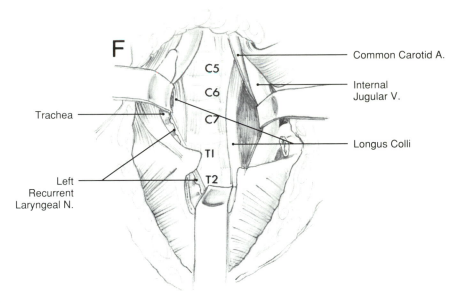

FIG 7–27 (cont.).
F, the carotid sheath with its contents is retracted laterally, the trachea and esophagus and left recurrent laryngeal nerve are retracted medially, and the aorta and innominate artery and vein are gently retracted distally. This exposes the prevertebral fascia of the lower three cervical and upper two thoracic vertebrae. (Modified from Sundaresan N, Shah J, Feghall JG: A transsternal approach to the upper thoracic vertebrae. *Am J Surg* 1984; 148:473–477.)

the midline and the skin edges retracted (Fig 7–28). With use of electrocautery an incision is made into the nuchal fascia, staying in the midline. The trapezius muscle, which is confluent with the nuchal fascia, is mobilized bilaterally and retracted. The ligamentum nuchae is incised in the midline down to the tips of the spinous processes. The deep muscle layer is dissected off the spinous processes subperiosteally.

If the more cranial portion of the cervical spine is to be exposed, the insertions of the rectus capitis posterior major and oblique capitis inferior muscles from the C2 spinous processes are resected, with care taken to avoid injury to the greater occipital nerve, suboccipital nerve, and more importantly, the vertebral artery. When the posterior arch of C1 is exposed the dissection must not extend more than 1.5 cm from the midline and should be maintained in the subperiosteal plane. At the same time it is important to avoid unnecessary force on the posterior arch of C1, as it may be rather mobile and weak, especially in patients with rheumatoid arthritis.

If exposure to the posterior occiput is desired, sharp dissection is used to expose the external occipital protuberance. The dissection is carried laterally subperiosteally. If fixation of the occiput is required, two small drill holes are placed 5 to 7 mm from the foramen magnum and 5 to 7 mm from the midline. The posterior atlanto-occipital ligament is then dis-

sected off the posterior lip of the foramen magnum. Meticulous technique is used to separate the dura from the inner table of the posterior occipital bone. Fixation wires can then be passed through the drill holes caudally, exiting through the foramen magnum.

The goal may be to achieve fixation of C1-C2. In this case, the superficial exposure is carried out as described above, with proximal muscles dissected off the posterior elements in a subperiosteal plane. The dissection must not be extended laterally more than 1.5 cm on the posterior arch of C1. The medial aspect of the C2-C3 facet joint is exposed by lateral dissection. The atlantoaxial ligament between C1 and C2 and the ligamentum flavum between C2 and C3 are removed. The dura is separated from the undersurface of the lamina. Sublaminar wires may then be passed, with great care taken not to injure the dura or subdural structures. Fusion then can be carried out in either a Gallie- or Brooks-type technique.

Magerl has described a method of fusing C1-C2 by transarticular screw fixation, which can be accomplished even if there is a defect in the posterior ring of C1. This is carried out through a posterior approach with exposure from the occiput to C7. The facet joints of C1-C2 are opened. Approximately 5 mm of the inferior articular processes of C1 is exposed, and Kirschner wires are driven into the pro-

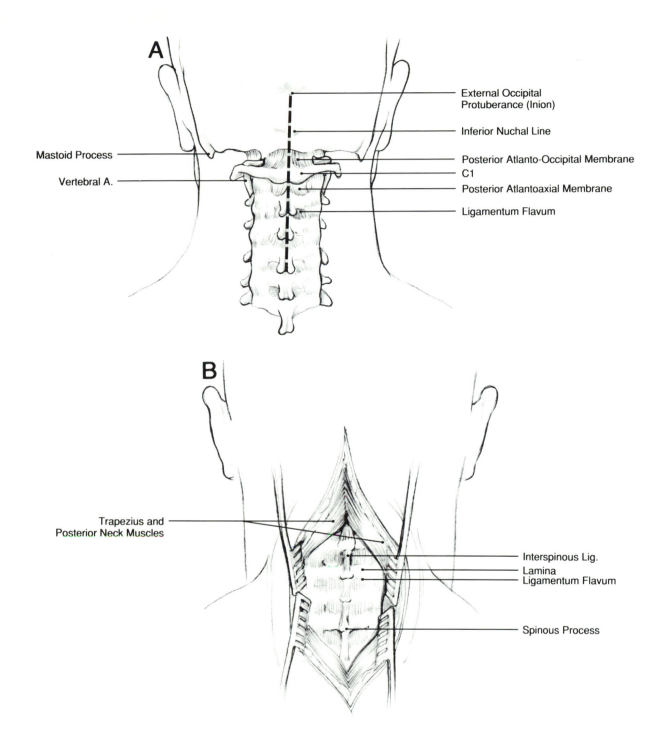

A

External Occipital
Protuberance (Inion)

Inferior Nuchal Line

Mastoid Process

Posterior Atlanto-Occipital Membrane

C1

Vertebral A.

Posterior Atlantoaxial Membrane

Ligamentum Flavum

B

Trapezius and
Posterior Neck Muscles

Interspinous Lig.
Lamina
Ligamentum Flavum

Spinous Process

FIG 7–28.
Posterior approach. **A,** midline skin incision may extend from the external occipital protuberance (inion) as far distally as required. **B,** the ligamentum nuchae has been incised in the midline and retracted with the trapezius and paracervical muscles, which have been dissected off the spinous processes and laminae subperiosteally.   *(Continued.)*

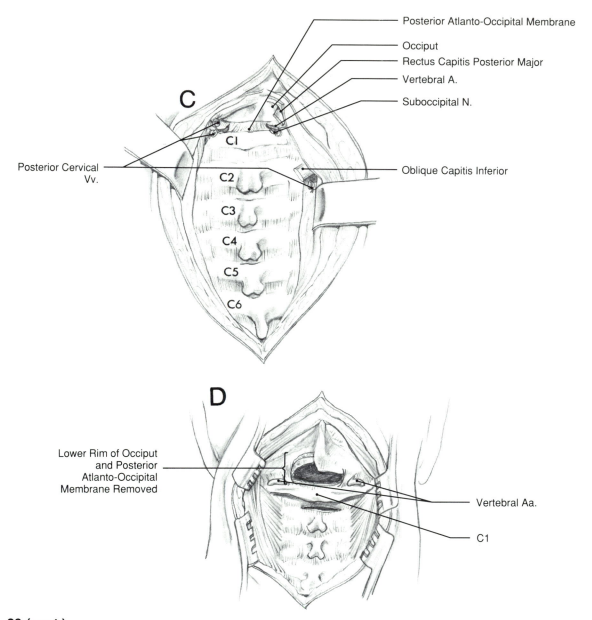

FIG 7–28 (cont.).
C, the insertions of the rectus capitis posterior major and oblique capitis inferior muscles from the C2 spinous process are resected to expose the proximal cervical spine. Care must be taken to avoid injury to the suboccipital nerve and vertebral artery. **D,** exposure of the posterior occiput and removal of a portion of its lower rim, together with the posterior atlanto-occipital membrane and a portion of the atlantoaxial membrane, in preparation for occipital-cervical fusion.

(Continued.)

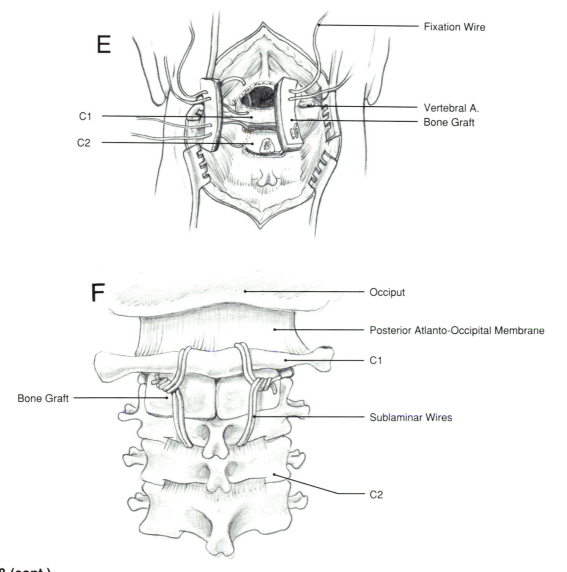

FIG 7–28 (cont.).
E, fixation of occiput to C2 with fixation wires and bone graft. **F,** atlantoaxial arthrodesis by the wedge compression method.

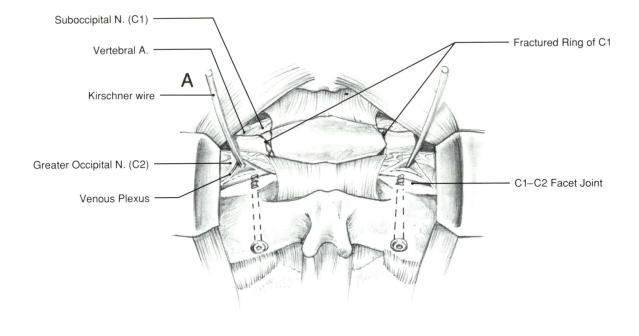

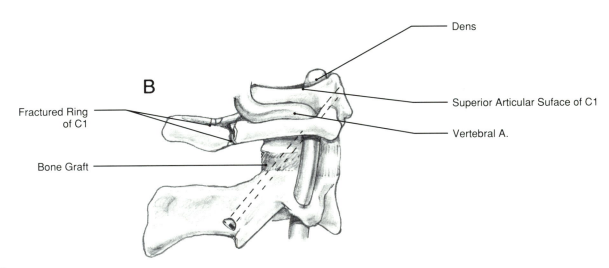

FIG 7–29.
C1-C2 fusion by transarticular screw fixation. Note defect in ring of C1. **A,** posterior view of exposed C1 and C2. Kirschner wires inserted into the inferior articular processes and gently pulled cranially to retract the greater occipital nerve and accompanying venous plexus. This permits visualization of the C1-C2 facet joints. Screws are then inserted sagittally from caudal to cranial and can be visualized as they cross the joint. **B,** lateral view of C1 and C2 fixed with transarticular screw. The C1-C2 joint is packed with cancellous bone graft to obtain fusion. (Modified from Magerl F, Seemann P-S: Stable posterior fusion of the atlas and axis by transarticular screw fixation, in Kehr P, Weidner A (eds): *Cervical Spine I.* New York, Springer-Verlag, New York, 1987, pp 322–327).

cesses. Bending the Kirschner wires proximally will lift and retract the greater occipital nerve and associated veins cranially. Screws are then inserted in a sagittal, superior direction beginning at the lower edge of the inferior articular process of C2. The screws exit C2 at the posterior rim of its proximal ar-ticular surfaces and are directed into the lateral masses of C1. The direction of screw placement and final screw length are determined by image intensification. Care must be taken to place the screws within the lateral masses of C1 and C2 to avoid injury to the vertebral artery. Fusion is accomplished

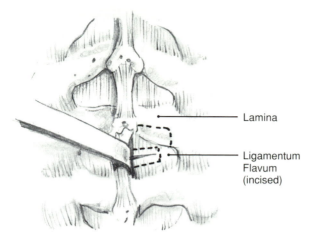

FIG 7–30.
Technique for disk excision. Incision in ligamentum flavum (surrounding *dashed line* indicates amount of ligamentum flavum to be removed). *Dashed line* on lamina indicates caudal portion of cranial lamina to be removed.

by placing cancellous bone graft into the denuded C1-C2 facet joints. A supplemental Gallie fusion can also be carried out if indicated (Fig 7–29).

Occasionally exposure of the lower posterior cervical spine is required. If the posterior elements are completely intact, the technic of spinous process wiring will provide adequate fixation. Dissection is carried down to the spinous processes. The paraspinal neck muscles are then dissected off the posterior elements in the subperiosteal plane. The lateral extent of the dissection will depend upon the purpose of the exposure. If surgery is being carried out for the purpose of posterior fusion without decompression, lateral exposure can be stopped at the facet joint and interspinous process wiring carried out as described by Rogers. When the posterior cervical approach is used for purposes of decompression, the ligamentum flavum can be sharply dissected off the superior margin of the more caudal lamina. Once this is accomplished, dissection can then be carried in a cranial direction and the ligamentum flavum and lamina excised with rongeurs (Fig 7–30). The lateral extent of the decompression can be carried to the medial border of the facet to decompress the spinal cord. However, if nerve root decompression is desired, it must extend laterally to include the medial portion of the facet joint at the desired level. Retraction on the nerve root should be minimized to prevent injury.

If fusion is required after laminectomy or the laminae and spinous processes have been destroyed by tumor, trauma, infection, or other inflammatory

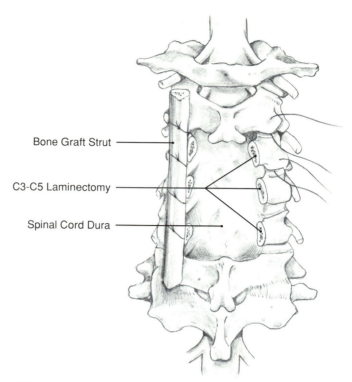

FIG 7–31.
Posterolateral fusion accomplished by facet joint wiring and bone strut. (Modified from Robinson RA, Southwick WO: Indications and technics for early stabilization of the neck in some fracture dislocations of the cervical spine. *South Med J* 53:565–579, 1960.)

processes, posterolateral facet joint fusion is the procedure of choice. Fixation can be achieved either by securing plates to the lateral masses with screws or facet joint wiring with a bone strut, as described by Robinson and Southwick (Fig 7–31).

BIBLIOGRAPHY

Alonso WA, Black P, Connor GH, et al: Transoral, transpalatal approach for resection of clival chordoma. *Laryngoscope* 1971; 81:1626–1631.

Apuzzo MLJ, Weiss MH, Hyden JS: Transoral exposure of the atlantoaxial joint. *J Neurosurg* 1978; 3:201–207.

Bailey RW, Badgley CE: Stabilization of the cervical spine by anterior fusion. *J Bone Joint Surg* 1960; 42A:565–594.

Bauer R, Kerschbaumer F, Poisel S: *Operative Approaches in Orthopedic Surgery and Traumatology.* New York, Thieme Medical Publishers Inc, 1987.

Brooks AL, Jenkins EB: Atlanto-axial arthrodesis by the wedge compression method. *J Bone Joint Surg* 1978; 60A:279–284.

Cauchoix J, Binet J: Anterior surgical approaches to the spine. *Ann R Col Surg Engl* 1957; 27:237–243.

Cloward R: *Ruptured cervical intervertebral discs.* Codman & Shurtleff, 1974.

de Andrade JR, McNab I: Anterior occipitocervical fusion using an extrapharyngeal approach. *J Bone Joint Surg* 1969; 51A:1621–1626.

Erickson LC, Greer RO: Ponticulus posticus: An anomaly of the first cervical vertebra as seen on the cephalometric head film. *Oral Surg Oral Med Oral Pathol* 1984; 57:230.

Fang HSY, Ong GB: Direct anterior approach to the upper cervical spine. *J Bone Joint Surg* 1962; 44A:1588–1604.

Gallie WE: Skeletal traction in the treatment of fractures and dislocations of the cervical spine. *Ann Surg* 1937; 106:770–776.

Grant JCB: *An Atlas of Anatomy,* ed 6. Baltimore, Williams & Wilkins Co, 1972.

Gray H: *Anatomy of the Human Body,* ed. 30. Philadelphia, Lea & Febiger, 1973.

Grodinsky M, Holyoke EA: The fasciae and fascial spaces of the head, neck and adjacent regions. *Am J Anat* 1938; 63:367–383.

Henry AK: *Extensile Exposure,* ed 2. Edinburgh, E & S Livingston, 1957.

Hodgson AR, Stock FE, Fang HSY, et al: Anterior spinal fusion: The operative approach and pathologic findings in 412 patients with Pott's disease of the spine. *Br J Surg* 1960; 48:172–178.

Hoppenfeld S: *Surgical Exposures in Orthopaedics: The Anatomical Approach,* ed 1. Philadelphia, J B Lippincott Co, 1984.

Louis R: *Surgery of the Spine.* Berlin, Springer-Verlag, 1982.

Magerl F, Seemann P-S: Stable posterior fusion of the atlas and axis by transarticular screw fixation, in Kehr P, Weidner A (eds): *Cervical Spine I.* New York, Springer-Verlag, New York, 1987, pp 322–327.

Meyer PR Jr (ed): *Surgery of Spine Trauma.* New York, Churchill Livingstone, Inc, 1989.

Moore KL: *Clinically Oriented Anatomy,* ed 2. Baltimore, Williams & Wilkins Co, 1985.

Netter FH: *The Ciba Collection of Medical Illustrations: Musculoskeletal System,* vol 8. Summit, NJ, Ciba-Geigy Corp, 1987.

Perry J: Surgical approaches to the spine, in Pierce D, Nichol V (eds): *The Total Care of Spinal Cord Injuries.* Boston, Little, Brown & Co, 1977, pp 53–79.

Riley LH Jr: Surgical approaches to the anterior structures of the cervical spine. *Clin Orthop Rel Res* 1973; 91:16–20.

Robinson RA, Smith GW: Anterolateral cervical disc removal and interbody fusion for cervical disc removal syndrome. *Bull Johns Hopkins Hosp* 1955; 96:223–224.

Robinson RA, Southwick WO: *AAOS Instructional Course Lectures,* vol XVII, *Surgical Approaches to the Cervical Spine.* St. Louis, C V Mosby Co, 1960, pp 299–330.

Robinson RA, Southwick WO: Indications and technics for early stabilization of the neck in some fracture dislocations of the cervical spine. *South Med J* 53:565–579, 1960.

Rogers WA: Fractures and dislocations of the cervical spine: An end result study. *J Bone Joint Surg* 1957; 39A:341–376.

Rogers WA: Treatment of fracture dislocation of the cervical spine. *J Bone Joint Surg* 1942; 24:245–258.

Rothman R, Simeone F: *The Spine,* ed 2. Philadelphia, W B Saunders Co, 1982.

Simmons EH, du Toit G: Lateral atlantoaxial arthrodesis. *Orthop Clin North Am* 1978; 9:1101–1114.

Southwick WO, Robinson RA: Surgical approaches to the vertebral bodies in the cervical and lumbar region. *J Bone Joint Surg* 1957; 39A:631–644.

Sundaresan N, Shah J, Feghall JG: A transsternal approach to the upper thoracic vertebrae. *Am J Surg* 1984; 148:473–477.

Verbiest H: Anterolateral operations for fractures and dislocations in the middle and lower parts of the cervical spine. *J Bone Joint Surg* 1969; 51A:1489–1530.

Watkins, RG: *Surgical Approaches to the Spine.* New York, Springer-Verlag, New York, 1983.

Whitesides TE Jr, Kelly RP: Lateral approach to the upper cervical spine for anterior fusion. *South Med J* 1966; 59:879–883.

Whitesides TE Jr, McDonald AP: Lateral retropharyngeal approach to the upper cervical spine. *Orthop Clin North Am* 1978; 9:1115–1127.

8

Thoracolumbosacral Spine

Marc A. Asher, M.D.
David P. Kraker, M.D.

ANATOMIC FEATURES OF THE THORACOLUMBOSACRAL SPINE

The function and accessibility of the thoracolumbosacral spinal column are strongly affected by the rib cage, abdomen, and ilia. Spinal cord and nerve function and accessibility are strongly influenced by their precise relationships with the alternating hard- and soft-tissue segments of the spinal column. This chapter stresses the anatomy of these relationships.

Bony Anatomy

There are usually twelve thoracic and five lumbar vertebrae (Fig 8–1). Each features an axial plane void, or spinal canal, bound ventrally by the vertebral body and dorsally by a bony arch. Embryologically each body is formed from adjacent somite halves, with postnatal growth occurring at the subchondral end-plates. The arch forms as two separate halves and consists of the spinous process, lamina, pars interarticularis, superior and inferior facet processes, and pedicles. Circumferential growth of the arch occurs primarily at the junction of the pedicle with the body (neurocentral synchondrosis).

Distinctive features of the thoracic vertebrae (Fig 8–2) include the oblique placement of the spinous processes, short pars interarticularis, horizontal orientation of the intervertebral facet joints, costal articular surfaces on the transverse processes and vertebral bodies, and bodies wider in the sagittal than the

coronal plane. The long axes of the pedicles are nearly parallel to the midsagittal plane. In both the coronal and sagittal planes the center of the pedicle is in line with the cranial edge of the transverse process.

Features distinctive of the lumbar vertebrae (Fig 8–3) are the relatively large and horizontal spinous processes, long pars interarticularis, intervertebral facet joint orientations more nearly parallel with the sagittal than the coronal plane, large superior facet processes topped by a mammillary process, and bodies wider in the coronal than the sagittal plane. From L1 to L5 the long axes of the pedicles become somewhat more convergent (dorsal to ventral) toward the midsagittal plane. The pedicle centers are in the same plane as the transverse process center line.

The sacrum (Fig 8–4) consists of five fused vertebrae and includes large lateral masses. These represent costal elements that develop with the upper three or more segments. Neural exit from the bony mass is provided by dorsal and ventral foramina, which are directly aligned in the coronal plane of the sacrum. By virtue of its bulk and trapezoidal shape, the sacrum is well-equipped to provide a base for the spine and broad attachments for the ilium.

Joints, Motion Segments, and Supporting Structures

Adjacent vertebrae are joined by a synostosis, the intervertebral disk, and two synovial joints, the

207

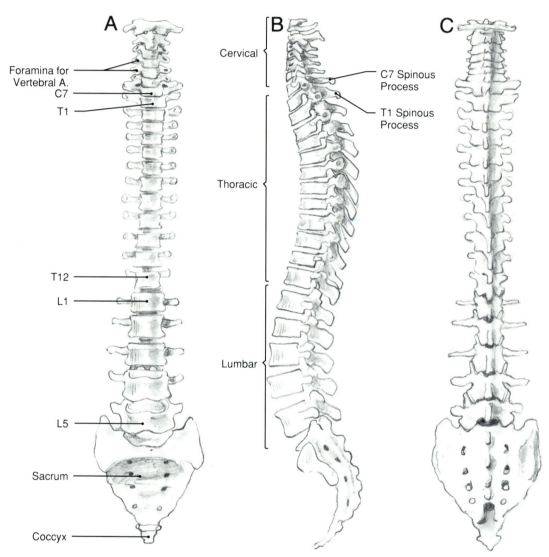

FIG 8–1.
Vertebral column. **A,** anteroposterior view. **B,** lateral view. **C,** posteroanterior view.

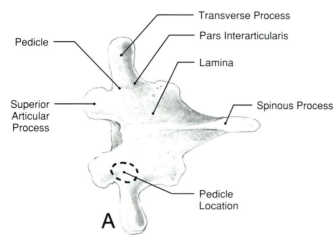

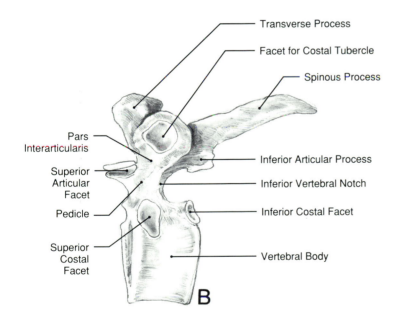

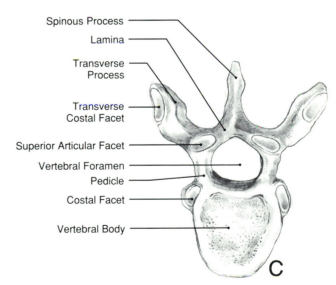

FIG 8–2.
Midthoracic vertebra. **A,** posteroanterior view; *dashed circle* indicates location of underlying pedicle. (Note vertebrae are oriented as visualized by the right-handed surgeon with the cephalad aspect of the vertebra to the left.) **B,** lateral view. **C,** axial view, from cephalad to caudad.

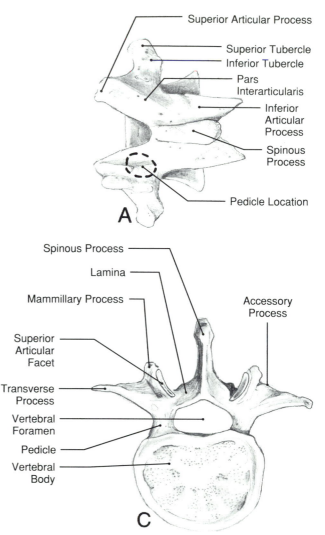

A

FIG 8–3.
Midlumbar vertebra. **A,** posteroanterior view; *dashed circle* indicates location of underlying pedicle. **B,** lateral view. **C,** axial view (from cephalad to caudad).

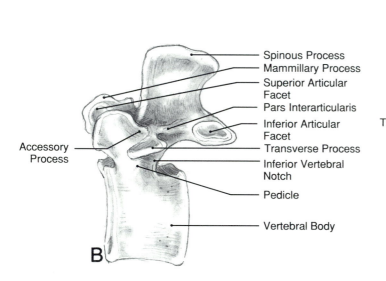

B

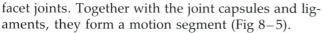

C

facet joints. Together with the joint capsules and ligaments, they form a motion segment (Fig 8–5).

The intervertebral disk is the primary axial load-transmitting articulation. It consists of cartilaginous end-plates, fibrocartilaginous outer ring (annulus fibrosis), and gelatinous center (nucleus pulposus). The fibers of the annulus are obliquely oriented and arranged in layers, with more ventral than dorsal layers.

The motion segment ligaments are extensive and include the supraspinous and interspinous ligaments, ligamentum flavum, intertransverse ligaments, and posterior and anterior longitudinal ligaments. The strongest of the dorsal ligaments, the ligamentum flavum, is of particular interest because of its proximity to the spinal canal and its vulnerability to the process of aging. Part of its uniqueness relates to its high (approximately 80%) content of elastic fibers that maintain it in constant tension.

In the thoracic spine each motion segment also has costovertebral and costotransverse articulations, which are synovial joints (Fig 8–6). The rib cage, of which these articulations are but a part, considerably limits thoracic spine motion, particularly in flexion and extension.

The lumbosacral and sacroiliac articulations are stabilized by strong ligaments (Fig 8–7). The lumbosacral and corporotransverse (transforaminal) ligaments are of particular interest, since they have been cited as a likely cause of the L5 nerve root tethering and entrapment that are associated with and hinder the reduction of spondylolisthesis.

Some motion occurs in all planes at each motion segment. In general, however, lumbar motion segments are best equipped for flexion and extension and thoracic motion segments for axial rotation. An exception is the L5–S1 articulation, where more rotation occurs than in any other motion segment in the

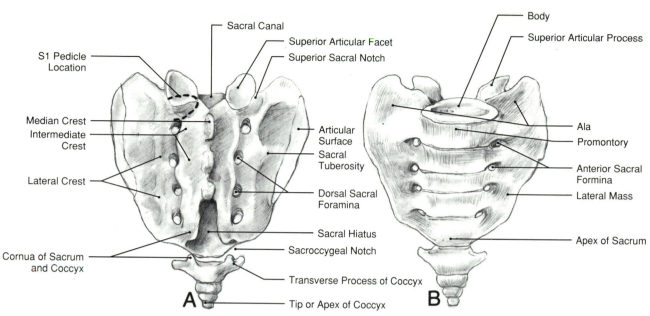

FIG 8–4.
Sacrum. **A,** posteroanterior view; *dashed semicircle* indicates location of underlying pedicle. **B,** anteroposterior view.

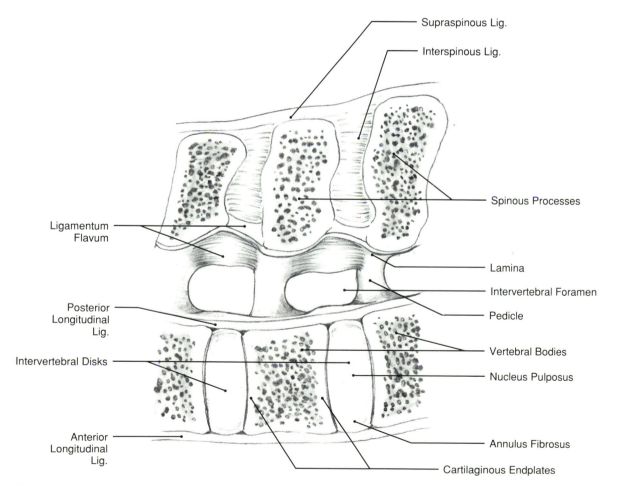

FIG 8–5.
Sagittal plane hemisection of two lumbar motion segments. Note ligamentum flavum is the roof of the intervertebral foramen.

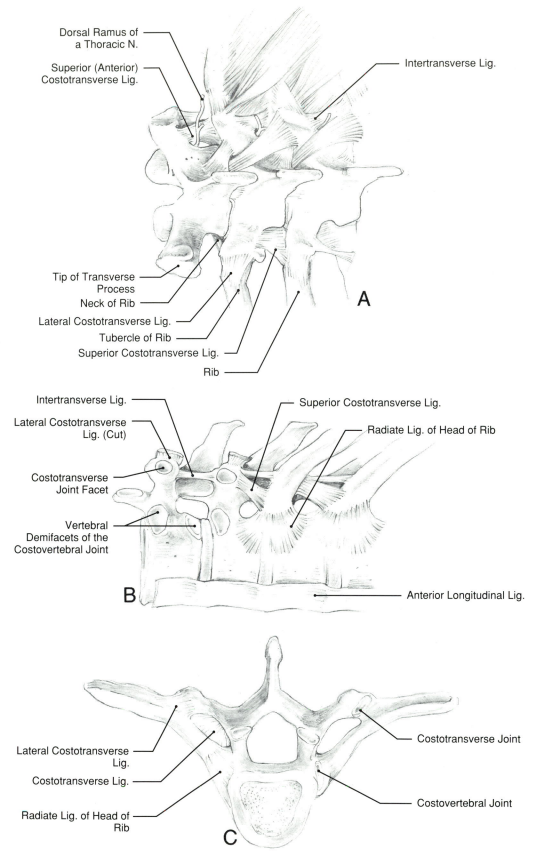

Dorsal Ramus of a Thoracic N.

Superior (Anterior) Costotransverse Lig.

Intertransverse Lig.

Tip of Transverse Process

Neck of Rib

Lateral Costotransverse Lig.

Tubercle of Rib

Superior Costotransverse Lig.

Rib

A

Intertransverse Lig.

Lateral Costotransverse Lig. (Cut)

Costotransverse Joint Facet

Vertebral Demifacets of the Costovertebral Joint

Superior Costotransverse Lig.

Radiate Lig. of Head of Rib

Anterior Longitudinal Lig.

B

Lateral Costotransverse Lig.

Costotransverse Lig.

Radiate Lig. of Head of Rib

Costotransverse Joint

Costovertebral Joint

C

FIG 8–6.
Segment of the thoracic spine (note costovertebral articulation). **A,** posteroanterior view. **B,** lateral view. **C,** axial view, from cephalad to caudad.

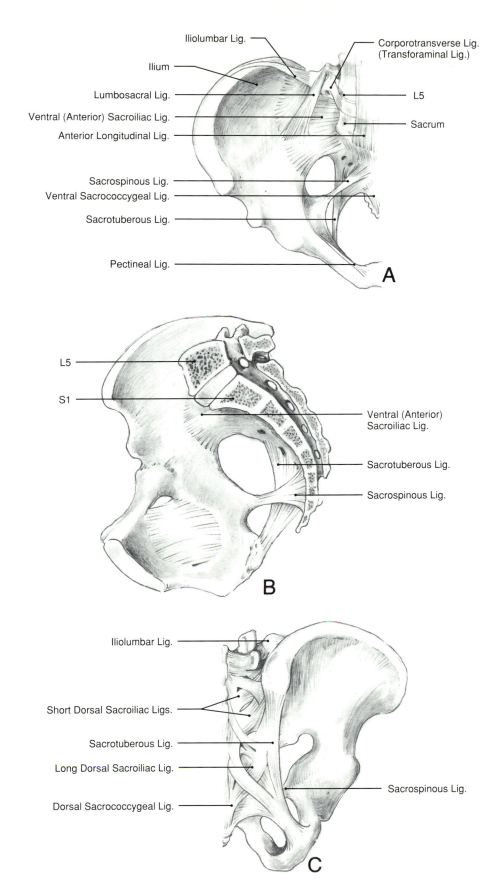

FIG 8–7.
L5-sacrum-iliac articulations. **A,** anteroposterior view. **B,** sagittal hemisection of sacrum. **C,** posteroanterior view.

lower thoracic or lumbar spine. Lateral bending range is similar for the thoracic and lumbar spine motion segments except at L5-S1, where it is markedly diminished.

Muscles

Muscles of the spine are primarily located dorsally. With some exceptions, most notably the psoas and quadratus lumborum, muscle forces acting ventrally affect the spine indirectly through the rib cage, abdomen, or investing fascia (Fig 8–8). The two major groupings of dorsal spine musculature are superficial (those outside the thoracolumbar fascia) and deep (those enclosed by the thoracolumbar fascia).

There are three layers of superficial muscles: (1) trapezius and latissimus dorsi; (2) levator scapulae and rhomboideus major and minor; and (3) serratus posterior superior and inferior (Fig 8–9). All originate from midline fascia and/or spinous processes except the levator scapulae, which originate from the transverse processes of the first three or four cervical vertebrae. The first two layers insert on and affect the shoulder and arm. The serrati insert on the upper and lower ribs and aid inspiration. All are innervated by branches from the ventral rami.

There are three major and one minor deep muscle groups. The major groups from dorsal to ventral are the splenius, erector spinae (sacrospinalis), and transversospinal. All have certain features in common: no one muscle spans the entire length of the spine and the origins are always caudal to the inser-

tions. To a greater or lesser extent they all extend, laterally bend, or rotate the spine. The predominant function is often apparent from the name. All are innervated by branches from the dorsal rami.

The splenius originates from the ligamentum nuchae and spinous processes from C7 and T1-6 (Fig 8–10). It divides into two parts: the capitis, which inserts on the skull, and the cervicis, which inserts on the posterior tubercle of the first two or three cervical vertebrae.

The erector spinae group has a broad tendinous origin from the T10 and lower spinous processes, median and lateral sacral crest, and iliac crest. As the group ascends, it divides into three columns (from lateral to medial) the iliocostalis, longissimus, and spinalis. Each column is subdivided on the basis of the major areas it spans. In general the muscle fascicles in each column span six to ten vertebral segments, with new fascicles originating as old ones insert. The iliocostalis inserts on the ribs and cervical transverse processes; the longissimus inserts on the upper ribs, cervical transverse processes, and mastoid process of the skull; and the spinalis inserts on the spinous processes of the upper thoracic vertebrae, the spinalis cervicis and capitis blending with the semispinalis.

As the name implies, the transversospinal group (inner layer of deep muscles of the back) originates on the transverse and articular processes and inserts on the spinous processes and skull (Fig 8–11). The four major divisions of the transversospinal muscles and their characteristics are as follows: (1) the semi-

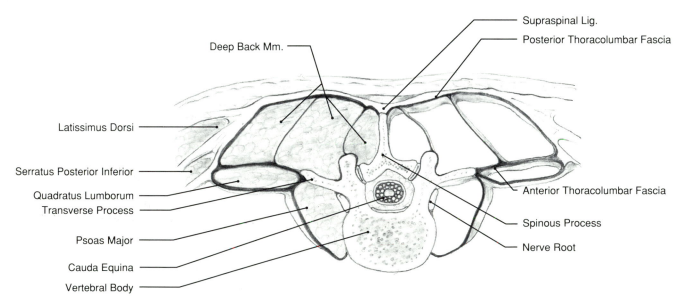

FIG 8–8.
Transverse section of the trunk at the upper lumbar spine. Note thoracolumbar fascia.

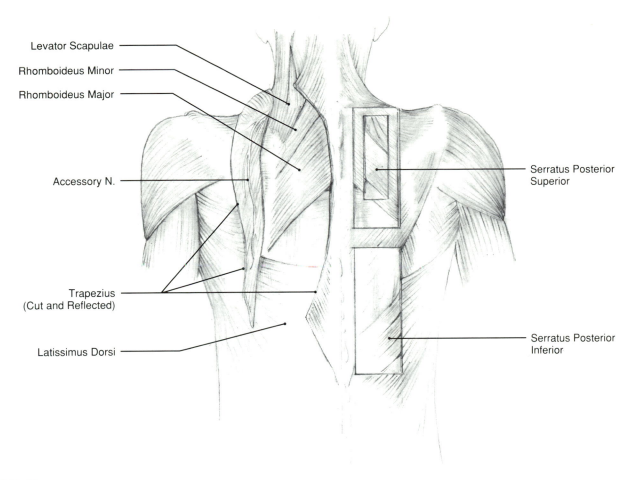

Levator Scapulae

Rhomboideus Minor

Rhomboideus Major

Accessory N.

Trapezius
(Cut and Reflected)

Latissimus Dorsi

Serratus Posterior
Superior

Serratus Posterior
Inferior

FIG 8–9.
Superficial muscles of the back. Note accessory nerve on undersurface of trapezius. (Cut-out boxes reveal underlying serratus posterior superior and serratus posterior inferior.)

spinalis muscles include thoracis, cervicis, and capitis portions, with each fascicle spanning four to six segments; (2) the multifidi are present the entire length of the spine, with each fascicle spanning two to four segments; (3) the rotatores, short and long portions, which span one or two motion segments (Fig 8–12); and (4) the suboccipital muscles (see cervical spine).

The minor deep muscles of the back include the interspinales, intertransversarii, and levatores costarum (see Fig 8–12). The interspinales are innervated by branches of the dorsal primary divisions of the spinal nerves and assist in extension of the vertebral column. The intertransversarii are innervated by branches of the dorsal and ventral primary divisions and assist in lateral bending of the vertebral column. The levatores costarum are supplied by the dorsal primary rami of the spinal nerves. They assist in inspiration.

The anterolateral muscles of the thoracolumbar

vertebrae include the quadratus lumborum and the psoas major and minor (Figs 8–8 and 8–13, A). The quadratus lumborum is a muscle of the posterior abdominal wall. It originates from the iliac crest, iliolumbar ligament, transverse processes of the lower three lumbar vertebrae, and anterior layer of the thoracolumbar fascia that lies immediately dorsal to it. The quadratus inserts onto the transverse processes of the upper lumbar vertebrae and the medial aspect of the twelfth rib. It is innervated by branches from the ventral rami of the four upper lumbar nerves and functions as a lateral flexor and extender of the spinal column. It also aids inspiration by fixing the lower ribs.

The psoas consists of two portions (major and minor) and arises from the anterolateral bodies of T12 to L5 and the transverse processes of L1 through L5. It inserts on the lesser trochanter of the femur. It is innervated by branches from the lumbar nerves, principally the first, second, and third. It is primarily

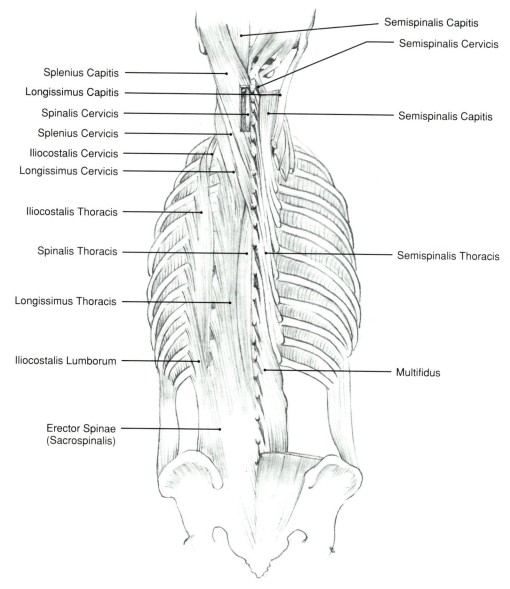

Splenius Capitis

Longissimus Capitis

Spinalis Cervicis

Splenius Cervicis

Iliocostalis Cervicis

Longissimus Cervicis

Iliocostalis Thoracis

Spinalis Thoracis

Longissimus Thoracis

Iliocostalis Lumborum

Erector Spinae
(Sacrospinalis)

Semispinalis Capitis

Semispinalis Cervicis

Semispinalis Capitis

Semispinalis Thoracis

Multifidus

FIG 8–10.
Outer two layers of the deep muscles of the back: splenius and erector spinae groups *(left labels)*, and outer two divisions of the transversospinal group *(right labels)*.

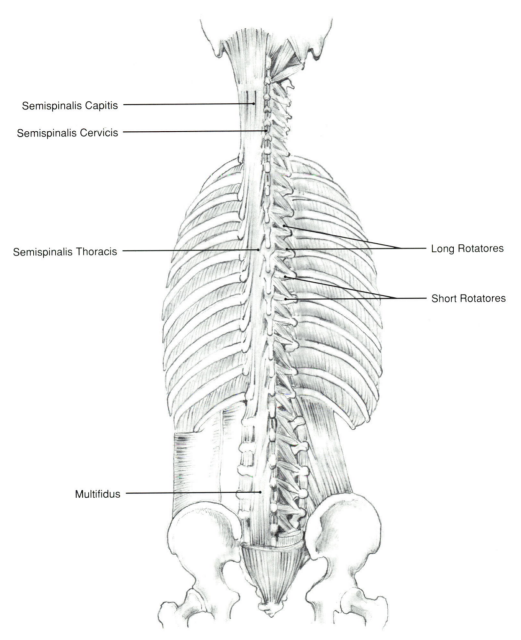

FIG 8–11.
Inner layer of deep muscles of the back (transversospinal group), except suboccipital muscles (see cervical spine).

DEEP BACK MUSCLES
(Inner Layer)

MINOR BACK MUSCLES

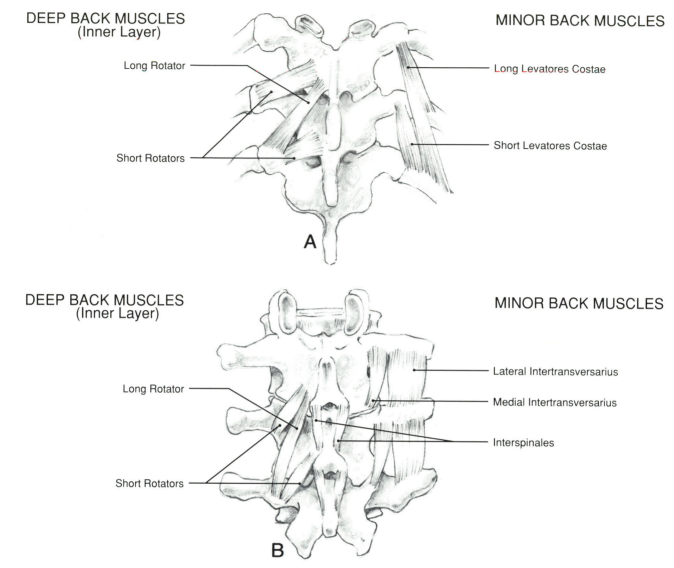

Long Rotator

Short Rotators

Long Levatores Costae

Short Levatores Costae

A

DEEP BACK MUSCLES
(Inner Layer)

MINOR BACK MUSCLES

Long Rotator

Short Rotators

Lateral Intertransversarius

Medial Intertransversarius

Interspinales

B

FIG 8–12.
Long and short rotators, a division of the inner layer of deep back muscles (left side of illustration), and minor muscles of the back (right side of illustration). **A,** thoracic region. **B,** lumbar region. Note levatores costarum muscles do not occur in the lumbar spine, and intertransversarius muscles do not occur in the thoracic spine.

a flexor of the thigh, but in circumstances of bilateral or unilateral overactivity or contracture it may produce lumbar hyperlordosis or scoliosis, respectively.

Both the quadratus lumborum and psoas are covered ventrally by the transversalis fascia (Fig 8–13, B). Between this portion of the transversalis fascia and peritoneum are three potential spaces: the posterior retroperitoneal, bound by the transversalis fascia and posterior renal fascia; the perinephric, bound by the anterior and posterior layers of the renal (Gerota's) fascia; and the anterior retroperitoneal space, bound by the posterior parietal peritoneum and anterior renal fascia. The retrofascial space is

dorsal to the transversalis fascia and contains the psoas muscle.

Neurologic Structures

The spinal cord begins at the medulla oblongata and ends as the conus medullaris at vertebral level L1-2. In its course through the vertebral canal the spinal cord disperses and receives twelve thoracic, five lumbar, and five sacral paired (right and left) dorsal and ventral nerve roots. The paired roots then enter the intervertebral foramina, just below the pedicle of the same-numbered vertebral level

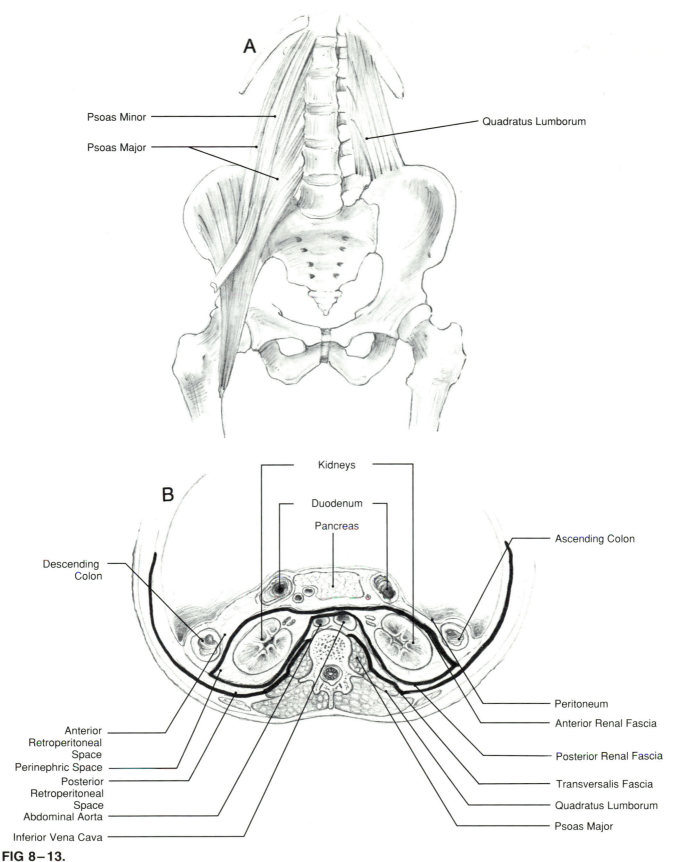

A, Psoas Minor

Psoas Major

Quadratus Lumborum

B, Kidneys

Duodenum

Pancreas

Descending Colon

Ascending Colon

Anterior Retroperitoneal Space

Perinephric Space

Posterior Retroperitoneal Space

Abdominal Aorta

Inferior Vena Cava

Peritoneum

Anterior Renal Fascia

Posterior Renal Fascia

Transversalis Fascia

Quadratus Lumborum

Psoas Major

FIG 8–13.
A, anterolateral muscles of the spine. **B,** transverse section at L2 showing the fascia and fascial spaces dorsal to the peritoneal sac and ventral to the vertebra.

(i.e., the T12 nerve roots exit just below the T12 pedicle) (Fig 8–14).

Three membranes cover and protect the spinal cord (Fig 8–15). The innermost is the pia mater. It is inseparably adherent to the spinal cord and invests its arteries and veins. At the spinal cord's termination the pia mater continues distally as a fibrous band, the filum terminale. The outermost protective layer is the tough dura mater. It begins at the foramen magnum from the cranial dura and ends at S1, where it becomes the coccygeal ligament. This dural ligament covers the filum terminale, and together they end by attaching to the periosteum of the coccyx. At each segmental level the dura mater evagi-

nates laterally with the spinal nerve roots to end just beyond the dorsal root ganglion, which is at the level of the vertebral pedicle. The intermediate covering of the spinal cord is the arachnoid. It follows the limits of the dura mater, separated from it by a small space. Additional protection for the cord is provided by the small, triangular denticulate ligaments between the nerve roots. These segmentally attach the pia and spinal cord laterally to the dura mater by piercing the arachnoid membrane.

The dorsal and ventral roots join just beyond the dorsal root ganglion to form the spinal nerve. Almost immediately the spinal nerve divides again to form the dorsal and ventral primary rami. The small

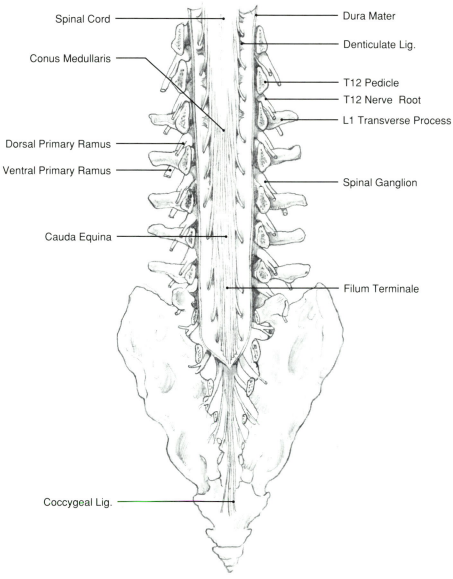

FIG 8–14.
Dorsal view of the thoracolumbosacral portion of the spinal canal, depicting spinal cord and nerve roots.

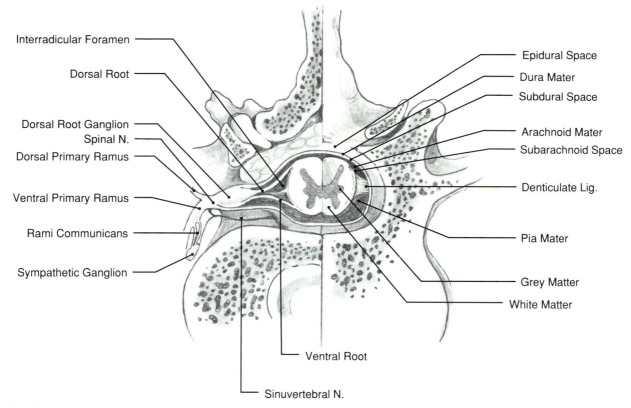

Interradicular Foramen

Dorsal Root

Dorsal Root Ganglion
Spinal N.
Dorsal Primary Ramus

Ventral Primary Ramus

Rami Communicans

Sympathetic Ganglion

Epidural Space
Dura Mater
Subdural Space

Arachnoid Mater
Subarachnoid Space

Denticulate Lig.

Pia Mater

Grey Matter
White Matter

Ventral Root

Sinuvertebral N.

FIG 8−15.
Cross section of the spinal cord in the spinal canal at the level of the foramen on the left side of the drawing and the pedicle on the right side of the drawing.

sinuvertebral nerve (recurrent spinal meningeal) promptly branches from the ventral primary rami and, after being joined by a branch from a gray rami communicans, reenters the spinal canal ventral to the nerve root.

The rami communicans (white) next branch from the ventral primary rami of T1 through L2 or L3 and join the sympathetic chain. Branching from the sympathetic chain are grey rami communicans, which join the ventral and dorsal primary rami at each level, and splanchnic nerves that continue to form the visceral plexuses and ganglia, of which the superior hypogastric plexus is one. This plexus overlies the bifurcation of the abdominal aorta (more to the left than right) and the junction of the common iliac veins near the sacral promontory (Fig 8−16).

The dorsal primary rami of both the thoracic and lumbar spinal nerves pass between the transverse processes of the vertebrae alongside the pars interarticularis. They divide into medial and lateral branches to supply the deep muscles of the back and the adjacent joints and ligaments (Fig 8−17). The medial branches terminate as cutaneous endings above the midthoracic level, whereas the lateral

branches provide cutaneous endings below this level.

The ventral rami of spinal nerves T2-6 course in the intercostal space below the main intercostal vessels and between the intercostal muscles. The ventral rami of T7-11 (thoracoabdominal nerves) travel between the intercostal muscles, pass behind (dorsal to) the costal cartilage, and continue between the transversalis and internal oblique muscles to innervate the abdominal muscles and skin. They end as sensory branches with T10 at the level of the umbilicus. The subcostal nerve (ventral ramus of spinal nerve T12) also provides motor branches to the abdominal muscles and cutaneous innervation to the area of the mons pubis.

The ventral rami of the lumbar nerves exit from the spinal column behind the psoas to form the lumbar plexus. They emerge as a series of nerves: the iliohypogastric (L1, sometimes combined with T12); ilioinguinal (L1); genitofemoral (L1-2); lateral femoral cutaneous (L1 to L3); the obturator (L2 to L4); the accessory obturator (L3-4); and femoral (L2 to L4) nerves (Fig 8−18). The ventral rami of L4 and L5 join to form the lumbosacral trunk, which enters the pel-

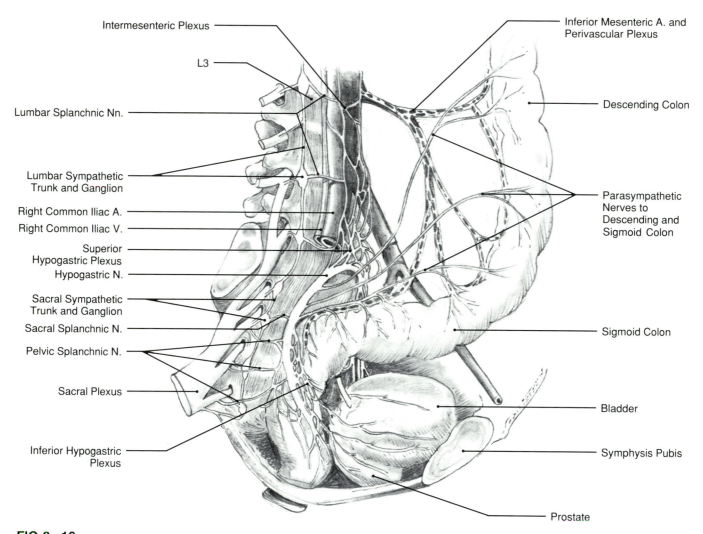

FIG 8–16.
Hypogastric plexus. (Modified from Woodburne RT: *Essentials of Human Anatomy.* New York, Oxford University Press, 1957.)

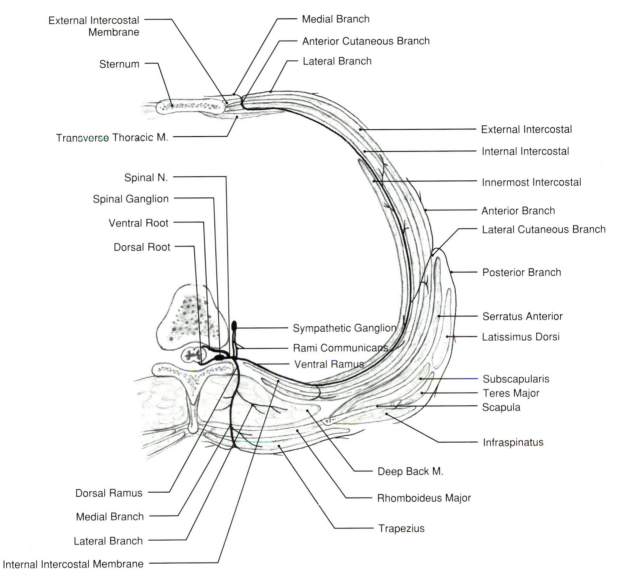

FIG 8–17.
An intercostal nerve in relation to its surrounding structures.

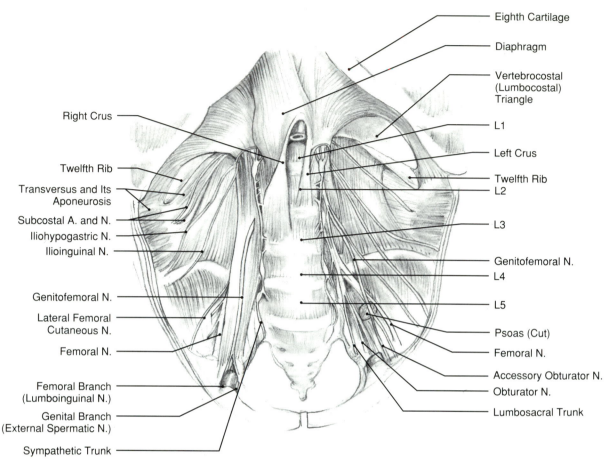

Eighth Cartilage

Diaphragm

Vertebrocostal (Lumbocostal) Triangle

L1

Left Crus

Twelfth Rib
L2

L3

Genitofemoral N.
L4

L5

Psoas (Cut)

Femoral N.

Accessory Obturator N.
Obturator N.

Lumbosacral Trunk

Right Crus

Twelfth Rib

Transversus and Its Aponeurosis

Subcostal A. and N.
Iliohypogastric N.
Ilioinguinal N.

Genitofemoral N.

Lateral Femoral Cutaneous N.

Femoral N.

Femoral Branch (Lumboinguinal N.)

Genital Branch (External Spermatic N.)

Sympathetic Trunk

FIG 8–18.
Posterior wall of the abdomen.

vis and, along with the ventral rami of the sacral nerves, forms the sacral plexus (Fig 8–19).

Arteries

The spinal cord receives two arterial blood supplies, the longitudinal and segmental. The longitudinal supply is from the anterior and posterior spinal arteries. The anterior spinal artery is formed by the union of two small branches from the vertebral arteries on the floor of the skull. Two posterior spinal arteries arise as small branches from the vertebral or posteroinferior cerebellar arteries (Fig 8–20, A). Though these spinal arteries may traverse the entire length of the spinal cord, they supply sufficient blood for only the superior cervical segments of the spinal cord. The segmental arterial system supplies the remainder of the cord.

The segmental arterial supply arises at various levels from dorsal branches of the costovertebral trunk of the subclavian, the posterior intercostals, and the lumbar branches of the aorta. The iliolumbar artery arises from the internal iliac. In the thorax, for example, a dorsal branch of a posterior intercostal further divides into a muscular branch (which continues dorsally with the dorsal rami of the spinal nerve) and a spinal branch (which enters the intervertebral foramen, generally ventral to the dorsal root ganglion and ventral spinal root) (Fig 8–20, B). Just inside the intervertebral foramen the spinal branch further divides into three tributaries: (1) a posterior central branch to the floor of the vertebral canal; (2) a prelaminar branch to the underside of the lamina and ligamentum flavum; and (3) a radicular branch that pierces the dural sac and anastomoses with the anterior or posterior spinal arteries. These radicular branches are also known as medullary feeders. They do not occur at every level, averaging four to five anterior and nine posterior for the thoracolumbar spine.

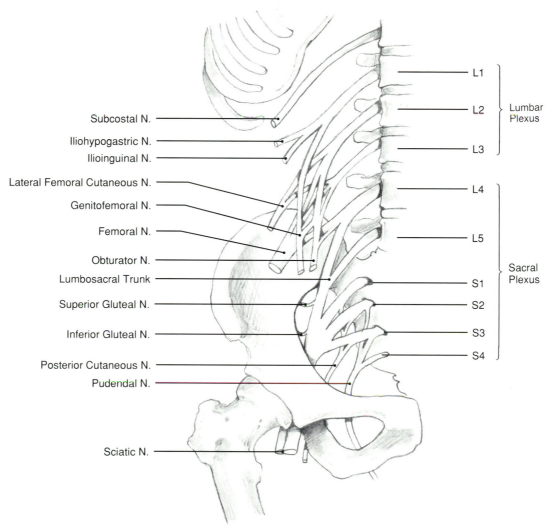

Subcostal N.

Iliohypogastric N.

Ilioinguinal N.

Lateral Femoral Cutaneous N.

Genitofemoral N.

Femoral N.

Obturator N.

Lumbosacral Trunk

Superior Gluteal N.

Inferior Gluteal N.

Posterior Cutaneous N.

Pudendal N.

Sciatic N.

L1

L2

L3

L4

L5

S1

S2

S3

S4

Lumbar Plexus

Sacral Plexus

FIG 8–19.
Lumbar and sacral plexuses.

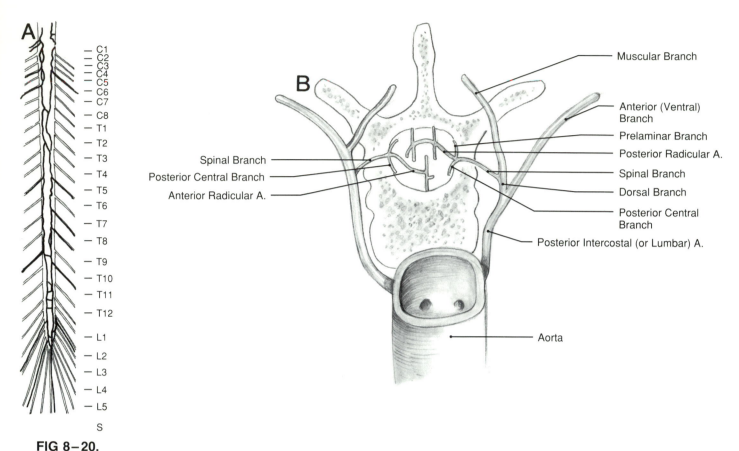

FIG 8–20.
Arterial supply to the spinal canal and cord. **A,** Posterior longitudinal system. Posterior radicular arteries *(dark lines)* shown entering at several levels. (Redrawn from Dommissee GF: *The Arteries and Veins of the Human Spinal Cord and Brain.* New York, Churchill Livingstone, Inc, 1975.) **B,** segmental system in thoracic region.

A giant anterior medullary feeder, the artery of Adamkiewicz, may or may not be present on either side at any level from T7 to L4. Most commonly, however, it is present on the left side between T7 and L4.

Veins

The spinal column is drained by an extensive venous complex. The spinal cord itself is drained by six longitudinal veins: the anteromedian, the posteromedian, two posterolateral (one on each side), and two similarly paired anterolateral veins. These in turn are segmentally drained by anterior and posterior radicular veins that combine and exit the dura to join the anterior and posterior internal venous plexuses of the vertebrae (Fig 8–21, A).

The vertebral bodies are drained by basivertebral veins that drain into the large anterior internal longitudinal plexuses by means of transverse anastomoses (Figs 8–21, B and C). These plexuses lie outside the dura. They freely connect with the less distinct posterior internal longitudinal venous plexuses and the intervertebral veins that exit the intervertebral foramina.

The vertebral column is also drained by the posterior and anterior external venous plexuses. The former anastomose with the internal plexuses and intervertebral vein. The latter anastomose with the basivertebral and intervertebral veins. Taken together, the internal and external venous plexuses are known as Batson's plexus.

The intervertebral veins drain into the segmental veins, which, depending upon the level, eventually drain into the azygos, hemiazygous, accessory hemiazygous, inferior vena cava, or common iliac vein (Fig 8–22). The iliolumbar vein, the only segmental vein draining into the common iliac vein, is short and directly overlies the anterolateral aspect of the L5-S1 disk, a fact of surgical importance (Fig 8–23).

The cisterna chyli, which eventually drains into the junction of the left subclavian and internal jugu-

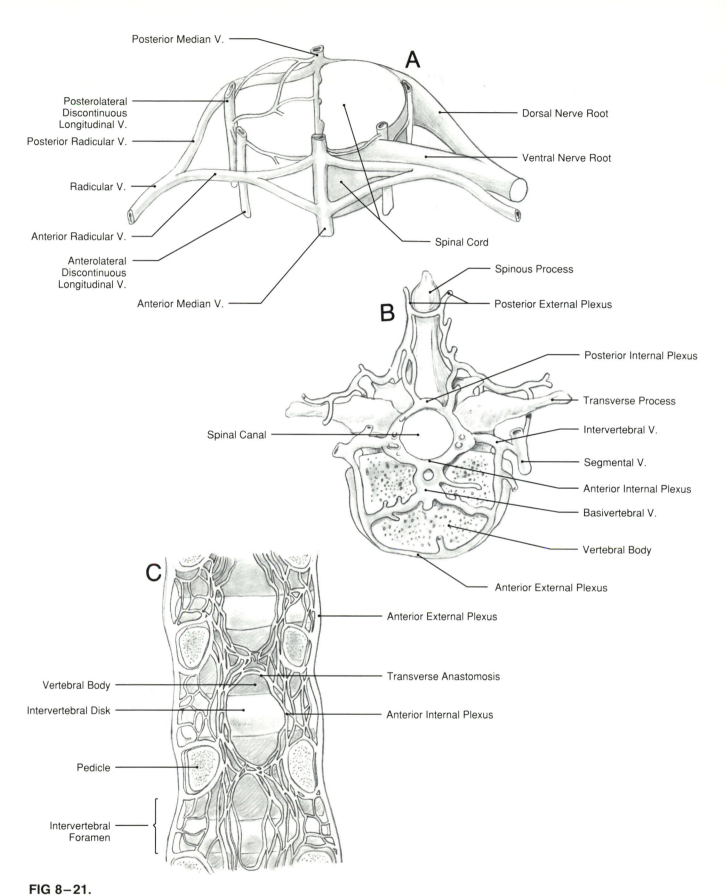

FIG 8–21.
Venous drainage of the spinal column. **A,** venous drainage of the spinal cord. **B,** axial view of venous drainage of a vertebral body. The internal and external venous plexuses are collectively known as Batson's plexus. **C,** coronal view of the anterior internal venous plexus.

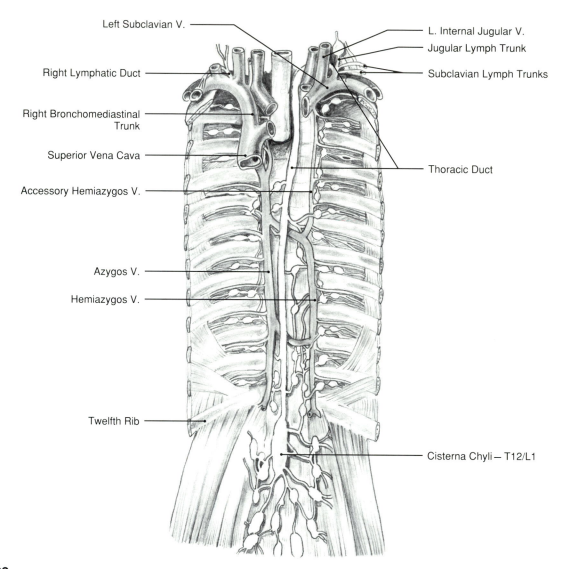

Left Subclavian V.

Right Lymphatic Duct

Right Bronchomediastinal
Trunk

Superior Vena Cava

Accessory Hemiazygos V.

Azygos V.

Hemiazygos V.

Twelfth Rib

L. Internal Jugular V.

Jugular Lymph Trunk

Subclavian Lymph Trunks

Thoracic Duct

Cisterna Chyli — T12/L1

FIG 8–22.
Anteroposterior view of the thoracic and upper lumbar spine illustrating the segmental venous drainage system, cisterna chyli, and thoracic duct. (For purposes of orientation, the right ventricle of the heart, which has been removed, lies at the level of the seventh rib.)

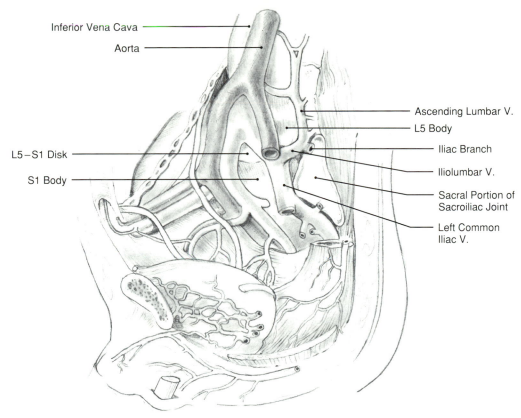

Inferior Vena Cava

Aorta

Ascending Lumbar V.

L5 Body

Iliac Branch

L5–S1 Disk

Iliolumbar V.

S1 Body

Sacral Portion of
Sacroiliac Joint

Left Common
Iliac V.

FIG 8–23.
An oblique view of the left common iliac vein and iliolumbar vein. Note relationship of iliolumbar vein to L5-S1 disk.

lar veins via the thoracic duct, lies in the interval between the inferior vena cava and vertebral column at the thoracolumbar junction (see Fig 8–22).

SURGICAL APPROACHES TO THE THORACOLUMBOSACRAL SPINE

General anesthesia is usually preferred. Neurological monitoring is aided by limiting pharmacological paralysis. The patient should have some response to nerve stimulus and an anesthetic combination that allows the wake-up test to be performed. Unless contraindicated, moderate hypotension with a mean systolic pressure of approximately 60 to 75 mm Hg is desirable. Body temperature should be preserved by warming and humidification of inhalation mixtures and elevation of room temperature as necessary.

Local anesthesia is preferred for percutaneous approaches and may be used for diskectomy (even

at times for osteotomy, such as in ankylosing spondylitis). Spinal anesthesia may be used for lumbar laminectomy. These techniques offer the advantage of more direct monitoring of neurological function.

Pertinent radiographs should be displayed on view boxes in the operating room. In particular it is important to be aware of any congenital abnormalities, such as spina bifida occulta or transitional vertebra, that may make level identification difficult.

Dorsal Approaches

The prone position on longitudinal chest rolls is the most versatile position for the dorsal approaches (Fig 8–24, A). It provides some decompression of the abdominal contents, introduces the least distortion to the spine, provides some stability following extensive osteotomies, and is the least obstructive to intraoperative radiography. To aid lumbar exposure by opening the interlaminar spaces or to accommodate fixed kyphotic deformity, the table may be partially flexed (Fig 8–24, B). The major disadvantage of

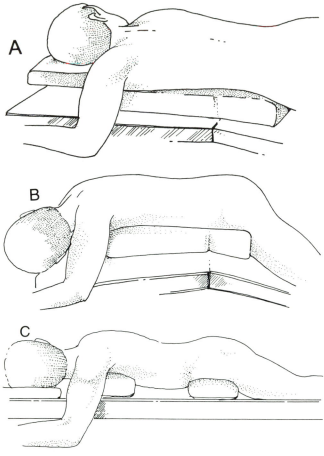

FIG 8–24.
Patient positioned prone on longitudinal chest rolls. **A,** with table flat. **B,** with table partially flexed. **C,** transverse placement of chest rolls to aid thoracolumbar and lumbar kyphosis correction.

the prone position on longitudinal chest rolls is incomplete abdominal decompression. Transverse placement of the chest rolls may be helpful in treatment of burst fractures of the lumbar spine and thoracolumbar junction (Fig 8–24, C).

A commonly used alternative is the Relton-Hall frame, which provides more effective abdominal decompression (Fig 8–25). Disadvantages are increased skin pressure concentrations at the support pads, increased upper thoracic kyphosis and decreased lumbar lordosis, instability following extensive osteotomy, and some obstruction to radiography, especially C-arm fluoroscopy.

For limited midline exposures of the lower lumbar spine, as for diskectomy, the kneeling position offers maximum abdominal decompression (Fig 8–26). The knee-chest position should be avoided because it may impede circulation in the lower extremities and result in myoglobin release. The kneel-

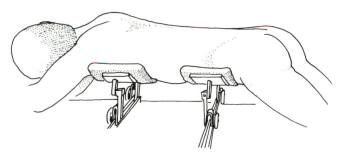

FIG 8–25.
Patient in prone position on Relton-Hall frame. When instrumenting the lower lumbar and lumbosacral spine, the hips should be extended.

ing position also provides interlaminar opening comparable to the flexed position with elongated chest rolls. Disadvantages include flattening of lumbar lordosis (making proper sagittal plane alignment with spinal instrumentation difficult), tensing of the paraspinal muscles (making lateral exposure more difficult), and elimination of posteroanterior radiograph control. The kneeling position should probably be avoided for longer operations and for elderly patients, as lactic acid build-up and release may be sufficient to cause cardiac arrhythmia when the position is terminated.

In each of these positions, shoulder abduction is limited to 90 degrees in order to avoid stretching of the brachial plexus.

In operations on the upper thoracic spine and cervicothoracic junction, stabilization of the head with skull tongs or clamps and placement of the arms alongside the patient's trunk allows better access (Fig 8–27).

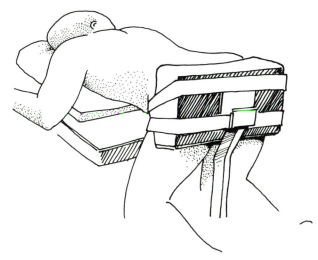

FIG 8–26.
Patient in prone-kneeling position (90 degree hip and knee flexion).

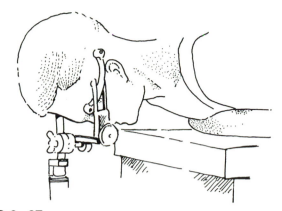

FIG 8–27.
Patient in prone position, with head supported by skull tongs and arms at the side.

Finally, the lateral position may be utilized for combined procedures requiring simultaneous dorsal and ventral exposure. Some prefer it for hemilaminotomy (Fig 8–28).

Midline Extensile Approaches

Dorsal midline incisions are the ultimate in extensile exposure. It is desirable to prepare and drape an area larger than the anticipated operative field.

Incision.—The approximate level to be exposed is identified using the iliac crest, the lower rib cage, and the prominent C7 spinous process as guides (Fig 8–29). When precise incision placement is required, as for microdiskectomy, a preincision localizing radiograph is required. To ensure a straight midline incision, a string held taut between C7 and S2 is helpful as an incision guide. With severe coronal plane spine deformity, a variable amount of deviation toward the apex is necessary. The initial incision extends just through the dermis (Fig 8–30). From this point electrocautery dissection is used almost exclusively. The incision is then deepened through the subcutaneous tissue to expose the tips of the spinous processes, which show as a longitudinal white line, the supraspinous ligament. This is

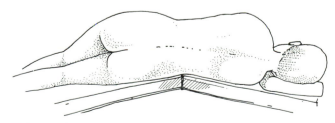

FIG 8–28.
Lateral position for operation on the lumbar spine by posterior approach.

readily apparent in the lumbar region of the spine. In the thoracic region the superficial muscles of the back may tend to overlap, thus obscuring the midline. This is especially true in a deformed spine. Tensing of these muscles with a self-retaining retractor and proceeding from caudad to cephalad, being careful not to incise these muscles, help ensure a clean exposure of the supraspinous ligament.

The ligament is then incised with electrocautery. In children, the apophyses are split with a knife.

At this point precise radiographic localization of the anatomical level is desirable. Posteroanterior exposure is usually preferred, unless prohibited by the patient's position. If the T12 level is to be included in the exposure (and the twelfth rib is present) an alternative method of level confirmation is to postpone precise level identification until the medial aspect of the twelfth rib can be exposed. In any event it is undesirable to subperiosteally strip any more of the spine than is needed.

Spinous Processes, Lamina, and Facets (Fig 8–31).—These midline structures are exposed subperiosteally. An elevator is used to retract the deep back muscles and electrocautery to elevate the periosteum and detach muscular origins and insertions. Brisk bleeding from the dorsal external vertebral venous plexus is usually encountered and controlled with electrocautery. The insertions of the thoracospinal muscles onto the inferior edge of the spinous processes and laminae are particularly tenacious. Exposure of the inferior facet process occurs with exposure of the outer reaches of the lamina. In the lumbar spine, exposure of the superior facet process, if needed, is done by following the lamina onto the pars and facet process. At the outer edge of the pars interarticularis, the muscular branch from the dorsal spinal artery and the dorsal ramus will be encountered. They can be preserved if further dissection laterally is not required.

For orientation it is advisable to locate the center of the pedicle mentally. It lies below the base of the superior facet process (see bony anatomy).

Exposure is now wide enough for laminotomy, laminectomy, and dorsal and/or facet arthrodesis. If arthrodesis is being performed, any remaining interspinous ligament as well as the facet capsules are removed with curettes and rongeurs.

Transverse Processes.—For intertransverse arthrodesis or extraforaminal exploration, further exposure of the transverse process is necessary.

The transverse processes are best exposed by

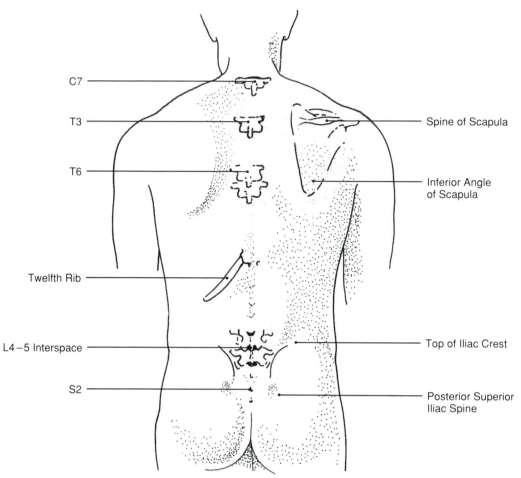

FIG 8–29.
Dorsal surface topography. Note landmarks corresponding to vertebral levels (e.g., top of iliac crest and L4-5 interspace).

following their middorsal surface laterally with electrocautery and transecting the overlying transversospinal muscles (Fig 8–32). The transverse process is further exposed by sweeping the electrocautery subperiosteally cephalad and caudad. Bleeding from the dorsal external vertebral venous plexus is expected, and is controlled by electrocautery.

The muscular branch of the dorsal spinal artery and the dorsal ramus are divided and the cut portions of the transversospinal muscle retracted or re-

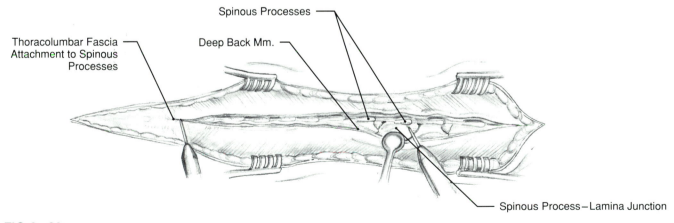

FIG 8–30.
Dorsal midline approach: incision through tips of the spinous processes.

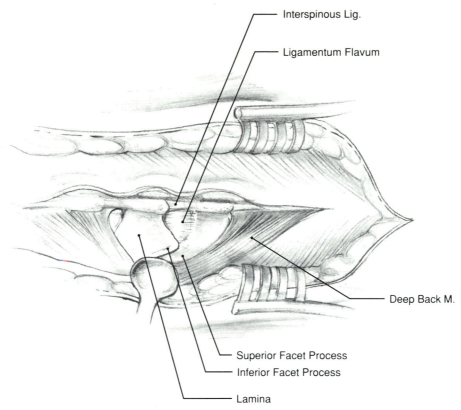

FIG 8–31.
Dorsal midline approach: spinous process through facet joint.

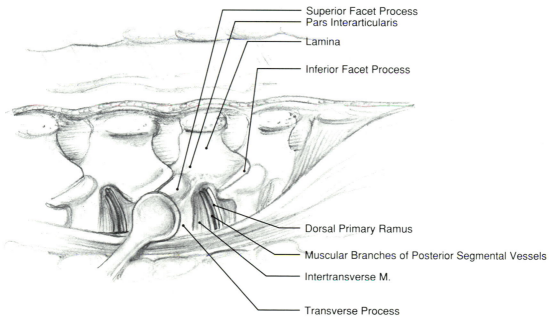

FIG 8–32.
Dorsal midline approach: transverse process and intertransverse gutter.

sected to expose the intertransverse gutter. The latter can be accomplished by lifting the muscle with a rongeur or large tissue forceps and cutting with electrocautery.

Sacrum.—There are some special considerations for exposing the sacrum (Fig 8–33). The lamina may be quite thin (or even partially missing) and easily penetrated. The dorsal branch of the segmental vessels exiting the dorsal foramina directly enters the substance of the multifidus. Adequate exposure of the L5–S1 facet and superior sacral notch can usually be obtained with preservation of the dorsal rami. When needed, exposure lateral to the dorsal foramina is best accomplished by lifting the multifidus and, with electrocautery, transecting a distance above (dorsal to) the dorsal foramen. This leaves a cuff of tissue around the dorsal foramen, which allows easier control of bleeding with electrocautery. It is important to remember that sacral exposure is usually more difficult in males than females because of the relatively narrow interiliac crest distance in males.

Spinal Canal: Hemilaminotomy.—Entry to the spinal canal is gained through the ligamentum flavum near the midline, avoiding laceration of the dura and venous plexuses. Many technics are acceptable. One is to thin the ligamentum flavum at the midline with a succession of small rongeur bites (Fig 8–34, A). Entry may be completed by making

additional small rongeur bites or grasping the thinned ligamentum flavum edge and making a shallow incision through the remaining fibers (Fig 8–34, B). Inside the canal, the change in color between the thinned ligamentum flavum (yellow) and epidural fat (white) is readily apparent. The underside of the ligamentum flavum is then palpated with an angled elevator to separate it from the posterior internal venous plexus and dura. These structures may be further separated by gently passing a small cotton surgical patty into the epidural space. The ligamentum flavum is grasped, lifted laterally, and incised along the superior and inferior lamina.

The interlaminar opening is then enlarged by isolation and removal of portions of the inferior and lateral edges of the cephalad lamina, as well as the underlying ligamentum flavum.

Limited access to the floor of the spinal canal is now possible. The nerve root (L5 for L4–5 laminotomy) is generally located by gentle probing along the lateral wall of the canal and retraction lateral toward the midline (Fig 8–34, C). An alternative method is lateral retraction of the epidural fat. If difficulty is encountered in locating the nerve, the L5 pedicle should be located with a probe. This may require removal of some of the medial edge of the superior facet. The nerve may then be identified by gentle sliding of the probe down the medial wall of the pedicle. Bleeding from the internal vertebral plexus may be encountered and should be controlled with bipolar cautery. Thrombin-soaked gel-

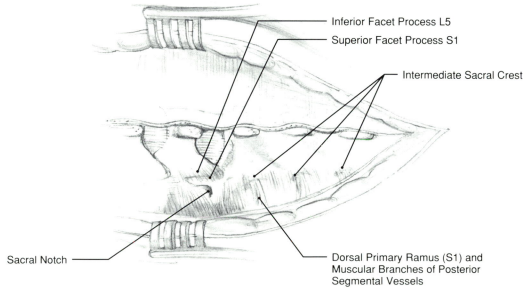

FIG 8–33.
Sacrum: exposure of the alae and area lateral to the dorsal foramen.

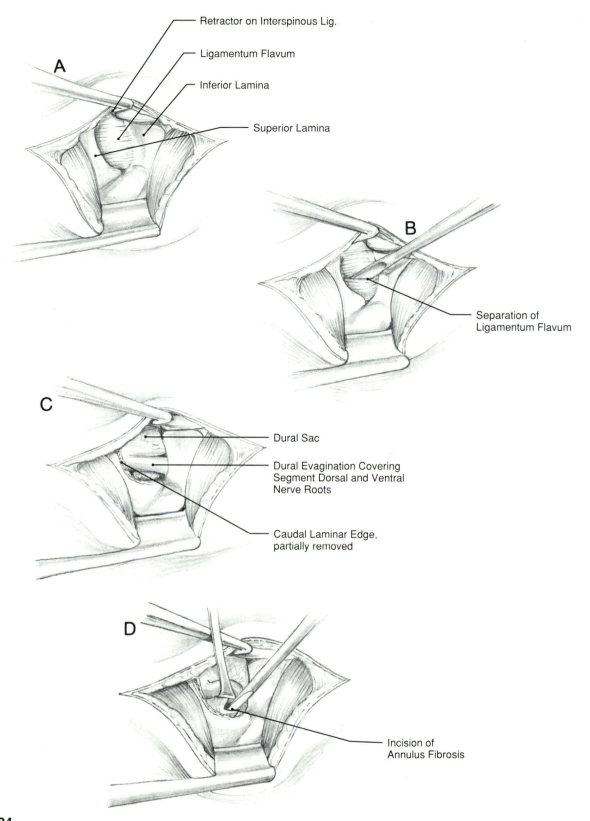

Retractor on Interspinous Lig.

Ligamentum Flavum

Inferior Lamina

Superior Lamina

Separation of
Ligamentum Flavum

Dural Sac

Dural Evagination Covering
Segment Dorsal and Ventral
Nerve Roots

Caudal Laminar Edge,
partially removed

Incision of
Annulus Fibrosis

FIG 8–34.
Hemilaminotomy approach to the spinal canal. **A,** exposed, thinned ligamentum flavum. **B,** ligamentum flavum incision. **C,** exposed spinal canal. **D,** root retraction and incision of annulus fibrosis.

foam on a cotton-type surgical patty or oxidized cellulose may also be helpful. These maneuvers expose the annulus fibrosis (Fig 8–34, D).

Spinal Canal: Laminotomy and Laminectomy.— Wider exposure of the spinal canal, including the subarticular zone, may be accomplished by bilateral laminotomy (Fig 8–35). This may be done by leaving the interspinous ligament and spinous process intact or, as is usually done if exposure of this extent is needed, removing the inferior portion of the spinous process and midline lamina. Additional exposure may be obtained by undercutting the remaining inferior edge of the lamina and inferior facet process. The ligamentum flavum attaches at this site, which in the elderly is a common site of osteophyte formation. The undercutting technique involves identifying the bone-ligamentum flavum layer and the dura. If clearance allows, a bone punch is used to remove overlying bone and ligament (flavum). If clearance does not allow, the bone is osteotomized, then removed with a curette. If such internal decompression cannot be expected to provide adequate canal decompression, laminectomy is needed. This may be accomplished with a rongeur, usually beginning at the inferior edge of the lamina, or lateral osteotomy of the lamina, with the lamina removed in one piece.

Removing the medial edge of the superior facet joint with its underlying ligamentum flavum, using the same undercutting techniques, may afford still wider exposure.

Foraminotomy.—These same bone and ligament removal technics may also enlarge the foramen by undercutting the entire width of the facet joint and removing the ligamentum flavum from its lateral attachment on the outer edge of the foramen (Fig 8–36). Eventually the extraforaminal region is entered.

Facetectomy.—Occasionally, removal of the entire facet is necessary to expose and decompress the foraminal canal. Rarely, part or even all of a pedicle may require removal. Facetectomy may also help provide adequate exposure of the posterolateral floor of the spinal canal (for example, to facilitate posterior lumbar interbody fusion) (Fig 8–37). If the facet joint is removed, restabilization is usually necessary.

Extraforaminal Approach.—Exposure of the extraforaminal region alone is provided by incision and removal of the intertransverse ligament. Intertransverse ligament exposure may be done from the midline (Fig 8–38, A) or by retraction of the midline incision and development of the plane between the multifidus and longissimus (Figs 8–38, B to D). Because of the obliquity and interblending of the muscular fibers, this is an indistinct interval. Bipolar coagulation is sometimes necessary to control bleeding from the muscular branches of the dorsal branch of the segmental arteries and the extensive venous plexus. The remainder of the dorsal ramus, which will have been divided in the approach to the pos-

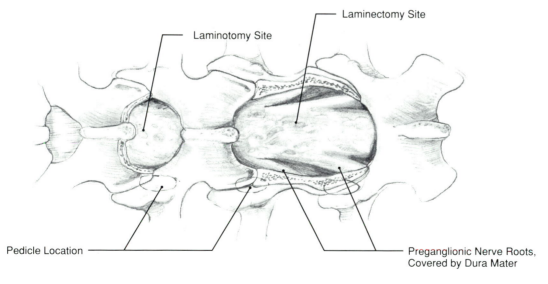

Laminotomy Site

Laminectomy Site

Pedicle Location

Preganglionic Nerve Roots, Covered by Dura Mater

FIG 8–35.
Laminotomy and laminectomy: sequence showing progressive dorsal exposure of the spinal canal by bilateral laminotomy (left portion of illustration) and laminectomy (right portion of illustration).

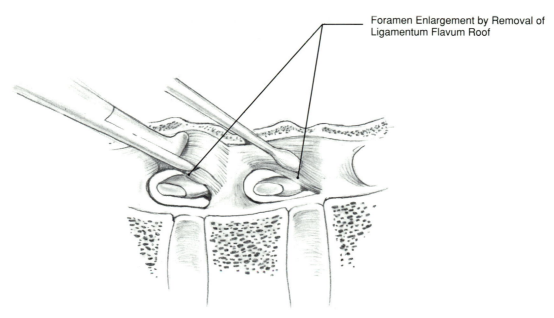

FIG 8–36.
Foraminotomy.

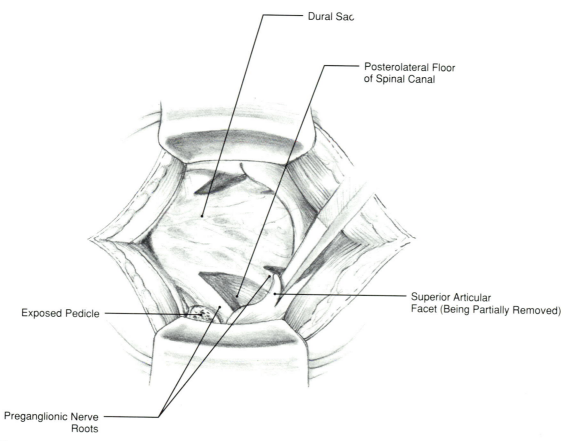

FIG 8–37.
Facetectomy with exposure of the posterolateral floor of the spinal canal.

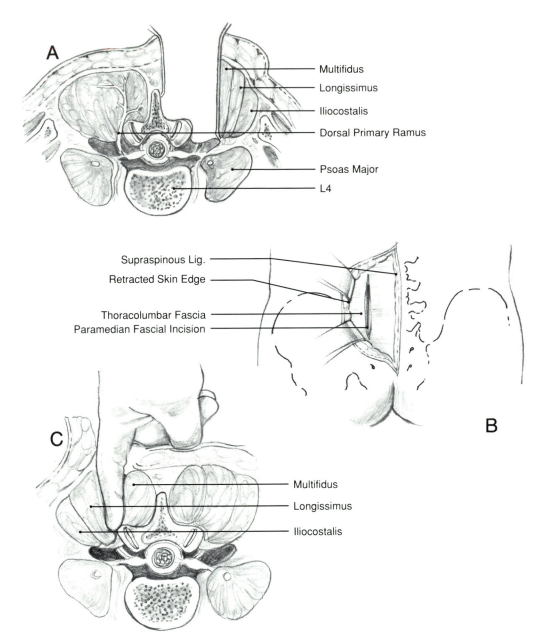

FIG 8–38.
Direct extraforaminal approach. **A,** midline approach. **B** and **C,** paramedian approach between the multifidus and longissimus
muscles.   *(Continued.)*

terolateral space, will also likely be noted. The outer
edge of the superior facet may be removed to facilitate exposure. The ventral ramus traverses the lower
portion of the intertransverse space, and the intervertebral disk is directly below it (Fig 8–38, E).

Transpedicular Approach.—The transpedicular
approach exposes the interior of the vertebral body,
intervertebral disk, and floor of the spinal canal. The
approximate entry site to the pedicle canal is identi-

fied by locating the confluence of the superior facet
process, transverse process, and pars interarticularis, a site recently referred to as the force nucleus
(Fig 8–39, A). The cortex is removed to expose the
underlying cancellous bone. This bone is then removed with a succession of curettes to allow identification of the cortical walls of the pedicle. Staying
within these walls and curetting ventrally allow entry to the vertebral body. The cancellous bone of the
body may be removed by curetting. Bleeding from

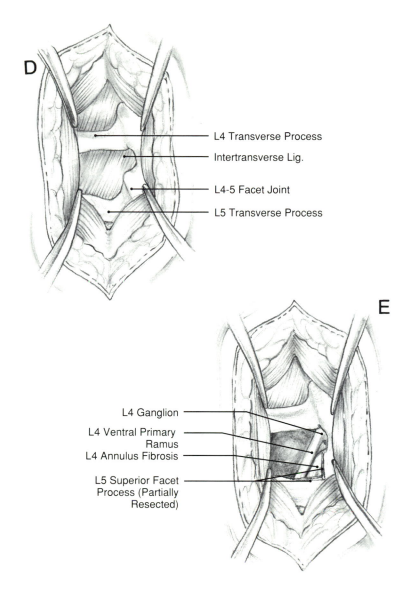

FIG 8–38 (cont.).

D, exposure of intertransverse ligament. **E,** exposure of the nerve root and intervertebral disk following removal of the intertransverse ligament and the outer edge of the superior facet. (Redrawn from Zindrick MR, Wiltse LL, Rauschning W: Disk herniations lateral to the intervertebral foramen, in White AH, Rothman RH, and Ray CD (eds): *Lumbar Spine Surgery.* St Louis, CV Mosby Co, 1987.)

the basivertebral plexus may be profuse and can be controlled with bone wax pushed into the pedicle entry site. Usually the approach is bilateral. The cephalad disk may be exposed by curetting through the pedicle in a cephalad direction (Figs 8–39, B and C).

For central canal decompression and/or osteotomy, the angle of approach may be dropped from relatively vertical to more horizontal by osteotomy of the transverse process and subperiosteal removal of the outer wall of the pedicle. The superior and inferior pedicle walls may likewise be removed. Finally,

the medial cortical wall of the pedicle is removed to expose the spinal canal. Removal of the pedicle medial wall exposes the posterior cortex of the vertebral body. Throughout the exposure meticulous subperiosteal dissection is necessary to minimize bleeding from the muscular branch of the dorsal spinal artery, its branches, and the anterior internal venous plexuses.

Posterior Ilium and Sacroiliac Joint.—A midline lumbosacral incision exposes these posterolateral structures. The skin is elevated and the plane be-

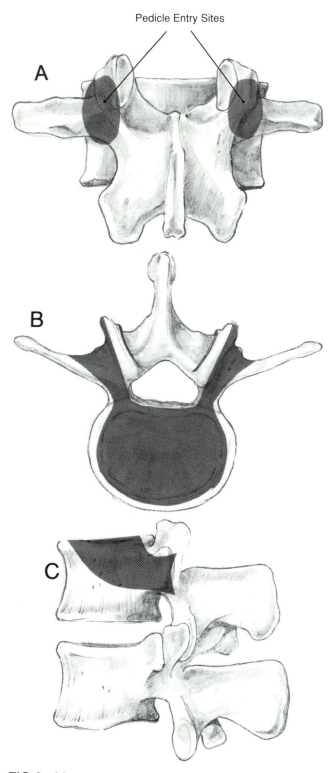

Pedicle Entry Sites

A

B

C

FIG 8–39.
Transpedicular approach. **A,** site of identification, entry, and enlargement of the pedicle intermedullary canal. **B,** axial view of the removed bone. **C,** sagittal view of the removed bone. (Redrawn from Heinig CF: Eggshell procedure, in Lugue E (ed): *Segmental Spinal Instrumentation.* Thorofare, New Jersey, Slack, 1984, pp 221–234.)

tween the loose connective tissue and lumbodorsal fascia developed. In this manner the posterior superior and inferior iliac spines and iliac crest are exposed (Fig 8–40, A). This is easier in males than females, in whom the posterior iliac crests are more widely separated. For direct exposure of the posterior iliac crest a supplemental paramedian incision just lateral to the posterior superior iliac spine is advisable (Fig 8–40, B). This helps protect the cluneal nerves from injury.

The outer table of the ilium is exposed by incision of the gluteal fascia and gluteus maximus muscle just below their origin and subperiosteally stripping of the outer table of the ilium. The sciatic notch is identified by subperiosteal dissection distal to the posterior inferior iliac spine. On the outer table of the ilium is a large nutrient foramen; bleeding from this area can be controlled with soft tissue electrocautery and bone wax. During bone graft removal, care is exercised to avoid penetrating the sacroiliac joint.

The reflected gluteal muscle and fascia are closed in a liquid-tight fashion with running layers of suture, usually two. Again, caution must be used to avoid the cluneal nerves that exit in the soft tissue directly over the crest. If they are injured, they should be gently tractioned, divided with electrocautery, and allowed to retract.

To expose the sacroiliac joint, the origins of the erector spinae muscle are mobilized from the iliac crest and separated from the medial portion of the crest by subperiosteal electrocautery dissection.

Posterior Rib Exposure.—Partial posterior rib removal may be desirable to treat rib cage deformity and/or procure a bone graft. The ribs arising from T5 through T10 are usually involved. It is usually best to preserve the eleventh and twelfth ribs to help preserve chest wall contour.

The cutaneous branches of the dorsal rami are best preserved by a paramedian incision over the apex of the rib deformity. However, to avoid a second incision, the midline incision is usually used. The cutaneous branches of the dorsal rami should be protected when possible. When sacrifice is necessary to obtain exposure, the cutaneous nerve should be gently tractioned, cut with electrocautery near its exit from the deep spinal musculature, and allowed to retract into the musculature. Any obvious distal remnant is excised.

From the midline incision the origins of the superficial back muscles (trapezius, latissimus dorsi, and rhomboids) are separated from the supraspinous ligament and the thin (at this point) thoracolumbar fascia that overlies the deep back muscles. Entry to this plane is facilitated by beginning caudally, where the thoracolumbar fascia is more distinct. Although somewhat difficult to establish in the midline, the plane between the superficial and deep muscles soon becomes apparent. This plane should be developed until the outer edge of the iliocostalis is reached. The indistinct interval between the iliocostalis and longissimus is then developed (Fig 8–41, A). Electrocautery is used to dissect these muscles from the ribs. Dissection continues to the tips of the transverse processes. Care is taken to preserve lateral branches of the dorsal rami.

The periosteum overlying the rib is then incised by electrocautery and the rib exposed by subperiosteal dissection (Fig 8–41, B). The rib is then resected from the posterior axillary line to just medial to the apex. The remaining medial portion of the rib should be removed, flush with the transverse process. Special caution is necessary in stripping the parietal pleura near the midline since it is quite thin. If the pleura is entered, it should be sutured and the suture tied while the lung is expanded. A chest tube should be inserted before or after closure.

Deep closure is accomplished with a running suture for the periosteal opening of the rib bed. The iliocostalis and longissimus edges are loosely reapproximated. A catheter for closed suction is placed

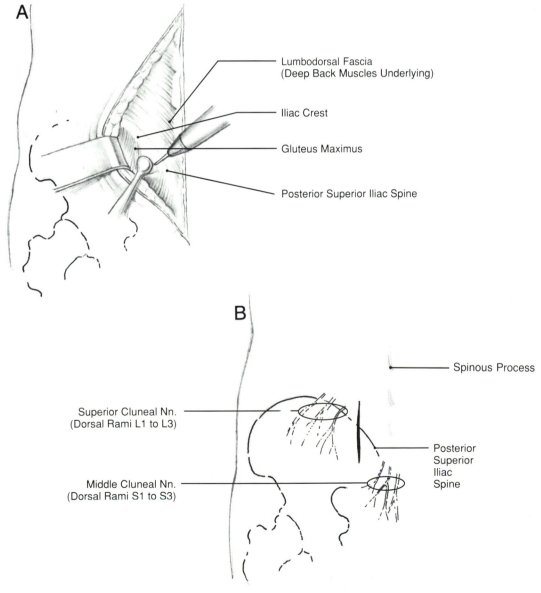

FIG 8–40.
Exposure of the iliac crest from the midline. **A,** midline incision and exposure. **B,** paramedian incision.

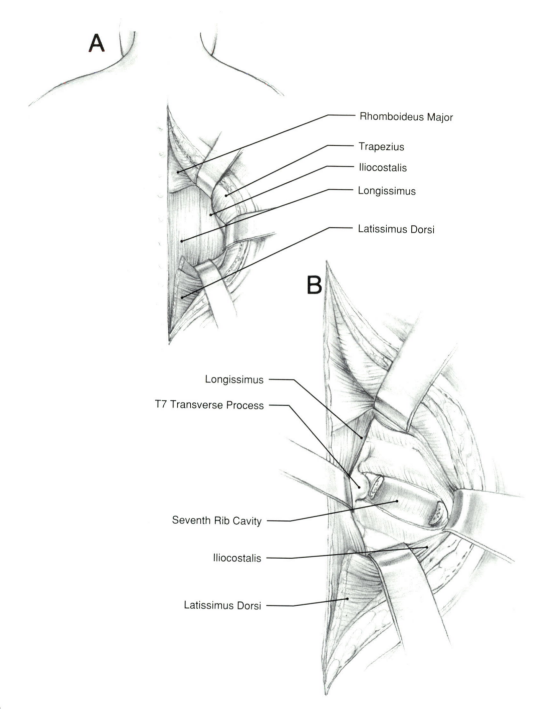

FIG 8–41.
Posterior rib exposure. **A,** dorsal exposure of the rib cage. **B,** removal of posterior portion of the rib.

in the interval between the deep and superficial muscle layers of the back. The origin of the superficial muscles is sutured to the midline fascia of the same side.

Closure.—Methods of closure vary slightly under diverse circumstances, at different levels, and among surgeons. In the lumbar spine, following ex-

tensive bilateral posterolateral dissection, a large potential dead space exists. This can be partially obliterated by closure of the remaining muscles of the deep back with loose nonstrangulating sutures. If instrumentation has been inserted, these sutures may be run under it. The midline fascial layer, represented by the divided half of the supraspinous ligament, is closed with interrupted sutures. In the lumbar spine these may be passed through the tip of the spinous processes. Unless laminectomy or osteotomy has been performed, liquid-tight closure of this same layer is accomplished with running resorbable sutures. If bleeding is minimal and closure is liquid-tight, postoperative closed suction is not needed; otherwise, a suction catheter is placed over the fascial closure. A catheter is also placed if the ilium is exposed from the midline or ribs are exposed. The subcutaneous tissues are closed with running resorbable sutures that pass through the deep dermis on the exit portion of the suture pass. The skin is usually closed with subcuticular resorbable sutures but sometimes with staples.

Dorsolateral Approaches

Thoracic Spine Approaches

Percutaneous Approach (T2 to T9).—A percutaneous approach may sometimes be used for biopsy of the thoracic spine vertebral bodies from T2 through T9. However, this is more difficult in the thoracic than the lumbar spine. Also, biopsy of a thoracic disk is generally impossible because of the overlying articular head of the rib. For these reasons, open transpedicular biopsy may be preferred.

The patient is positioned prone. Either biplanar fluoroscopy or computed tomography is necessary. Local anesthesia is used. Intravenous access with a large catheter should be provided, and anesthesia standby should be considered. Unless contraindicated by disease and location, the spine is approached from the right.

The biopsy path begins 4 cm (minor variation may be necessary because of body habitus) from the midline and between the transverse processes. It projects at a 35-degree angle toward the midsagittal plane and passes superiorly to the rib (Fig 8–42). This path passes in the same plane as the rib neck and enters the vertebral body at the base of the pedicle. During needle advancement, the patient is monitored for signs of nerve root irritation and gentle aspiration is maintained to monitor for chest cavity, vascular, or dural entry. If any of these occur, the needle is withdrawn. Once bone is reached, the biopsy needle is advanced 1 cm into the vertebral body. Overall, the needle should not be advanced more than 7 cm.

Costotransversectomy Approach.—This approach exposes the lateral spinal canal, thoracic disks, and lateral aspect of the vertebral body.

Although the patient may be positioned prone and a paramedian incision made, the semiprone po-

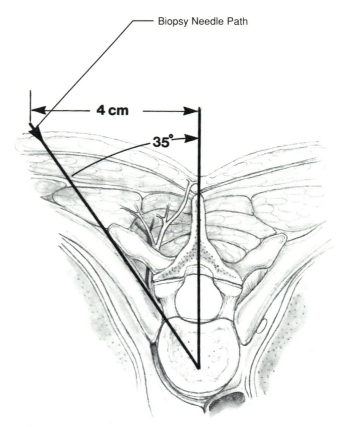

FIG 8–42.
Percutaneous approach to the thoracic spine (T2-9) (not drawn to scale).

sition and oblique incision are preferred (Fig 8–43, A)

The rib to be resected depends upon the structure to be approached. It is important to remember that the articular surface of the rib overlies the intervertebral disk between the body of the same number as the rib and the body above.

Following incision, the superficial back muscles may be divided in the direction of the incision or split in the direction of their fibers (Fig 8–43, B). The deep back muscles (iliocostalis and longissimus) and transversospinal muscles overlying the transverse process may then be divided in line with the rib and transverse process to be resected. Alternatively, the interval between the iliocostalis (laterally) and the longissimus (medially) may be developed by dissection.

The rib is then exposed subperiosteally; it is remembered that the pleura is quite thin medially. The rib from the apex to the tip of the transverse process is resected (Fig 8–43, C). The transverse process is cut with a rongeur and removed from the remaining rib head by incision of the costotransverse ligament.

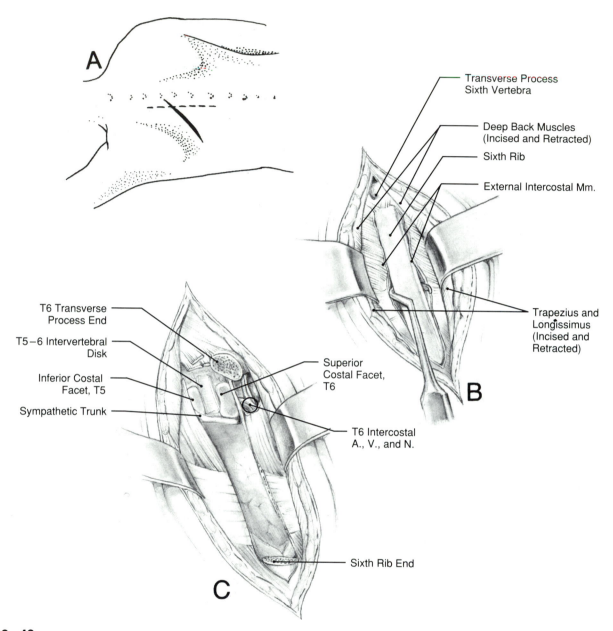

FIG 8–43.
Costotransversectomy. **A,** semiprone position and incision options (oblique incision: *solid line;* paramedian incision: *dashed line*). **B,** rib exposure. **C,** rib resection and disk exposure.

The rib head is then freed from its capsular attachment and disarticulated.

The neurovascular bundle associated with the unresected rib above and that associated with the resected rib are identified by developing the space between the intercostal muscles. The intervertebral disk and the pedicle just below it are identifiable and can be exposed subperiosteally. The vascular supply of this area is ample; however, bleeding can be controlled with bipolar electrocautery. Exposure of the spinal canal, if needed, is facilitated by pedicle resection.

Lumbar Spine Approaches

Percutaneous Approach (T10 to L5).—Patient position and anesthesia are the same as for thoracic biopsy.

For T10 through L3 biopsy, the entry path begins about 6.5 cm from the midline, even with the superior edge of the transverse process for disk biopsy and the inferior edge of the transverse process for body biopsy (Fig 8–44, A). The path projects at a 35-degree angle toward the midsagittal plane. The entry instrument may be a trochar or a 16- or 18-gauge spinal needle. During passage the patient is

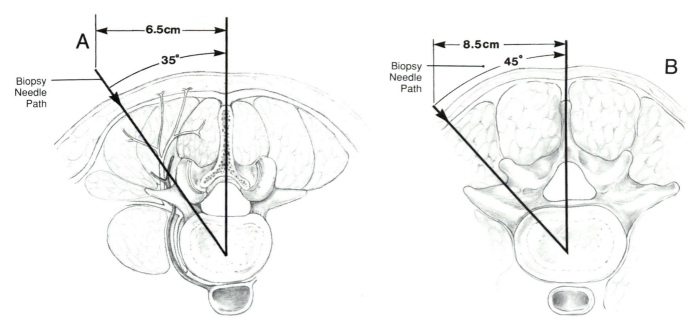

FIG 8–44.
Percutaneous approach to the lower thoracic and lumbar spine (T10 to L5). **A,** upper lumbar spine. **B,** lower lumbar spine (not drawn to scale).

monitored for nerve root irritation. If it occurs, entry is stopped and the instrument withdrawn and redirected. For L4 or L5 biopsy the entry path begins about 8.5 cm from the midline and projects at a 45-degree angle toward the midsagittal plane (Fig 8–44, B).

Ventrolateral and Ventral Approaches

Transthoracic Approach to Thoracic Spine (Third Through Ninth Ribs)

Upper, as opposed to lower, thoracic spine exposure is complicated somewhat by the presence of the scapula, trapezius, latissimus dorsi, rhomboids, and serratus anterior. Their relevant anatomy is shown in Figure 8–45, A and B.

The patient is positioned in the lateral decubitus position. The side of exposure is usually dictated by the focus of disease or deformity (Fig 8–45, C). If the side is optional, the right-sided approach (left lateral decubitus position) is better from T2 to T7 or T8, as the heart, aortic arch, and thoracic aorta make approach from the left somewhat more difficult.

For exposure through the third or fourth rib, a hockey-stick incision curving somewhat under the level of the scapula is made. The T1-T2 disk space can be reached through a third rib approach anteriorly, but only with difficulty.

The superficial back muscles (latissimus dorsi, trapezius, and rhomboids) are divided as close as

possible to their origins (Fig 8–45, D and E). This necessitates some development of the skin flap distally. The angle of the scapula is then retracted to expose the rib cage. To avoid denervation of the serratus anterior muscle (long thoracic nerve), this muscle is incised as near to its origin on the ribs (upper eighth or ninth) as possible. The third or fourth rib, whichever is desired, is then identified. This is done by counting both upward from the twelfth rib and downward from the first rib, which can be palpated under the retracted scapula and rhomboid major, which has been partially divided. The periosteum overlying the rib is incised (Fig 8–45, F). Dorsally this incision will pass through the serratus posterior superior, as well as the underlying deep back muscles (iliocostalis and longissimus). The rib is then exposed subperiosteally and removed from as near the costal cartilage as possible to the transverse process.

If a vascularized rib graft is planned, exposure of the rib is different. Rather than the periosteum, the cephalad (superior) interosseous muscles are incised (by electrocautery) at their attachment to the rib. The rib is then separated from its costal cartilage. The caudal (inferior) interosseous muscles are then divided about 3 to 4 cm caudal to the rib. The dorsal (proximal) portion of the rib (rib angle to transverse process) is then exposed subperiosteally. Care is taken to protect the interosseous vessels. The exposed rib is then osteotomized with a rib cutter. It is essential that the segmental vessels of this level not

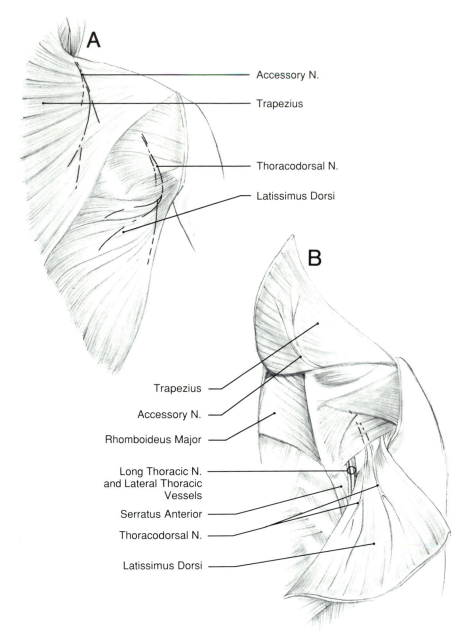

FIG 8–45.
Thoracotomy. **A** and **B,** relative anatomy of the trapezius, latissimus dorsi, rhomboids, serratus anterior, and their nerve supply.   *(Continued.)*

be ligated during subsequent exposure. Thus, for grafting above a curve apex of about T5, vascularized rib graft should be taken from two to three levels below the apex. For curves with apices below T5, the graft should be taken two to three levels above the apex.

Exposure through lower thoracotomies is similar, except that the incision is placed directly over the rib to be excised and retraction of the scapula is not necessary (Fig 8–45, C). Because of the angle of

the ribs, it is necessary to enter through a rib one or two levels cephalad to the cephalic end of the operative field. The extent of rib excision is from as close to the costal cartilage as possible, to the transverse process.

The pleural cavity is then entered by incision of the rib bed, with care taken to protect the underlying lung (Fig 8–45, G). The rib bed incision is best made relatively cephalad, thus leaving a better cuff of tissue at the caudal edge and providing protection

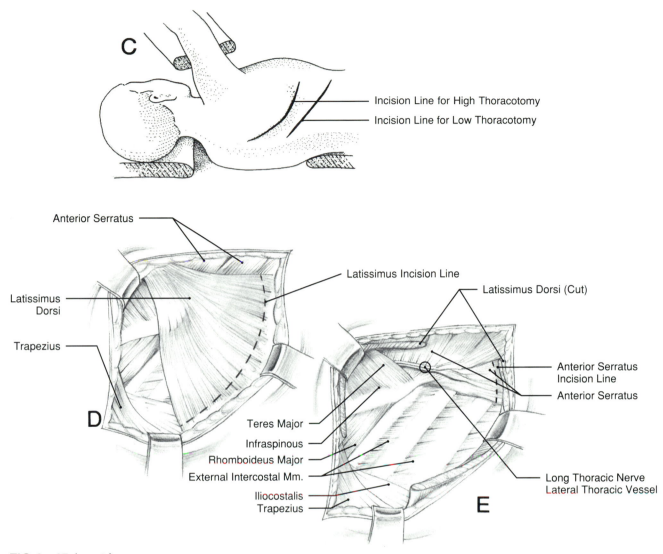

FIG 8–45 (cont.).
C, skin incision for high and low thoracotomy. **D,** latissimus dorsi incision *(dashed line).* **E,** serratus incision *(dashed line).*
(Continued.)

for the neurovascular bundle during closure. The lung is then allowed to collapse, and the rib cage is opened with a rib spreader.

The parietal pleura invests the spinal column, which is readily seen under it. The disks present as ridges and the bodies as valleys. The segmental vessels, which are under the parietal pleura, are over the bodies. The overlying parietal pleura is elevated and incised. Care is taken to protect the underlying segmental vessels.

The loose connective tissue plane underlying the prevertebral parietal pleura is then developed to expose the segmental vessels (Fig 8–45, H). If these vessels must be divided for exposure, they should be mobilized and divided some distance ventrally

from the intervertebral foramen. This helps protect the intersegmental arterial anastomoses present at any level of the intervertebral foramina.

Before closure, a chest tube is placed at approximately the T10-11 interspace in the midaxillary line. Closure is begun by reapproximating the prevertebral parietal pleura with running, locking, resorbable suture. The remaining ribs are approximated with pericostal sutures of doubled No. 1 chromic catgut. Suture placement between the inferior rib and its underlying neurovascular bundle may be done first and accomplished by subperiosteal passage of the needle next to the rib. This may decrease the incidence of intercostal pain. Usually the suture is placed so as to include most of the intercostal

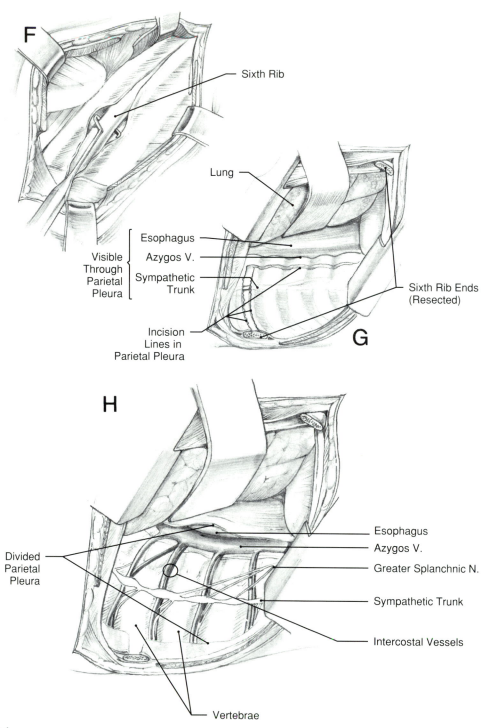

F

Sixth Rib

Lung

Esophagus

Azygos V.

Visible
Through
Parietal
Pleura

Sympathetic
Trunk

Sixth Rib Ends
(Resected)

Incision
Lines in
Parietal Pleura

G

H

Divided
Parietal
Pleura

Esophagus

Azygos V.

Greater Splanchnic N.

Sympathetic Trunk

Intercostal Vessels

Vertebrae

FIG 8–45 (cont.).
F, rib exposure. **G,** pleural cavity entry. (Note incision line in parietal pleura may be extended on undersurface of rib as shown.) **H,** spinal column exposure. (Redrawn from Bauer R, Kerschbaumer F, Poisel S: *Operative Approaches in Orthopedic Surgery and Traumatology.* Stuttgart, Thieme, 1987.)

muscles caudal to (below) the rib. Excluding the neurovascular bundle cephalad (above) is not difficult. After placement (but not tying) of the pericostal sutures, the intercostal gap is partially closed with the rib approximator and the intercostal muscles sutured with a running, locking, resorbable stitch. The ribs are then further approximated and the pericostal sutures tied. The divided muscle planes are then closed in layers with running suture.

Thoracolumbar Spine Approach

The side of approach is determined by the pathologic condition. If optional, the left side is generally preferred, because the aorta, with its firmer wall, is easier to mobilize than the vena cava. In addition, there is less interference from the spleen and liver. However, two precautionary notes are in order. First, the giant anterior medullary feeder artery (Adamkiewicz), when present, is more common on the left. Second, implants applied from the left to the ventral surface of the spine may threaten major vascular structures.

The presence and location of the thoracoabdominal nerves (intercostal nerves 7 to 11) dictate placement of the incision line for the thoracoabdominal exposure (Figs 8–46, A and B). To avoid abdominal wall denervation, it is best to incise between the thoracoabdominal nerves and, when distal extension is needed, transect the segmentally innervated rectus and proceed across the opposite rectus if necessary. Another means of extension is to proceed down the midline linea alba, remembering that the aponeurosis of the internal oblique muscle is not divided in the lower one fourth of the abdominal wall. This transition is known as the arcuate line of the rectus sheath, and below this point the internal and external abdominal obliques, as well as the transverse abdominis aponeurosis, pass ventrally to the rectus abdominis muscle (Fig 8–46, B). In any event, it is desirable to avoid distal pararectus extension along the outer edge of the rectus sheath (linea semilunaris), as this interrupts segmental innervation of the rectus muscle.

The patient is placed in a lateral decubitus position but allowed to rotate posteriorly 10 to 20 degrees (Fig 8–46, C). The incision is begun just lateral to the midline over the proximal portion of the rib to be excised (usually the ninth or tenth) and follows the direction of the rib ventrally toward the abdominal midline (toward the umbilicus in the case of the tenth rib).

The thoracic exposure for this approach is the same as for the transthoracic approach.

Over the abdomen the external abdominal oblique muscle and, medially, its fascia are incised in the direction of the skin incision. The internal oblique and transversalis muscles and fascia are divided at their attachment to the costal cartilage, which is also incised (Fig 8–46, D). Digital palpation through this small opening, beginning on the undersurface of the rib cage, allows ready entry into the subdiaphragmatic retroperitoneal space below the anterolateral and lateral abdominal wall. This exposure is progressively enlarged by alternately continuing the incision of the diaphragm (about 1 cm from the chest wall) and stripping the peritoneum from the undersurface of the transversalis fascia. The internal oblique and transversalis layers are usually mobilized together and, when sufficiently cleared of the peritoneum, divided (Fig 8–46, E). If the peritoneal cavity is entered, the edges are approximated with running 2-0 resorbable suture.

The retroperitoneal contents, including the ureter and spleen or liver, are mobilized toward the midline. The retroperitoneal space contains a fibrofatty layer of varying thickness. This is mobilized by digital dissection and division of the fibrous connections as needed. This fibrofatty tissue is mobilized near the posterior abdominal wall to provide entry into the posterior retroperitoneal space and expose the transversalis fascia overlying the quadratus lumborum and psoas muscles. During this dissection, care is taken to protect not only the iliohypogastric and ilioinguinal nerves, which exit the interval between these two muscles, but also the genitofemoral nerve as it exits through the substance of the psoas muscle at about the midlumbar spine (Fig 8–46, F).

The parietal pleura over the thoracic spine is incised and mobilized as described for the thoracic exposure. The lumbar disk (elevations) and bodies (depressions) may be palpated and even visualized under a thin layer of fibrofatty tissue. The aorta (left side), and particularly the vena cava (right side), can be readily palpated and seen. The medial border of the psoas is visible over the anterolateral aspect of the bodies. Along the medial border of the psoas major, the sympathetic trunk is both palpable and visible. The bodies and disks are further exposed by division of the overlying transversalis fascia and mobilization of the medial border of the psoas, along with the sympathetic trunk, in a lateral direction. This mobilization necessitates transection of some or all of the lumbar splanchnic nerves passing from the sympathetic ganglia to join the celiac intermesenteric and superior hypogastric plexus. Transecting these nerves does not seem to be detrimental, as the plex-

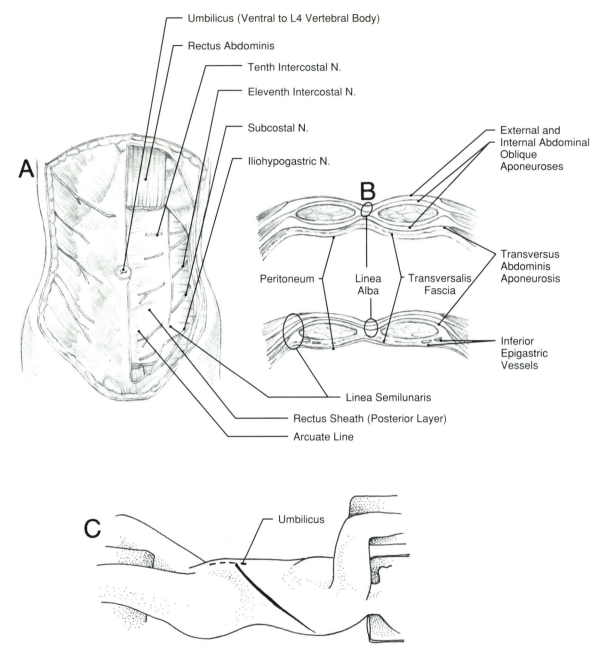

FIG 8–46.
Thoracolumbar exposure. **A,** relative abdominal wall anatomy. **B,** cross-section of the rectus sheath above *(top)* and below *(bottom)* the arcuate line. **C,** position and skin incision *(dashed line* indicates distal extension). *(Continued.)*

uses obtain splanchnic branches from the opposite side and from the more proximal plexuses, which are supplied by the greater (T5-9 or 10) and lesser (T9-11) splanchnic nerves.

Further exposure of the spinal column anteriorly requires mobilization of the crus of the diaphragm from its ventral origin on the vertebral bodies, L1 and L2 on the left and L1 to L3 on the right. At least one large segmental vessel usually passes under the

crus. If more anterior body exposure is desired, the space between the vertebral bodies and great vessels may be developed. Exposure beyond the midline almost certainly requires ligation of the segmental vessels. To protect the interforaminal anastomoses, this should be done away from the intervertebral foramen, near the anterolateral aspect of the bodies. For disk excision only it is desirable to preserve the segmental vessels, especially the larger ones. This can-

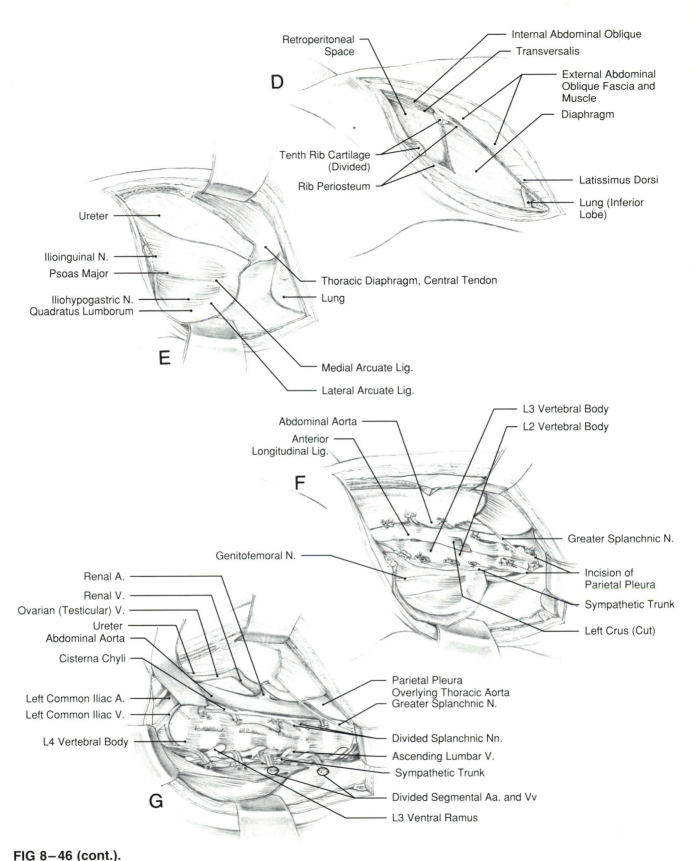

FIG 8–46 (cont.).

D, entry into the pleural cavity and retroperitoneal space. **E,** exposure of the pleural cavity and retroperitoneal space. **F,** exposure of the anterior surface of the spine. **G,** reflection of the psoas and exposure of the ventral rami and base of the pedicles. (Modified from Bauer R, Kerschbaumer F, Poisel S: *Operative Approaches in Orthopedic Surgery and Traumatology.* Stuttgart, Thieme, 1987.)

not be done if intersegmental implants are to be inserted.

In mobilization of the psoas from its vertebral body origins, it is important to remember that the lumbar ventral rami enter the psoas substance almost immediately after exiting the intervertebral foramen. With continued reflection of the psoas, the ventral rami eventually become visible along with the base of the pedicle (Fig 8–46, G). Removal of the pedicle provides visualization of the spinal canal.

Closure is begun by placement of a chest tube in the midaxillary line from about the eighth and ninth rib interspace or lower. The tube is positioned posteriorly in the thoracic cavity, extending to the upper thoracic levels. The crus is then reattached. The parietal pleura is closed with a running resorbable suture. The reflected edge of the psoas muscle is brought back toward its origin, with sutures placed into the periosteum overlying the vertebral bodies. The overlying transversalis fascia is generally too thin to close. The diaphragm may be reattached with a running long-life resorbable suture, which may be interrupted on two or three occasions, or with interrupted sutures. Before diaphragmatic closure is completed, abdominal wall closure is begun with running, long-life resorbable suture placed in the internal oblique-transversalis layer. The internal oblique-transversalis layer must be palpated on its undersurface to be sure there are no abdominal wall deficiencies that could lead to herniation. Just before the costal cartilage is reapproximated, the remainder of the diaphragm is closed. The chest portion of the incision is closed as for thoracic exposure, as described previously. The external oblique layer of muscle and fascia is closed with a running, long-life resorbable suture. This muscle is in essentially the same layer as the latissimus dorsi. Subcutaneous tissues and skin edges are closed.

Twelfth Rib Subdiaphragmatic Approach to the Lumbar Spine

Considerations of side of approach are the same as for thoracoabdominal exposure.

A 45-degree oblique position is used (Fig 8–47, A). The spine incision begins just lateral to the midline dorsally and extends obliquely towards the midline at a point about one third of the distance from the umbilicus to the pubis.

Following incision of the external oblique and latissimus dorsi muscles, the tips of the eleventh and twelfth ribs can be readily palpated. The twelfth rib is further exposed by incision of the serratus posteroinferior and the underlying iliocostalis and longus muscles. These are incised along the direction of the rib from the costal cartilage anteriorly to the transverse process posteriorly. Rib periosteum is then incised near the upper edge of the rib, allowing rib exposure. The rib's cartilaginous tip is avulsed by lifting, and the rib is removed back to the end of the transverse process. The costal cartilage is lifted and the adjacent attached internal abdominal oblique and transversalis muscles, as well as the ventral rib periosteum and peripheral diaphragm, are incised. In this manner, the retroperitoneal space below the diaphragm (Fig 8–47, B) and extrapleural space above the diaphragm (Fig 8–47, C) are entered.

The retroperitoneal portion of the exposure is the same as the thoracoabdominal exposure. Distal extension, as described for the lumbar retroperitoneal approach, provides access to the entire lumbar spine.

Further development of the extrapleural portion of the approach provides exposure of the thoracolumbar junction, i.e., T12 body, T12 disk, and L1 body. Extrapleural exposure is best accomplished by stripping the pleural sac from its peripheral attachment to the diaphragm. The parietal pleural reflection is then carefully stripped from its attachment to the undersurface of the periosteum of the rib, moving in a caudad to cephalad direction. Once it is separated from the parietal pleura, the deep rib periosteum is incised. As the pleura may be quite adherent to the periosteum, it may be necessary to divide the periosteum near its inferior or caudal edge (Fig 8–47, D).

The twelfth rib can usually be removed while the integrity of the pleural cavity is preserved. This is very difficult with the eleventh rib. However, following twelfth rib removal and extrapleural exposure as described, further access to the thoracolumbar junction may be gained by eleventh rib resection, leaving its underlying periosteum intact.

If the pleural cavity is entered, it should be closed in an airtight manner with running, locking suture. The lung should be expanded before the suture is tied. This will sometimes obviate the need for a chest tube, a need that can be monitored postoperatively with chest radiographs. Alternatively, a chest tube can be placed before the patient is moved from the operating table.

Further exposure of the spinal column is done in the same manner as thoracolumbar exposure. Reflection of the psoas major muscle is easiest if begun over the intervertebral disks, because its origin is more secure there and the segmental vessels lie over the vertebral bodies. Even though the segmental

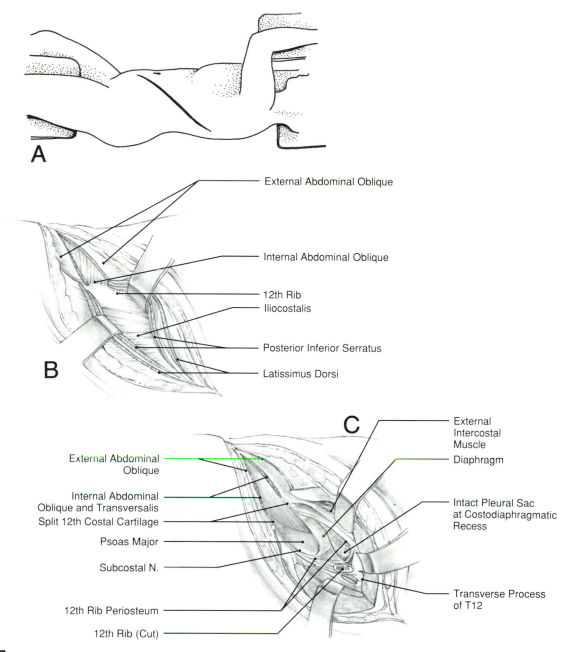

External Abdominal Oblique

Internal Abdominal Oblique

12th Rib
Iliocostalis

Posterior Inferior Serratus

Latissimus Dorsi

External
Intercostal
Muscle

External Abdominal
Oblique

Diaphragm

Internal Abdominal
Oblique and Transversalis

Split 12th Costal Cartilage

Intact Pleural Sac
at Costodiaphragmatic
Recess

Psoas Major

Subcostal N.

Transverse Process
of T12

12th Rib Periosteum

12th Rib (Cut)

FIG 8–47.
Subdiaphragmatic approach to the lumbar spine with removal of the twelfth rib. **A,** position and skin incision. **B,** entry into the retroperitoneal space. **C,** exposure of extrapleural space. *(Continued.)*

vessels have been ligated and tied near the midline, further mobilization dorsally may result in bleeding, which can be controlled by further ligation or vascular clips.

Exposure of the ventral primary rami and pedicle may require sacrifice of some of the sympathetic trunk. This causes a temporary increase in temperature of the ipsilateral leg and foot, but does not appear to cause any long-term problems.

Spinal canal exposure is now possible (Fig 8–47, E). This involves careful removal of the disks on either side of the abnormal vertebral body, removal of cancellous bone from the middle and posterior thirds of the vertebral body, removal of adjacent cephalad and caudal vertebral end-plates and pedicle, and, lastly, removal of the posterior wall of the vertebral body. Visualization aids protection of the nerve root(s) and dural sac. Removal of the cancel-

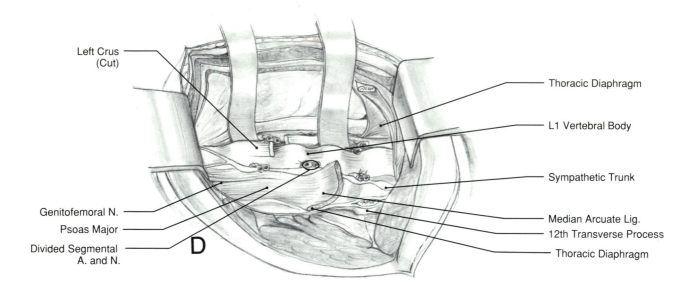

Left Crus (Cut)

Thoracic Diaphragm

L1 Vertebral Body

Sympathetic Trunk

Genitofemoral N.

Psoas Major

Divided Segmental A. and N.

Median Arcuate Lig.

12th Transverse Process

Thoracic Diaphragm

D

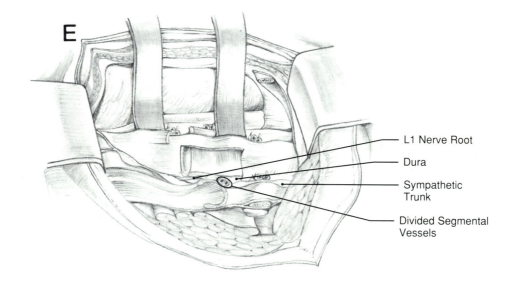

E

L1 Nerve Root

Dura

Sympathetic Trunk

Divided Segmental Vessels

FIG 8–47 (cont.).
D, diaphragm transected. **E,** exposure of the spinal canal. (Modified from Bauer R, Kerschbaumer F, Poisel S: *Operative Approaches in Orthopedic Surgery and Traumatology.* Stuttgart, Thieme, 1987.)

lous bone from the body before canal exposure eliminates, or at least diminishes, blood loss from the basivertebral plexus. During cancellous bone removal, bleeding from the plexus, which may be brisk, can be controlled by packing with bone wax. Cancellous bone removal, including cephalad and caudad subchondral end-plate removal, further provides a void to receive the posterior wall of the vertebral body. During canal exposure, bipolar coagulation of the internal venous plexus, and at times the spinal branch of the segmental artery, is often necessary.

Closure is similar to that of the thoracolumbar

incision, except that there are no remaining ribs to approximate. To avoid incisional concavity, layer closure of at least the outer layer of the rib periosteum and of the iliocostalis-longissimus and serratus posteroinferior is necessary.

Lower Lumbar Spine Approaches

Retroperitoneal Approach.—Unless determined by the disease process being treated, approach from the left is preferred. Mobilization of the major vessels overlying the lower lumbar spine is easier from the left.

The patient is placed in semisupine position with the operative side elevated 20 to 30 degrees. The distal end of the incision is located at or near the abdominal midline, midway between the umbilicus and pubis. This point is directly over the L5-S1 junction and midway between the subcostal and iliohypogastric nerves. The incision then extends obliquely posteriorly in a line midway between the iliac crests and the twelfth rib. Proximal extension toward the dorsal midline provides access to the midlumbar spine. Distal extension, whether by midline division of the linea alba or continuation of the incision across the midline rectus sheath and underlying rectus, provides access to the lumbosacral junction (Fig 8–48, A).

The external and internal oblique muscles are di-

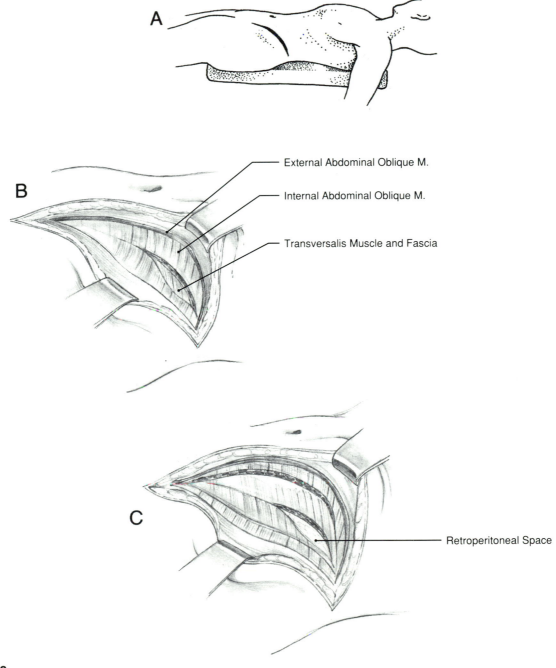

FIG 8–48.
Retroperitoneal exposure of the lumbar spine. **A,** position and skin incision. **B,** incision of the external and internal oblique muscles. **C,** posterolateral entry into the retroperitoneal space. *(Continued.)*

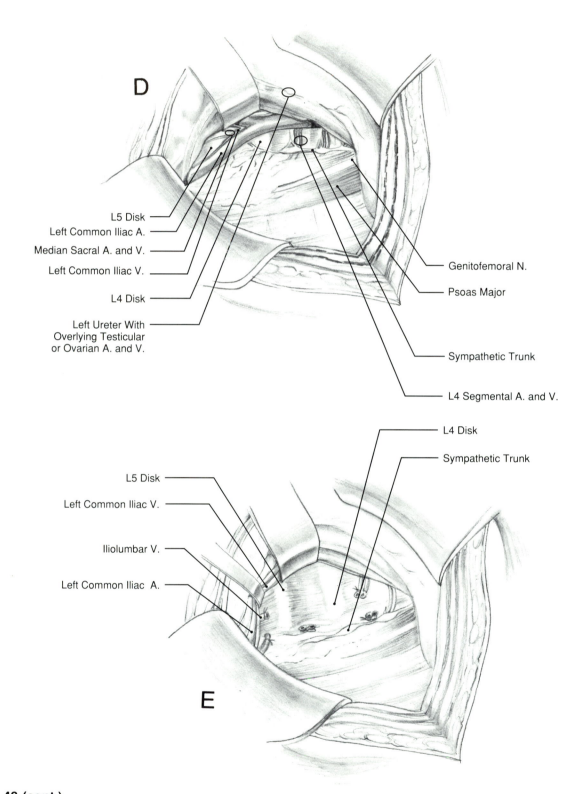

D

L5 Disk

Left Common Iliac A.

Median Sacral A. and V.

Left Common Iliac V.

L4 Disk

Left Ureter With
Overlying Testicular
or Ovarian A. and V.

Genitofemoral N.

Psoas Major

Sympathetic Trunk

L4 Segmental A. and V.

L4 Disk

Sympathetic Trunk

L5 Disk

Left Common Iliac V.

Iliolumbar V.

Left Common Iliac A.

E

FIG 8–48 (cont.).
D, visualization of the spine and adjacent structures. **E,** exposure after ligation of the iliolumbar vein and segmental vessels, allowing retraction of the left common iliac vessels.

vided in line with the skin incision (Fig 8–48, B). Incision of the transversalis muscle begins at the dorsal (proximal) end of the incision, as entry into the retroperitoneal space is easier because of an interval layer of fat (Fig 8–48, C). The transversalis is divided ventrally to the edge of the rectus sheath (linea semilunaris). If distal extension is planned or needed, the external and internal oblique aponeuroses overlying the rectus muscle are divided to the midline, and the rectus is transected. Distal incision of the linea alba may then be performed as needed, or extension across the midline may be used. As the linea semilunaris is approached, the inferior epigastric vessels will likely be encountered. They are clamped and tied as necessary to provide adequate exposure.

The retroperitoneal space is enlarged and the retroperitoneal contents mobilized to the right to expose the abdominal aorta and its bifurcation into the common iliac arteries (Fig 8–48, D). The testicular or ovarian artery and vein overlying the ureter will be seen. The common iliac veins and their junction to form the inferior vena cava will be seen underlying the aorta. Overlying the aorta is the superior hypogastric plexus.

Approach to the spine between the great vessels and psoas requires mobilization and ligation of the segmental vessels (Fig 8–48, E). Over the bodies of L3 and L4 this is relatively easy. The anterolateral approach to the L5 body and L5-S1 disk space is blocked by the common iliac vein, which is tethered by the short, rather large, iliolumbar vein (see Fig 8–23). Mobilization and ligation of this vessel are necessary for distal exposure. Once the iliolumbar vein is ligated, however, the common iliac artery and vein can be elevated to expose as far as the L5-S1 disk space.

An alternative for L5-S1 exposure is to mobilize the preaortic soft tissue, which includes the superior hypogastric plexus, and to expose the L5-S1 junction directly anteriorly by identifying and ligating the median sacral artery and vein. This allows a more direct approach to the anterior aspect of the L5-S1 disk space but may increase the risk of hypogastric plexus disruption. This may rarely lead to retrograde ejaculation.

Closure is same as for the lumbar portion of the thoracolumbar approach.

Transperitoneal Approach.—The patient is positioned supine. Either a midline or a Pfannenstiel incision may be used (Fig 8–49, A). If limited access to no more than the L4-5 and L5-S1 disk is needed, and cosmesis is desired, the curved Pfannenstiel incision, located centrally about 8 cm above the pubic symphysis, may be used. The upper portion of the incision is then raised as a full-thickness flap. This allows midline incision of the linea alba. Care is taken to identify and protect the dome of the bladder at the inferior portion of the incision.

The midline incision, which begins about 5 cm above the umbilicus and ends about 5 cm above the pubis, is preferred because it allows for extensile exposure. Following incision of the linea alba (Fig 8–49, B), the transversalis fascia and peritoneum are incised (Fig 8–49, C). The omentum and abdominal contents are then mobilized proximally. The urinary bladder will be palpated distally. In this manner the posterior peritoneum is exposed (Fig 8–49, D). The posterior peritoneum is carefully elevated and incised to protect the underlying fibers of the superior hypogastric plexus (Fig 8–49, E). This plexus is mobilized as seems appropriate, usually from right to left. The median sacral artery and vein are identified and ligated (Fig 8–49, F).

The L5-S1 disk is approached immediately below the bifurcation of the aorta and the junction of the common iliac veins. The left common iliac vein tends to overlie the L5-S1 disk and, for best protection, should be mobilized and gently retracted intermittently with a vessel loop.

Depending upon the configuration of the patient, approach to the L4-5 disk may be either lateral to the aorta and vena cava or between the common iliac arteries to the left and the vena cava to the right (Fig 8–49, G). The segmental vessels should be mobilized and tied. Exposure may be continued proximally to visualize the L3-4 disk space, but will need to be carried out between the aorta and vena cava to protect the inferior mesenteric artery, which branches at the L3 level.

The posterior peritoneum is closed with a running suture. The hypogastric plexus is avoided. The anterior peritoneum is closed with a running suture. The rectus sheath is closed with interrupted sutures.

Anterior Iliac Crest Approach

Although it is remote to the spine, exposure of the iliac crest may be necessary for the purpose of obtaining bone graft.

An oblique incision is made just below the crest of the ilium from just lateral to the anterior superior iliac spine to about the junction of the anterior one third and posterior two thirds of the crest (Fig 8–50, A). The external oblique muscle, which overlaps the upper portion of the iliac crest, is mobilized proxi-

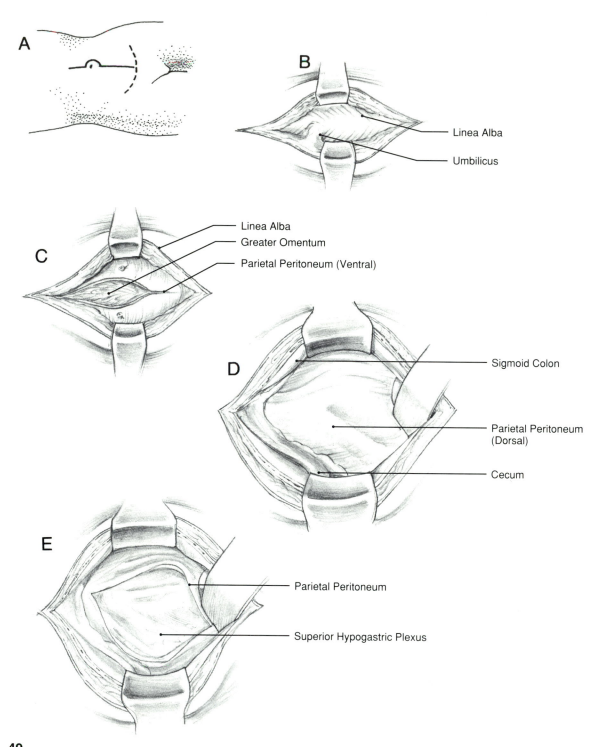

FIG 8–49.
Anterior transperitoneal exposure of the lower lumbar spine and lumbosacral junction (*solid line* = midline incision; *dashed line* = Pfannenstiel incision). **A,** position and skin incision. **B,** exposure of the linea alba. **C,** splitting of the peritoneum after division of the linea alba. **D,** visualization of the posterior peritoneal layer. **E,** incision of the posterior peritoneum.

(Continued.)

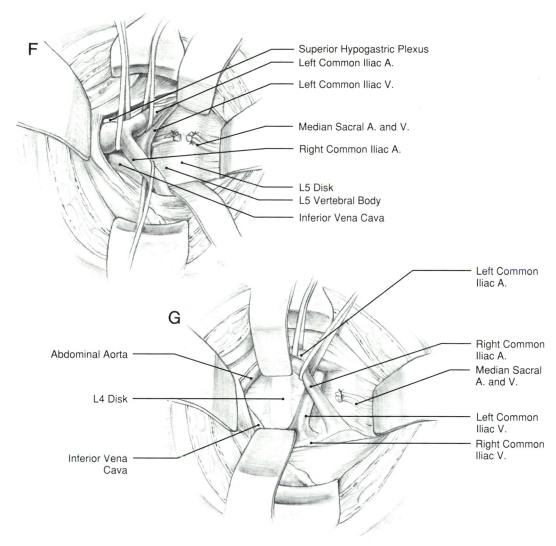

FIG 8–49 (cont.).
F, exposure of the sacral promontory. **G,** exposure of the fourth lumbar vertebra and L4-5 disk. (Modified from Bauer R, Kerschbaumer F, Poisel S: *Operative Approaches in Orthopedic Surgery and Traumatology.* Stuttgart, Thieme, 1987.)

mally by electrocautery dissection of the superficial portion of its insertion on the iliac crest (Fig 8–50, B). Small sensory nerves (lateral cutaneous branches of the hypogastric and subcostal nerves) may be encountered. If they cannot be protected, they should be gently tractioned, divided with electrocautery adjacent to their exit points, and allowed to retract into the external oblique muscle. With the outer external oblique elevated, the gluteus medius fascia and muscle are incised directly below the top of the crest. A small cuff of soft tissue is left attached to the crest to aid closure. The outer table is exposed by subperiosteal dissection (Fig 8–50, C).

If exposure of the inner table alone is desired,

fascial and periosteal attachments just below the medial edge of the iliac crest are incised and subperiosteal dissection is performed (Fig 8–50, D).

If exposure of both tables is needed, the periosteum overlying the crest can be divided and subperiosteal dissection accomplished on both the inner and outer tables. In children the cartilaginous iliac apophysis should be incised with a scalpel and preserved as much as possible, as it is split. Need for removal of the top of the crest may be avoided by removal of a rectangular bicortical graft (Fig 8–50, E). This avoids any unpleasant change in crest contour.

During closure the fascial and muscular layers should be securely reattached with running locking

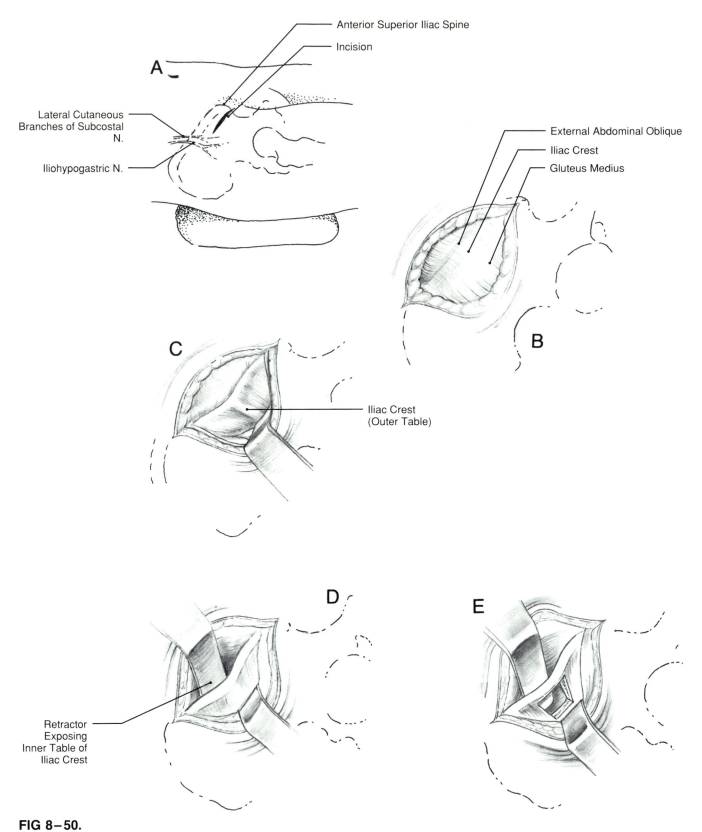

FIG 8–50.
Exposure of the anterior iliac crest. **A,** skin incision. **B,** external oblique mobilization. **C,** outer table. **D,** inner table. **E,** removal of bicortical graft.

sutures. The external oblique overlap is secured over the deeper incision.

BIBLIOGRAPHY

Altemeier WA, Alexander JW: Retroperitoneal abscess. *Arch Surg* 1961; 83:512–524.

Asher MA, Strippgen WE: Anthropometric studies of the human sacrum relating to dorsal transsacral implant designs. *Clin Orthop* 1986; 203:48–62.

Bauer R, Kerschbaumer F, Poisel S: *Operative Approaches in Orthopedic Surgery and Traumatology.* Stuttgart, Thieme, 1987.

Bogduk N, Twomey LT: *Clinical Anatomy of the Lumbar Spine.* New York, Churchill Livingstone, Inc, 1987.

Bohlman HH, Freehafer A, Dejak J: The results of treatment of acute injuries of the upper thoracic spine with paralysis. *J Bone Joint Surg* 1985; 67:360–369.

Bradford DS, Lonstein JE, Moe JH, et al: *Moe's Textbook of Scoliosis and Other Spinal Deformities,* ed 2. Philadelphia, WB Saunders Co, 1987.

Brown JE, Nordby EJ, Smith L: *Chemonucleolysis.* Thorofare, Slack, NJ, 1985.

Capener N: The evolution of lateral rachotomy. *J Bone Joint Surg* 1954; 36B:173–179.

Crenshaw AH: *Campbell's Operative Orthopaedics,* ed 7. St Louis, CV Mosby Co, 1987.

Dommissee GF: *The Arteries and Veins of the Human Spinal Cord and Brain.* New York, Churchill Livingstone, 1975.

Glossary of Spinal Terminology. Chicago, American Academy of Orthopaedic Surgeons, 1985.

Golub BS, Silverman B: Transforaminal ligaments of the lumbar spine. *J Bone Joint Surg* 1969; 51A:947–956.

Grant JCB: *Grant's Atlas of Anatomy,* ed 5. Baltimore, Williams & Wilkins Co, 1962.

Gray H: *Anatomy of the Human Body,* ed 30. Philadelphia, Lea & Febiger, 1973.

Hadley LA: *Anatomico-Roentgenographic Studies of the Spine.* Springfield, Ill, Charles C Thomas, Publisher, 1964.

Heinig CF: Eggshell procedure, in Luque E (ed): *Segmental Spinal Instrumentation.* Thorofare, Slack, NJ, 1984, pp 221–234.

Hodgson AR, Stock FE: Anterior spine fusion. *Br J Surg* 1956; 44:266–275.

Hodgson AR, Stock FE, Fang HSY, Ong GB: Anterior spine fusion. *Br J Surg* 1960; 48:172–178.

Hollinshead WH: *Anatomy for Surgeons. Vol 3: The Back and Limbs,* ed 2. New York, Harper & Row, 1969.

Hoppenfeld S, deBoer P: *Orthopaedics: The Anatomic Approach.* Philadelphia, JB Lippincott Co, 1984.

Leong JCY: Anterior interbody fusion, in Lin PM, Gill K (eds): *Lumbar Interbody Fusion.* Rockville, Md, Aspen Publishing Co, 1989, pp 133–148.

Lombard JS: The lumbosacral ligament, cited by Wiltse L: The intervertebral foramina, in Watkins RG, Collis JS (eds): *Lumbar Discectomy and Laminectomy.* Rockville, MD, Aspen Publishing Co, 1987, pp 211 and 213.

Louis R: *Surgery of the Spine.* Berlin, Springer-Verlag, 1983.

McAfee PC, Bohlman HH, Yuan HA: Anterior decompression of traumatic thoracolumbar fractures with incomplete neurological deficit using a retroperitoneal approach. *J Bone Joint Surg* 1985; 67A:89–104.

McMinn RMH, Hatchings, RT: *Color Atlas of Human Anatomy.* Chicago, Year Book Medical Publishers, 1977.

Meyers MA: *Dynamic Radiology of the Abdomen: Normal and Pathologic Anatomy,* ed 2. New York, Springer-Verlag, New York, 1982.

Michelle AA, Krueger FJ: Surgical approach to the vertebral body. *J Bone Joint Surg* 1949; 31A:873–878.

Morrison AB: The levatores costarum and their nerve supply. *J Anat* 1954; 88:19.

Netter FH: *The Ciba Collection of Medical Illustrations. Vol 8: Musculoskeletal System. Part I: Anatomy, Physiology, and Metabolic Disorders.* Summit, NJ, Ciba-Geigy Corp, 1987.

Ottolenghi CE: Diagnosis of orthopaedic lesions by aspiration biopsy. *J Bone Joint Surg* 1955; 37A:443–464.

Ottolenghi CE: Aspiration biopsy of the spine. *J Bone Joint Surg* 1969; 51A:1531–1544.

Rathke FW, Schlegel KF: *Surgery of the Spine.* Stuttgart, Thieme, 1979.

Rohen JW, Yokochi C: *Color Atlas of Anatomy: A Photographic Study of the Human Body.* Tokyo, Igaku-Shoin, 1984.

Rothman RH, Simeone FA: *The Spine,* ed 2. Philadelphia, WB Saunders Co, 1982.

Simons GW, Sty JR, Starshak RJ: Retroperitoneal and retrofascial abscesses. *J Bone Joint Surg* 1983; 65A:1041–1058.

Steele HH: Rib resection and spine fusion in correction of convex deformity in scoliosis. *J Bone Joint Surg* 1983; 65A:920–925.

Steffee AD, Biscup RS, Sitkowski DJ: Segmental spine plates with pedicle screw fixation: A new internal fixation device for disorders of the lumbar and thoracolumbar spine. *Clin Orthop* 1986; 203:45–53.

Thron AK: *Vascular Anatomy of the Spinal Cord.* New York, Springer-Verlag, New York, 1988.

Transfeldt E, Bradford DS, Robinson D, Heithoff K: The cause of neurologic deficit in acute spondylolisthesis (listhetic crisis) and in reduction of grades III-V spondylolisthesis. *Orthop Trans* 1987; 11:112.

Watkins RG: *Surgical Approaches to the Spine.* New York, Springer-Verlag, New York, 1983.

White AA, Panjabi MM: The basic kinematics of the human spine: A review of past and current knowledge. *Spine* 1978; 3:12–20.

Williams PL, Warwick R: *Gray's Anatomy,* ed 36. New York, Churchill Livingstone, Inc, 1980.

Woodburne RT: *Essentials of Human Anatomy.* New York, Oxford University Press, 1957.

Zindrick MR, Wiltse LL, Rauschning W: Disc herniations lateral to the intervertebral foramen, in White AH, Rothman RH, Ray CD (eds): *Lumbar Spine Surgery.* St Louis, CV Mosby Co, 1987.

PART IV

Pelvis and Lower Limb

Overview

Frederick W. Reckling, M.D.

The pelvis (from the Greek *pyelos*, an oblong trough, or basin) supports and protects the lower abdominal organs and transmits forces from the head, arms, and trunk to the lower extremities. The pelvis also provides attachment for muscles of balance and locomotion (Fig IV–1).

The hip joint is the most structurally stable, yet mobile, joint in the body. In addition to transmitting large forces from the trunk and the ground, it plays a major role in locomotion. In addition it participates in elevating or lowering the body, as in climbing or in rising from a chair. With every step the hip abductors on the stance leg must create a force to balance about 85% of the body weight (head, arms, trunk, and opposite leg). The hip joint serves as a fulcrum during locomotion and therefore sustains more than twice the body weight with each step.

The thigh provides a conduit for neurovascular structures of the extremity, and the femur provides attachments for the muscles of locomotion. Forces are transmitted from the foot, leg, and knee to the hip via the femur.

The knee is a complex joint with three articulating surfaces, the medial tibiofemoral, lateral tibiofemoral, and patellofemoral. The knee can support the body in the erect position without muscle contraction. It participates in lowering and elevating the body weight during sitting, squatting, and climbing. It also permits rotation of the body when the individual turns on a planted foot. In walking, the normal knee reduces energy expenditure by decreasing the vertical and lateral axial oscillations of the center of gravity of the body while sustaining vertical forces equal to two to four times body weight. The varied functions of the knee—to withstand large forces, provide great stability, and at the same time provide great range of motion—is achieved by a unique combination of bony and soft tissue anatomy. The bony architecture provides mobility while stability is achieved by an intricate combination of muscles, ligaments, and cartilage. Industrial and sporting injuries to the stabilizing structures of the knee occur frequently due to the large torque forces acting on the long lever-arms of the femur and tibia.

The forces of the foot and ankle are transmitted proximally to the knee via the leg. The leg provides attachment for the muscles that move the foot and ankle and stabilize the knee. The leg provides passage for the neurovascular structures that supply the foot and ankle.

The ankle connects two unequal lever-arms, the leg and the foot. The larger lever-arm, the leg, consists of two parallel bones (tibia and fibula) that act as an integrated unit. The smaller bone, the fibula, serves primarily as a buttress at the ankle joint to prevent lateral translation of the talus. The fibula bears only a small portion of the force transmitted by the femur, estimated to be approximately one sixth of body weight. The larger tibia conveys most of the body weight directly to the talus and acts as a solid lever in ankle injuries.

The foot serves as the body's link to its environment and as such provides the body with part of the proprioceptive feedback to sustain gait. The foot begins each step as a flexible structure and completes it as a rigid lever. The foot completes the triad (unparalleled cerebral cortical development, unique vocalization apparatus, and adaptation of lower limb structures for bipedal gait) that distinguishes man from other mammals.

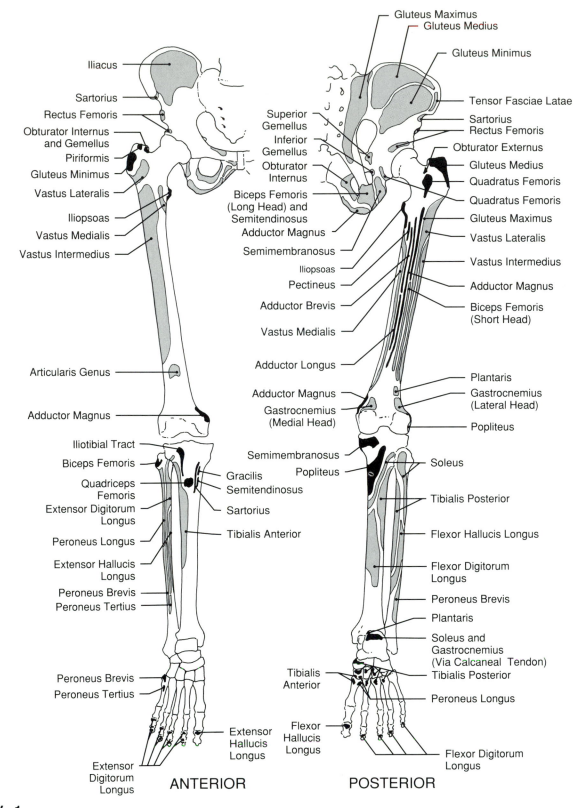

Iliacus

Sartorius

Rectus Femoris

Obturator Internus and Gemellus

Piriformis

Gluteus Minimus

Vastus Lateralis

Iliopsoas

Vastus Medialis

Vastus Intermedius

Articularis Genus

Adductor Magnus

Iliotibial Tract

Biceps Femoris

Quadriceps Femoris

Extensor Digitorum Longus

Peroneus Longus

Extensor Hallucis Longus

Peroneus Brevis

Peroneus Tertius

Peroneus Brevis

Peroneus Tertius

Extensor Hallucis Longus

Extensor Digitorum Longus

Superior Gemellus

Inferior Gemellus

Obturator Internus

Biceps Femoris (Long Head) and Semitendinosus

Adductor Magnus

Semimembranosus

Iliopsoas

Pectineus

Adductor Brevis

Vastus Medialis

Adductor Longus

Adductor Magnus

Gastrocnemius (Medial Head)

Semimembranosus

Popliteus

Gracilis

Semitendinosus

Sartorius

Tibialis Anterior

Tibialis Anterior

Flexor Hallucis Longus

Gluteus Maximus

Gluteus Medius

Gluteus Minimus

Tensor Fasciae Latae

Sartorius

Rectus Femoris

Obturator Externus

Gluteus Medius

Quadratus Femoris

Quadratus Femoris

Gluteus Maximus

Vastus Lateralis

Vastus Intermedius

Adductor Magnus

Biceps Femoris (Short Head)

Plantaris

Gastrocnemius (Lateral Head)

Popliteus

Soleus

Tibialis Posterior

Flexor Hallucis Longus

Flexor Digitorum Longus

Peroneus Brevis

Plantaris

Soleus and Gastrocnemius (Via Calcaneal Tendon)

Tibialis Posterior

Peroneus Longus

Flexor Digitorum Longus

ANTERIOR

POSTERIOR

FIG IV–1.
Origins *(gray-shaded areas)* and insertion *(dark areas)* sites of muscles of the pelvis and lower limb. Anterior and posterior views.

9

Pelvis and Acetabulum

Frederick W. Reckling, M.D.
Melvin P. Mohn, Ph.D.

ANATOMICAL FEATURES OF THE PELVIC RING AND ACETABULUM

Severe injuries to the pelvis and its contents are second only to those of the skull in terms of mortality and morbidity. In the past, surgery to expose and stabilize complex fractures of the pelvis was undertaken rarely and reluctantly due to the complex anatomy of this region. Recently enthusiasm has increased for treatment of pelvic fractures with open reduction and internal stabilization, particularly pelvic fractures with hip joint involvement. Early, secure fixation of these fractures will allow more rapid mobilization of such severely injured patients and provide better long-term functional results. This chapter is heavily weighted toward management of fractures of the pelvis and acetabulum, but the anatomy and surgical approaches described apply to tumor management and reconstructive work as well. Because of the continuity of the hip joint with the pelvic structures, some of the approaches involving the pelvis will be found in the Hip chapter.

Bony Anatomy and Ligamentous Structures

The bony pelvis and ligaments protect the pelvic viscera, support the vertebral column, and provide attachment for the muscles of locomotion. The bones that form the bony pelvis (the sacrum and coccyx posteriorly and the innominate bones laterally and anteriorly) articulate with one another to form a complete ring (Fig 9–1). In the infant each innominate bone consists of three separate bones (ilium, ischium, and pubis), which are fused in the adult.

The ilium forms the superior portion of the innominate bone. The anterolateral projections of the ilium, referred to as the wings, or ala, give rise to extensive muscle attachments. The most inferior portion of the ilium, known as the body, forms the superior portion of the acetabulum.

The posteromedial surfaces of the ilia articulate with the sacrum to form the sacroiliac joints. These articulations are reinforced by very strong ligaments (Fig 9–2). The anterior or ventral sacroiliac ligaments are relatively thin and lie across the front of the joints. The dorsal or posterior ligaments are strong and blend with the even stronger interosseous sacroiliac ligaments. This posterior sacroiliac ligamentous complex (posterior sacroiliac and interosseous sacroiliac ligaments) prevents posterior displacement of the pelvic ring on the sacrum. Considered from the other point of view, this ligamentous complex prevents anterior displacement of the sacrum and axial skeleton on the pelvis during weight bearing and at the same time allows slight rotatory motion at the sacroiliac joints during gait.

The pelvis is also tethered together by strong ligaments (sacrotuberous ligaments) running from the sacrum to the ischial tuberosity (Fig 9–3). These ex-

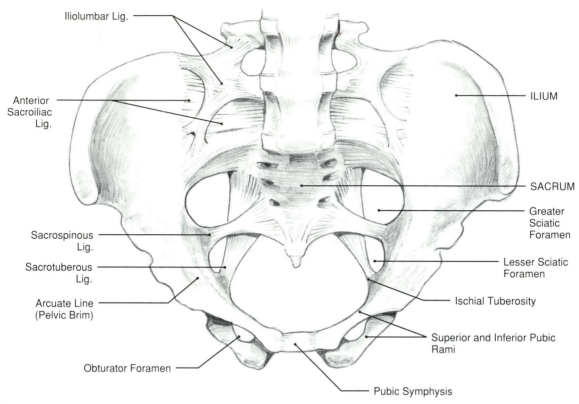

FIG 9–1.
Bony pelvis and ligaments.

tremely strong ligaments, positioned in the vertical plane, resist vertical shearing forces applied to the hemipelvis. The sacrospinous ligaments run from the lateral edge of the sacrum to the ischial spine. They are very strong and resist diastasis of the sacrum and ilium.

The ligaments running from the lumbar vertebrae to the ilium are referred to as iliolumbar ligaments. They pass laterally from the transverse process of the fourth and fifth lumbar vertebrae to the posterior part of the iliac crest. These ligaments resist the tendency of the vertebrae to dislocate anteri-

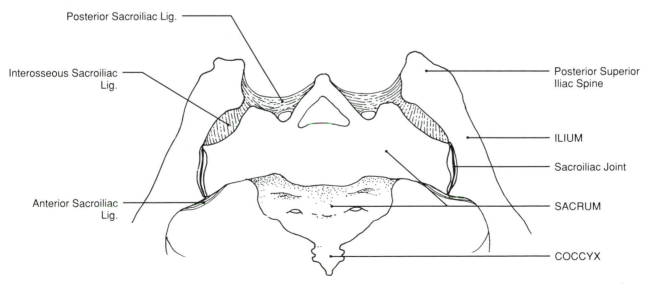

FIG 9–2.
Sacroiliac ligaments.

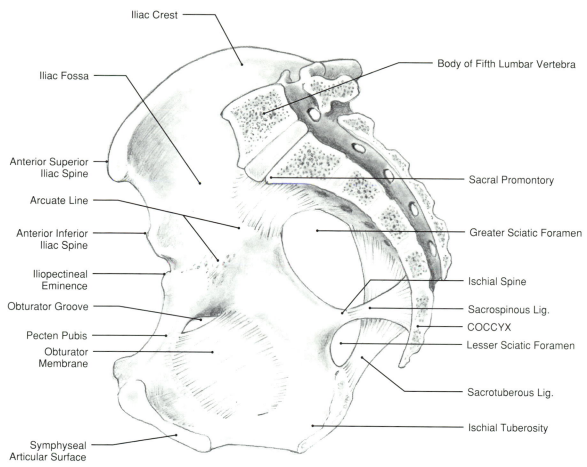

Iliac Crest

Iliac Fossa

Anterior Superior
Iliac Spine

Arcuate Line

Anterior Inferior
Iliac Spine

Iliopectineal
Eminence

Obturator Groove

Pecten Pubis

Obturator
Membrane

Symphyseal
Articular Surface

Body of Fifth Lumbar Vertebra

Sacral Promontory

Greater Sciatic Foramen

Ischial Spine

Sacrospinous Lig.

COCCYX

Lesser Sciatic Foramen

Sacrotuberous Lig.

Ischial Tuberosity

FIG 9–3.
Bony hemipelvis. Note sacrotuberous and sacrospinous ligaments.

orly due to the oblique plane of the base of the sacrum.

The ischium forms the most posterior and inferior portion of the innominate bone (Fig 9–4). Its body forms the posterior half of the lower two thirds of the acetabulum. Its anterior projection (ramus) forms the posterior and inferior walls of the obturator foramen and continues forward to join the pubis. The large posterior expansion of the ischium is known as the ischial tuberosity. A projection on the posterosuperior aspect known as the ischial spine separates the greater sciatic notch superiorly from the lesser sciatic notch inferiorly.

The pubis forms the anterior and inferior portions of the innominate bone. The superior pubic ramus forms the anterior half of the inferior two thirds of the acetabulum. The inferior ramus curves posteriorly and inferiorly to join the ischial ramus, and it forms the inferior wall of the obturator foramen. All three innominate components contribute to the socket (acetabulum) for reception of the femoral head. The pubes are united anteriorly in a symphy-

sis strengthened by a heavy fibrocartilaginous disk and strong symphyseal ligaments.

In order to understand the bony anatomy of the acetabulum, one should not think of the acetabulum simply as the socket for the femoral head but consider the bony masses that limit and support the acetabulum (Fig 9–5). Viewed laterally the acetabulum may be considered as contained within the open arms of an inverted Y formed by two columns of bone (the anterior and posterior columns). The longer anterior, or iliopubic, column runs obliquely downward, inward, and anteriorly from the anterior part of the superior iliac crest to the pubic symphysis. The shorter posterior column, voluminous and thick, runs caudally from the head of the angles of the greater sciatic notch to the ischial tuberosity. (Note that the posterior column is not usually considered to include the posterior aspect of the ilium.) The posterior column converges with the anterior column just above the acetabulum. The summit of the angle is filled with compact bone that constitutes the roof of the acetabulum and forms the keystone

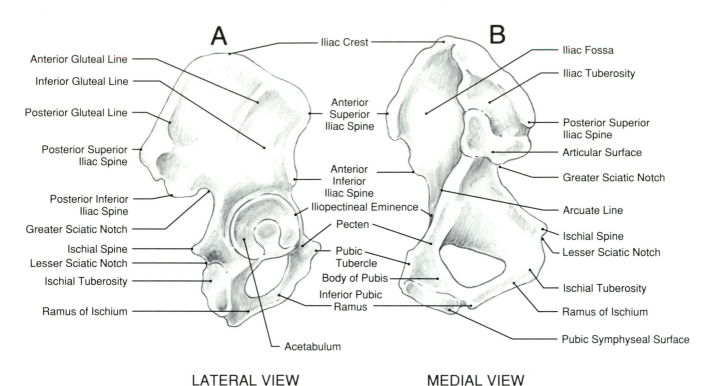

Anterior Gluteal Line
Inferior Gluteal Line
Posterior Gluteal Line
Posterior Superior Iliac Spine
Posterior Inferior Iliac Spine
Greater Sciatic Notch
Ischial Spine
Lesser Sciatic Notch
Ischial Tuberosity
Ramus of Ischium

Iliac Crest
Anterior Superior Iliac Spine
Anterior Inferior Iliac Spine
Iliopectineal Eminence
Pecten
Pubic Tubercle
Body of Pubis
Inferior Pubic Ramus
Acetabulum

Iliac Fossa
Iliac Tuberosity
Posterior Superior Iliac Spine
Articular Surface
Greater Sciatic Notch
Arcuate Line
Ischial Spine
Lesser Sciatic Notch
Ischial Tuberosity
Ramus of Ischium
Pubic Symphyseal Surface

LATERAL VIEW   MEDIAL VIEW

FIG 9–4.
Innominate bone. **A,** lateral view. **B,** medial view.

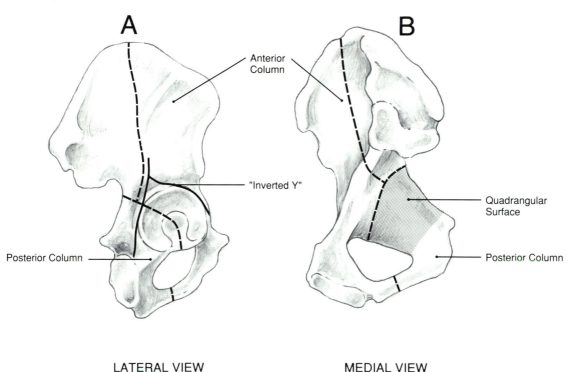

Anterior Column
"Inverted Y"
Posterior Column
Quadrangular Surface
Posterior Column

LATERAL VIEW   MEDIAL VIEW

FIG 9–5.
Acetabulum and supporting anterior and posterior bony columns *(dashed lines).* **A,** lateral view. The acetabulum is contained within the open arms of an inverted Y *(solid lines).* The stem of the Y and its anterior arm are formed by the anterior column, while the posterior arm represents the posterior column. **B,** Medial view. Note quadrilateral surface *(shaded area).*

of the arch. The area of the posterior column referred to as the quadrilateral surface represents the inner aspect of the body of the ischium. The midportion of the posterior column cranial to the ischial spine is quite thin. Misdirected transacetabular screws in this region often penetrate the joint (see Fig 9–8). The rim, or lip, of the acetabulum is referred to as the wall of the acetabulum.

Vascular Anatomy

In 60% of the patients who die as the result of pelvic fracture, death is due to related hemorrhage. The vascular anatomy of the pelvis is so extensive and complex that it can be thought of as a "vascular sink." Surgeons who deal with pelvic trauma and operate in this area must be familiar with its vascular anatomy.

Arteries

The main arterial supply to the pelvis is from the internal iliac (hypogastric) artery, which begins at the bifurcation of the common iliac artery opposite the sacroiliac articulation, crosses the pelvic brim or inlet, and follows a short, curved course about 4 cm toward the greater sciatic notch (Fig 9–6). The pattern of its branches is somewhat variable, but in most people it branches into ventral and dorsal divisions that supply the wall of the pelvis, pelvic viscera, buttocks, genital organs, and part of the medial thigh. The distribution of the various branches may be grouped into visceral, ventral parietal, and dorsal parietal.

The umbilical artery is a remnant of the fetal umbilical artery. It gives off the superior and middle vesical arteries, which supply the apex and fundus portions of the bladder. The inferior vesical artery arises from the internal iliac or by a common stem with the middle rectal artery. It supplies the fundus and neck of the bladder, the prostate, and the seminal vesicles in males. In females the uterine artery arises from the medial surface of the internal iliac and supplies the cervix and a portion of the vagina. The middle rectal artery supplies the rectum, anasto-

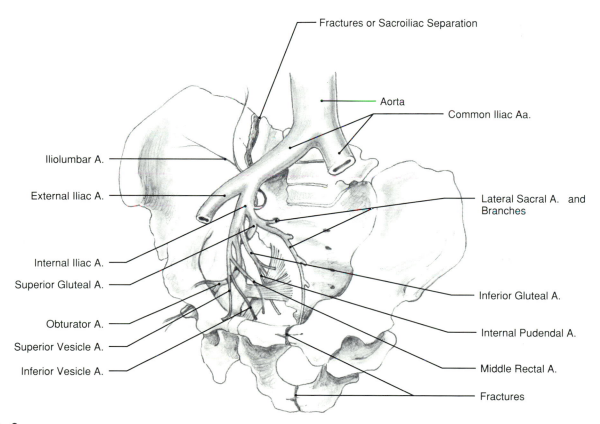

FIG 9–6.
The internal iliac artery and its branches. Note the vulnerability of the iliolumbar, lateral sacral, and superior gluteal arteries with an injury to the sacroiliac complex. The obturator and internal pudendal arteries are vulnerable with fractures of the pubic rami and injuries of the symphysis. (Modified from Brotman S, Soderstrom CA, Oster-Granite M, et al: Management of severe bleeding in fractures of the pelvis. *Surg Gynecol Obstet* 1981; 153:823.)

mosing with the inferior vesicle and superior and inferior rectal arteries. The obturator artery usually arises from the ventral or medial surface of the internal iliac artery and runs ventrally on the lateral wall of the pelvis. Inside the pelvis, it gives off branches to the inner pelvic wall, bladder, and pubis. Outside the pelvis it divides into anterior and posterior branches at the margin of the obturator foramen.

The internal pudendal artery, which supplies the perineum and external genitalia, passes caudally toward the inferior border of the greater sciatic notch to emerge from the pelvis between the piriformis and coccygeus. It then crosses the ischial spine to enter the perineum via the lesser sciatic notch.

The inferior gluteal artery passes through the lower portion of the greater sciatic foramen below the piriformis to supply the gluteus maximus muscle and skin of the buttock and upper posterior thigh. It also communicates with vessels of the thigh to form the so-called "cruciate anastomosis" (see Hip chapter).

The iliolumbar artery is a branch of the posterior division of the internal iliac that turns upward to the medial border of the psoas major muscle to supply the iliacus and psoas muscles, as well as the bone in that area. Two or three lateral sacral arteries usually also arise from the posterior division of the internal iliac. These vessels pass medially and dorsally to enter the anterior sacral foramina, and they eventually supply the skin and muscles of the dorsum of the sacrum.

The superior gluteal artery is the largest branch of the internal iliac and appears to be its direct continuation. It is a short artery that runs dorsally to pass out of the pelvis through the greater sciatic notch, just above the superior border of the piriformis muscle, and supply the gluteus medius and minimus muscles. The superior gluteal artery is especially subject to shearing forces because of the way it angulates as it passes out of the pelvis and because it lies in contact with the bone at the sciatic notch.

Veins

The venous drainage of the pelvis is extensive, and the fact that the veins are arranged in plexuses closely applied to the pelvic walls and viscera puts them at great risk of injury as a result of pelvic fractures (Fig 9–7). In addition, these plexuses are not easily displaced and, being thin-walled, cannot retract like their arterial counterparts. Much of the

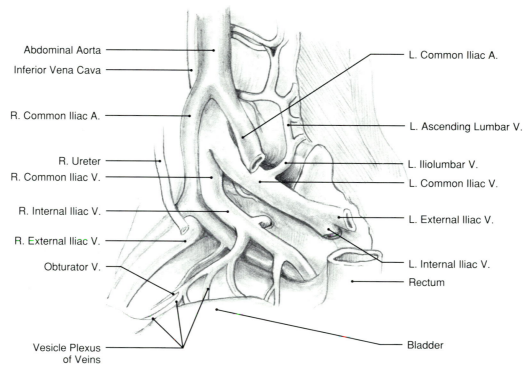

FIG 9–7.
Veins of the pelvis.

extraperitoneal hemorrhage that follows pelvic fractures is probably due to injury to the venous plexuses.

The common iliac veins are the distal continuation of the inferior vena cava at its bifurcation. They are formed by the union of the internal and external iliac veins ventral to the sacroiliac articulation. The right common iliac is shorter than the left. It runs vertically and ascends dorsally and then laterally to the right common iliac artery. The left common iliac vein is longer and more oblique in its course. It is first situated on the medial side of the corresponding artery and then dorsal to the right common iliac artery. Both common iliac veins usually receive iliolumbar and lateral sacral veins.

Keating et al. have shown in anatomic and radiographic studies that vascular structures (the internal iliac vessels and branches) are vulnerable to injury when transacetabular screws are used to stabilize pelvic fractures or fixate acetabular components in total hip arthroplasty. The danger area is a pie-shaped section of the acetabulum formed by an arc drawn from the midportion of the superior dome to the superior border of the transverse acetabular ligament. If possible this region should be avoided when transacetabular screws are placed (Fig 9–8).

Lumbosacral Plexus

Pelvic fractures and associated iliosacral dislocations may cause a stretching force to nerves of the lumbosacral plexus. Because of their proximity to the sacroiliac joint, the fourth and fifth lumbar and first sacral nerve roots are more vulnerable and most frequently injured (Fig 9–9). It is estimated that over 50% of patients with double vertical (Malgaigne) pelvic fractures have persistent neurological damage. The lumbosacral nerve plexus is derived from the anterior rami of the T12–S4 spinal nerves. A branch of the L4 root crosses the fifth lumbar transverse process; L5 crosses and grooves the ala of the sacrum where it is joined by the branch of L4 just described to form the lumbosacral trunk. The upper four anterior sacral rami leave the anterior sacral foramina, grooving the lateral mass of the sacrum. The

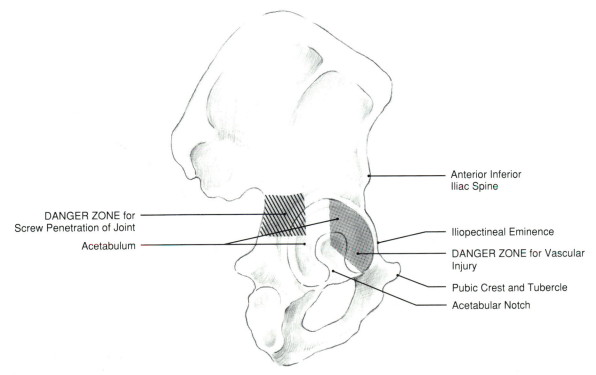

FIG 9–8.
Shaded areas of acetabulum indicate danger zones. *Diagonal lines* represent thin area of posterior column. Misdirected screws utilized to stabilize acetabular fractures in this area may penetrate the hip joint. *Stippled area* delineates danger zone due to possibility of injury to the iliac vessels and branches with placement of transacetabular screws during fracture fixation or total hip arthroplasty. (Adapted from Keating EM, Ritter MA, Faris PM: Structures at risk from medially placed acetabular screws. *J Bone Joint Surg* 1990; 72A: 509–511.)

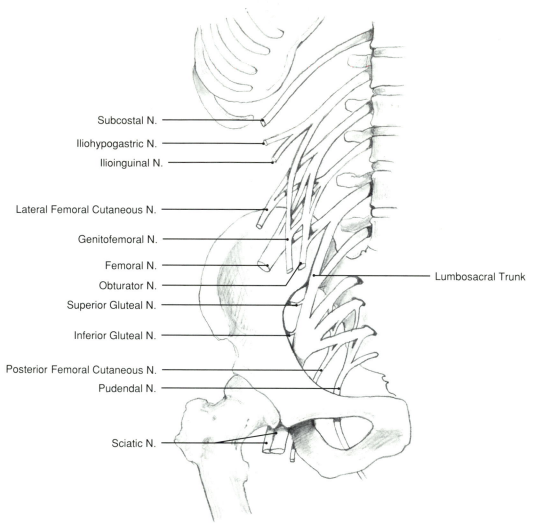

Subcostal N.

Iliohypogastric N.

Ilioinguinal N.

Lateral Femoral Cutaneous N.

Genitofemoral N.

Femoral N.

Obturator N.

Superior Gluteal N.

Inferior Gluteal N.

Posterior Femoral Cutaneous N.

Pudendal N.

Sciatic N.

Lumbosacral Trunk

FIG 9–9.
Lumbosacral plexus.

lumbosacral trunk unites with the S1 sacral root anterior to the sacroiliac joint, and they in turn unite with S2, S3, and S4 to form the sciatic nerve. The sciatic nerve is the largest branch of the lumbosacral plexus. It leaves the pelvis through the greater sciatic foramen between the lower border of the piriformis and the ischial border of the sciatic notch. Its two divisions, the tibial and peroneal, are loosely held together. The nerve is commonly injured in pelvic trauma, especially in posterior dislocation of the hip with or without acetabular fracture. The peroneal division is the most prone to injury and least likely to recover. The pudendal nerve (S2 to S4) escapes the pelvis through the greater sciatic foramen between the piriformis and coccygeus, just medial to the sciatic nerve. The superior gluteal nerve (L4, L5,

and S1) and its artery and veins leave the pelvis by winding around the greater sciatic notch above the piriformis. Although the artery may be injured by trauma, injury to the nerve is uncommon. However, in posterior approaches to the hip joint, particularly for the management of acetabular fractures, the nerve is in jeopardy. This is because application of a pelvic fixation plate may require excessive retraction and stretch the nerve. The inferior gluteal nerve (L5, S1, and S2) exits the pelvis beneath the piriformis and behind the sciatic nerve to supply the gluteus maximus. The femoral, obturator, and posterior femoral cutaneous nerves, and other cutaneous branches derived from the lumbosacral plexus, are discussed in the chapters on the thoracolumbosacral spine, hip, and thigh.

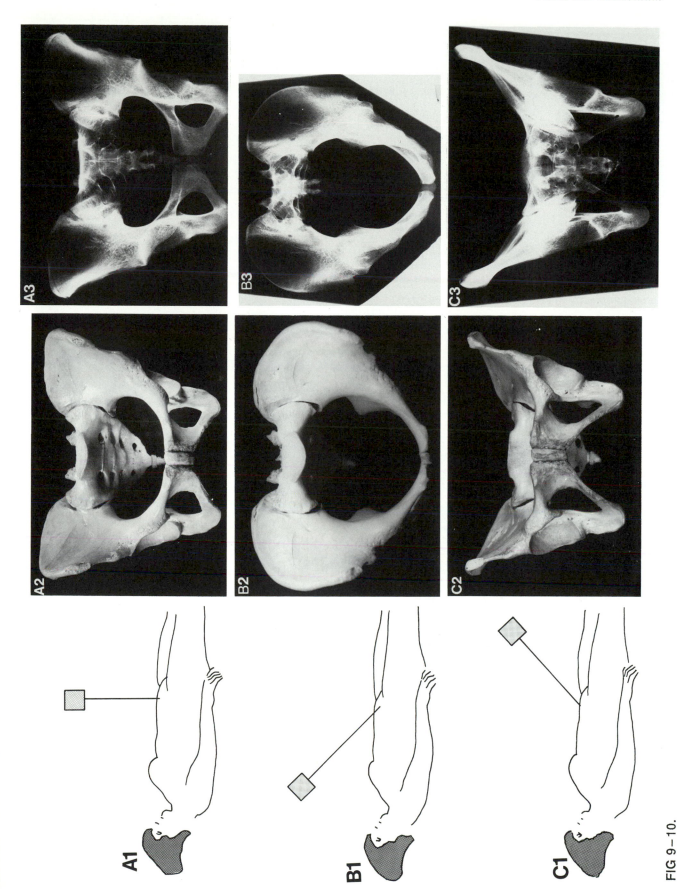

FIG 9–10.
Radiographic examination of bony anatomy of the pelvis. **A**, routine anterior view of pelvis. *(1)* direction of x-ray beam; *(2)* photograph of bony pelvis; *(3)* radiograph of bony pelvis. **B**, inlet view of pelvis. *(1)* Direction of x-ray beam; *(2)* photograph of bony pelvis; *(3)* radiograph of bony pelvis. **C**, outlet view of pelvis. *(1)* Direction of x-ray beam; *(2)* photograph of bony pelvis; *(3)* radiograph of bony pelvis.

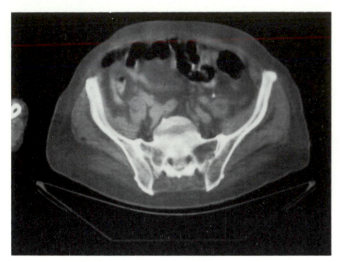

FIG 9–11.
Computed tomography of an intact pelvis at the level of the sacroiliac joint.

Viscera

The overall incidence of bladder and urethral injuries associated with pelvic fractures is 13%. The incidence of gastrointestinal injuries is relatively low, but when bowel disruption occurs it is potentially very serious. Readers should consult standard anatomy texts to review the visceral contents of the pelvis.

Roentgenographic Anatomy

In this chapter we emphasize surgical anatomy and approaches to deal with fractures of the pelvis and acetabulum. In order to understand the fracture patterns, one must understand the radiographic anatomy of the pelvis and acetabulum.

Pelvis

Three anterior radiographic projections are valuable in assessing injuries or other abnormalities of the bony pelvis (Fig 9–10). The routine anteroposterior view of the pelvis is in reality an oblique view because the plane of the true pelvic brim lies oblique to the axis of the trunk. This view is valuable for general assessment but does not clearly define anterior or posterior displacement or proximal or distal migration of the hemipelvis. To assess posterior displacement or inward or outward rotation of the anterior pelvis, an inlet view is helpful. This projection is taken with the patient supine and the x-ray beam

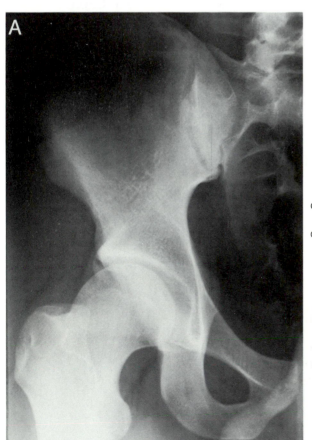

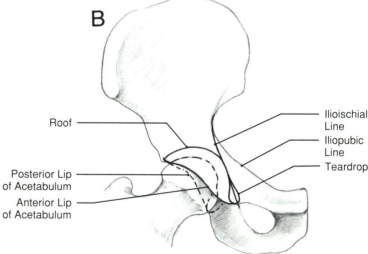

FIG 9–12.
Radiologic landmarks of the acetabulum. **A,** standard anteroposterior radiograph of right hip. **B,** diagram showing radiologic landmarks of the acetabulum: anterior lip, posterior lip, and roof of the acetabulum; ilioischial line; iliopubic line (brim of the true pelvis); teardrop.

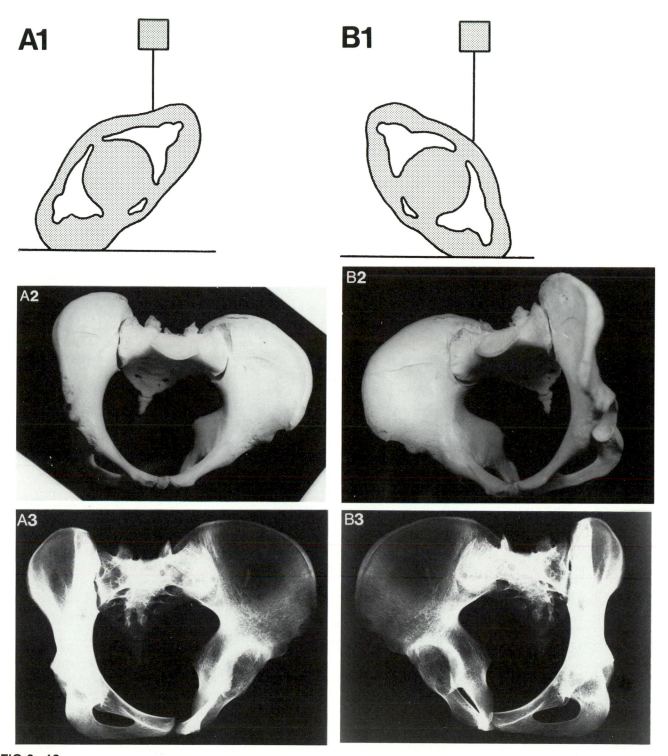

FIG 9–13.
Radiographic anatomy of the acetabulum (Judet views). **A,** obturator oblique view. *(1)* Position of patient to evaluate injury to *right* hemipelvis (viewed cranial to caudal). Patient is supine but rolled 45 degrees *away* from the side of injury. The entire anterior column, the posterior lip of the acetabulum, and the entire obturator ring are well visualized in this view. *(2)* Photograph of bony pelvis; *(3)* radiograph of bony pelvis. **B,** iliac oblique view. *(1)* Position of patient to evaluate injury to *right* hemipelvis (viewed cranial to caudal). Patient is supine but rolled 45 degrees *toward* the side of injury. The posterior column, anterior lip of the acetabulum and iliac wings are well visualized in this view. *(2)* Photograph of bony pelvis; *(3)* radiograph of bony pelvis.

directed from the head to the midpelvis at an angle of approximately 40 degrees to the plate. The tangential view, which is made with the patient supine and the x-ray beam directed from the feet to the symphysis at an angle 40 degrees to the plate, is helpful to evaluate for superior displacement of the hemipelvis. It will also show superior or inferior displacement of the anterior portion of the pelvis.

Computed tomography (CT) has proven useful in evaluating the bony anatomy of patients with pelvic fractures, particularly when the injury involves the sacroiliac complex (Fig 9–11).

Acetabulum

Four radiographic views are necessary for assessment of the acetabulum. The first is a standard anteroposterior view of the pelvis to detect possible injuries of the opposite side. The second, a standard anteroposterior view centered on the involved hip, provides excellent visualization of the landmarks, including the anterior and posterior lips of the acetabulum, acetabular roof, ilioischial line, iliopubic line (brim of the true pelvis), and teardrop (Fig 9–12). The teardrop ("tranentropfen") is a radiographic landmark that can serve as a reference point. The internal limb of the teardrop is formed by the outer wall of the obturator groove, which merges posteriorly with the outline of the quadrilateral surface of the ischium. The bottom of the teardrop is the acetabular notch, which forms the superior border of the obturator foramen. The external limb of the teardrop is tangential to part of the surface of the outer aspect of the cotyloid fossa.

Two radiographic views (obturator oblique and iliac oblique) as described by Judet are very helpful in assessment of acetabular and pelvic column fractures. The obturator oblique view is centered on the involved hip with the patient supine but rolled 45 degrees away from the side of injury. This superimposes the anterior and posterior iliac spines but spreads out the obturator foramen (Fig 9–13). The entire anterior column (iliopectineal brim) is well visualized on this view, as is the posterior lip of the acetabulum and the entire obturator ring. The iliac oblique view is centered on the involved hip with the patient supine but rolled 45 degrees toward the affected side. This spreads out the iliac wing. The posterior column is visualized well on this view, as are the anterior lip of the acetabulum and iliac wing.

CT is very effective in analysis of acetabular fractures (Fig 9–14).

Using reconstruction CT, it is possible to characterize the three-dimensional nature of these injuries.

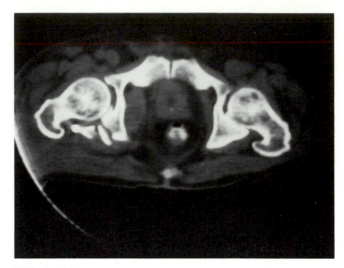

FIG 9–14.
Computed tomography of right acetabulum (viewed caudal to cranial). Note fracture of posterior wall and column with intraarticular bony fragments.

This technique has been especially useful in evaluating two-column fractures, assessing the integrity of the acetabular dome and quadrilateral surface, identifying the stable fragment, and determining the presence or absence of loose fragments in the hip joint (Fig 9–15).

Classification of Acetabular Fractures

Several classifications of acetabular fractures have been described based on their anatomic, radiographic, and prognostic features. All of the classifications have stressed the importance of the integrity of the superior and posterior articulating surfaces of the acetabulum. Letournel has proposed a detailed and inclusive classification of acetabular fractures (Table 9–1). In this classification, acetabular fractures are divided into two large groups: elementary and associated fractures. Elementary fractures include those in which part or all of one column of the acetabulum has been detached. There are five elementary forms: fractures of the posterior wall of the acetabulum; fractures of the posterior column; fractures of the anterior wall of the acetabulum; fractures of the anterior column; and transverse fractures. Associated fractures include at least two of the elementary forms listed. There are five principal associations: T-shaped fractures (transverse fractures with a split of the ischiopubic fragment, which may run vertically through the obturator foramen or backward through the ischium, sparing the obturator foramen); fractures of the posterior column and

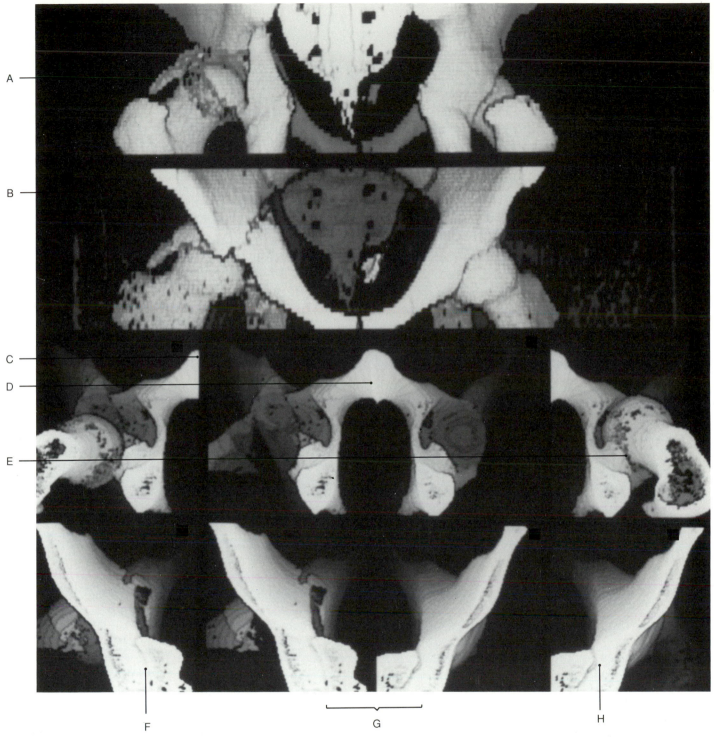

FIG 9–15.
Multiple surface shaded three-dimensional views of an acetabular fracture, reconstructed from computed tomography examination. These studies simulate what could be seen if the lower half of the pelvis and upper parts of the hips could be viewed directly, with no overlying soft tissues. The lines on the surfaces are contour lines, which improve appreciation of depth. **A,** *posterior* view of the pelvis shows the orientation of the fracture in the posterior column of the *left* acetabulum, as well as loss of integrity of the posterior bony rim. **B,** anterior plane of the pelvis shows the orientation of the fracture in the anterior column. **C,** looking upward into the left hip demonstrates the posterior and lateral displacement of the femoral head. **D,** side-by-side comparison of both hips, looking upward with the femurs removed. The comminution and displacement of the fragments of the acetabular roof can best be appreciated on this view. The concentric rings visible on the normal right side show the normal concavity of the roof of the acetabulum. The lateral half of the left acetabular roof has been fragmented. Two large pieces are displaced away from the acetabulum. At least two smaller fragments are visible within the acetabulum adjacent to the posterior inferior rim. **E,** the normal right hip looking upward, for comparison to **C.** The spots overlying the femoral head are artifacts of three-dimensional reconstruction. **F,** top down view of left hip, which shows fracture line traversing the quadrilateral quadrangular surface. **G,** top down view of both halves of pelvis with hips removed. **H,** top down view of normal right hip is for comparison to **F.** (Courtesy of John M. Bramble, M.D., and Mark D. Murphey, M.D., Dept. of Radiology, University of Kansas Medical Center.)

TABLE 9-1.

Classification of Acetabular Fractures

I. Elementary Fractures
   1. Posterior wall
   2. Posterior column
   3. Anterior wall
   4. Anterior column
   5. Transverse fractures
II. Associated Fractures (include at least two elementary fractures)
   1. T-shaped fractures (transverse fracture with split of the ischiopubic fragment)
   2. Fractures of posterior column and posterior acetabular wall
   3. Transverse and posterior wall fractures
   4. Fracture of anterior wall or column associated with hemitransverse fracture posteriorly
   5. Fracture of both columns

(Adapted from Letournel E, Judet R: *Fractures of the Acetabulum.* Berlin, Springer-Verlag, 1981.)

posterior acetabular wall; transverse and posterior fractures; fracture of the anterior column or anterior wall, associated with a hemitransverse fracture posteriorly; and fracture of both columns.

SURGICAL APPROACHES TO THE PELVIC RING AND ACETABULUM

Bone Graft from Ilium

One of the most common sources of bone graft is the iliac crest. Autogenous cancellous, cortical, or full-thickness grafts can be readily obtained from this area. The rare complication of sacroiliac joint subluxation can be prevented by avoiding the stabilizing ligaments and violating the sacroiliac joint itself. The greatest quantity of bone is found in the posterior half of the iliac crest.

An incision is made which parallels the posterior two thirds of the ilium (Fig 9–16). If the incision is made too far anteriorly the lateral femoral cutaneous nerve can be injured as it passes under the inguinal ligament in the region of the anterior superior iliac spine. The subcutaneous tissues are divided by sharp dissection to expose the iliac crest. The gluteal fascia is incised and the muscles stripped subperiosteally from the outer table of the ilium. In a child the incision is made in the iliac apophysis down to the bone, and then dissection carried out subperiosteally. The muscles are stripped from the iliac crest and dissected subperiosteally with wide reflection of the tissue to expose the majority of the outer

table of the posterior ilium. If desired, bone from the inner table may be obtained by stripping the abdominal muscles and the iliacus from the ilium. Bone is obtained with the use of an osteotome or gouge. Care is taken to leave a rim of bone 2 cm around the greater sciatic notch to avoid injury to the structures passing through it (sciatic nerve, superior and inferior gluteal nerves and vessels).

Approach to the Pubic Symphysis

Exposure to the pubic symphysis is sometimes required for stabilization of pubic diastasis or fractures, tumor resection, or treatment of osteomyelitis. Before the pubis is approached surgically a Foley catheter should be placed transurethrally to decompress the urinary bladder and aid in locating the urethra by palpation. Most surgeons prefer a low transverse curvilinear (Pfannenstiel) incision located about 2 cm superior to the pubic rami (Fig 9–17). The heads of the rectus abdominis are resected off the superior pubic rami if trauma has not already done so. The dissection is carried laterally along both superior pubic rami for 4 to 5 cm. If wider exposure is necessary, the intercrural fibers formed by the aponeurosis of the external oblique muscle are incised parallel with the inguinal ligament, and the spermatic cord(s) (round ligaments in females) are identified and gently retracted. By subperiosteal dissection the obturator foramina are identified and partially exposed medially. The catheterized urethra is palpated out of the way and the symphysis brought together with the use of a tenaculum. Fixation is achieved with a reconstruction plate applied superiorly and/or anteriorly across the symphysis. If there are associated unilateral or bilateral pubic rami fractures, the approach can be extended laterally for greater exposure (see ilioinguinal approach). The rectus abdominis and external oblique aponeuroses are carefully repaired during closure.

Approaches to the Posterior Pelvis and Sacroiliac Joints

Posterior Approach to Single Sacroiliac Joint

The sacroiliac joint can be approached posteriorly through an incision that begins at the posterior superior iliac spine and courses distally and slightly medially to the caudal border of the joint (Fig 9–18). The gluteus maximus is dissected off the superior portion of the ilium. The paraspinous muscle group is elevated off the sacrum. Ideally the dissection is carried distally enough that a finger can be intro-

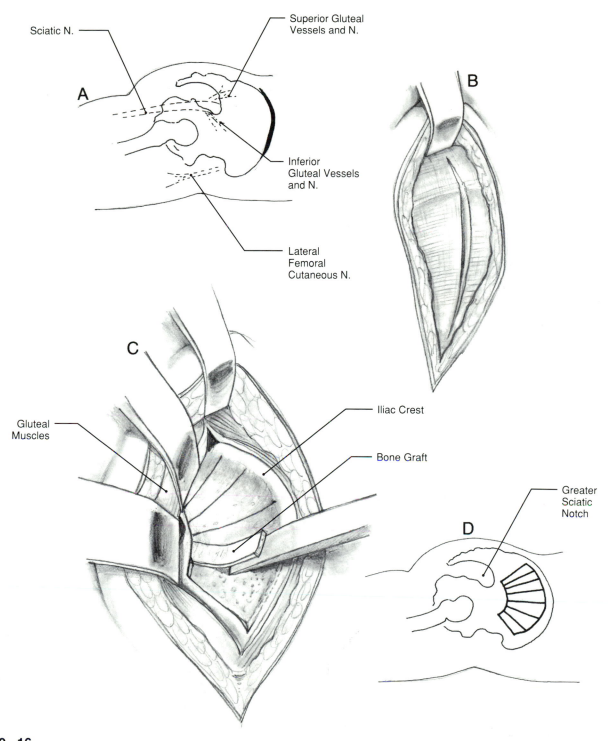

FIG 9–16.
Bone graft from ilium. **A,** skin incision. **B,** fascial incision. **C,** gluteal muscles reflected and bone graft obtained from outer table of the ilium. **D,** preferred sites for obtaining bone graft. Note rim of bone remaining around greater sciatic notch.

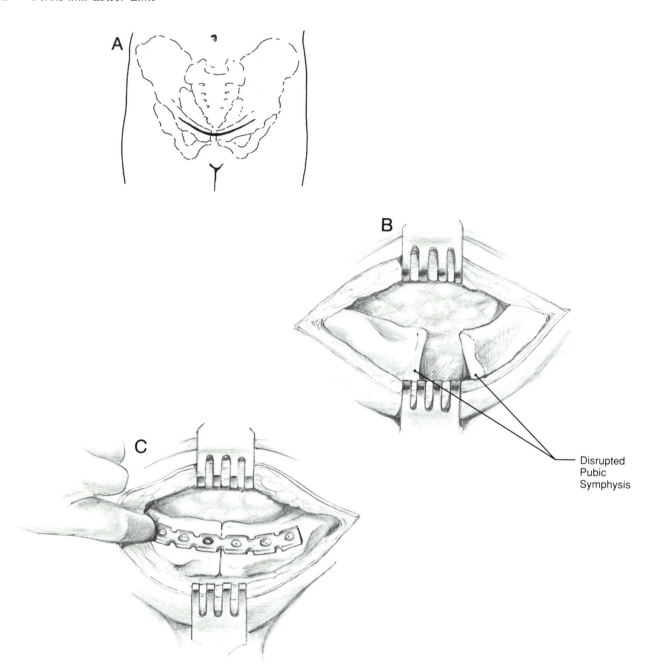

FIG 9–17.
Approach to the pubic symphysis. **A,** skin incision. **B,** disrupted pubic symphysis exposed by reflecting the rectus abdominis and soft tissue from the symphysis. **C,** symphysis approximated and stabilized with a reconstruction plate and screws.

duced through the sciatic notch. This is done to palpate the inferior aspect of the sacroiliac joint and assess the reduction of the joint or associated fracture.

Bilateral Approach to Sacroiliac Joints

Complex disruptions of the pelvic ring with unstable dislocation or fracture-dislocation of both sacroiliac joints may require stabilization. An extensile surgical approach as described by Mears may be utilized for this purpose. This approach can be accomplished through a straight transverse incision, which can then be tailored to fit the particular situation (Fig 9–19). If exposure of the sciatic notch is necessary to explore the sciatic nerve, the incision is curved distally. If the iliac crest needs to be exposed, the incision is curved proximally. The incision is centralized

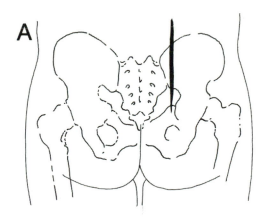

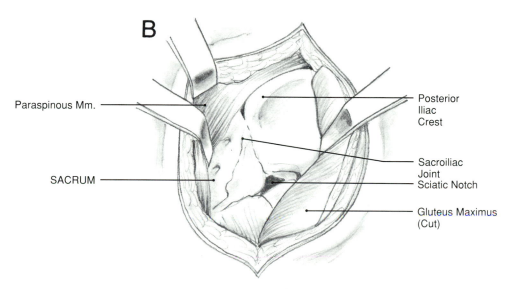

Paraspinous Mm.

Posterior
Iliac
Crest

Sacroiliac
Joint
Sciatic Notch

SACRUM

Gluteus Maximus
(Cut)

FIG 9–18.
Posterior approach to sacroiliac joint. **A,** skin incision. **B,** superior origin of gluteus maximus incised and reflected laterally, and paraspinous muscles reflected medially.

at the midpoint of the sacrum. It is carried directly through the deep fascia. Osteotomies of those portions of the iliac spines which project posterior to the sacrum will allow lateral reflection of the gluteus maximus and provide a flat surface on which to apply a fixation plate. Elevation of the paraspinous muscle group off the sacrum and osteotomies of the spines of the sacrum permit "tunneling" of the muscles and insertion of a double cobra plate, or in small individuals, a contoured reconstruction plate. The plate is attached to the ilium by screws, which also penetrate the sacral ala. Bone grafts to facilitate fracture healing can be readily obtained from the posterior ilium.

Sea-gull Approach

Jacobs and Montesano have described a so-called "sea-gull" approach to the posterior pelvis and sacroiliac joints. This approach has been useful in the management of sacral fractures, posterior sacroiliac joint lesions, and sacral canal compromise. It is called the sea-gull approach because the outline of the skin incision has the appearance of a sea-gull in flight.

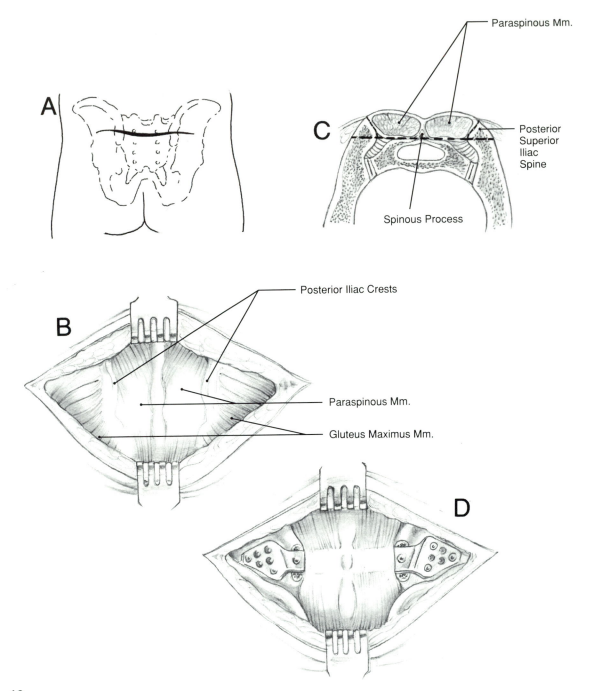

FIG 9–19.
Bilateral approach to sacroiliac joints. **A,** skin incision. **B,** exposure of posterior iliac crests with attached gluteus maximus muscles and paraspinous muscle group. **C,** diagram showing resection plane *(dashed line)* of posterior ilium and dorsal vertebral spine and plane for tunneling below the paraspinous muscle group. **D,** application of contoured fixation plate on the posterior pelvis. (Adapted from Mears DC, Rubash HE: *Pelvic and Acetabular Fractures.* Thorofare, NJ, Slack, 1986, pp 220–221.)

The bilaterally symmetric incision begins in the midline at the most caudal sacral level desired and proceeds laterally (Fig 9–20). Just lateral to the posterior superior iliac crest, the incision curves craniad, staying lateral and inferior to the iliac crests. The

dissection is carried down through skin and subcutaneous tissue. The paraspinous muscle group is detached from its caudal insertion into the sacrum and iliac crest to allow retraction cranially. The gluteal muscles are subperiosteally reflected off the poste-

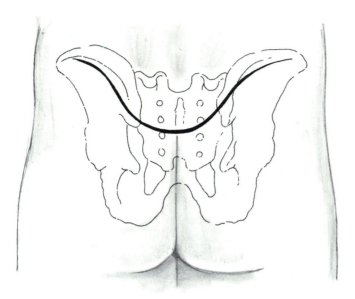

FIG 9–20.
Sea-gull skin incision for approach to the posterior pelvis and sacroiliac joints.

rior ilium bilaterally. Three myocutaneous flaps are thus created: two are gluteal, and the third is a wide midline lumbosacral flap that extends distally from a proximal base.

Approach to Posterior Acetabular Wall and Posterior Pelvic Column

The goal of treatment of acetabular fractures should be the same as that of all fractures involving diarthrodial joints, that is, anatomical reduction and early joint motion. This goal is often difficult to realize because of the inability to obtain adequate reduction by closed methods and because of the complexities of surgical exposure for open reduction procedures.

Fractures involving the posterior lip (posterior wall) of the acetabulum may be approached through a standard Gibson or Osborne incision, which splits the gluteus maximus along the direction of its fibers (see Hip chapter).

Kocher-Langenbeck Approach

Posterior column fractures are best approached through an extended Kocher-Langenbeck exposure (Fig 9–21). This approach is performed with the patient in lateral decubitus or prone position on a fracture table with the knee flexed to 45 degrees. This position relaxes the sciatic nerve, which is at risk during the procedure.

The incision begins at the superior border of the greater trochanter and curves proximally toward the

posterior superior iliac spine. In most instances the incision is carried to within 6 to 8 cm of the spine, but if the fracture involves the superior portion of the posterior column, the incision may have to be carried as far as the posterior superior iliac spine. The closer the incision approaches to the posterior superior iliac spine, the greater the risk to the superior gluteal neurovascular structures. The inferior branch of the incision extends 15 to 20 cm vertically on the outer face of the thigh. The fascia lata is divided vertically and the aponeurotic incision continued upward to split the fibers of the gluteus maximus. This process separates the upper third of the gluteus maximus, which receives its blood supply from the superior gluteal artery, from the lower two thirds, which is supplied by the inferior gluteal vessels. The gluteus maximus is innervated solely by the inferior gluteal nerve, and if the muscle is split too far medially, the nerve trunks innervating the superior one third of the gluteus maximus may be injured. This should be avoided if possible.

The subgluteal bursa is opened and divided at the level of the trochanter, and the margins of the gluteus maximus are retracted. This exposes the deep layer of muscles (short external rotators) and the femoral insertion of the gluteus maximus. This plane of dissection is developed to the level of the intertrochanteric crest of the femur, near the quadratus femoris insertion. This muscle is followed medially to locate the sciatic nerve. The nerve is traced throughout its course up to the sciatic notch and freed from any bone fragments or hematoma. Dividing the femoral insertion of the gluteus maximus while ligating branches of the posterior circumflex femoral vessels allows greater mobilization of the gluteus maximus to provide wider exposure. If the short external rotator muscles (piriformis, gemelli, and obturator internus) are intact, they should be divided through their tendinous insertions. Sutures should be placed near the cut ends, which are then wrapped over the nerve for further protection. If it becomes necessary to gain access to the ischial tuberosity it is preferable to strip the origin of the quadratus femoris from the ischium rather than divide the muscle itself. This avoids unnecessary bleeding from the complex of vessels in this area (cruciate anastomosis—see Hip chapter).

After the external rotators are divided, stripping of the capsule and periosteum will expose the posterior pelvic column. As stripping is continued, the anterior border of the sciatic notch and the ischial spine will come into view. It is important to remember that the sciatic nerve rests directly against the

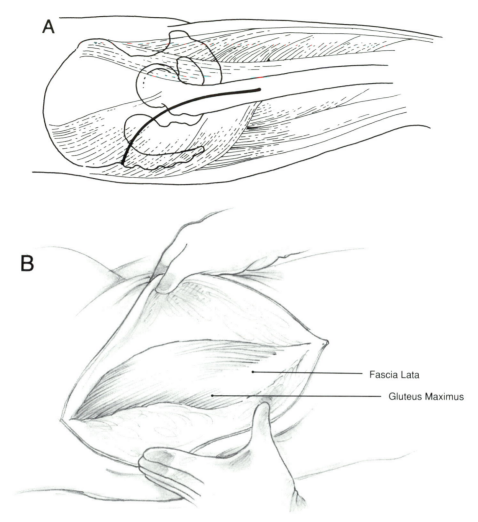

FIG 9–21.
Kocher-Langenbeck approach to the posterior acetabular wall and posterior pelvic column. **A,** skin incision. **B,** exposure of gluteus maximus fascia and fascia lata.
(Continued.)

bony edge of the greater sciatic notch and must be carefully maneuvered out of the way. Lifting the obturator internus opens the underlying bursa in its extrapelvic part. This maneuver affords access to the lesser sciatic notch and beyond to the inner wall of the pelvis. In distal dissection it is essential to stay in the subperiosteal plane, again to avoid injury to the sciatic nerve. By this approach the entire posterior column, including the greater and lesser sciatic notches and ischial spine, can be exposed and the retroacetabular (quadrilateral) pelvic surface palpated. Trochanteric osteotomy with retraction of the hip abductors craniad can also be carried out if greater exposure is required.

Again, the dangers in this approach are to the sciatic nerve and the superior gluteal nerve and vessels, particularly if the dissection is carried medially as far as the posterior superior iliac spine. Great care must be taken with the placement of retractors, especially in the region of the sciatic notch.

Triradiate Transtrochanteric Approach to the Pelvis and Acetabulum

Senegas has described a transtrochanteric surgical approach to expose complex acetabular fractures that involve both the anterior and posterior columns. Mears has modified the approach using a triradiate incision (Fig 9–22). This approach is helpful in exposing almost the entire pelvis, except for the most inferior portion of the anterior column and pubic symphysis. It is designed to provide extensive exposure to the lateral aspect of the pelvis without threatening the blood supply (superior and inferior

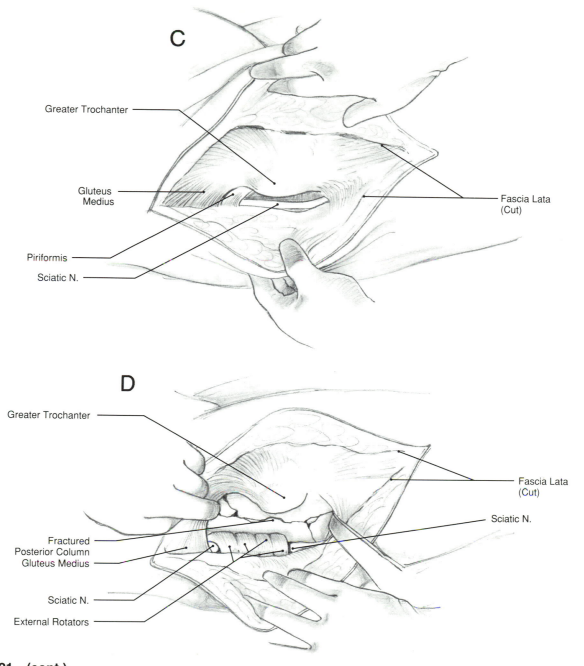

FIG 9–21   (cont.).
C, fascia lata incised. **D,** external rotators detached at their insertion and reflected over the sciatic nerve. Exposure of fractured posterior column.

gluteal vessels) of the abductor muscles. This exposure can begin as the Kocher-Langenbeck posterior approach and, if necessary, be converted to the triradiate exposure by addition of the anterior limb.

The patient is placed in a full lateral position on a conventional operating table. Routine preparation and draping are undertaken from the anterior to posterior midline. The extremity is draped free to permit intraoperative manipulation. The superficial landmarks for the incision are the anterior and posterior superior iliac spines and greater trochanter. The longitudinal limb of the triradiate incision extends distally from the greater trochanter for about 8 cm. The proximal extensions of the incision course in posterosuperior and anterosuperior directions, respectively. The angles of the flaps thus formed are

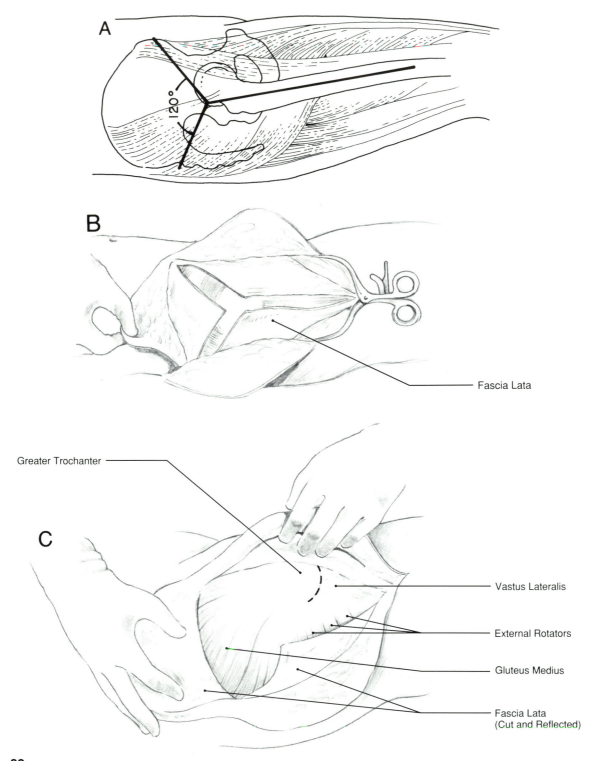

FIG 9–22.
Triradiate transtrochanteric approach. **A,** triradiate skin incision. **B,** fascial incision in line with skin incision. **C,** site *(dashed line)* for trochanteric osteotomy. *(Continued.)*

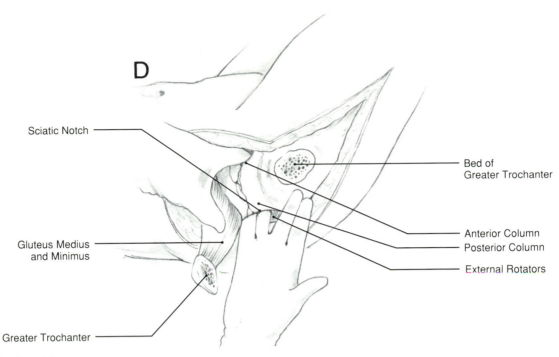

Sciatic Notch

Gluteus Medius
and Minimus

Greater Trochanter

Bed of
Greater Trochanter

Anterior Column
Posterior Column

External Rotators

D

FIG 9–22 (cont.).

D, the greater trochanter has been osteotomized and the attached gluteal muscles retracted proximally. The short external rotators have been removed from the proximal femur, exposing the posterior (ischiopubic) column. The fascia lata and myofascia of the tensor fasciae latae have been incised from the anterior superior iliac spine, exposing the anterior (iliopubic) column. A transverse fracture involving both the anterior and posterior columns is completely exposed. (Adapted from Mears DC, Rubash HE: *Pelvic and Acetabular Fractures.* Thorofare, NJ, Slack, 1986.)

approximately 120 degrees. The posterosuperior limb projects toward the posterior superior iliac spine for 6 to 8 cm, while the anterosuperior limb continues across to the anterior superior iliac spine, avoiding the lateral femoral cutaneous nerve. The distal longitudinal limb of the incision is extended down to the fascia lata, which is divided.

The anterior fascial incision is made directly below the anterior skin incision. Through the posterior limb of the incision, the myofascia of the gluteus maximus is incised and the muscle bluntly split in line with its fibers. Care is taken to avoid injury to the inferior gluteal nerve and inferior and superior gluteal vessels. On the lateral aspect of the proximal femur, the attachments of the gluteus medius and vastus lateralis are identified. A transverse incision is made between them, down to the bone, in the region of the vastus ridge. After predrilling for subsequent screw reattachment the greater trochanter is osteotomized and reflected craniad with the attached gluteus medius and minimus. Next, the short external rotators of the hip are excised from their attachments to the proximal femur as far distally as the midportion of the quadratus femoris. The vessels of the cruciate anastomosis (see Hip chapter)

must be cauterized. The rotators are reflected posteriorly to allow visualization of the underlying posterior column and the adjacent capsule of the hip joint.

During the dissection, the hip capsule and its vessels are carefully preserved. With the gluteus medius and minimus reflected superiorly, the lateral pelvis and most of the acetabulum are approached by elevation of the periosteum. By sharp and blunt dissection, the posterior column is exposed, starting at the greater sciatic notch. Blunt retractors are inserted with great care into the greater sciatic notch to maintain exposure of the posterior column. The abductor muscle mass can be anchored superiorly and posteriorly with two Steinmann pins inserted into the ilium. The superior gluteal vessels in the abductor muscle mass are carefully protected.

The distal portion of the posterior column can be exposed to the level of the ischial tuberosity by sharp incision of the origin of the hamstring muscles. The sacrotuberous ligament may be incised to facilitate exposure, but this maneuver may compromise one of the few remaining stabilizing elements of the pelvis.

For exposure of the anterior column, the fascia

lata and myofascia of the tensor fasciae latae are incised from the anterior superior iliac spine to the greater trochanter. The anterior border of the tensor fasciae latae is sharply incised from the fascia so that the muscle can be retracted superiorly and posteriorly along with the cutaneous flap. The anterior margin of the tensor fasciae latae and the gluteus minimus are incised from the ilium. Subperiosteal elevation of the gluteus medius and minimus is undertaken anteriorly to posteriorly; these muscles are then elevated from the capsule of the hip joint, which is carefully preserved. Care must be taken to preserve the superior gluteal nerve and vessels. For greater exposure to the anterior column the sartorius and rectus femoris can be detached from their origins. The lateral femoral cutaneous nerve should be protected as this is done.

Extensive pelvic fractures often present with tears in the capsule of the hip joint. If tears are not present, a small incision may be made in the superior aspect of the capsule, adjacent to the acetabulum, to permit access to the hip joint. An incision in this area is less apt to damage the blood supply to the femoral head. Visualization of the joint is necessary to verify anatomical reduction and, more significantly, to identify and remove osteochondral fragments from within the hip joint.

Approaches to Anterior Acetabular Wall and Anterior Pelvic Column

Fractures involving only the anterior wall of the acetabulum can be approached through a Smith-Petersen incision (see Hip chapter). Some anterior column fractures can be approached through a Smith-Petersen or Watson-Jones incision (see Hip chapter). However, if the fracture pattern is extensive, complex, and distal to the iliopectineal brim, an ilioinguinal approach, as described by Letournel, may be required. This approach allows access to almost the entire inner aspect of the innominate bone from the sacroiliac joint to the pubic symphysis. The anatomy encountered during this approach is complex. Surgeons are strongly advised to carry out this procedure in the dissection laboratory before using it in a clinical situation.

Ilioinguinal (Letournel) Approach

Before this approach is begun an indwelling Foley catheter is placed and the perineal area completely shaved and prepared. Draping should allow placement of a lateral traction pin through the greater trochanter, which may be required to facilitate fracture reduction. Distal femoral traction may

also help to obtain fracture reduction. The patient is operated upon in the supine position. The incision follows the anterior two thirds of the iliac crest. From the anterior superior iliac spine it curves in a slightly concave direction and extends medially as far as the midline. The incision terminates about two fingerbreadths above the pubic symphysis (Fig 9–23). In the proximolateral portion of the incision the lateral femoral cutaneous nerve will be encountered and should be protected.

The sheet muscles of the abdomen are stripped from the iliac crest in one layer and elevated in continuity with the iliacus muscle. This exposes the iliac fossa as far back as the sacroiliac joint and pelvic brim. The aponeurosis of the external oblique muscle is incised from the anterior superior iliac spine to as far as the midline, passing 2 cm above the superficial ring of the inguinal canal. The inferior lip of the external oblique muscle is then elevated to expose the origin of the muscular portion of the internal oblique and transversus abdominis muscles. These muscles are carefully separated from the inguinal ligament; the muscles themselves are not cut but rather their fibrous tendinous zone of origin from the inguinal ligament. This leaves a linear tendinous fringe of 2 mm to 3 mm in breadth, comprising 1 mm of the inguinal ligament itself, which facilitates repair during wound closure. Incising the origins of the internal oblique and transversus abdominis muscles at the inguinal ligament allows direct access to the psoas sheath, which at this level adheres to the inguinal ligament. The sheath itself is opened transversely and its medial limit located. With the finger used as a guide, the medial surface of the iliopectineal fascia is freed of lymph-containing tissue adjacent to the femoral sheath.

The iliopectineal fascia is dissected down to the iliopectineal eminence. From there, the attachment of the iliopectineal fascia to the bone is progressively divided along the brim of the true pelvis. This offers access to the true pelvis and its quadrilateral surface. The iliopsoas muscle, femoral nerve, and lateral femoral cutaneous nerve are gathered in an umbilical tape or Penrose drain. In the inner part of the field, a second tape is placed around the round ligament (spermatic cord in males), which is displaced. In the inner part of the incision, the transversalis fascia and the common insertion of the internal oblique and transversus abdominis muscles (conjoined tendon, or falx inguinalis) are incised a few millimeters from their insertion on the pubis, thus opening the retropubic space.

If it is necessary to work as far medially as the

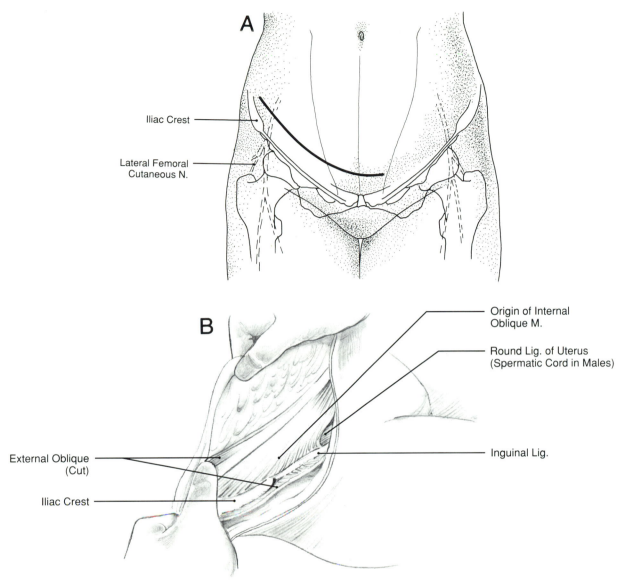

FIG 9–23.
Ilioinguinal (Letournel) approach to the anterior acetabular wall and anterior pelvic column. **A,** the skin incision extends along the anterior two thirds of the iliac crest to the anterior superior iliac spine, then curves distally and medially to reach the midline 2 cm above the pubic symphysis. Note lateral femoral cutaneous nerve. **B,** external oblique aponeurosis incised from the anterior superior iliac spine to the midline, passing 2 cm above the superficial ring of the inguinal canal.

(Continued.)

pubic symphysis, the rectus abdominis muscle is divided 1 to 2 cm from its insertion. The external iliac vessels are now mobilized. Prior to retraction of the external iliac vessels a careful look is made to identify the obturator artery and nerve. The obturator artery usually arises from the internal iliac artery but at times (up to 30%) may arise from the inferior epigastric artery. If this anomalous "abnormal" obturator artery is present, it must be clamped and ligated to avoid avulsion or traction injury and subsequent

bleeding. The external iliac vessels must be isolated with the finger to conserve the surrounding tissue, which contains deep lymphatics. These vessels are encircled by a third umbilical tape. The structures passing beneath the inguinal ligament, having thus been isolated in their separate tapes, are mobilized transversely. It is between them that the pelvic bone can be reached. One or two Steinmann pins driven into the ilium in front of the sacroiliac joint can serve as abdominal retractors. Once the fracture has been

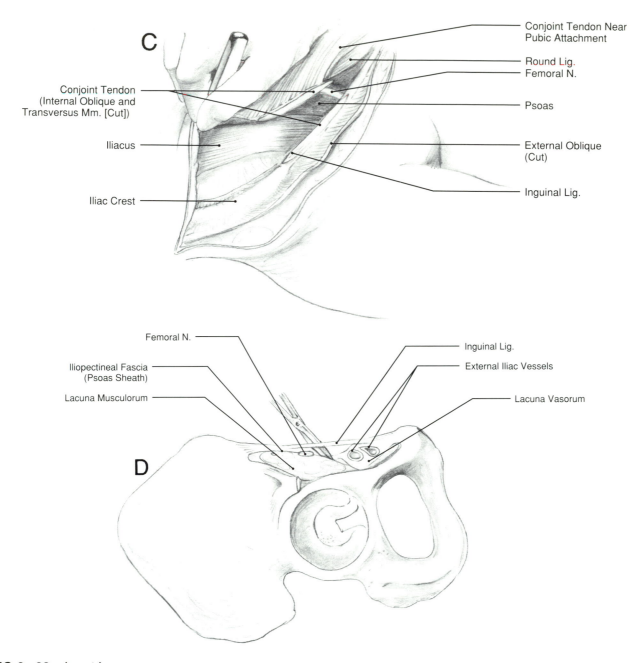

FIG 9–23 (cont.).
C, the conjoined tendon (internal oblique and transversalis abdominis) is incised from the outer half of the inguinal ligament, leaving 2 to 3 mm of inguinal ligament with the conjoined tendon for subsequent reapproximation. **D,** division of the iliopectineal fascia. Care is taken to protect the lacuna vasorum. Note the iliopectineal fascia (psoas sheath) separates the lacuna musculorum (which contains the iliopsoas, femoral nerve, and lateral femoral cutaneous nerve) from the lacuna vasorum (which contains the external iliac vessels and lymphatics).   *(Continued.)*

completely exposed, reduction and internal fixation can be carried out.

Extended Iliofemoral Approach

The extended iliofemoral approach, as described by Letournel, has been used to gain simultaneous exposure to the anterior and posterior columns of the pelvis and the external iliac wall. This approach allows posterior reflection of the muscles innervated by the superior and inferior gluteal neurovascular structures. The procedure is carried out with the patient in the lateral decubitus position on an ortho-

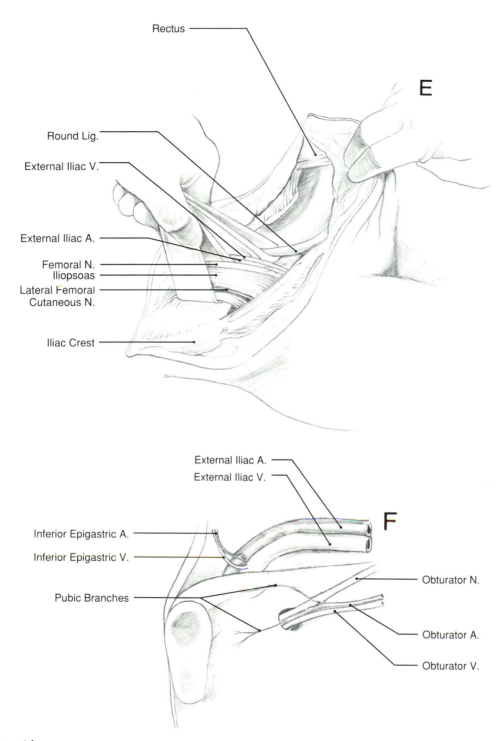

FIG 9–23   (cont.).
E, the iliopsoas muscle has been freed from the pelvic brim by finger and subperiosteal dissection and, together with the femoral and lateral femoral cutaneous nerve, retracted with a Penrose drain. A second sling (Penrose drain) is placed around the round ligament (spermatic cord in males). After the obturator artery is located and identified and the absence or presence of an anomaly determined, the external iliac vessels are freed up by blunt finger dissection. The associated deep lymphatic tissue is preserved as much as possible. A third sling is then placed around the external iliac vessels. **F,** normal obturator artery. Note that the obturator artery, which is a branch of the internal iliac artery, together with the corresponding vein and nerve, passes through the obturator groove at the posterior border of the pubic ramus.   *(Continued.)*

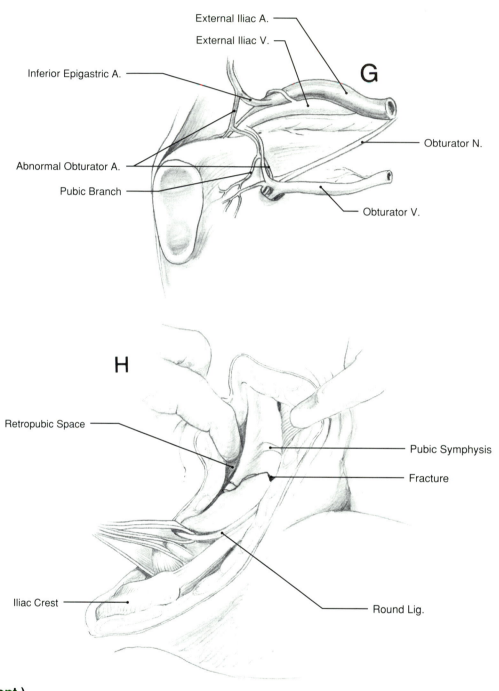

FIG 9–23 (cont.).
G, abnormal obturator artery. In up to 30% of individuals the obturator artery arises from the inferior epigastric instead of the internal iliac artery. If present it must be identified, clamped, and ligated. **H,** with mobilization of the structures within the Penrose drains and subperiosteal dissection, the entire anterior pelvic column can be exposed for fracture reduction and fixation. (Adapted and modified from Letournel E, Judet R: *Fractures of the Acetabulum.* Berlin, Springer-Verlag, 1981.)

paedic operating table with a support column between the thighs and distal femoral skeletal traction applied to the involved side.

A skin incision is made in the form of an inverted J, beginning at the posterior superior iliac spine and carried anteriorly along the iliac crest as far as the anterior superior iliac spine (Fig 9–24). The incision is then curved distally and directed toward the outer border of the patella halfway down the thigh. The gluteal fascia is excised along the iliac

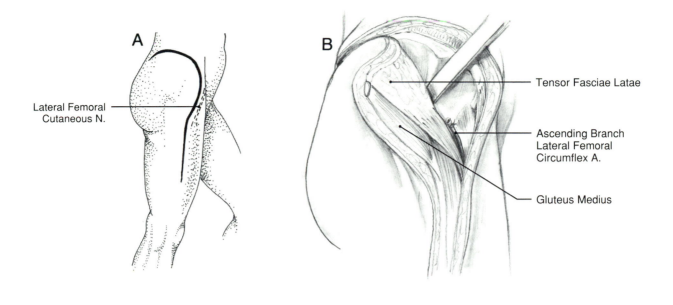

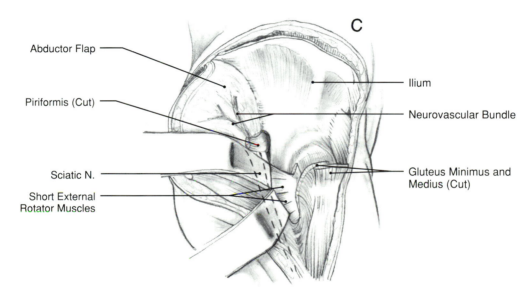

FIG 9–24.
Extended iliofemoral approach. **A,** skin incision. **B,** gluteus medius and minimus and tensor fasciae latae muscles are progressively detached from the iliac wing. The ascending branch of the lateral femoral circumflex artery is identified, clamped, and ligated. **C,** the tendons of the gluteus medius and minimus are incised just proximal to their insertion on the greater trochanter. The abductor muscle flap is lifted from the outer ilium. Care is taken to preserve the neurovascular bundle.

(Continued.)

crest, and the muscles (tensor fasciae latae and gluteus medius and minimus) are subperiosteally reflected from the iliac wing. The lateral femoral cutaneous nerve lies anteromedial to the dissection and should not be disturbed. The fascia lata is split in line with the skin incision. The ascending branch of

the lateral femoral circumflex artery is clamped, ligated, and divided. Bleeding from the nutrient vessels in the outer wing of the ilium is controlled with bone wax. The fat overlying the hip joint is stripped off. The gluteus medius and minimus are divided near their attachment on the greater trochanter, with

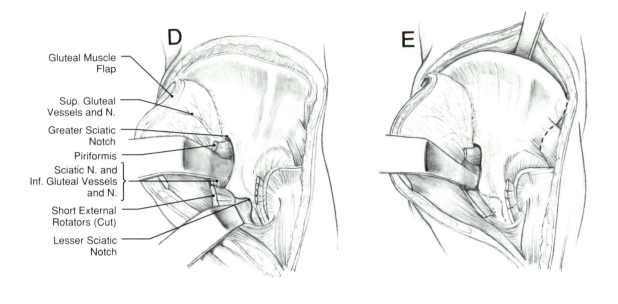

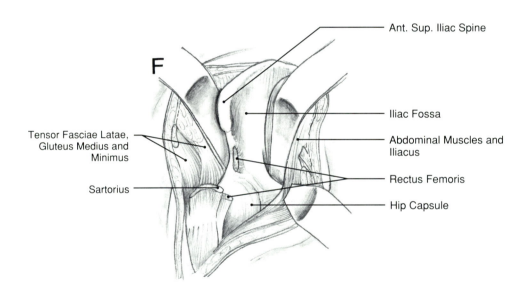

FIG 9–24   (cont.).
D, the short external rotators of the hip are incised at their femoral insertions and retracted posteriorly. The sciatic nerve is protected. This allows exposure of the entire posterior column. **E,** the sartorius and rectus femoris are removed from their origins *(dashed line)*. **F,** (medial view) exposure of the iliac fossa, pelvic brim, and anterior rim of the acetabulum. (Adapted and modified from Letournel E, Judet R: *Fractures of the Acetabulum.* Berlin, Springer-Verlag, 1981.)

a cuff of tendon left for subsequent reattachment. The large muscle flap thus created, consisting of the gluteus medius, gluteus minimus, tensor fasciae latae, and neurovascular bundles, is then lifted from the ilium and retracted posteriorly. The short external rotators are detached from their trochanteric insertion. These muscles are then carefully retracted posteriorly over the sciatic nerve, which affords some protection.

Opening the bursa under the obturator internus allows access to the lesser sciatic notch and thus to the interior of the true pelvis. The ischium, as far distally as the tuberosity, can be exposed by subperiosteal dissection. The whole of the posterior column of the pelvis is thus exposed. The entire external wing of the ilium is also exposed, as well as the anterior column as far distally and medially as the iliopectineal eminence. Division of the origins of the rectus femoris and retraction of the iliopsoas will allow exposure as far as the lateral aspect of the superior pubic ramus. Thus, all but the very distal portion of the anterior column of the pelvis can be exposed with this approach.

Modified Extensile Iliofemoral Approach

Reinert, et al. have described a modification of the extended iliofemoral approach of Letournel. It has been advocated for exposure to treat T-type and complex transverse fractures, fractures that involve both columns of the pelvis, and nonunions. This modification utilizes a T-shaped skin incision with large flaps and osteotomies of the iliac crest, greater trochanter, and anterior superior iliac spine. The operative exposure creates an abductor muscle flap, which is hinged on the superior gluteal muscular bundles at the sciatic notch in the manner described by Letournel. Because the approach interrupts the communicating vascular supply to the abductor muscles (cruciate anastomosis), patency of the superior gluteal artery is an absolute prerequisite. Reinert recommends a preoperative arteriogram to verify

that the superior gluteal artery is intact. Theoretical advantages of this approach are that it allows fixation of fractures from both sides of the iliac wing and the skin incision allows utilization of a standard posterior approach with conversion to extensile exposure if necessary. It is also thought that osteotomy of the greater trochanter is more apt to heal firmly than soft tissue reapproximation of the gluteus medius and minimus. Furthermore, it is suggested that later reconstructive procedures, such as bone grafting, arthrodesis, or arthroplasty, can be readily carried out if this initial approach to the pelvic fracture has been used.

The operative procedure is carried out with the patient in the lateral decubitus position and the involved extremity draped out free. A skin incision is made 1 cm distal and parallel to the iliac crest from the anterior to the posterior superior iliac spine (Fig 9–25). A second incision is made laterally along the proximal third of the thigh parallel to the femoral shaft. It is continued cranially over the tip of the tro-

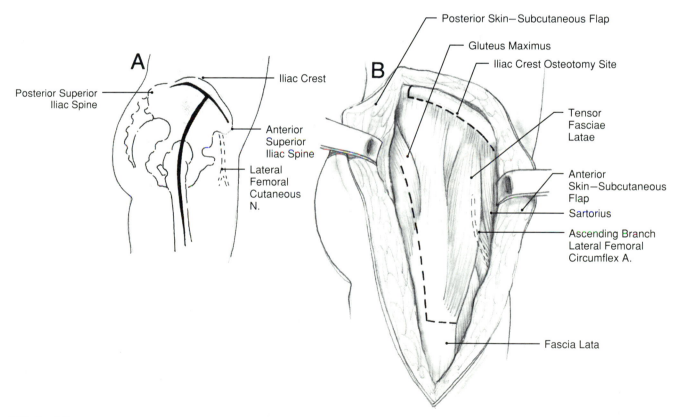

FIG 9–25.
Modified extensile iliofemoral approach. **A,** skin incision. **B,** gluteal fascia is split from proximal to distal *(vertical dashed line)* along the fibers of the gluteus maximus distally. Fascia lata is transected *(transverse dashed line)* distal to the termination of the tensor fasciae latae muscle. The tensor fasciae latae muscle is separated from the sartorius and rectus muscles and mobilized. The ascending branch of the lateral femoral circumflex artery is identified and carefully ligated and divided. (Reanastomosis of this vessel may be required should the vascular supply to the abductor flap, i.e., the superior gluteal artery, be damaged.) *(Continued.)*

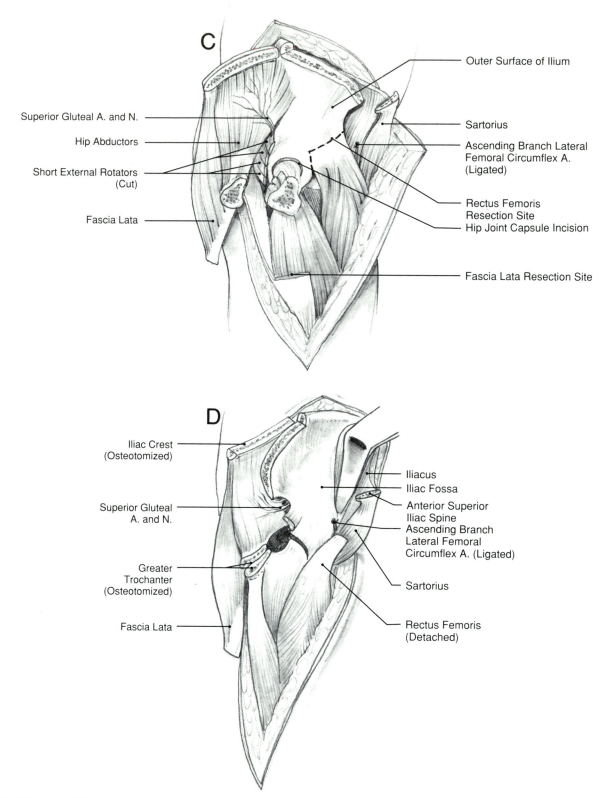

FIG 9–25 (cont.).
C, osteotomy of the anterior iliac crest and retraction with attached sartorius. Osteotomy of iliac crest preserving attachment of abductor muscles. Abductor mass is elevated subperiosteally. Standard trochanteric osteotomy is carried out. Heads of rectus femoris are to be detached from their origins *(dashed line)*. **D,** the inner table of the ilium is exposed by dissection of abdominal muscles and iliacus subperiosteally.

(Continued.)

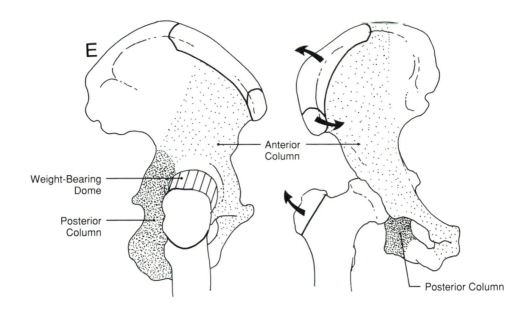

Weight-Bearing
Dome

Posterior
Column

Anterior
Column

Posterior Column

LATERAL VIEW   ANTERIOR VIEW

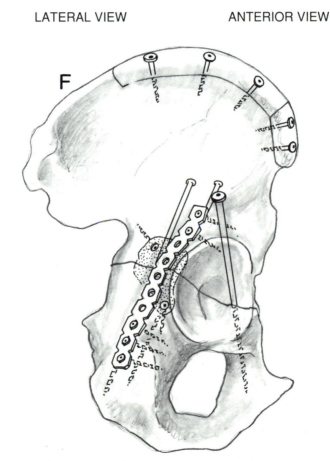

FIG 9–25   (cont.).
E, schematic diagram indicating osteotomies and the direction of retraction *(arrows)* of the osteotomized bone with attached musculature. *Lightly stippled area* represents anterior pelvic column and *heavily stippled area* represents posterior column. **F,** schematic diagram of pelvic fracture reconstruction utilizing lag screws and reconstruction plate. The osteotomies have been reapproximated and secured with screws. (Drawn after Reinert CM, Bosse MJ, Poka A, et al: A modified extensile exposure for the treatment of complex or malunited acetabular fractures. *J Bone Joint Surg* 1988; 70A: 329–337.)

chanter, curving gently in an anterior direction to intersect with the initial incision at a 90-degree angle. Anterior and posterior skin flaps are then created by sharp dissection of the subcutaneous tissue from the deep fascia. Development of the anterior flap allows access to the anterior superior iliac spine and the interval between the tensor fasciae latae and sartorius. Identification and preservation of the lateral femoral cutaneous nerve is carried out. The posterior flap is developed only enough to allow a standard posterior approach to the hip. For this the gluteal fascia is split proximally and the gluteus maximus fibers divided bluntly until branches of the inferior gluteal neurovascular bundle are encountered.

The hip is then flexed 45 degrees and abducted. The fascia lata is opened from the trochanter distally along the femoral shaft to the distalmost portion of the tensor fasciae latae. For increased posterior exposure the tendinous insertion of the gluteus maximus on the linea aspera is partially released. Distally the interval between the sartorius and tensor fasciae latae is defined. The fascia lata is transected at its junction with the tensor fasciae latae muscle. This muscle is separated from the sartorius and rectus and freed up anteriorly, posteriorly, and deeply. In the proximal portion of this dissection the ascending branch of the lateral femoral circumflex artery will be encountered and should be carefully ligated and divided. This is an important step, because reanastomosis of this vessel might be necessary if the vascular supplies to the abductor flap via the superior gluteal vessels are damaged during the operation.

At this point an incision is made in the periosteum along the superior aspect of the iliac crest. The incision commences 2 cm posterior to the anterior superior iliac spine and extends for the length of the exposed crest. The abdominal and iliacus muscles are dissected off the iliac crest for 10 to 15 cm. The interval between the origin of the sartorius and tensor fasciae latae is identified. The anterior superior iliac spine is then osteotomized. This fragment, with the attached sartorius and inguinal ligament, is retracted medially, as are the abdominal muscles and the iliacus.

Further subperiosteal dissection of the iliacus exposes the inner part of the ilium as far as the greater sciatic notch. At this point a tricortical portion of the posterior and middle iliac crest measuring 10 to 12 cm in length and approximately 1.5 cm in height is osteotomized. The osteotomy begins at the inner surface of the crest, with the attachment of the abductor muscles to the osteotomized fragment preserved. The abductor muscle mass is then elevated subperiosteally from the outer surface of the ilium,

and a standard trochanteric osteotomy is performed. The entire abductor muscle mass is separated from the hip capsule and the inferior portions of the ilium and gently retracted posteriorly with the trochanter. The superior gluteal neurovascular structures are preserved as they exit from the sciatic notch. Excising the external rotators from their trochanteric attachment exposes the superior aspect of the posterior column. The quadratus femoris muscle should be left intact and the medial femoral circumflex vessel spared. It is important to identify and protect the sciatic nerve during this part of the procedure. Hematoma and small fracture fragments compromising the nerve should be removed. If further exposure anteriorly is required, the direct and reflected heads of the rectus femoris can be released to increase access to the anterior column.

The capsule is opened at the lip of the acetabulum. This allows exposure of the hip joint itself, assessment for any intraarticular fragments, and reduction of the articular surface. Further exposure to the joint itself can be obtained by inserting a large Schanz screw into the region of the greater trochanter and retracting the trochanter with a T-handled universal chuck. The ilium can be exposed down to the sciatic notch on its inner and outer surfaces if the dissection is continued distally and the quadratus femoris and origins of the hamstrings resected from the posterior surface of the ischium. The fracture pattern can be assessed and the fractures debrided and internally fixed with lag screws and/or fixation plates.

Antibiotics should be used during and after the procedure. Adequate suction and drainage should be maintained for at least 36 hours and perhaps longer, depending upon the amount and persistence of drainage. Some means of preventing postoperative heterotopic ossification about the dissection sites should be considered.

Hemipelvectomy

Hemipelvectomy (hindquarter amputation, ilioabdominal amputation, transiliac amputation) is most often done as ablative cancer surgery. In rare instances, it may be the only method of controlling hemorrhage in patients with severe pelvic trauma. Specially tailored flaps may be required in certain cancer operations. However, hemipelvectomy utilizing a posterior flap composed of skin and subcutaneous tissue overlying the buttock muscles, primarily gluteus maximus, is the most commonly used method. This technic is described here.

A Foley catheter should be inserted and, when

possible, the patient prepared preoperatively with cleansing enemas. The anus is stitched closed for the duration of the procedure. The patient is positioned on the operating table in the lateral position with the sound side downward. The entire lower extremity on the affected side is prepared and draped to allow intraoperative manipulation. The skin incision is begun at the pubic tubercle and extended superiorly and laterally along the inguinal ligament to the ante-

rior superior iliac spine and then swung posteriorly along the iliac crest (Fig 9–26). The abdominal muscles and inguinal ligament are detached from the iliac crest, and the iliac fossa is opened between the peritoneum and iliacus muscle. The inferior epigastric vessels are ligated and divided. The inguinal ligament and rectus abdominis insertion are dissected near the pubis, and the spermatic cord (males) is retracted medially. The retropubic space of Retzius is

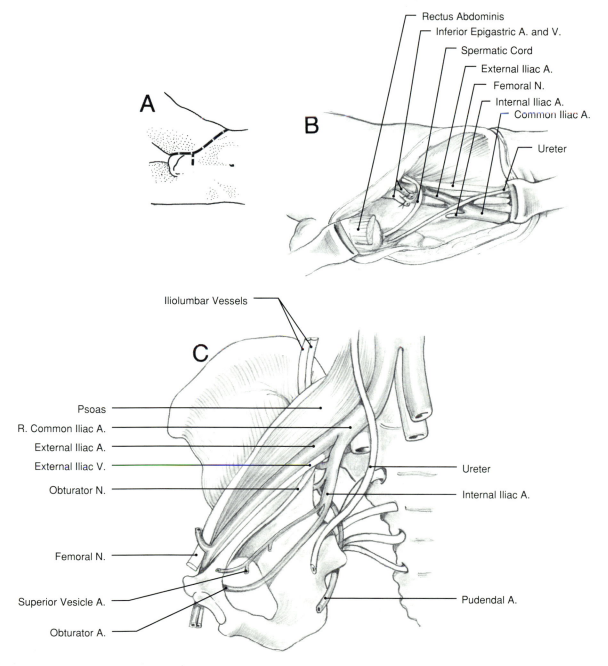

FIG 9–26.
Hemipelvectomy. **A,** anterior skin incision. **B,** rectus abdominis transected and retracted. Inferior epigastric vessels ligated. **C,** schematic drawing of regional neurovascular structures. *(Continued.)*

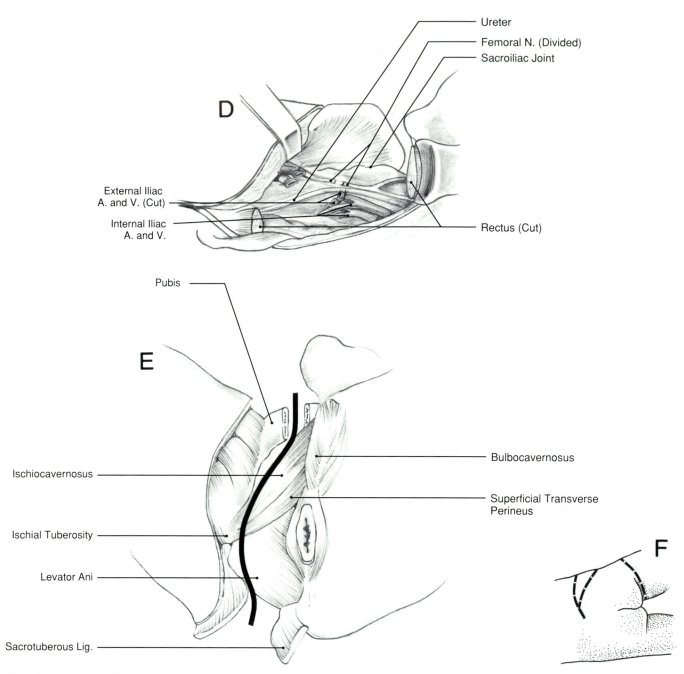

FIG 9–26   (cont.).
D, ligation of major vessels at desired level (see text). E, perineal dissection. F, posterior skin incision.

(Continued.)

opened and the bladder retracted into the pelvis. The major vessels must then be ligated. There is some leeway as to the optimum level of vessel ligation. If resection of the ilium is to be carried far enough posteriorly that the gluteus maximus will not be retained in the posterior flap, the common iliac vessels are ligated, which results in less bleeding. If, however, the gluteus maximus is to be included in the posterior flap, it is best to ligate and divide the external iliac vessels and femoral nerve and retain the internal iliac vessels. These vessels supply the muscle and subcutaneous fat of the posterior flap. The limb is then widely abducted and the incision carried inferiorly and laterally from the pubic tubercle along the pubic and ischial rami to the ischial tuberosity. The rami are exposed subperi-

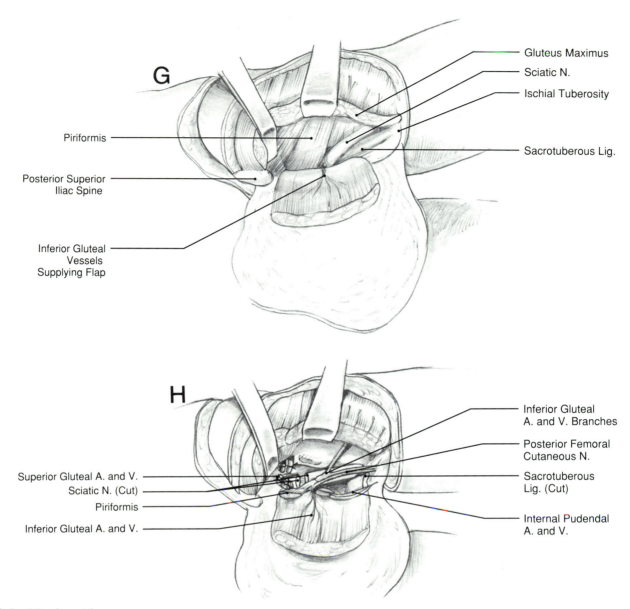

FIG 9–26 (cont.).
G, gluteus maximus divided in line with skin incision, elevated, and retracted posteriorly. **H,** piriformis divided, sciatic nerve and superior gluteal vessels ligated and divided. Inferior gluteal vessels preserved.
(Continued.)

osteally, and the ischiocavernosus and corpus cavernosus are elevated from the bony surfaces. The urogenital diaphragm is also reflected off the ischiopubic ramus. The pubic symphysis is then divided.

The posterior portion of the dissection is begun by extending the anterior incision over the crest of the ilium to the posterior superior iliac spine. At this point, the incision is turned abruptly laterally and distally to the greater trochanter and then posteriorly in the gluteal crease to join the perineal part of the incision. The gluteus maximus is divided in line with the skin incision. Elevation of this flap of mus-

cle, subcutaneous fat, and skin brings the gluteus medius and sciatic nerve into view. The piriformis muscle and the sciatic, posterior femoral cutaneous, pudendal, and superior gluteal nerves are divided. The internal pudendal artery and vein are ligated. The superior and inferior gluteal vessels are preserved as much as possible to maintain the blood supply to the gluteal flap. The ilium is then transected just anterior to the sacroiliac joint with a Gigli saw. This is done by placing the saw through the greater sciatic notch and anteriorly over the iliac crest. The sacrotuberous and sacrospinous ligaments

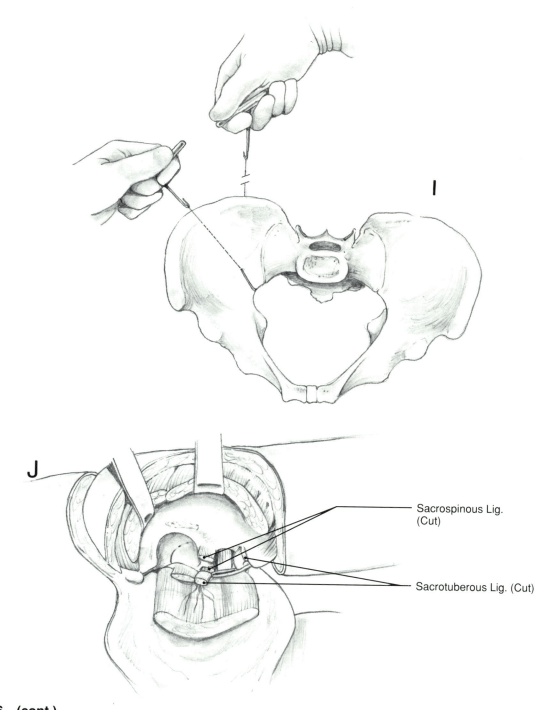

FIG 9–26   (cont.).
I, transection of ilium. **J,** sacrotuberous and sacrospinous ligaments divided.

(Continued.)

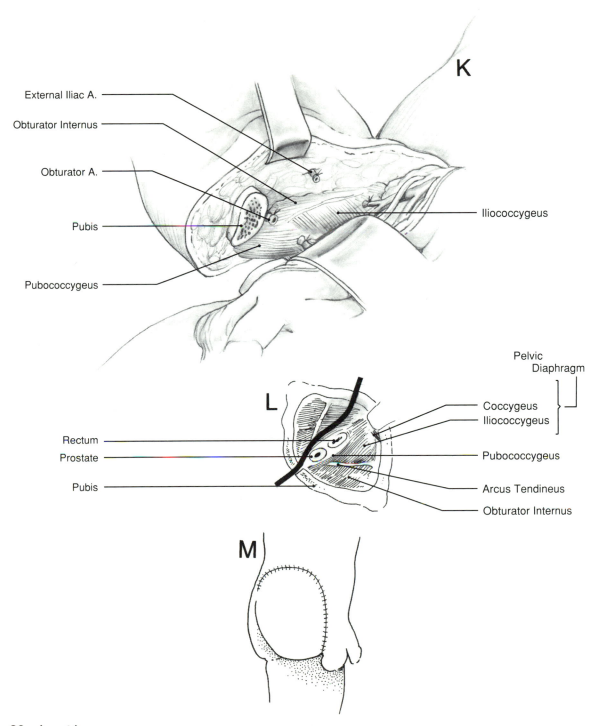

K

External Iliac A.

Obturator Internus

Obturator A.

Pubis

Pubococcygeus

Iliococcygeus

L

Pelvic Diaphragm

Coccygeus
Iliococcygeus

Rectum

Prostate

Pubis

Pubococcygeus

Arcus Tendineus

Obturator Internus

M

FIG 9–26   (cont.).
K, external rotation of the limb allows wide intrapelvic exposure. Obturator vessels are ligated. **L,** cross-section viewing into the pelvis (from cephalad to caudad) depicts transection *(solid line)* of levator ani portion of pelvic diaphragm. **M,** flap closure. (Modified from Slocum DB: *An Atlas of Amputations.* St Louis, CV Mosby Co, 1949.)

are divided. The levator ani portion of the pelvic diaphragm (pubococcygeus and iliococcygeus muscles) is divided near the midline. External rotation of the limb now allows wide intrapelvic exposure. The obturator vessels and nerve are ligated and divided, and the psoas muscle is transected at the level of the sacroiliac joint. The entire lower extremity is then removed. The gluteus maximus flap is swung anteriorly and sutured to the rectus abdominis and psoas muscles. Prior to wound closure, deep and subcutaneous drains are placed.

BIBLIOGRAPHY

Brotman S, Soderstrom CA, Oster-Granite M, et al: Management of severe bleeding in fractures of the pelvis. *Surg Gynecol Obstet* 1981; 153:823.

Clark SS, Prudencio RF: Lower urinary tract injuries associated with pelvic fractures: Diagnosis and management. *Surg Clin North Am* 1972; 52:183.

Crenshaw AH: *Campbell's Operative Orthopaedics*, ed 7. St Louis, CV Mosby Co, 1987.

Eckardt JJ: Modified hemipelvectomy utilizing an anteromedial vascularized myocutaneous flap, in Tronzo RG (ed.): *Surgery of the Hip Joint*, vol 2, ed 2. New York, Springer-Verlag New York, 1987, pp 61–72.

Grant JCB: *An Atlas of Anatomy*, ed 6. Baltimore, Williams & Wilkins Co, 1972.

Gray H: *Anatomy of the Human Body*, ed 30. Philadelphia, Lea & Febiger, 1973.

Jacobs RR, Montesano, PX: The sea-gull approach to the posterior pelvis. *Techniques Orthop* 1990; 4:65–66.

Judet R, Judet J, Letournel E: Fractures of the acetabulum. *J Bone Joint Surg* 1964; 46A:1615.

Kane WJ: Fractures of the pelvis, in Rockwood CA, Green DP (eds): *Fractures*. Philadelphia, JB Lippincott Co, 1975, pp 905–1001.

Keating EM, Ritter MA, Faris PM: Structures at risk from medially placed acetabular screws. *J Bone Joint Surg* 1990; 72A:509–511.

King D, Steelquist J: Transiliac amputation. *J Bone Joint Surg* 1943; 25:351–367.

Letournel E: Acetabulum fractures: Classification and management. *Clin Orthop Rel Res* 1980; 151:81–106.

Letournel E, Judet R: *Fractures of the Acetabulum*. Berlin, Springer-Verlag, 1981.

Mack LA, Harley JD, Winquist RA: CT of acetabular fractures: Analysis of fracture patterns. *AJR* 1982; 138:407.

Matta JM, Letournel E, Browner BD: Surgical management of acetabular fractures, in Anderson LD (ed): *Instructional Course Lectures*, vol 35. St Louis, CV Mosby Co, 1986, pp 382–397.

Mears DC, Rubash HE: Extensile exposure of the pelvis. *Contemp Orthop* 1983; 6:21.

Mears DC, Rubash HE: *Pelvic and Acetabular Fractures*. Thorofare, NJ, Slack, 1986.

Moore KL: *Clinically Oriented Anatomy*, ed 2. Baltimore, Williams & Wilkins Co, 1985.

Netter FH: *The Ciba Collection of Medical Illustrations: Musculoskeletal System*, vol 8. Summit, NJ, Ciba-Geigy Corp, 1987.

Peltier LF: Complications associated with fractures of the pelvis. *J Bone Joint Surg* 1965; 47A:1060–1069.

Pennal GF, Davidson J, Garside H, Plewes J: Results of treatment of acetabular fractures. *Clin Orthop Rel Res* 1980; 151:115–123.

Pennal GF, Tile MD, Waddell JP, Garside H: Pelvic disruption: Assessment and classification. *Clin Orthop Rel Res* 1980; 151:12–21.

Pritchard DJ: Tumors, in Tronzo RG (ed): *Surgery of the Hip Joint*, vol II, ed 2. New York, Springer-Verlag New York, 1987, pp 31–60.

Reckling FW: Pelvic and acetabular fractures. In Goldsmith HS, Denton JR (eds): *Practice of Surgery, Orthopedics*, vol 2. Philadelphia, Harper & Row, 1984.

Reinert CM, Bosse MJ, Poka A, et al: A modified extensile exposure for the treatment of complex or malunited acetabular fractures. *J Bone Joint Surg* 1988; 70A: 329–337.

Rothenberger DA, Fischer RP, Perry JF: Major vascular injuries secondary to pelvic fractures: An unsolved clinical problem. *Am J Surg* 1978; 136:660.

Schatzker J, Tile M: *The Rationale of Operative Fracture Care*. New York, Springer-Verlag New York, 1987.

Senegas J, Liorzou G, Yates M: Complex acetabular fractures: A transtrochanteric lateral surgical approach. *Clin Orthop Rel Res* 151:107–114, 1980.

Slocum DB: *An Atlas of Amputations*. St Louis, CV Mosby Co, 1949.

Tile M: *Fractures of the Pelvis and Acetabulum*. Baltimore, Williams & Wilkins Co, 1984.

Wagman LD, Terz, JJ: Hemipelvectomy and translumbar amputation. In Moore WS, Malone JM (eds): *Lower Extremity Amputation*. Philadelphia, WB Saunders Co, 1989.

Wasielewski RC, Cooperstein LA, Kruger MP, et al: Acetabular anatomy and the transacetabular fixation of screws in total hip arthroplasty. *J Bone Joint Surg* 1990; 72A:501–509.

10

Hip and Thigh

Frederick W. Reckling, M.D.
Melvin P. Mohn, Ph.D.

ANATOMIC FEATURES OF THE HIP AND THIGH

Although both the hip and shoulder are ball-and-socket joints, the hip joint differs because of certain characteristics that increase its strength and stability at the expense of mobility. The head of the femur forms more than half a sphere, unlike the humeral head, which forms only a small fraction of a sphere. The femoral head is more deeply embedded in the acetabular socket than the humeral head in the glenoid. The fibrous capsule of the hip joint is particularly strong compared with that of the shoulder joint. The muscles that cross the hip joint, instead of inserting close to the femoral head, insert some distance from it, thus providing more leverage strength.

Bony Anatomy

The hip joint is the articulation of the femoral head with the acetabulum (Fig 10–1). Because the neck of the femur is only three quarters the equatorial diameter of the head, a large range of motion is possible before the femoral neck impinges on the acetabulum.

Acetabulum

(See also pelvis chapter)

The bony acetabulum is deepened by a fibrocartilaginous lip, the acetabular labrum, which is attached to its rim. The labrum is discontinued in the lower part of the acetabulum (acetabular notch), but the ring is completed by a heavy fibrous band known as the transverse ligament of the acetabulum. The transverse ligament is attached only at its ends; the proximal portion does not reach the bottom of the notch. This forms a foramen through which the acetabular artery travels. This artery gives branches to the ligament of the head of the femur. The ligament of the head of the femur (also known as the ligamentum teres) originates from both sides of the acetabular notch and the floor of the acetabular fossa deep to the transverse ligament. From this origin, the ligament passes medially and upward around the head of the femur and attaches to the upper part of the fovea of the femoral head. The ligament is covered by a thin layer of synovium, which also covers the fat in the acetabular fossa.

Proximal End of Femur

The proximal end of the femur includes the head, neck, and greater trochanter (Fig 10–2). The head is nearly spherical and displays a small rough end, the fovea. The head joins the neck of the femur at the epiphyseal line. The neck joins the shaft at an angle of 125 to 135 degrees. The angle between the plane of the femoral condyles and the axis of the femoral neck (anteversion) is approximately 14 degrees in an adult. The greater trochanter is a large traction apophysis for insertion of the abductors. It overhangs the expanded junction of the neck and shaft to form the trochanteric fossa. Posteriorly a

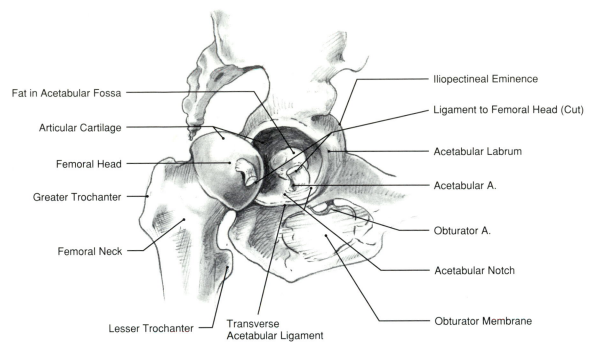

Fat in Acetabular Fossa

Articular Cartilage

Femoral Head

Greater Trochanter

Femoral Neck

Lesser Trochanter

Transverse Acetabular Ligament

Iliopectineal Eminence

Ligament to Femoral Head (Cut)

Acetabular Labrum

Acetabular A.

Obturator A.

Acetabular Notch

Obturator Membrane

FIG 10–1.
Articulation of the hip joint.

prominent intertrochanteric crest connects the greater trochanter to the lesser trochanter, which projects from the posteromedial aspect of the proximal femoral shaft. A small quadrate tubercle is located midway along the intertrochanteric crest. Anteriorly the greater and lesser trochanters are joined by a thin intertrochanteric line.

Femoral Shaft

The femoral shaft is tubular in shape and slightly bowed anteriorly below the trochanters. This fact is taken into consideration in the design of intramedullary nails. The femoral shaft is smooth, with the exception of a prominent posterior midshaft longitudinal ridge, the linea aspera, which has roughened medial and lateral lips. The linea aspera lips diverge proximally and distally. Proximally, the medial lip runs obliquely forward below the lesser trochanter, becoming continuous with the intertrochanteric line. The lateral lip runs upward, ending in the posterior gluteal tuberosity. Distally, the lips of the linea aspera separate above the condyles. They are referred to as the medial and lateral supracondylar lines, and between them lies the smooth popliteal surface of the femur. Another prominent bony landmark on the posterior surface of the femur is the pectineal line, which extends distally from the lesser trochanter. The pectineal line lies between the gluteal tuberosity and the upper part of the medial

lip of the linea aspera. The shaft of the femur is surrounded by and gives attachment to a large number of muscles.

Hip Joint Ligaments

Three areas of marked thickening of the longitudinal fibers of the hip capsule are considered hip ligaments: the iliofemoral, ischiofemoral and pubofemoral ligaments (Fig 10–3). The iliofemoral ligament is thick and one of the strongest ligaments in the body. It is triangular, with its apex attached to the body of the ilium between the anterior inferior iliac spine and the rim of the acetabulum. Its base is attached along the intertrochanteric line of the femur. The ligament resembles an inverted Y and is referred to as the Y ligament of Bigelow. It occupies the anterior aspect of the hip joint and strongly resists hyperextension at the hip joint.

The ischiofemoral ligament, the thinnest of the three, arises from the body of the ischium behind and below the acetabulum. It attaches to the upper and posterior part of the femoral neck at the junction with the greater trochanter. The ischiofemoral ligament resists forced internal rotation of the hip. A small, thin band of circular capsular fibers forms the so-called zona orbicularis, located medial to the intertrochanteric crest posteriorly.

The third ligament, the pubofemoral ligament,

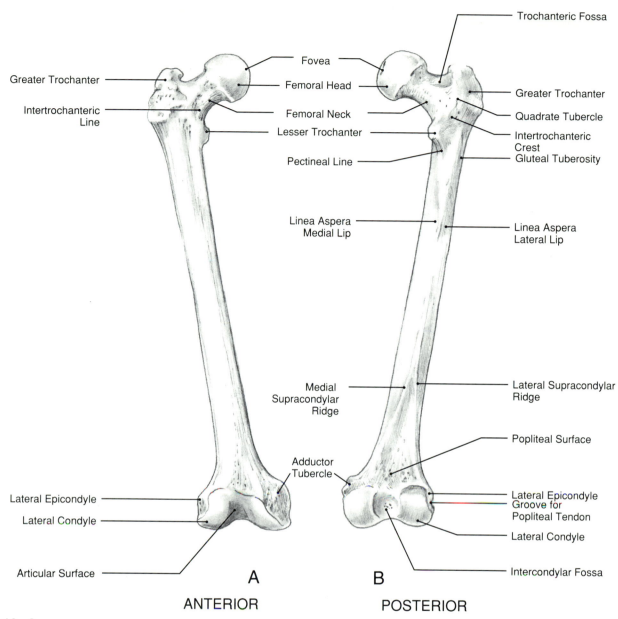

FIG 10–2.
Femur. **A,** anterior view. **B,** posterior view.

arises from the body of the pubis close to the acetabulum and the adjacent part of the superior ramus of the pubis. It passes directly in front of the lower part of the head of the femur and attaches to the lower surface of the femoral neck.

Synovial Membrane

The synovial membrane of the hip joint is in direct contact with the fibrous capsule surrounding the joint (Fig 10–4). Proximally the membrane attaches to the acetabular rim. It also passes over the inner surface of the transverse acetabular ligament, covers the fat extending inward from the floor of the acetabular notch, and attaches to the edges of the acetabular fossa. In doing so it covers the ligament of the femoral head (ligamentum teres). Distally, the synovial membrane and capsule extend anteriorly, superiorly, laterally, inferiorly, and medially to the base of the femoral neck. Therefore this portion of the neck is intracapsular. Posteriorly the membrane and capsule reach less far distally, only to the region of the zona orbicularis. Thus the lower third of the posterior femoral neck is extracapsular. When the

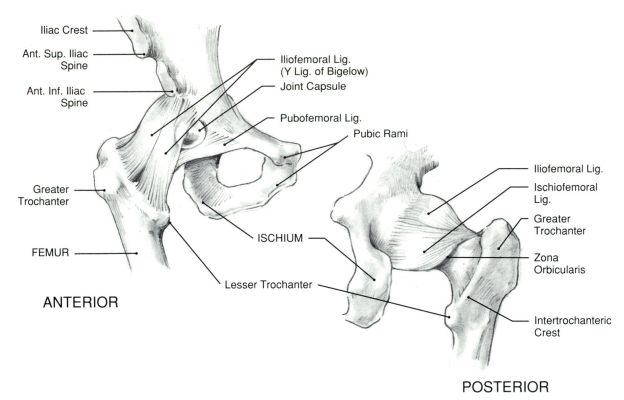

ANTERIOR

Iliac Crest

Ant. Sup. Iliac Spine

Ant. Inf. Iliac Spine

Greater Trochanter

FEMUR

Iliofemoral Lig. (Y Lig. of Bigelow)

Joint Capsule

Pubofemoral Lig.

Pubic Rami

ISCHIUM

Lesser Trochanter

POSTERIOR

Iliofemoral Lig.

Ischiofemoral Lig.

Greater Trochanter

Zona Orbicularis

Intertrochanteric Crest

FIG 10–3.
Ligaments of the hip joint.

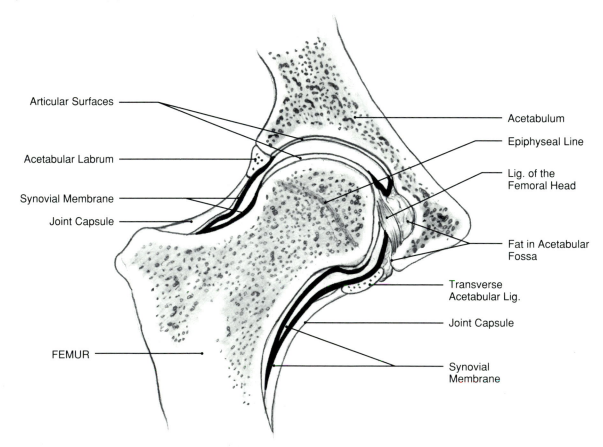

Articular Surfaces

Acetabular Labrum

Synovial Membrane

Joint Capsule

FEMUR

Acetabulum

Epiphyseal Line

Lig. of the Femoral Head

Fat in Acetabular Fossa

Transverse Acetabular Lig.

Joint Capsule

Synovial Membrane

FIG 10–4.
Synovial membrane *(dark lines)* of the hip joint.

synovial membrane reaches the neck of the femur, it is reflected back proximally along the neck as far as the epiphyseal line and the articular cartilage covering the head. Some of the inner fibers of the fibrous capsule of the hip are also reflected inwardly upon the neck. Because these inner fibers are not uniform in their reflection they form retinacula, that is, projections of fibrous capsule covered by synovial membrane. The vessels for the neck and head of the femur are located in these retinacula and therefore are called retinacular vessels (Fig 10–5).

Arteries of the Hip Joint

The blood supply to the hip joint (Figs 10–5 and 10–6) is derived from arteries in the area, namely the medial and lateral femoral circumflex, obturator, and superior and inferior gluteal arteries. In addition there is often a contribution from the first perforating branch of the profunda (deep) femoris. The arteries to the head and the major portion of the neck are derived from both femoral circumflex vessels and, to a variable extent, from an acetabular branch of the obturator artery. This obturator arterial branch passes through the acetabular notch to supply the soft tissue in the acetabular fossa. It accompanies and supplies the ligamentum teres. Though the intracapsular portion of the upper end of the femur is supplied by the femoral circumflex arteries, the extracapsular part of the upper end of the femur is supplied by the inferior gluteal and first perforating arteries, as well as the circumflex vessels. This arterial complex is referred to as the cruciate anastomosis. When the circumflex vessels pierce the fibrous capsule of the hip joint at its attachment to the femur and run upward toward the head on the surface of the neck, they are known as retinacular vessels. They are vulnerable to disruption with an intracapsular hip fracture.

Nerves to the Hip Joint

The hip joint is supplied by several nerves, and the innervation is variable (Fig 10–7). The nerve supply to the hip usually includes branches of the femoral and obturator nerves, the accessory obturator nerve when present, and at times the superior gluteal nerve and nerve to the quadratus femoris.

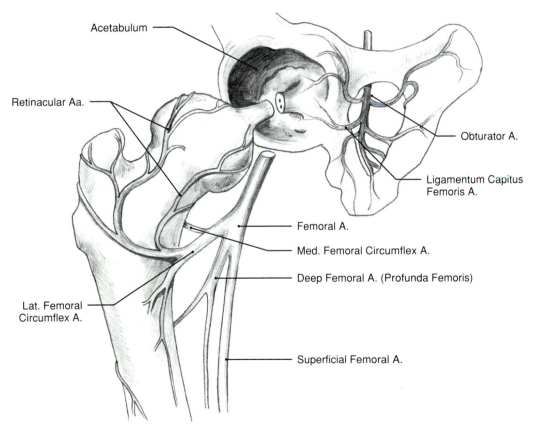

FIG 10–5.
Arterial supply to the femoral head and neck (anterior view).

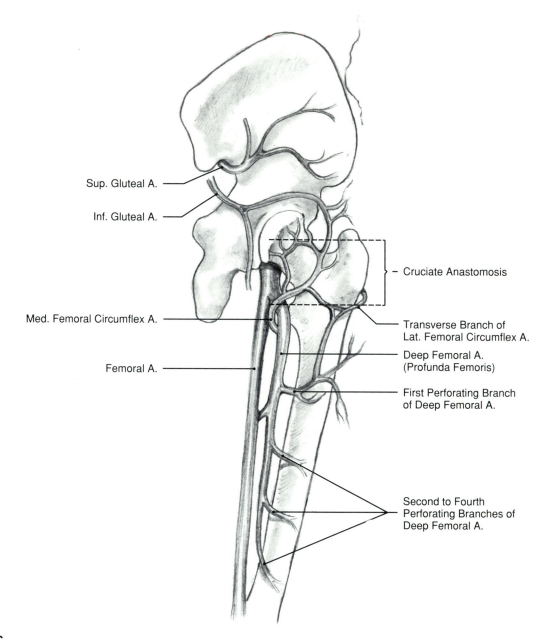

Sup. Gluteal A.

Inf. Gluteal A.

Med. Femoral Circumflex A.

Femoral A.

Cruciate Anastomosis

Transverse Branch of
Lat. Femoral Circumflex A.

Deep Femoral A.
(Profunda Femoris)

First Perforating Branch
of Deep Femoral A.

Second to Fourth
Perforating Branches of
Deep Femoral A.

FIG 10–6.
Arterial supply (posterior view) to the extracapsular part of the upper end of the femur (cruciate anastomosis). The cruciate anastomosis of the thigh is composed of anastomotic branches of the inferior gluteal, the medial and lateral femoral circumflex artery, and the first perforating artery of the deep femoral (profunda femoris) artery.

The femoral branches are distributed largely to the region of the iliofemoral ligament and the posterosuperior part of the capsule in the region of the ischiofemoral ligament. Branches of the obturator and/or accessory obturator nerve also are distributed to the region of the pubofemoral ligament. Branches of the superior gluteal nerve innervate the superolateral portion of the capsule, and a branch from the

nerve to the quadratus femoris goes to the sparsely innervated posterior part of the capsule.

Muscles of the Hip and Thigh

The hip joint is surrounded by thick, broad muscle groups that all play a role in the stability and support of the hip joint and in locomotion. A total of

ANTERIOR

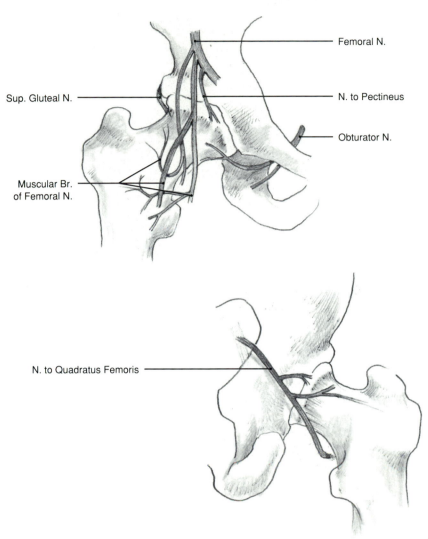

Sup. Gluteal N.

Femoral N.

N. to Pectineus

Obturator N.

Muscular Br.
of Femoral N.

N. to Quadratus Femoris

POSTERIOR

FIG 10–7.
Usual pattern of nerve supply to the hip joint.

21 individual muscles span the hip joint. Of these, 13 are one-joint muscles, attaching to the ilium and femur. Six span the hip and the knee, attaching the ilium and ischium to the tibia or fibula. One muscle runs from the lumbar vertebrae to the femur, and one (or two if the gluteus maximus is included) goes from the sacrum to the femur.

Although many muscles about the hips have more than one direction of action, it is convenient and practical to group them according to their main function, that is, flexion, extension, abduction, adduction, and external rotation. Muscles of the anterior thigh primarily function as knee extensors, and the posterior thigh muscles function as knee flexors.

For the most part the individual muscles in each functional group for the hip and knee are innervated by branches of the same nerve. The design of surgical approaches to the hip joint and femur takes advantage of this fact, and thus these approaches are between muscle groups and in internervous planes whenever possible (Tables 10–1 and 10–2).

Hip Flexors

The hip flexors include the sartorius, rectus femoris, iliopsoas, and pectineus (Figs 10–8 and 10–9). They are supplied by the femoral nerve. The pectineus sometimes is supplied also by the obturator nerve or an accessory obturator nerve.

TABLE 10–1.

Functional Grouping of Muscles Spanning Hip Joint

Muscle	Nerve	Principal Group Function
Sartorius	Femoral	Flexion
Rectus femoris		
Iliopsoas		
Pectineus*		
Adductor longus	Obturator	Adduction
Adductor brevis		
Adductor magnus**		
Gracilis		
Obturator externus		
Semitendinosus	Sciatic	Extension
Semimembranosus		
Biceps femoris		
Gluteus maximus	Inferior gluteal	
Gluteus medius	Superior gluteal	Abduction
Gluteus minimus		
Tensor fasciae latae		Not precisely known
Piriformis	S1, S2	External rotation
Gemellus superior	Nerve to obturator	
Obturator internus	internus	
Gemellus inferior	Nerve to quadratus	
Quadratus femoris	femoris	

*Sometimes the accessory obturator or obturator also supplies the pectineus.
**The adductor magnus also receives innervation from the sciatic.

The sartorius is a long straplike muscle that runs obliquely across the anteromedial aspect of the thigh. It originates from the anterior superior iliac spine and runs downward and medially in a superficial position to the medial surface of the thigh. It passes across the knee somewhat behind the axis of motion. Below the knee it angles anteriorly, and its tendon attaches on the proximal part of the medial surface of the tibia, anterior and proximal to the insertion of the gracilis and semitendinosus.

The rectus femoris arises by two tendons, the larger rounded straight tendon arising from the anterior inferior iliac spine and a thinner flattened tendon, the so-called reflected tendon, arising from the ilium just above the acetabulum. A few fibers may arise from the anterior hip joint capsule. These tendons converge, and as the muscle fibers move distally they combine with the fibers of the vastus lateralis, intermedius, and medialis to become the so-called quadriceps femoris, which inserts on the patella.

The iliopsoas (see Fig 10–8) represents the confluence of two distinct muscles, the iliacus and psoas major. The iliacus is a fanshaped muscle that arises from the inner surface of the wing of the ilium. The psoas major arises from the side of the vertebral column, from the lower borders of the twelfth thoracic to the upper borders of the five lumbar vertebrae. The psoas major narrows as it runs along the lateral brim of the pelvis, and behind the inguinal ligament it blends with the iliacus muscle. The iliopsoas crosses the hip joint anteriorly, forms a part of the floor of the femoral triangle, and inserts on the lesser trochanter of the femur (see Fig 10–14).

The pectineus arises from the superior pubic ramus, forms part of the floor of the femoral triangle, and inserts by a broad thin tendon onto the medial femur, distal to the lesser trochanter. In addition to its primary function as a hip flexor, it may be a weak adductor of the thigh.

Hip Adductors

The hip adductors (see Figs 10–8 and 10–9) span the anteromedial aspect of the joint. The muscles constituting this group are the adductor longus, adductor brevis, adductor magnus, gracilis, and ob-

TABLE 10–2.

Grouping of Hip Joint–Spanning Muscles According to Innervation

Nerve	Lumbosacral Plexus Divisions	Muscles	Principal Function	Other Functions
Superior gluteal	Dorsal L4, L5 S1	Gluteus medius Gluteus minimus Tensor fasciae latae	Abduction	Flexion, internal and external rotation
Femoral	Dorsal L2 L3 L4	Iliopsoas Pectineus* Sartorius Rectus femoris	Flexion	Adduction, internal and external rotation
Obturator	Ventral L2 L3 L4	Pectineus* Adductor longus Adductor brevis Adductor magnus** Gracilis Obturator cxternus	Adduction	Extension, flexion, internal and external rotation
Sciatic	Ventral L4 L5 S1 S2 S3 Dorsal same except S3	Biceps femoris Semitendinosus Semimembranosus Adductor magnus**	Extension	Adduction, internal rotation
N. to obturator internus	L5, S1, S2	Obturator internus Superior gemellus	External rotation	
N. to quadratus femoris	L4, L5, S1	Quadratus femoris Inferior gemellus	External rotation	
Inferior gluteal	L5, S1, S2	Gluteus maximus	Extension	External rotation
N. to piriformis	S1, S2	Piriformis	External rotation	

*Sometimes the accessory obturator or obturator also supplies the pectineus.
**Adductor magnus receives dual innervation.

turator externus. All are innervated by the obturator nerve. In addition, the lower posterior portion of the adductor magnus is innervated by the sciatic nerve.

The adductor longus is the most anterior of the adductor muscles in the upper part of the thigh. It arises by a strong tendon from the front of the pubis just below the pubic tubercle and inserts onto the medial lip of the linea aspera between the attachments of the vastus medialis and adductor magnus. It lies medial to the pectineus and contributes to the floor of the femoral triangle. The adductor longus and sartorius converge at the apex of the femoral triangle (see Fig 10–16) and form the upper part of the floor of the adductor canal.

The gracilis (see Fig 10–9) is a long straplike muscle on the medial side of the thigh. It arises from the lower part of the body of the pubis close to the symphysis and from an upper part of the inferior ramus. Below the knee its thin tendon curves forward and expands to insert onto the medial surface of the tibia, below the medial condyle and between the insertions of the sartorius and semitendinosus. These three tendons form the so-called pes anserinus, or "goosefoot" (see knee chapter). The anserine bursa, located between the three associated tendons and the tibia, may become painful and distended due to acute or chronic trauma to the medial aspect of the knee. The gracilis is innervated by the anterior branch of the obturator nerve. It adducts and medially rotates the thigh and flexes the hip if the knee is kept from flexing. It also flexes and medially rotates the leg.

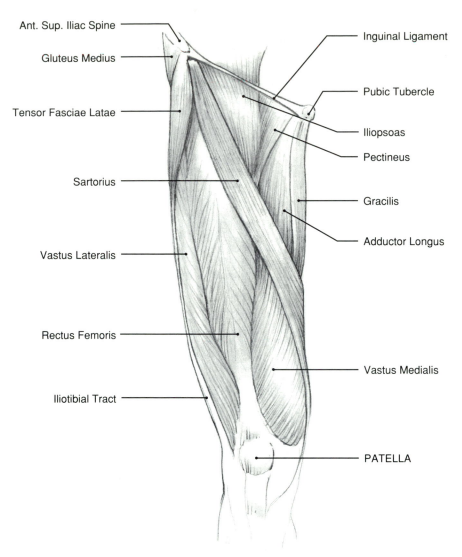

Ant. Sup. Iliac Spine

Gluteus Medius

Tensor Fasciae Latae

Sartorius

Vastus Lateralis

Rectus Femoris

Iliotibial Tract

Inguinal Ligament

Pubic Tubercle

Iliopsoas

Pectineus

Gracilis

Adductor Longus

Vastus Medialis

PATELLA

FIG 10–8.
Hip flexors (sartorius, rectus femoris, iliopsoas, and pectineus) and knee extensors—quadriceps complex—(rectus femoris, vastus medialis, vastus lateralis, and vastus intermedius, not shown).

The adductor brevis (Fig 10–10) is located deep to the pectineus and arises as a relatively broad tendon from the body and inferior ramus of the pubis. It inserts onto the upper half of the linea aspera in a line running proximally from this point toward the lesser trochanter.

The adductor magnus (see Fig 10–10) is a very large muscle. It arises from the lower part of the inferior pubic ramus and from the entire length of the ramus of the ischium as far as the lower part of the ischial tuberosity. The fibers that arise more anteriorly insert on the upper part of the linea aspera and on a portion of the femur above this as far as the insertion of the quadratus femoris. The intermediary fibers insert along the remainder of the length of the

linea aspera. The fibers that arise most posteriorly insert on nearly the entire length of the medial supracondylar line (medial lower lip of the linea aspera) and onto the adductor tubercle at the lower border of the medial epicondyle. Just proximal to the adductor tubercle the muscle insertion is interrupted by the tendinous or adductor hiatus, a gap that allows the femoral vessels to enter into the popliteal fossa. The adductor magnus may be divided functionally, if not anatomically, into two distinct parts. The upper and more anterior component is referred to as the adductor portion. The more posterior fibers and those which insert lower are referred to as the hamstring or sciatic portion.

The obturator externus (see Fig 10–10) is the

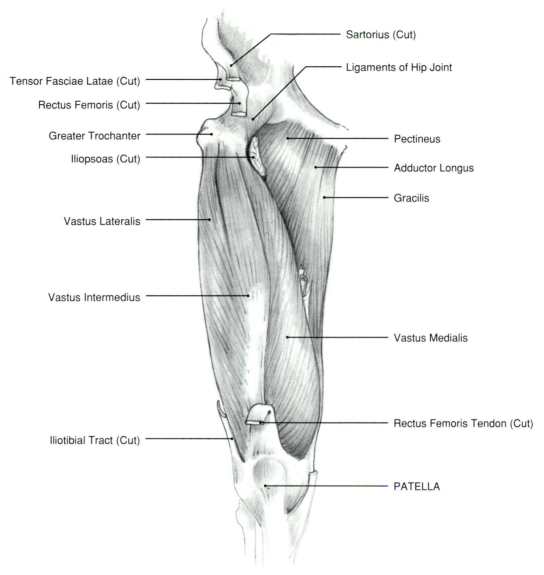

Sartorius (Cut)

Ligaments of Hip Joint

Tensor Fasciae Latae (Cut)

Rectus Femoris (Cut)

Greater Trochanter

Pectineus

Iliopsoas (Cut)

Adductor Longus

Vastus Lateralis

Gracilis

Vastus Intermedius

Vastus Medialis

Rectus Femoris Tendon (Cut)

Iliotibial Tract (Cut)

PATELLA

FIG 10–9.
Adductor longus and gracilis (hip adductors that lie superficial to the remainder of the hip adductors).

deepest muscle of the adductor group. It arises from the external surface of the obturator membrane and the external surface of the pubis and ischium around the obturator foramen. Its fibers converge to resemble an inverted cone as the muscle passes below the capsule of the hip joint. The obturator externus then turns upward across the lower part of the back of the hip joint and inserts into the trochanteric fossa. The nerve supply to the obturator externus is provided by a direct branch of the obturator nerve or its posterior branch. Although the obturator externus is considered an adductor of the thigh, it is primarily an external rotator.

Hip Extensors

Hip extension is accomplished primarily by the large, complex gluteus maximus and the hamstring muscles.

The gluteus maximus (Fig 10–11) is a large, coarse-fibered muscle that runs diagonally downward and laterally. It arises from the outer surface of the ilium behind the posterior gluteal line and more extensively from the dorsal surface of the sacrum and adjacent sacrotuberous ligament. The insertion of the gluteus maximus has two parts, a superficial and a deep one. The anterior three quarters of the muscle gives rise to superficial tendinous fibers that continue the downward and lateral direction of the

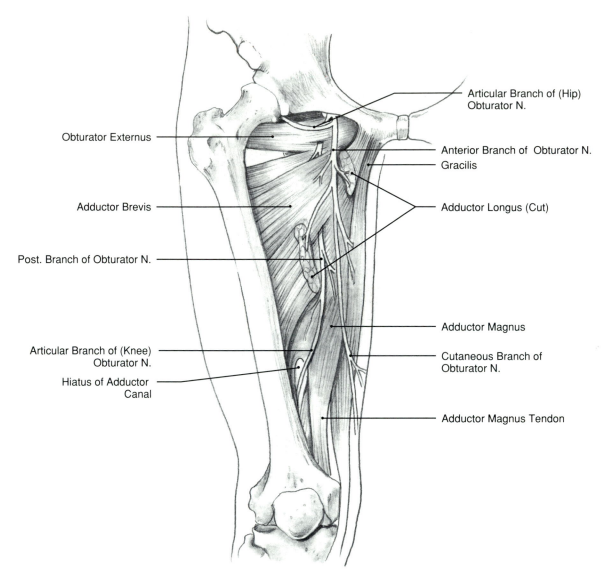

Obturator Externus

Adductor Brevis

Post. Branch of Obturator N.

Articular Branch of (Knee) Obturator N.

Hiatus of Adductor Canal

Articular Branch of (Hip) Obturator N.

Anterior Branch of Obturator N.

Gracilis

Adductor Longus (Cut)

Adductor Magnus

Cutaneous Branch of Obturator N.

Adductor Magnus Tendon

FIG 10–10.
Deeper layer of hip adductors (adductor brevis, adductor magnus and obturator externus). Note distribution and branches of the obturator nerve.

muscle. They cross the greater trochanter to insert into the fascia lata and contribute to the iliotibial tract. Much of the lower portion of the gluteus maximus inserts onto the gluteal tuberosity of the femur. However some of its fibers also attach to the fascia lata and lateral intermuscular septum. The main action of the gluteus maximus is hip joint extension, as in walking up stairs. The muscle is innervated by the inferior gluteal nerve.

The deep hip extensors are the so-called hamstring muscles, which include the semitendinosus, biceps femoris, semimembranosus, and that part of the adductor magnus which arises from the ischial tuberosity and inserts onto the adductor tubercle (see Fig 10–11). Except for the short head of the biceps, these muscles arise from the ischial tuberosity, and they are innervated by the tibial component of the sciatic nerve. The short head of the biceps arises from the distal femur (Fig 10–12) and is innervated by the common peroneal component of the sciatic nerve.

The semitendinosus muscle arises from the posteromedial surface of the distal part of the ischial tuberosity (see Figs 10–11 and 10–12). Its insertion forms part of the tendon complex (sartorius, gracilis, and semitendinosus) sometimes referred to as the pes anserinus, which inserts onto the proximal tibia (see Knee chapter).

The semimembranosus muscle arises by a long,

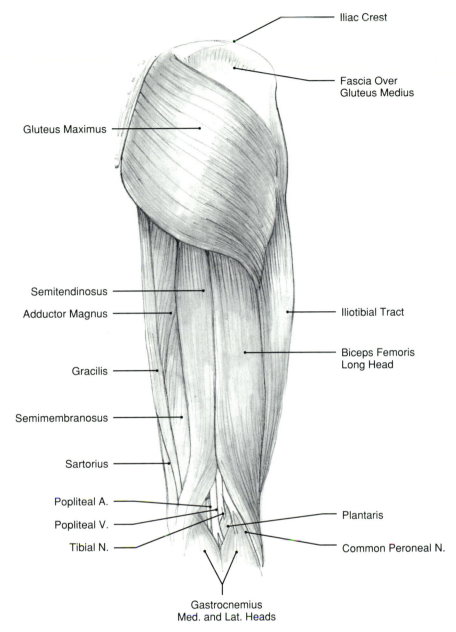

Iliac Crest

Fascia Over
Gluteus Medius

Gluteus Maximus

Semitendinosus

Adductor Magnus

Iliotibial Tract

Biceps Femoris
Long Head

Gracilis

Semimembranosus

Sartorius

Popliteal A.

Popliteal V.

Plantaris

Tibial N.

Common Peroneal N.

Gastrocnemius
Med. and Lat. Heads

FIG 10–11.
Hip extensors (gluteus maximus and hamstrings—which include the semitendinosus, biceps femoris, semimembranosus, and a portion of the adductor magnus).

flat tendon from the upper and outer impression on the tuberosity of the ischium (see Figs 10–11 and 10–12). The insertion of the muscle at the knee is rather complex (see Knee chapter). It ends mainly in the horizontal groove on the posteromedial aspect of the medial condyle of the tibia, but a prominent reflection from here forms the oblique popliteal ligament of the knee joint capsule. Other fibers extend from the tendon to the tibial collateral ligament and into the fascia of the popliteus muscle.

The biceps femoris muscle has two origins (see

Figs 10–11 and 10–12). The long head arises in combination with the semitendinosus muscle from the lower and medial portions of the ischial tuberosity and the lower part of the sacrotuberous ligament. The short head arises from the lateral lip of the linea aspera of the femur, the proximal two thirds of the supracondylar line, and the lateral intermuscular septum. The muscle fibers of the short head join the tendon of the long head to form the heavy, round tendon that forms the lateral margin of the popliteal fossa.

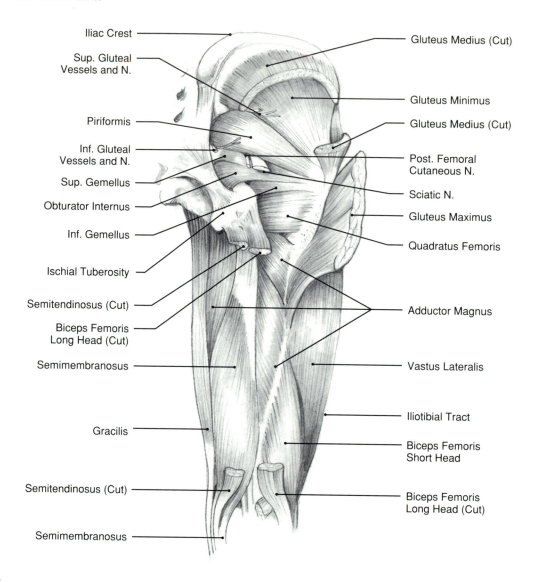

FIG 10–12.

Hip abductors and deep layer of hip extensors. Hamstrings, biceps femoris and semitendinosus have been resected to show deeper layer (semimembranosus and hamstring portion of the adductor magnus). Hip abductors include gluteus medius, gluteus minimus, and tensor fasciae latae. Short external rotators of the hip are piriformis, superior gemellus, obturator internus, inferior gemellus, and quadratus femoris.

Hip Abductors

The hip abductor muscles lie largely in the lateral and posterior regions. They include the gluteus medius, gluteus minimus, and tensor fasciae latae (Figs 10–12 and 10–13). The gluteus medius muscle arises from the external surface of the ilium between the anterior and posterior gluteal lines and from the gluteal aponeurosis. Its tendon inserts into the posterosuperior angle of the greater trochanter of the femur and onto the diagonal ridge on its lateral surface. It is a strong abductor of the hip. It is supplied by the superior gluteal nerve, which is accompanied by branches of the superior gluteal vessels.

The gluteus minimus muscle underlies the gluteus medius and arises from the ilium between the anterior and inferior gluteal lines. It inserts onto the anterosuperior aspect of the greater trochanter. In addition to abducting the femur, the minimus and medius participate in medial rotation of the thigh. In stance phase these muscles stabilize the pelvis, preventing its collapse toward the unsupported side.

The tensor fasciae latae muscle is enclosed between two layers of fascia. It arises from the anterior part of the external lip of the iliac crest, the outer surface of the anterior superior spine of the ilium, and the notch below the spine. It inserts into the ili-

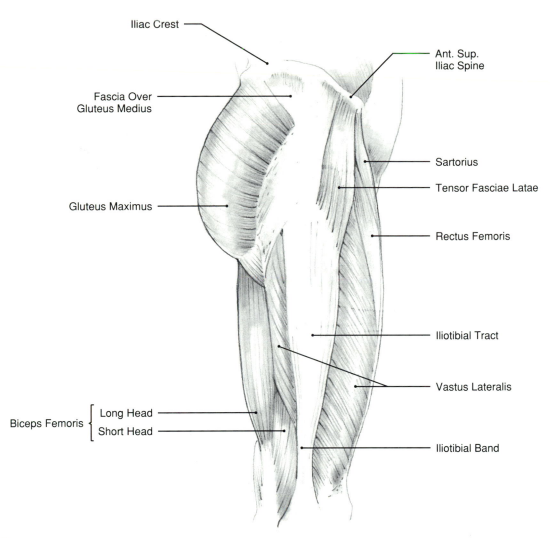

Iliac Crest

Ant. Sup.
Iliac Spine

Fascia Over
Gluteus Medius

Sartorius

Tensor Fasciae Latae

Gluteus Maximus

Rectus Femoris

Iliotibial Tract

Vastus Lateralis

Biceps Femoris { Long Head
Short Head

Iliotibial Band

FIG 10–13.
Superficial layer of muscles of lateral hip and thigh.

otibial tract. The tensor fasciae latae assists in flexion, abduction, and medial rotation of the thigh. It may also aid in stabilizing the femur on the tibia. The superior gluteal nerve ends in the tensor fasciae latae, and blood is supplied by the superior gluteal artery.

Short External Rotators of the Hip

The deep muscles of the posterolateral aspect of the hip consist of the short external rotators, which include the piriformis, obturator internus, superior gemellus, inferior gemellus and quadratus femoris muscles (see Fig 10–12).

The piriformis arises primarily from the central surface of the second through fourth sacral vertebrae and the posterior inferior spine of the ilium. It passes through the greater sciatic foramen and in-

serts into the posterior upper surface of the greater trochanter. It is supplied by branches of the first and second sacral nerves, which enter the pelvic surface of the muscle directly. The piriformis is an important anatomical landmark. The superior gluteal neurovascular structures exit the pelvis above the muscle and the inferior gluteal neurovascular structures and sciatic nerve below it.

The obturator internus muscle arises from the entire bony margin of the obturator foramen (with the exception of the obturator groove), the inner surface of the obturator membrane, and the pelvic surface of the innominate bone behind and above the obturator foramen. The fibers of the muscle converge as they exit the pelvis through the lesser sciatic foramen. At the level of the lesser sciatic notch the muscle turns 90 degrees to move laterally and horizontally and inserts on the medial surface of the greater trochanter of the femur, just above the trochanteric fossa. The obturator internus is considered a lateral rotator of the thigh, but it also has some abduction capability. Its nerve supply is derived from L5, S1, and S2. The same nerve also supplies the superior gemellus muscle. The superior and inferior gemellus (twins) muscles are small muscles that lie parallel to the tendon of the obturator internus. The superior gemellus arises from the ischial spine and the inferior gemellus from the ischial tuberosity adjacent to the lesser sciatic notch. The tendon of the obturator internus muscle receives the superior gemellus tendon along its superior border and the inferior gemellus tendon along its inferior border. These tendons merge just as they insert on the greater trochanter.

The quadratus femoris muscle is a thick, quadrilateral muscle located distal to the inferior gemellus. It arises from the upper part of the lateral border of the ischial tuberosity and inserts on the quadrate line of the femur. This muscle is a strong external rotator of the thigh. Its nerve supply is from L4, L5, and S1. This nerve also supplies the inferior gemellus.

Anterior Thigh Muscles (Knee Extensors)

The knee extensor muscles are located in the anterior aspect of the thigh (see Figs 10–8 and 10–9) and are collectively known as the quadriceps femoris muscle. They consist of the rectus femoris, vastus medialis, vastus lateralis, and vastus intermedius. Their tendons merge together to insert onto the proximal patella.

The rectus femoris muscle, as its name implies, runs straight down the thigh. The muscle arises from two heads: the straight head arises from the anterior inferior iliac spine and the reflected head from the anterior lip of the acetabulum, plus a few fibers from the anterior aspect of the hip joint capsule.

The vastus medialis muscle arises from entire extent of the medial lip of the linea aspera and distal half of the intertrochanteric line and from the medial intermuscular septum. The tendon inserts into the tendon of the rectus femoris as well as the superomedial border of the patella and the medial condyle of the tibia.

The largest component of the quadriceps femoris muscle is the vastus lateralis. It takes its origin from the femur by a broad aponeurosis attached to the upper part of the intertrochanteric line, the anterior

and inferior borders of the greater trochanter, the gluteal tuberosity and adjacent portion of the lateral lip of the linea aspera, and the entire length of the lateral intermuscular septum. The tendon of insertion is attached to the superolateral border of the patella and lateral condyle of the tibia.

The vastus intermedius muscle arises from the femoral shaft, the lower half of the lateral lip of the linea aspera, and the lateral intermuscular septum. Its fibers terminate in a superficial aponeurosis, which blends with the deep surface of the tendon of the rectus femoris and with the vastus medialis and lateralis muscles. All of the muscles of the quadriceps femoris complex are supplied by the femoral nerve.

Posterior Thigh Muscles (Hamstrings)

The posterior thigh muscles (hamstrings) function to flex the knee (see Knee chapter).

Femoral Triangle

The femoral triangle is located in the upper third of the front of the thigh and contains the femoral vessels and nerves (Fig 10–14). It is bound laterally by the medial border of the sartorius, medially by the medial border of the adductor longus, and superiorly by the inguinal ligament. Its roof is formed by the deep fascia lata of the thigh and the superficial cribriform fascia. Its floor is formed by the iliopsoas, pectineus, and adductor longus. There is a deep groove in the floor of the femoral triangle between the iliopsoas and pectineus muscles through which the medial circumflex femoral artery passes to the back of the thigh. The femoral artery is a continuation of the external iliac and passes under the inguinal ligament medial to the femoral nerve. The femoral vein lies medial to the femoral artery and in this region receives the greater saphenous vein. The femoral nerve descends under the inguinal ligament in the groove between the iliacus and psoas major muscles. In the triangle it divides into most of the muscular and cutaneous branches. Only the saphenous nerve and one of the nerves to the vastus medialis muscle continue into the adductor canal of the thigh. The femoral artery and vein are covered by the femoral sheath for about 3 cm beyond the inguinal ligament. Here the extraperitoneal connective tissue to the abdomen extends between the vessels and forms three compartments, a lateral one for the artery, a middle one for the vein, and a medial one

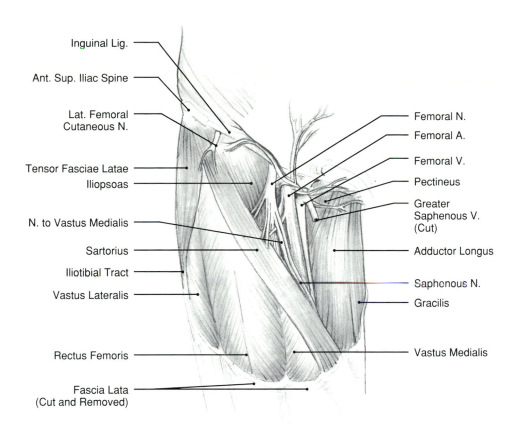

Inguinal Lig.

Ant. Sup. Iliac Spine

Lat. Femoral
Cutaneous N.

Tensor Fasciae Latae

Iliopsoas

N. to Vastus Medialis

Sartorius

Iliotibial Tract

Vastus Lateralis

Rectus Femoris

Fascia Lata
(Cut and Removed)

Femoral N.

Femoral A.

Femoral V.

Pectineus

Greater
Saphenous V.
(Cut)

Adductor Longus

Saphenous N.

Gracilis

Vastus Medialis

FIG 10–14.
Femoral triangle and contents.

for more deep inguinal nodes and fat. The medial compartment is converted into the femoral canal, and its abdominal opening is the femoral ring.

Arteries of the Thigh and Gluteal Region

Femoral Artery

The femoral artery (Fig 10–15) is the continuation of the external iliac artery. It is found largely in the femoral triangle and descends through the midregion of the thigh within the adductor, or subsartorial, canal. The adductor canal (Fig 10–16) conducts the femoral artery together with the femoral vein and one or two nerves through the middle third of the thigh. The canal begins about 15 cm below the inguinal ligament at the apex of the femoral triangle, where the sartorius muscle crosses the adductor longus muscle, and ends at the upper limit of the adductor hiatus. Distally a separation in the tendinous insertion of the adductor magnus muscle (adductor hiatus) allows the femoral vessels to descend posteromedially toward the back of the knee. The branches of the femoral artery are the superficial epigastric, superficial circumflex iliac, external pudendal, deep femoral, and descending genicular ar-

teries. The first three branches are primarily related to the lower abdominal wall and are not described here.

Deep Femoral Artery

The deep femoral artery (profunda femoris) is the largest branch of the femoral artery (Fig 10–17). It arises from the lateral side of the femoral artery about 5 cm below the inguinal ligament. It quickly dives into the thigh as it descends, lying behind the femoral artery and femoral vein on the medial side of the femur. It crosses the tendon of the adductor brevis muscle and at its lower border passes deep to the tendon of the adductor longus muscle. There it ends as the fourth perforating artery in the lower third of the thigh. In the femoral triangle the deep femoral artery gives rise to the medial and lateral circumflex femoral arteries and branches to the adductor muscles. It also provides three perforating branches in the thigh.

The medial circumflex femoral artery (see Figs 10–5 and 10–6) arises from the medial and posterior aspects of the deep femoral artery. The medial circumflex femoral artery runs deep in the femoral triangle between the pectineus and iliopsoas muscles and

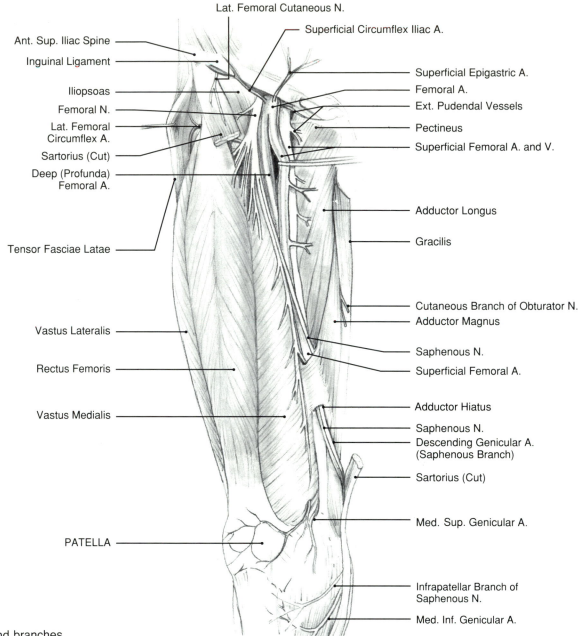

FIG 10-15.
Femoral artery and branches.

under the neck of the femur to reach the back of the thigh and hip. An acetabular branch of this artery may enter the hip joint beneath the transverse ligament of the acetabulum. Muscular branches supply the adductor brevis and adductor magnus muscles.

The lateral femoral circumflex artery (see Figs 10–5 and 10–6) arises from the lateral side of the deep femoral artery and passes laterally between the sartorius and rectus femoris muscles. It then divides into ascending, transverse, and descending branches to supply the anterior thigh muscles. The ascending branch passes upward beneath the tensor fasciae latae muscle to anastomose with the branches of the superior gluteal artery. The transverse branch enters the vastus lateralis muscle, wraps around the femur below the greater trochanter, and anastomoses with the medial femoral circumflex, inferior gluteal, and first perforating arteries on the posterior aspect of the thigh. This arterial arrangement is referred to as the cruciate anastomosis (see Fig 10–6). An articular artery for the hip joint may arise from any of the branches. The descending branch of the lateral fem-

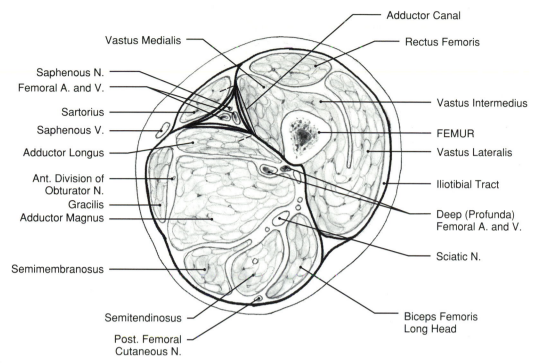

FIG 10–16.
Cross section of thigh. Note adductor canal and contents (femoral artery and vein and saphenous nerve).

oral circumflex artery passes superficial to the vastus lateralis muscle, together with a branch of the femoral nerve to this muscle. This branch anastomoses with the descending genicular branch of the femoral artery and the lateral superior genicular branch of the popliteal artery near the superior border of the patella.

The perforating arteries (see Figs 10–6 and 10–17), usually three in number, arise from the posterior surface of the deep femoral artery. They pierce the insertion of the adductor muscles directly against the linea aspera of the femur to reach the posterior compartment of the thigh. The deep femoral artery ends as the fourth perforating artery.

The descending genicular artery (see Fig 10–15) arises from the femoral artery just before the latter passes through the adductor hiatus and immediately divides into saphenous and articular branches (see Knee chapter).

Obturator Artery

The obturator artery is a branch of the internal iliac artery (see Fig 10–5). It may also arise as a branch of the inferior epigastric as the "abnormal obturator artery" (see Pelvis chapter). The obturator artery leaves the pelvis via the obturator canal and immediately divides into anterior and posterior branches. These supply the pectineus and obturator externus muscles and give branches to the adductor brevis and adductor magnus muscles. The posterior branch gives off an acetabular artery, which enters the hip joint through the acetabular notch and provides a small artery of the ligamentum teres and head of the femur.

Gluteal Arteries

The superior gluteal artery is a branch of the internal iliac artery (Figs 10–6 and 10–18). It emerges from the pelvis above the piriformis muscle and then divides into a superficial branch to the gluteus maximus muscle and a deep branch to the intermuscular plane between the gluteus medius and gluteus minimus muscles. An upper radical of this branch supplies the gluteus medius, gluteus minimus, and tensor fasciae latae muscles and reaches as far as the anterior superior iliac spine. A lower branch is directed toward the greater trochanter of the femur and supplies the gluteal muscles surrounding the hip joint.

The inferior gluteal artery, also a branch of the internal iliac artery, leaves the pelvis below the piriformis muscle and provides large muscular branches to the gluteus maximus muscle and the muscles arising from the ischial tuberosity (see Fig 10–18). A

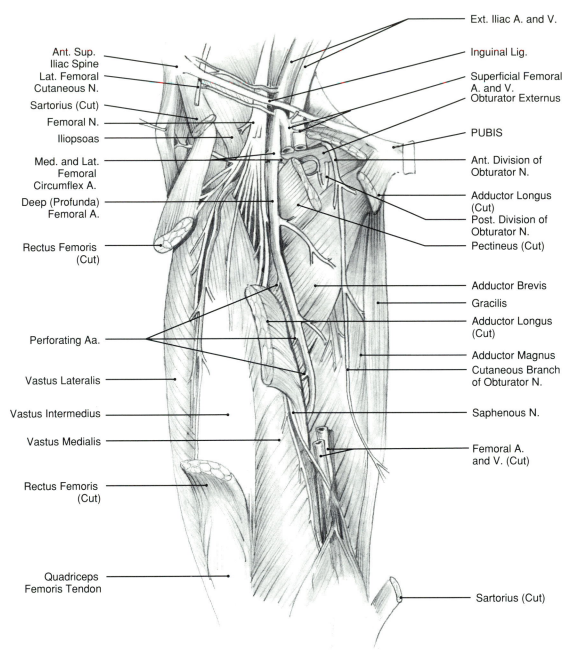

Ant. Sup.
Iliac Spine
Lat. Femoral
Cutaneous N.

Sartorius (Cut)

Femoral N.

Iliopsoas

Med. and Lat.
Femoral
Circumflex A.

Deep (Profunda)
Femoral A.

Rectus Femoris
(Cut)

Perforating Aa.

Vastus Lateralis

Vastus Intermedius

Vastus Medialis

Rectus Femoris
(Cut)

Quadriceps
Femoris Tendon

Ext. Iliac A. and V.

Inguinal Lig.

Superficial Femoral
A. and V.
Obturator Externus

PUBIS

Ant. Division of
Obturator N.

Adductor Longus
(Cut)
Post. Division of
Obturator N.
Pectineus (Cut)

Adductor Brevis

Gracilis

Adductor Longus
(Cut)

Adductor Magnus
Cutaneous Branch
of Obturator N.

Saphenous N.

Femoral A.
and V. (Cut)

Sartorius (Cut)

FIG 10–17.
Deep dissection of anterior thigh. Note deep femoral artery (profunda femoris artery) and its branches.

branch descends across the short lateral rotator muscles of the hip and participates in the cruciate anastomosis of the buttock and the back of the upper thigh (see Fig 10–6).

Nerves of the Gluteal Region and Thigh

Nerves of the Gluteal Region

The largest nerve in the gluteal region is the sciatic nerve (see Fig 10–18). In fact it is the largest in

the body. It actually consists of two nerves, the common peroneal and tibial, which are bound together. In most instances the sciatic nerve arises from the fourth and fifth lumbar and the first, second, and third sacral nerves. It emerges from the pelvis at the lower border of the piriformis muscle and enters the thigh in the hollow between the ischial tuberosity and the greater trochanter of the femur. It continues down the posterior aspect of the thigh and, at the apex of the popliteal fossa, divides into the tibial and

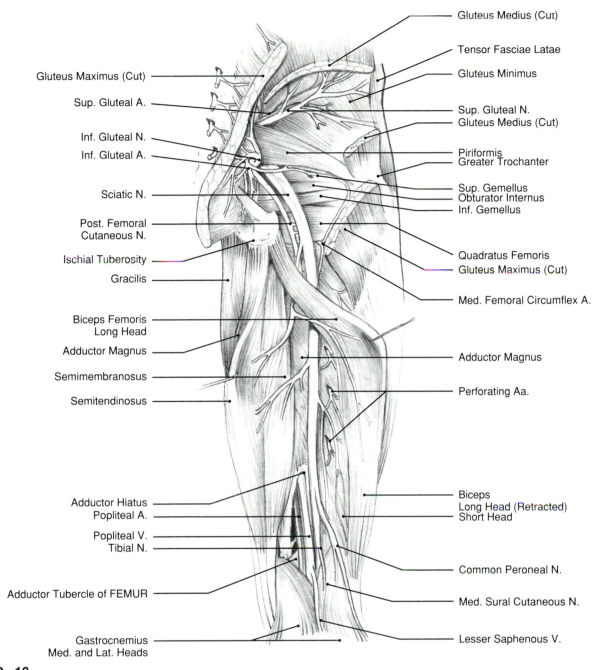

FIG 10–18.
Structures in the deep aspect of the buttock. Note superior and inferior gluteal vessels and nerves and their relationship to the piriformis muscle and sciatic nerve.

common peroneal portions. In approximately 10% of individuals the nerve divides higher. Occasionally the tibial and common peroneal nerves arise independently from the sacral plexus but pursue closely related courses until they reach the apex of the popliteal fossa. In some instances the sciatic nerve may supply an articular branch, which perforates the posterior part of the hip joint capsule.

Below the quadratus femoris muscle two branches of the tibial division of the sciatic nerve arise from its medial side to supply the hamstring muscles of the thigh. The proximal branch innervates the long head of the biceps femoris muscle and the upper portion of the semitendinosus. The distal branch supplies the lower portion of the semitendinosus and semimembranosus muscles and the ischial portion of the adductor magnus muscle. The tibial nerve continues its vertical course at the back of the knee and into the leg.

The nerve to the short head of the biceps femoris muscle arises from the lateral side of the sciatic nerve (common peroneal division of the sciatic nerve) in the middle third of the thigh. The common peroneal nerve descends in close relationship to the posterior aspect of the tendon of the biceps femoris along the upper lateral margin of the popliteal space and into the leg, curving around the neck of the fibula.

The nerve to the piriformis muscle has separate contributions from S1 and S2 and enters the piriformis at its pelvic surface.

The superior gluteal nerve arises from the posterior branches of L4, L5, and S1 and exits from the pelvis above the piriformis muscle. Beneath the gluteus maximus and gluteus medius muscles the nerve accompanies the superior gluteal vessels anteriorly over the surface of the gluteus minimus muscle. The superior gluteal nerve supplies the gluteus medius and minimus muscles and ascends beyond them to the tensor fasciae latae (see Fig 10–18).

The inferior gluteal nerve is formed from the posterior branches of L5, S1, and S2 and passes from the pelvis below the piriformis muscle. It enters the deep surface of the gluteus maximus muscle and is the *only* nerve to supply the gluteus maximus (see Fig 10–18).

The nerve to the quadratus femoris and inferior gemellus is formed from the anterior branches of L4, L5, and S1. In the gluteal region it is beneath the sciatic nerve and travels over the back of the ischium anterior to the gemellus muscles and the tendon of the internal obturator muscle. It gives articular branches to the hip joint (see Fig 10–7) and a branch to the inferior gemellus muscle. It ends in the anterior surface of the quadratus femoris muscle.

The nerve to the obturator internus and superior gemellus muscles is formed from the anterior branches of L5, S1, and S2. In the gluteal region it is inferomedial to the sciatic nerve. It crosses and innervates the superior gemellus muscle via a small branch. The nerve then continues, crosses the ischial spine, enters the lesser sciatic foramen, and eventually terminates in the pelvic surface of the muscle.

The posterior femoral cutaneous nerve exits through the sciatic notch with the sciatic nerve. In the gluteal region it lies along the medial side of the sciatic nerve and descends in the midline of the thigh (see Fig 10–18). It provides perineal branches that are cutaneous in the perineum and posterior scrotum.

Femoral Nerve

The femoral nerve is the largest branch of the lumbar plexus (see Fig 10–14). It is formed from the posterior divisions of the ventral rami of the second, third, and fourth lumbar nerves, and passes inferolaterally through the psoas major muscle. It then runs between the psoas major and iliacus and supplies both. It enters the thigh beneath the inguinal ligament and lies lateral to the femoral vascular sheath in the femoral triangle. Articular branches are given off to the hip joint (see Fig 10–7). Muscular branches of the femoral nerve innervate the pectineus, sartorius, and quadriceps femoris muscles. The nerve to the pectineus muscle arises at the level of the inguinal ligament. The nerve to the sartorius enters the upper two thirds of the muscle (see Fig 10–14). The branches to the muscles of the quadriceps femoris group enter these muscles proximally in the thigh.

The femoral nerve also provides several cutaneous branches to the anterior thigh. The saphenous nerve is the largest and longest of these femoral branches. It arises at the femoral triangle and descends through it on the lateral side of the femoral vessels to enter the adductor canal.

The lateral femoral cutaneous nerve is formed from L2 and L3. After emerging from the lateral border of the psoas major muscle, it passes obliquely over the iliacus. It courses toward the anterior superior iliac spine and enters the thigh, passing beneath or through the lateral end of the inguinal ligament (see Fig 10–14). The lateral femoral cutaneous nerve supplies the skin and fascia on the anterolateral surface of the thigh. Injury to this nerve may result in painful dysesthesias known as meralgia paresthetica.

Obturator Nerve

The obturator nerve is formed from the anterior divisions of the ventral rami of L2, L3, and L4. These branches unite within the posterior part of the iliopsoas muscle, forming a nerve that descends through this muscle to emerge from its medial border opposite the lower end of the sacroiliac joint. The nerve passes laterally and downward over the sacral ala and pelvic brim into the lesser pelvis. It then curves anteroinferiorly to follow the lateral pelvic wall, reaching the obturator groove at the upper part of the obturator foramen. The obturator nerve, together with the obturator vessels, travels through this groove and foramen (see Fig 10–7) to enter the thigh. Here it immediately divides into anterior and posterior branches (see Fig 10–10). The anterior branch courses anterior to the obturator externus and adductor brevis muscles and posterior to the pectineus and adductor longus muscles. It gives off articular branches to the hip joint and occasionally a branch to the pectineus muscle, as well as muscular branches to the adductor longus, gracilis, and adductor brevis muscles. The posterior branch of the obturator nerve pierces the anterior part of the obturator externus and innervates it. The nerve then passes distally between the adductor brevis and adductor magnus muscles and divides into two branches, which supply the upper part of the adductor magnus and at times the adductor brevis. A small branch exits from the lower part of the adductor magnus, travels through the hiatus of the adductor canal in conjunction with the femoral artery, and continues to the knee joint. The posterior branch of the obturator nerve supplies fibers to the femoral and popliteal vessels. It terminates by piercing the oblique popliteal ligament and supplying the articular capsule, cruciate ligaments, and synovial membrane of the knee joint. The fact that the posterior branch of the obturator nerve can have filaments to the hip as well as the knee may explain the well-known clinical observation that hip pathology sometimes presents as knee pain and, conversely, knee pathology as hip and anterior thigh pain.

SURGICAL APPROACHES TO THE HIP

Anterior Approaches

The hip joint can be approached anteriorly to carry out a variety of procedures such as open reduction of congenital hip dislocation; pelvic osteotomy, hip arthrodesis, hemiarthroplasty and total hip replacement. A number of eponyms (Smith-Petersen, Callahan, Luck, Fahey, Sutherland, and Rowe) have been applied to these approaches. Despite different skin incisions, all of the approaches have the common feature of dissection in an internervous plane. This plane lies between the sartorius muscle (supplied by the femoral nerve) and the tensor fasciae latae muscle (supplied by the superior gluteal nerve) in the superficial dissection, and between the rectus femoris muscle (supplied by the femoral nerve) and the gluteus medius muscle (supplied by the superior gluteal nerve) in the deep dissection. These approaches are carried out with the patient in supine position with a small bolster under the sacroiliac joint to elevate the hip off the operating table.

The skin incision begins at the junction of the anterior and middle thirds of the iliac crest, runs anteriorly to the anterior superior iliac spine, and curves distally to end 6 to 8 cm below the base of the greater trochanter. In children a straight oblique incision (as described by Salter) in the inguinal area, paralleling the inguinal ligament, is preferred (Fig 10–19). The interval between the sartorius and tensor fasciae latae is identified 4 to 6 cm below the anterior superior iliac spine. The fascia is incised and the interval developed proximally and distally. Care is taken to identify and gently retract the lateral femoral cutaneous nerve medially. The lateral femoral cutaneous nerve most commonly passes over the sartorius muscle 2 to 3 cm below the anterior superior iliac spine. The ascending branch of the lateral femoral circumflex artery lies deep to the tensor fasciae latae. When the interval between the rectus femoris and gluteus medius is developed, this branch will be encountered and must be ligated. Care must be taken to correctly identify the plane between the rectus femoris and gluteus medius. If dissection is carried too far medially the neurovascular structures in the femoral triangle (see Fig 10–14) can be injured.

The tensor fasciae latae can be partially detached from its iliac origin to allow wider exposure of the rectus femoris and gluteus medius. The dissection should be well lateral to the femoral artery, which is readily palpable. The rectus femoris is detached from its origin on the anterior inferior iliac spine and acetabulum and reflected medially. The gluteus medius is retracted laterally. The iliopsoas may be attached to the inferior aspect of the joint capsule and can be released. Adduction and external rotation of the limb will put the capsule under tension. A longitudinal or T-shaped capsular incision will expose the femoral head and neck and allow hip dislocation by further adduction and external rotation of the limb.

For extensive exposure of the anterior pelvis the origins of the tensor fasciae latae, sartorius, and if necessary gluteus medius and minimus can be bluntly dissected off the outer wing of the ilium. This should be done subperiosteally to minimize bleeding; however, application of bone wax may be the only way to control the bleeding from vessels coming out of the exposed surface of the ilium. If necessary the dissection can readily be extended distally in a plane between the vastus lateralis and rectus femoris to expose the proximal shaft of the femur.

Lateral Approaches

Several lateral approaches to the hip have been described and/or modified by a number of surgeons

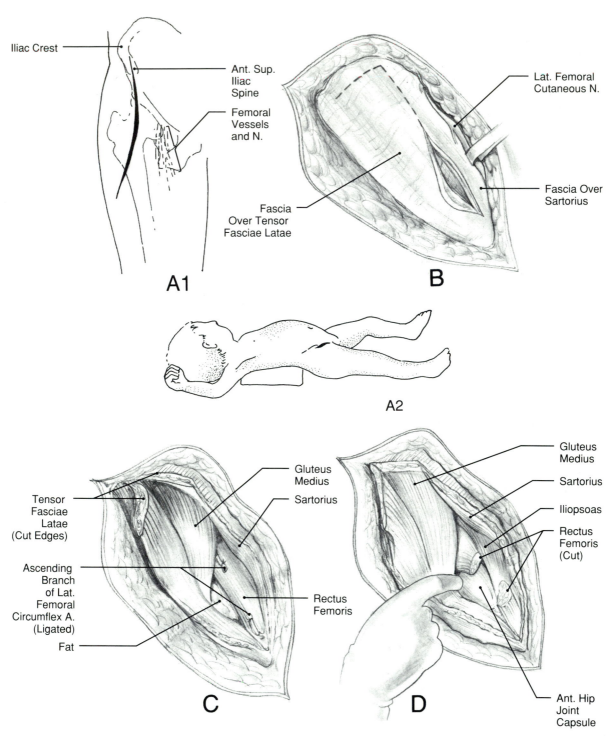

FIG 10–19.
Anterior approach to the hip joint. **A,** *(1),* skin incision (adult). Note location of femoral vessels and nerve. During deep dissection inappropriate placement of retractors could injure these structures. *(2),* skin incision (child). **B,** fascial incision begins 4 to 6 cm below the inguinal ligament in plane between the sartorius muscle and tensor fasciae latae muscle. The lateral femoral cutaneous nerve is identified and retracted medially. *Dashed lines* indicate extension of the fascial incision proximally and along the iliac crest, if needed, for wider exposure. **C,** the sartorius muscle is retracted medially, and the anterior portion of the tensor fasciae latae is cut and retracted laterally. The ascending branch of the lateral femoral circumflex artery is identified and ligated. The interval between the rectus femoris muscle and gluteus medius muscle is developed. **D,** resection of the rectus femoris muscle allows exposure of the anterior hip joint capsule.
(Continued.)

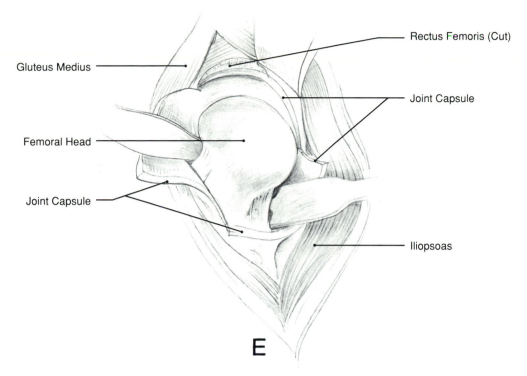

Gluteus Medius

Femoral Head

Joint Capsule

Rectus Femoris (Cut)

Joint Capsule

Joint Capsule

Iliopsoas

E

FIG 10–19 (cont.).

E, T-shaped capsular incision allows exposure of hip joint. Hip dislocated by adduction and external rotation of limb. Care must be taken in retracting the joint capsule and iliopsoas to avoid injury to the contents of the femoral triangle (femoral nerves and vessels).

(Ollier, Murphy, Brackett, Colonna, Watson-Jones, Burwell-Scott, Jergesen-Abbott, Harris, Hardinge, McFarland, and Osborne). In all of these approaches the deep dissection is carried out in the plane between the tensor fasciae latae and gluteus medius. This is not a true internervous plane because both the tensor fasciae latae and gluteus medius are innervated by the superior gluteal nerve. The dissections should stop short of damaging the main branch of the superior gluteal nerve, which passes from the gluteus medius to the tensor fascia latae about 3 cm below the iliac crest. The lateral approach to the hip is used extensively for procedures such as total hip replacement, hemiarthroplasty, and open reduction–internal fixation of femoral neck fractures.

The patient is placed in either supine or lateral decubitus position on the operating table. The skin incision starts approximately 5 cm behind the anterior superior iliac spine but level with it (Fig 10–20). The incision is continued down to the posterior aspect of the trochanter and then gently curved distally a few centimeters. The fascial incision is begun in the distal aspect of the wound and continued proximally. Care is taken to stay behind the palpable

posterior border of the tensor fasciae latae. Care is taken not to slice into the muscle belly of the tensor fasciae latae. The tensor fasciae latae is retracted anteromedially, and the portion of the gluteus medius overlying the hip joint is freed up by blunt dissection. A series of small vessels crossing the interval between the tensor fasciae latae and gluteus medius must be ligated or coagulated. A retractor is placed deep to the gluteus medius and the muscle retracted laterally and proximally to expose the superior margin of the joint capsule.

Further exposure is obtained by incising the origin of the anterior portion of the vastus lateralis at the vastus lateralis ridge of the greater trochanter and reflecting it inferiorly and laterally. The fat lying on the capsule is gently swept off by blunt dissection. External rotation of the limb puts the capsule on tension. The capsule is opened by an incision parallel to the femoral neck and another parallel to the rim of the acetabulum. The hip is dislocated at this point by flexion, adduction, and external rotation of the limb.

The lateral approach can be modified by three maneuvers to facilitate wider exposure to the hip joint. The anterior portion of the gluteus medius can

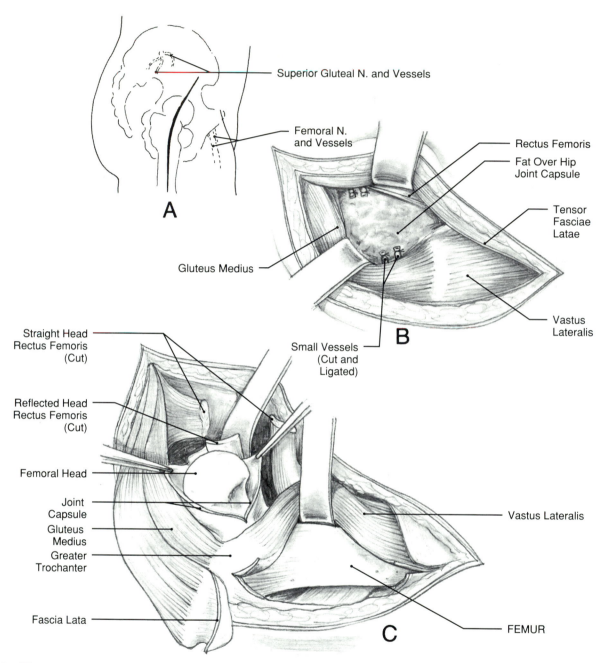

FIG 10–20.
Lateral approach to the hip joint. **A,** skin incision. Note superior gluteal nerve and vessels and femoral nerve and vessels. **B,** rectus femoris muscle retracted anteromedially and gluteus medius muscle posterolaterally. Small vessels found in this interval cauterized or ligated. **C,** rectus femoris heads of origin detached and retracted medially. Care is taken to avoid injury to the femoral vessels and nerves. Hip joint capsule opened and femoral head dislocated by flexion, adduction, and external rotation of the limb. The proximal femoral shaft can be exposed by splitting and retraction of the vastus lateralis muscle.

(Continued.)

be resected from the greater trochanter just above its insertion. This should be carefully reattached at the end of the procedure. Another widely practiced maneuver is trochanteric osteotomy (Fig 10–20,D). To accomplish this the osteotomy should be located at the base of the vastus lateralis ridge. The upper end of the osteotomy may be either intracapsular or extracapsular. The thickness of the osteotomized portion of bone varies depending on the procedure. The osteotomized trochanter, with the attached muscles

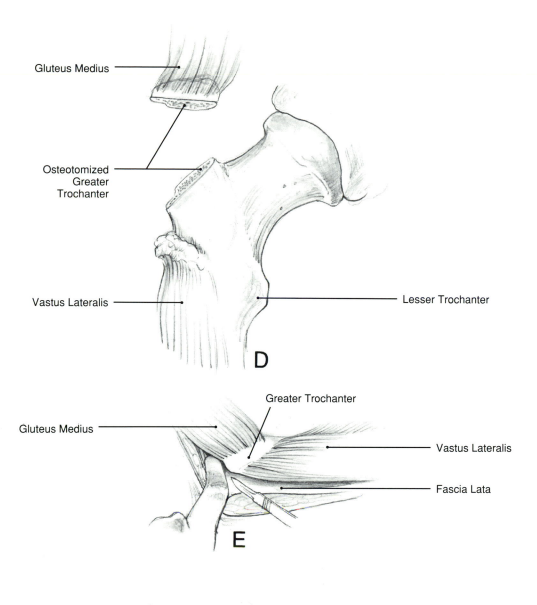

Gluteus Medius

Osteotomized Greater Trochanter

Vastus Lateralis

Lesser Trochanter

D

Greater Trochanter

Gluteus Medius

Vastus Lateralis

Fascia Lata

E

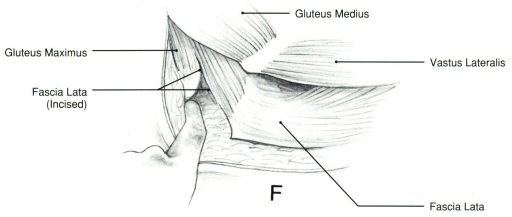

Gluteus Medius

Gluteus Maximus

Vastus Lateralis

Fascia Lata (Incised)

Fascia Lata

F

FIG 10–20   (cont.).
D, trochanter osteotomized to facilitate exposure. **E,** location for relaxation incision. **F,** relaxation incision in the fascia lata extended into fibers of gluteus maximus.

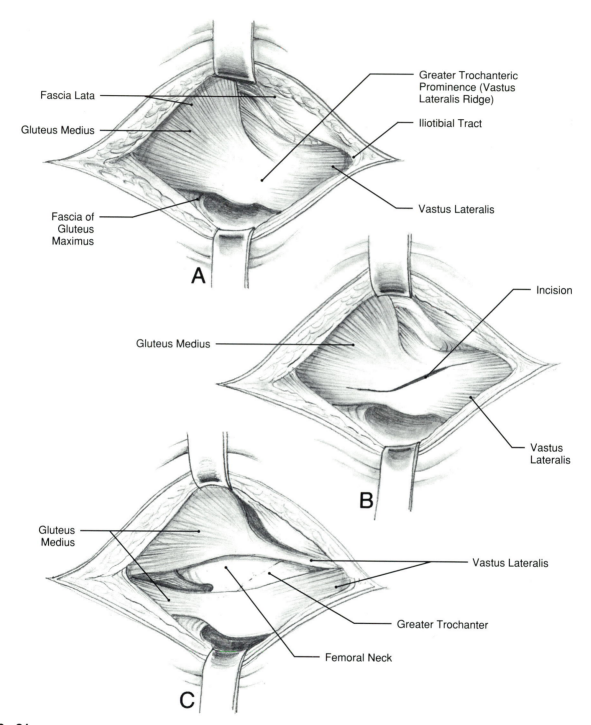

FIG 10–21.
Direct lateral approach to the hip joint. **A,** skin and fascia lata incised to expose gluteus medius and vastus lateralis complex.
B, an incision is made down to the bone of the trochanter, leaving the posterior third of the gluteus medius insertion undisturbed, and continuing obliquely across the trochanter, then distally in the vastus lateralis. **C,** exposure of greater trochanter.

(Continued.)

(gluteus medius and minimus), is retracted superiorly after being freed from the short external rotator insertions. The third maneuver (Fig 10–20,E and F) that can facilitate exposure is a short oblique incision in the fascia lata and gluteus maximus, as described by Harris. This allows room for the dislocated femoral head and greater trochanter. This incision is made at the level of the middle of the greater trochanter and extended medially and proximally into the gluteus maximus parallel to its fibers for a distance of about 4 cm.

McFarland and Osborne described a direct lateral approach to the hip that has been modified by Hardinge (Fig 10–21). The approach is based on the fact that the gluteus medius and vastus lateralis muscles are regarded as being in direct functional continuity through the thick periosteum covering the greater trochanter. This approach is unique in that it avoids the necessity for trochanteric osteotomy. Because the bulk of the gluteus medius muscle is preserved intact, it has been suggested that this approach permits early mobilization after surgery.

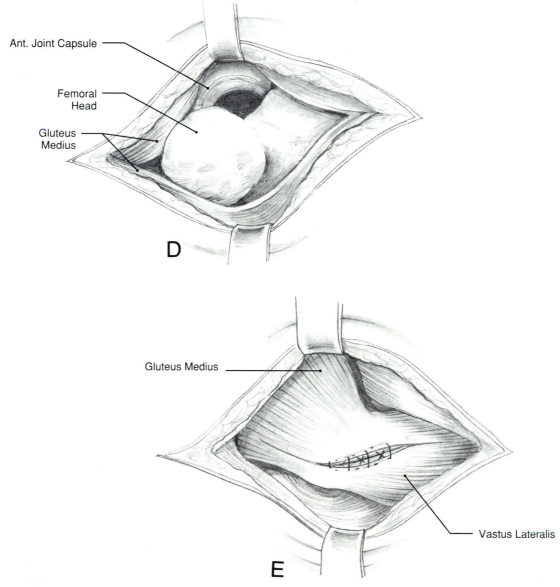

FIG 10–21 (cont.).
D, subperiosteal dissection and retraction of anterior two thirds of gluteus medius with underlying gluteus minimus and anterior joint capsule, as well as anterior portions of the vastus lateralis anteriorly to expose femoral head and neck. The hip is dislocated by flexion, adduction, and external rotation. **E,** meticulous approximation of the gluteus medius-vastus lateralis complex. (Modified from Hardinge K: The direct lateral approach to the hip. *J Bone Joint Surg* 1982; 64B:17–19.)

The patient is placed in supine or lateral decubitus position on the operating table. A straight lateral skin incision is made, centered over the greater trochanter, to expose the gluteal fascia and iliotibial band. These are divided in line with the skin incision along its entire length. In the proximal aspect of the wound the fascia lata is retracted anteriorly and the fascia of the gluteus maximus posteriorly. The prominent point of the vastus lateralis ridge is identified. At this point an incision is made down to the bone through the periosteum and fascia, leaving the posterior third of the gluteus medius insertion undisturbed on the trochanter. The incision is continued obliquely across the greater trochanter to the middle of the anterolateral aspect of the femur and 3 to 4 cm farther distally in the vastus lateralis, in line with the direction of its fibers. With a sharp knife the attachment of the anterior portion of the gluteus medius, the periosteum, and the tendinous junction of the gluteus medius, vastus lateralis, and origin of the vastus lateralis are peeled from the bone in one piece and retracted anteriorly. The tendon of the gluteus minimus is divided and retracted. This allows exposure of the hip joint capsule. The hip joint capsule is then opened to carry out the indicated procedure. During closure the capsule and gluteus minimus are meticulously sutured as one structure. The gluteus medius and vastus lateralis are returned to their original position and sutured to the undisturbed part of the vastus lateralis and gluteus medius.

Posterior Approach

In the last century at least twelve posterior surgical approaches or modifications of approaches to the hip have been described. The first description of the posterior approach to the hip was recorded by Von Langenbeck in 1874. This was modified by Kocher in 1887. The posterior approach to the hip allows easy, safe, and quick access to the joint. The approach has been widely used for hemiarthroplasty, total hip replacement, open reduction and internal fixation of periacetabular fractures, and drainage of the hip joint.

The skin incisions are essentially similar for the various posterior approaches, unlike the variety of skin incisions used in lateral and, to a lesser degree, anterior approaches. In all of the posterior approaches the skin is divided obliquely parallel to the fibers of the gluteus maximus at the superior border or along the upper fibers of the muscle. Another element of the incision extends distally from the region of the greater trochanter along the lateral proximal shaft of the femur for a variable distance. The deep dissection is accomplished by detachment of the short external rotators of the hip from their trochanteric attachment.

The procedure is carried out with the patient in the true lateral position. An incision is begun 5 cm distal and lateral to the posterior superior iliac spine and continued laterally and distally to the posterosuperior angle of the greater trochanter and then distally along the posterior border of the trochanter for 5 cm (Fig 10–22). The same skin incision can be made by flexing the hip to 90 degrees and making a straight longitudinal incision over the posterior aspect of the greater trochanter. This incision will curve when the hip is extended. The fascia lata is incised over the lateral aspect of the femur and the fibers of the gluteus maximus are split by blunt dissection. The gluteus maximus receives blood supply from the superior and inferior gluteal arteries, which enter the deep surface of the muscle. Splitting the muscle invariably causes some bleeding. If the splitting is done gently, the vessels may be identified and coagulated before they are cut across.

The fibers of the gluteus maximus and the deep fascia of the thigh are separated by retraction. This exposes the short external rotator muscles, which are attached to the upper part of the posterolateral aspect of the femur at the base of the trochanter. Internal rotation of the hip stretches the external rotator muscles, making their identification easier. Internal rotation of the hip also moves the rotators away from the sciatic nerve. The sciatic nerve exits through the greater sciatic notch below the piriformis muscle, lies over the external rotator muscles, then runs down the back of the thigh. The nerve should be located by palpation, but it is not necessary to dissect it free. If exposure of the sciatic nerve is desired, it can be accomplished by continuing the dissection proximally and medially. Caution should be taken to avoid injury to the superior and inferior gluteal vessels and nerves. The fat overlying the posterior hip joint is swept away from the external rotators. They are detached at their trochanteric insertion, reflected backward, and laid over the sciatic nerve to protect it during the procedure.

If necessary, the upper part of the quadratus femoris muscle, in addition to the short external rotators (piriformis, obturator internus, and gemelli), may be divided. There is an extensive blood supply to this region (cruciate anastomosis) (see Fig 10–6), and some of these vessels may require coagulation to prevent excessive bleeding. For further exposure the insertion of the gluteus maximus muscle can be detached from the upper femur. With the posterior

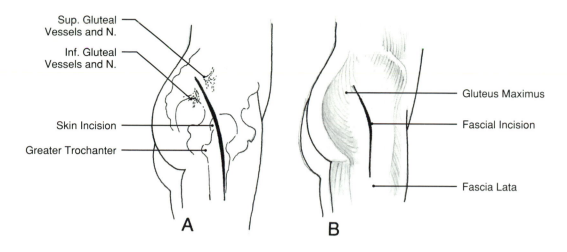

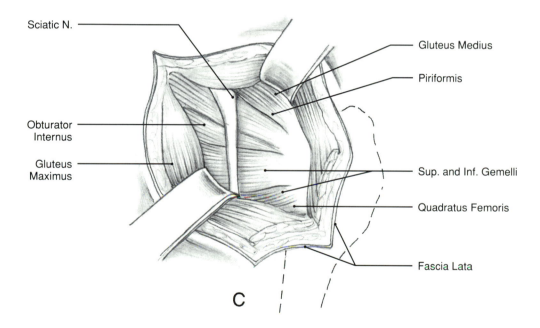

FIG 10–22.
Posterior approach to the hip joint. **A,** skin incision. Note superior and inferior gluteal vessels and nerves. **B,** fascial incision. **C,** exposure of external rotators with exposure of sciatic nerve. (When dissection is carried proximally and posteriorly, sciatic nerve is exposed, but ordinarily it is not necessary to obtain such wide exposure.) *(Continued.)*

aspect of the joint capsule fully exposed, the capsule is incised either with a longitudinal or T-shaped incision. Dislocation of the hip is achieved by flexion and internal rotation.

Medial Approach

Not commonly but occasionally the hip must be approached medially. This can be accomplished through an approach described by Ludloff in 1908.

This approach can be used for open reduction of congenital dislocation of the hip, biopsy and/or treatment of tumors of the femoral neck and medial aspect of the proximal shaft, and psoas release as well as obturator neurectomy. The procedure is carried out with the patient in supine position on an operating table with the affected hip flexed, abducted, and externally rotated (Fig 10–23). The superficial plane of dissection is between the adductor longus and gracilis and the deep dissection between

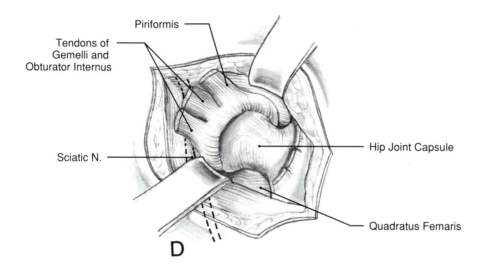

Piriformis

Tendons of
Gemelli and
Obturator Internus

Sciatic N.

Hip Joint Capsule

Quadratus Femaris

D

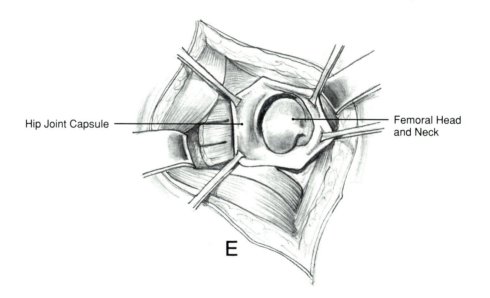

Hip Joint Capsule

Femoral Head
and Neck

E

FIG 10–22   (cont.).
D, resection and posterior reflection of short external rotators from their trochanteric insertion to protect underlying sciatic
nerve. **E,** incision in hip capsule.
(Continued.)

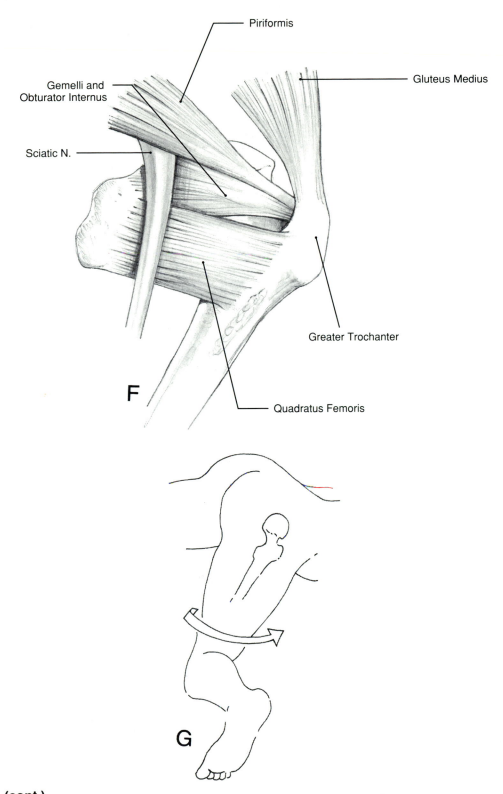

FIG 10–22 (cont.).
F, relationship of sciatic nerve to short external rotators. **G,** flexion and internal rotation to dislocate hip.

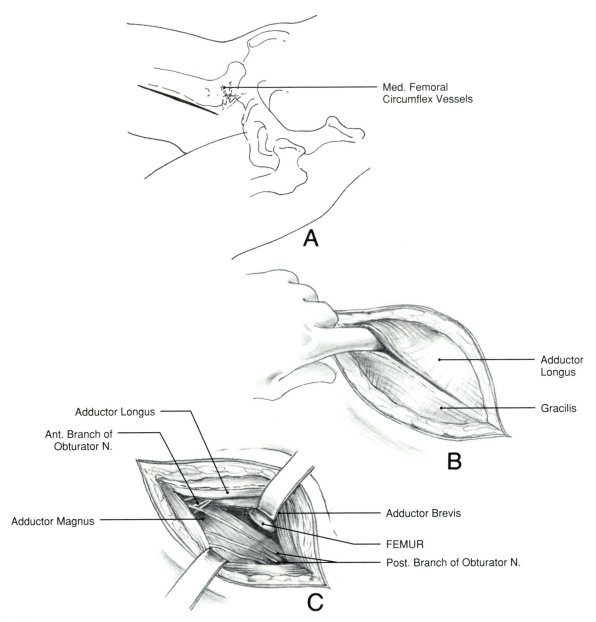

FIG 10–23.
Medial approach to the hip joint. **A,** skin incision with limb abducted, slightly flexed, and externally rotated. Note location of medial femoral circumflex vessels. **B,** fascia divided and plane between adductor longus and gracilis developed. **C,** deep dissection between adductor brevis and adductor magnus. Note branches of anterior division of the obturator nerve (lying on top of adductor brevis) and posterior division of obturator nerve (lying on top of the adductor magnus).

(Continued.)

the adductor brevis and adductor magnus. These are not truly internervous planes because all of these muscles are innervated by branches of the obturator nerve. However, they are supplied well proximal in the thigh, and the nerves should not be injured during the dissection. An incision is begun approximately 3 cm below the pubic tubercle and carried distally over the adductor longus. Superficial dissection identifies and develops the interval between the adductor longus and gracilis. The deep dissection is between the adductor brevis and adductor magnus, down to the lesser trochanter on the floor of the wound.

The structures at risk during this approach are the anterior and posterior divisions of the obturator nerve as well as the medial femoral circumflex ar-

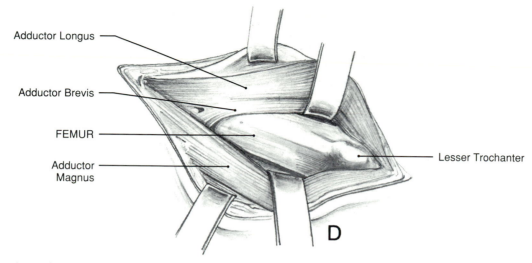

Adductor Longus

Adductor Brevis

FEMUR

Adductor
Magnus

Lesser Trochanter

D

FIG 10–23   (cont.).
D, exposure of proximomedial shaft of femur in the region of the lesser trochanter.

tery. As it exits the pelvis, the anterior division of the obturator nerve lies on top of the obturator externus. It runs down the medial aspect of the thigh between the adductor longus and adductor brevis, adhering closely to the latter (see Fig 10–10). This anterior branch supplies the adductor longus, adductor brevis, and gracilis in the thigh. The posterior division of the obturator nerve lies in the substance of the obturator externus, which it supplies. It then runs down the thigh on the adductor magnus and under the adductor brevis, supplying the adductor portion of the adductor magnus. The medial femoral circumflex artery passes medially around the psoas tendon between that structure and the pectineus to reach the posterior aspect of the hip joint capsule.

To deal with resistant congenital hip dislocations Mau, et al. have modified the Ludloff approach to perform an open reduction of the hip joint. This approach allows release of the contracted structures on the medial aspect of the hip, particularly the transverse acetabular ligament and the hip capsule itself. In this approach the deep dissection is carried out in the interval between the pectineus and iliopsoas. A drawback of this approach is that several branches of the medial circumflex artery and accompanying veins must be coagulated in the lateral corner of the wound in front of the pectineus muscle.

Hip Disarticulation

In dealing with cancer and, occasionally, severe trauma to the lower extremity, hip disarticulation may be required. As in other types of amputation the initial steps should be to secure control of the blood supply to the extremity. The procedure is begun with the patient in supine position with a bolster under the sacroiliac region of the involved extremity. An anterior racket-shaped incision is begun at the anterior superior iliac spine and then curved distally and medially almost parallel with the inguinal ligament to a point on the medial aspect of the thigh approximately 5 cm distal to the origin of the adductor muscles (Fig 10–24). The femoral artery and vein are identified, ligated, and divided along with the femoral nerve. The incision then traverses around the posterior aspect of the thigh about 5 cm distal to the ischial tuberosity and extends around the lateral aspect of the thigh approximately 8 cm distal to the base of the greater trochanter. From this point the incision is curved proximally to join the beginning of the incision just inferior to the anterior superior iliac spine.

The sartorius and rectus femoris muscles are detached from their iliac origin and reflected distally. The pectineus is transected approximately 1 cm from the pubis. External rotation of the limb brings the lesser trochanter and iliopsoas tendon into view. The iliopsoas tendon is divided at its insertion on the lesser trochanter. The adductor and gracilis muscles are divided at their origin from the pubis and the adductor magnus from the ischium. The plane between the pectineus and obturator externus and the short external rotators of the hip is exposed. The obturator artery is identified and carefully ligated. The obturator externus muscle is not divided at this point because the obturator artery may be inadvertently severed with the cut end retracting into the pelvis. This may lead to hemorrhage that is difficult

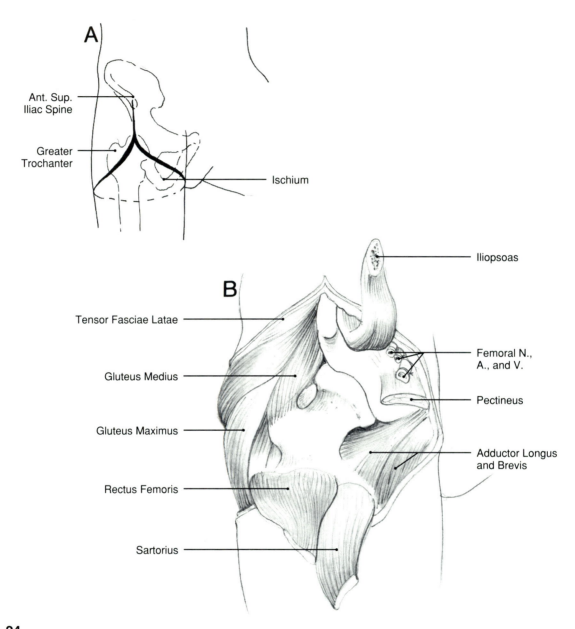

FIG 10–24.
Hip disarticulation. **A,** skin incision. **B,** ligation and division of the femoral vessels and nerve. Origins of sartorius and rectus femoris muscles detached and reflected distally. Resection of the pectineus at its origin and the iliopsoas at its insertion.

(Continued.)

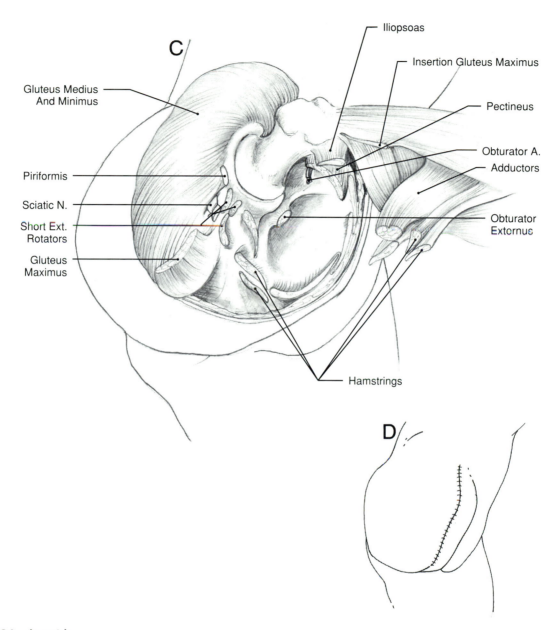

FIG 10–24 (cont.).
C, the adductors and gracilis are resected at their pubic origin. The hamstrings, including the adductor magnus, are resected from their ischial origin. The obturator artery is identified in the plane between the pectineus and obturator externus and carefully ligated. Internal rotation allows exposure and detachment with proximal reflection of the gluteus medius and minimus from their insertions on the greater trochanter. The fascia lata is divided along with the gluteus maximus through its distal fibers. The sciatic nerve is identified, ligated, and divided. The short external rotators are divided at their insertion and the hamstrings at their origin at the ischium. The hip capsule is opened and the ligament of the femoral head divided. **D,** the gluteal flap is brought forward and sutured to the remnants of the pectineus and adductor muscles, and the wound is closed. (Redrawn from Boyd HB: Anatomic disarticulation of the hip. *Surg Gynecol Obstet* 1947; 84:346.)

to control. The limb is next internally rotated. The gluteus medius and minimus muscles are detached from their insertions on the greater trochanter and retracted proximally. The fascia lata is divided, along with the most distal fibers of the gluteus maximus muscle. The gluteus maximus is retracted proximally. The sciatic nerve is identified, ligated to prevent bleeding from its associated ischiadic artery, and divided. The short external rotators of the hip, including the piriformis, gemelli, obturator internus, obturator externus, and quadratus femoris, are divided at their trochanteric insertion. The hamstring muscles are dissected off the ischial tuberosity. The hip joint capsule is incised and the ligamentum teres divided to complete the disarticulation. The large gluteal flap is brought anteriorly and sutured to the origin of the pectineus and adductor muscles.

SURGICAL APPROACHES TO THE THIGH (FEMUR)

The femur can be approached surgically from a number of directions, namely anteromedial, anterolateral, lateral, and posterolateral. These approaches are used to carry out procedures such as open reduction–internal fixation of fractures, drainage of osteomyelitis, biopsy or treatment of tumors, and corrective osteotomies. All of these approaches except the posterolateral require splitting a portion of the quadriceps femoris and thus are not carried out in a true internervous plane. However, because the nerve supply to the components of the quadriceps is given off high in the thigh, these approaches rarely result in quadriceps denervation. The femur can also be approached posteriorly. The posterior approach is particularly suited for exploration of the sciatic nerve.

Lateral Approach

The lateral approach to the femur is the approach most commonly used to deal with intertrochanteric hip fractures, pinning of slipped femoral capital epiphyses and/or femoral neck fractures, and internal fixation of shaft and supracondylar fractures. These procedures are usually carried out with the patient supine on a fracture table. An incision of the desired length is made over the lateral aspect of the thigh along a line from the greater trochanter to the lateral femoral condyle (Fig 10–25). The fascia

lata is split in line with the skin incision. The vastus lateralis and vastus intermedius are also split in line with the skin and fascial incisions. The vastus lateralis is then dissected off the shaft of the femur. The muscular branches of the perforating arteries from the profunda femoris will be encountered. If the dissection is performed bluntly these vessels are more readily identified and ligated. If the vessels are torn and not ligated, they will retract into the muscles of the posterior thigh and can cause significant blood loss.

Posterolateral Approach

Some surgeons have advocated a posterolateral approach (see Fig 10–25) to the femur with dissection between the vastus lateralis and lateral intermuscular septum because this procedure does not require splitting of the vastus intermedius. Also, in theory, this might be considered an internervous plane because the dissection is carried out between the vastus lateralis, supplied by the femoral nerve, and the hamstring muscles, supplied by the sciatic nerve. However, in reality, the vastus lateralis must be dissected off the anterior surface of the lateral intermuscular septum. This can rarely be done without leaving some denervated vastus lateralis fibers attached to the intermuscular septum.

A longitudinal skin incision is made along the posterolateral aspect of the thigh. The fascia is incised in line with the skin incision. The vastus lateralis is identified and dissected off the intermuscular septum and reflected anteriorly. The femur is then exposed by subperiosteal dissection. The perforating branches of the profundus femoris must be identified and ligated. If they are allowed to retract without ligation through the intermuscular septum they may cause significant bleeding.

Anterolateral Approach

The entire shaft of the femur can be exposed by an anterolateral approach, which can be readily extended into the hip joint if necessary. The approach requires splitting the vastus intermedius, and the postoperative formation of adhesions between the muscles of the quadriceps group may result in limited knee flexion. Dissection must therefore be done carefully and hemostasis obtained. Early knee motion should be encouraged postoperatively.

A skin incision is made over the anterolateral aspect of the thigh in a line between the anterior superior iliac spine and the lateral border of the patella (Fig 10–26). The length of the incision depends on

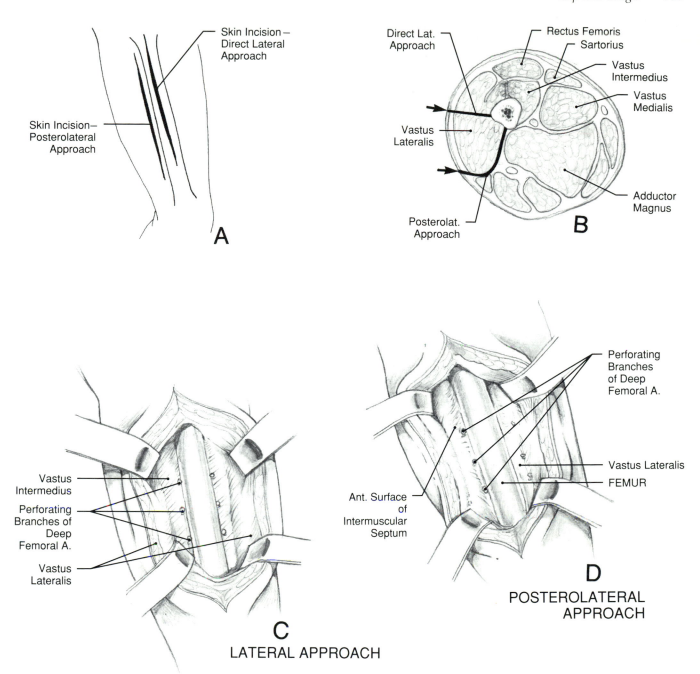

FIG 10–25.
Lateral and posterolateral approaches to the femur. **A,** skin incision for lateral and posterolateral approaches. **B,** cross section of the thigh depicting direct lateral approach to the femur by incision of the vastus lateralis and vastus intermedius in line with their fibers. Posterolateral approach along the lateral intermuscular septum is also shown. **C,** direct lateral approach through vastus lateralis and vastus intermedius. Note location of perforating branches of the deep femoral (profunda femoris) artery. **D,** posterolateral approach with dissection along the vastus lateralis and anterior surfaces of the lateral intermuscular septum. Again, note the perforating branches of the deep femoral (profunda femoris) artery.

the amount of exposure required. The fascia is incised and the dissection carried out between the lateral border of the rectus femoris and the medial border of the vastus lateralis. With retraction of the rectus femoris medially and the vastus lateralis laterally, the vastus intermedius is exposed and split in

the direction of its fibers. The femur is exposed by subperiosteal reflection of the vastus intermedius. In the proximal portion of the wound the nerve to the vastus lateralis will be encountered in the interval between the rectus femoris and vastus lateralis. This nerve should be protected. The descending branches

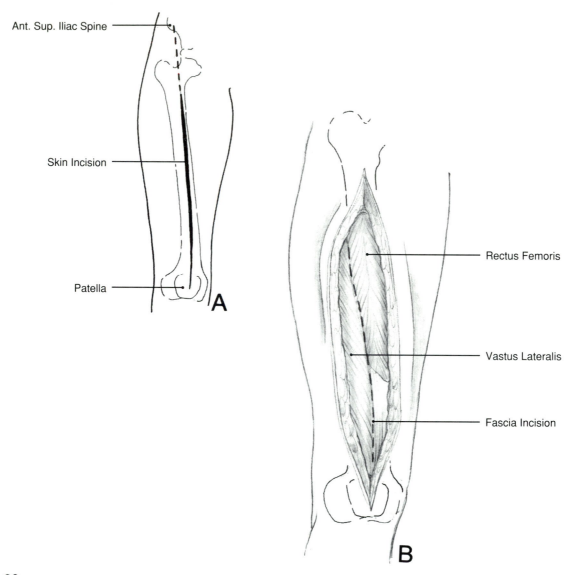

FIG 10–26.
Anterolateral approach to the femur. **A,** skin incision in line between the anterior superior iliac spine and the lateral border of the patella. Incision may be extended to approach the hip joint *(dashed line).* **B,** fascia incised *(dashed lines)* between rectus femoris and vastus lateralis and these muscles retracted.   *(Continued.)*

of the lateral femoral circumflex vessels will be also encountered in this area and must be ligated or cauterized. The incision can be extended proximally to expose the hip joint by dissection of the interval between the sartorius and tensor fasciae latae superficially and between the rectus femoris and gluteus medius in the deeper plane (see Anterior Hip Approach).

Anteromedial Approach

The anteromedial approach to the distal two thirds of the femur gives excellent exposure to deal

with fractures and infections and to carry out quadricepsplasty and corrective osteotomies. An incision is made on the anteromedial aspect of the thigh, over the interval between the rectus femoris and vastus medialis (Fig 10–27). The length of the incision depends on the amount of exposure required. The dissection is carried out between the vastus medialis and rectus femoris, both of which are supplied by the femoral nerve. Since these muscles are innervated by the femoral nerve proximally in the thigh, the nerve supply is not endangered. By retraction of the rectus femoris laterally and the vastus medialis medially the vastus intermedius is exposed. The vas-

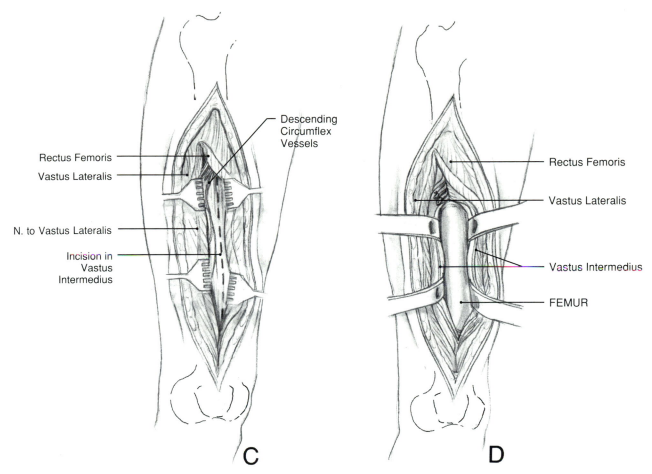

FIG 10–26 (cont.).
C, incision in vastus intermedius. Note nerve to vastus lateralis and descending branch of lateral femoral circumflex vessels.
D, exposure of femur by subperiosteal dissection and retraction of the split vastus intermedius.

tus intermedius is split in line with its fibers and dissected off the femoral shaft.

Posterior Approach to the Femur and/or Sciatic Nerve

There are very few indications to approach the femur posteriorly. This approach is most commonly used to explore the sciatic nerve. The approach is carried out with the patient lying prone. A skin incision is made in line from just distal to the gluteal fold to the proximal margin of the popliteal space, depending upon how much exposure is required (Fig 10–28). Care must be taken not to damage the posterior femoral cutaneous nerve, which lies under the deep fascia in the plane between the biceps femoris and semitendinosus muscles. Superficial dissection in the proximal portion of the wound is carried out by developing the plane between the biceps femoris and the lateral intermuscular septum overly-

ing the vastus lateralis. The long head of the biceps is reflected medially and the proximal femur exposed by subperiosteal dissection. If the plane of dissection is kept lateral to the biceps femoris, the sciatic nerve and its branches are not endangered. The short head of the biceps is identified and detached from its origin on the femur by sharp dissection. This allows further exposure to the posterior aspect of the femur.

In the distal half of the wound the long head of the biceps is retracted laterally to expose the sciatic nerve. Gentle lateral retraction on the sciatic nerve reveals the posterior aspect of the distal femur covered with periosteum. The femur itself is exposed by subperiosteal dissection. The short head of the biceps femoris is the *only* muscle supplied by the common peroneal nerve. This is important to know when electromyographic techniques are used to differentiate injury of the sciatic nerve (common peroneal component) from injury to the deep peroneal

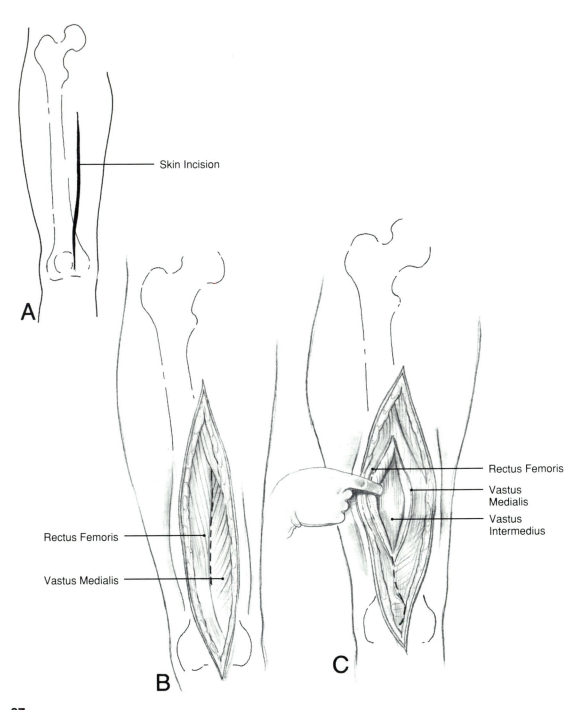

FIG 10–27.
Anteromedial approach to the femur. **A,** skin incision. **B,** fascia incised *(dashed line)* between the vastus medialis and rectus femoris. **C,** vastus medialis retracted medially and rectus femoris laterally. *(Continued.)*

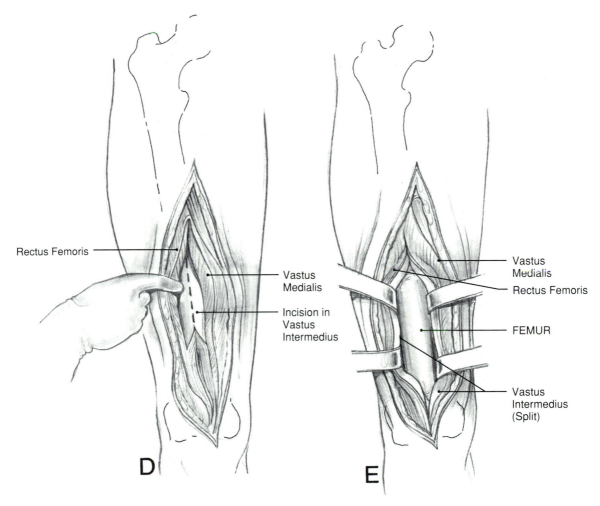

FIG 10–27 (cont.).
D, incision in vastus intermedius. **E,** subperiosteal dissection and retraction of split vastus intermedius exposes the femur.

nerve. Dissection in this area requires great care to identify the sciatic nerve and retract it gently laterally to avoid injury of the nerve itself.

Lateral Approach to the Posterior Surface of the Distal Femur

The posterior surface of the distal femur can be exposed by a lateral approach. This may be indicated in dealing with fractures of the distal femur. The approach is carried out with the knee slightly flexed. An incision is made along the superior edge of the iliotibial band and carried as far distally as the head of the fibula (Fig 10–29). The fascia immediately posterior to the iliotibial band is incised. Dissection of the short head of the biceps from the posterior surface of the lateral intermuscular septum allows access to the distal posterior aspect of the femur. Branches of the genicular vessels will be encountered and must be ligated and divided. The popliteal vessels are identified and retracted posteriorly. In the popliteal region the tibial nerve lies posterior to the popliteal vessels and the common peroneal nerve follows the posterior aspect of the biceps femoris. Care must be taken not to injure these structures.

Medial Approach to the Posterior Surface of the Femur and/or Femoropopliteal Vascular Structures

The medial approach to the distal femur may be used to treat fractures in this region and to explore the vascular structures in the distal thigh. The approach is carried out with the patient lying supine, the knee flexed, and the thigh externally rotated. The incision begins approximately 15 cm proximal to the adductor tubercle and continues along the ad-

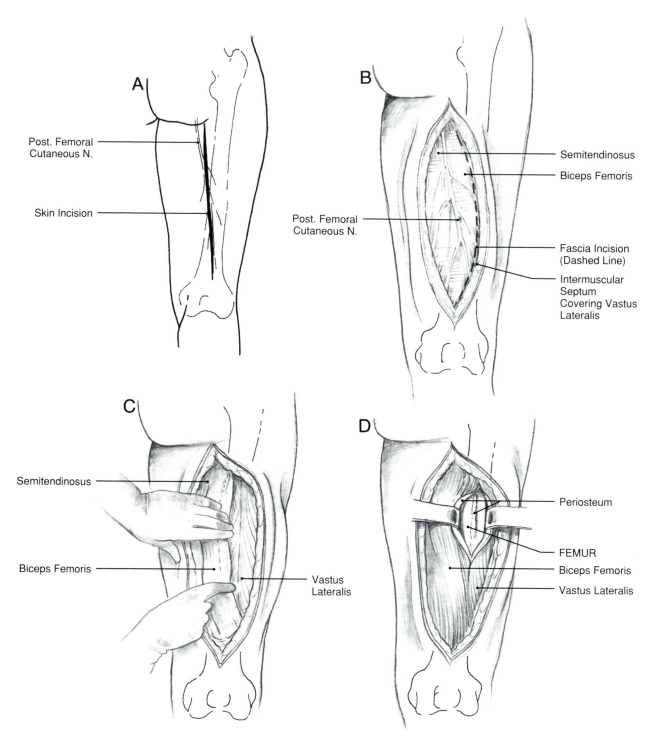

PROXIMAL DISSECTION

FIG 10–28.
Posterior approach to the femur and/or sciatic nerve. **A,** skin incision. Note posterior femoral cutaneous nerve. **B,** fascial incision *(dashed line)* between long head of biceps and intermuscular septum covering the vastus lateralis. Note nerve lying beneath fascia. **C,** long head of biceps femoris retracted medially. **D,** periosteal dissection allows exposure of proximal portion of femur.
(Continued.)

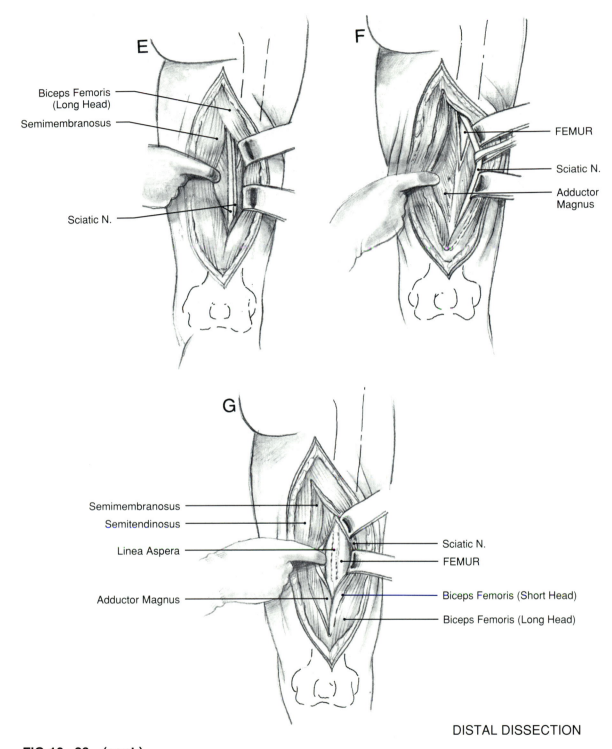

Biceps Femoris
(Long Head)

Semimembranosus

Sciatic N.

FEMUR

Sciatic N.

Adductor
Magnus

Semimembranosus

Semitendinosus

Linea Aspera

Adductor Magnus

Sciatic N.

FEMUR

Biceps Femoris (Short Head)

Biceps Femoris (Long Head)

DISTAL DISSECTION

FIG 10–28   (cont.).
E, in distal portion of wound the long head of the biceps femoris is retracted laterally to expose the sciatic nerve. **F,** gentle retraction of the sciatic nerve laterally allows exposure of distal portion of femur. **G,** resection of the short head of the biceps femoris from the femur allows greater exposure.

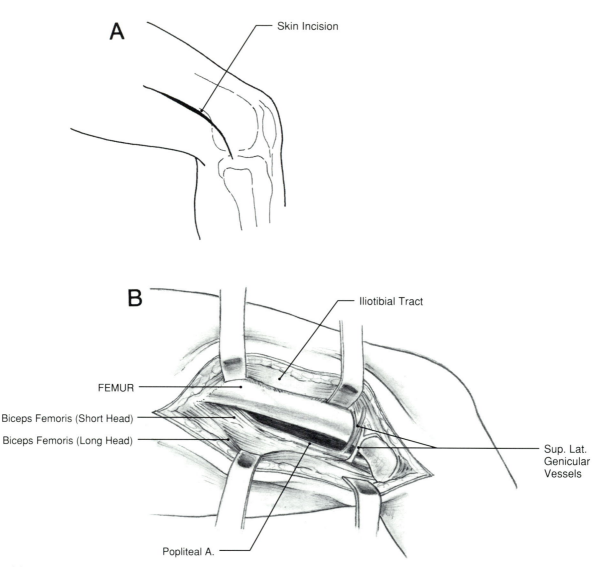

FIG 10–29.
Lateral approach to the distal femur. **A,** skin incision. **B,** fascia between the iliotibial tract and short head of the biceps is incised and the short head of the biceps detached from the lateral intermuscular septum and femur. Superior lateral genicular vessels are identified. These may require ligation.

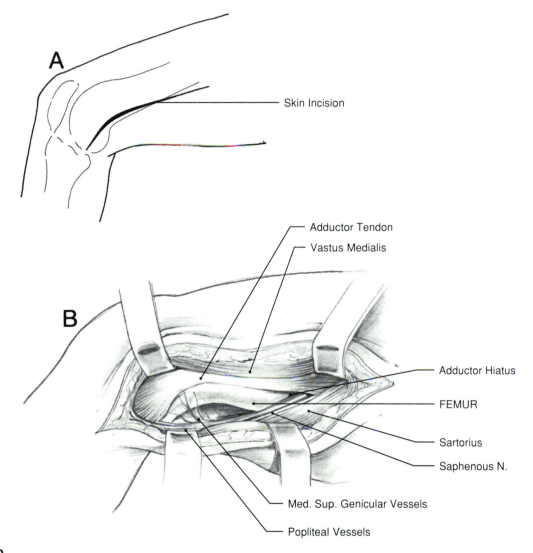

FIG 10–30.
Medial approach to the femur and femoropopliteal vascular structures. **A,** skin incision. **B,** plane between vastus medialis and sartorius developed. The vastus medialis is retracted anteromedially and the sartorius posteriorly. Note saphenous nerve, which should be gently retracted with the sartorius. The popliteal vessels are exposed after they emerge from the adductor canal. *(Continued.)*

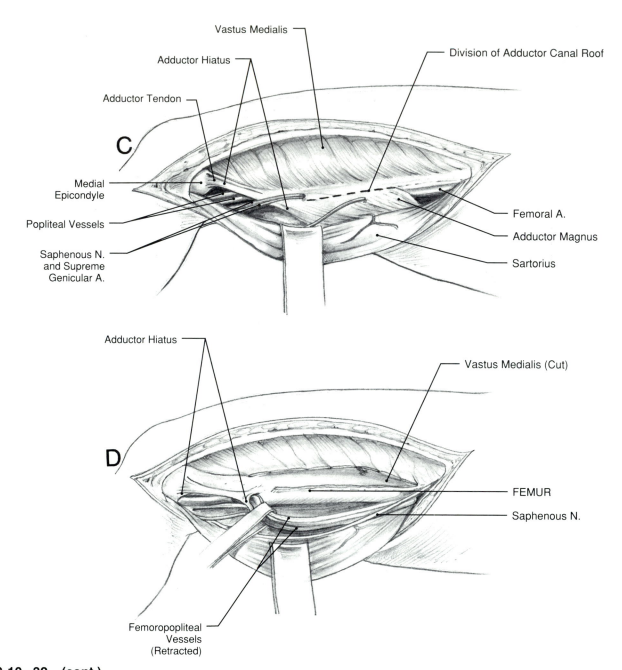

Vastus Medialis

Adductor Hiatus

Adductor Tendon

Division of Adductor Canal Roof

C

Medial Epicondyle

Popliteal Vessels

Saphenous N. and Supreme Genicular A.

Femoral A.

Adductor Magnus

Sartorius

Adductor Hiatus

Vastus Medialis (Cut)

D

FEMUR

Saphenous N.

Femoropopliteal Vessels (Retracted)

FIG 10–30 (cont.).
C, skin, fascial incisions, and dissection extended proximally to expose femoral vessels proximal to adductor hiatus. *Dashed lines* indicate where roof of the adductor canal will be dissected. **D,** retraction of femoropopliteal vessels and exposure of femur.

ductor tendon for a distance of 5 cm distal to the tubercle (Fig 10–30). The fascia is incised just posterior to the anterior edge of the sartorius. With the knee flexed the sartorius will fall posteriorly to expose the tendon of the adductor magnus muscle. Care must be taken to protect the saphenous nerve, which follows the sartorius on its deep surface. The thin fascia just posterior to the adductor magnus tendon is dissected free to expose the posterior surface of the femur and popliteal vessels at the popliteal space. If necessary to expose the femoral vessels proximal to the adductor hiatus, the roof of the adductor canal is incised. Gentle retraction of the vessels posteriorly will fully expose the distal femur.

BIBLIOGRAPHY

Aufranc OE: *Constructive Surgery of the Hip.* St. Louis, CV Mosby Co, 1962.

Banks SW, Laufman H: *An Atlas of Surgical Exposures of the Extremities.* Philadelphia, WB Saunders Co, 1968.

Bost FC, Schottstaedt ER, Larsen LJ: Surgical approaches to the hip joint. *Am Acad Orthop Surg Instr Course Lectures* 1954; 11:131.

Boyd HB: Anatomic disarticulation of the hip. *Surg Gynecol Obstet* 1947; 84:346.

Brackett EG: Study of the different approaches to the hip joint. *Boston Med Surg* 1912; CLXVI:235.

Burwell HN, Scott D: A lateral intermuscular approach to the hip joint. *J Bone Joint Surg* 1954; 36B:104.

Colonna PC: The trochanteric reconstruction operation for ununited fractures of the upper end of the femur. *J Bone Joint Surg* 1960; 42B:5.

Crenshaw AH (ed): *Campbell's Operative Orthopaedics,* ed 7 St Louis, CV Mosby Co, 1987.

Cubbins WR, Callahan JJ, Scuderi CS: Fractures of the neck of the femur. *Surg Gynecol Obstet* 1939; 68:87.

Fahey JJ: Surgical approaches to bones and joints. *Surg Clin North Am* 1949; 29:65.

Gibson A: Posterior exposure of the hip joint. *J Bone Joint Surg* 1950; 32B:183.

Gibson A: The posterolateral approach to the hip joint. *Am Acad Orthop Surg Instr Course Lectures,* 1953; 10:175.

Hardinge K: The direct lateral approach to the hip. *J Bone Joint Surg* 1982; 64B:17–19.

Harris WH: A new lateral approach to the hip joint. *J Bone Joint Surg* 1967; 49A:891.

Harris WH: A new approach to total hip replacement without osteotomy of the greater trochanter. *Clin Orthop Rel Res* 1975; 106:19–26.

Harty M, Joyce JJ: Surgical approaches to hip and femur. *J Bone Joint Surg* 1963; 45A:175.

Head WC, Mallory TH, Berklacich FM, et al: Extensile exposure of the hip for revision arthroplasty. *J Arthroplasty* 1987; 2:265–273.

Henry AK: *Extensile Exposure.* Edinburgh, E & S Livingstone, 1966.

Hoppenfeld S, deBoer P: The hip, in Hoppenfeld S, deBoer P (eds): *Surgical Exposures in Orthopaedics: The Anatomic Approach.* Philadelphia, JB Lippincott Co, 1984, pp. 301–356.

Hunter SC: Southern hip exposure. *Orthopedics* 1986; 9:1425–1428.

Jergensen F, Abbott LC: A comprehensive exposure of the hip joint. *J Bone Joint Surg* 1955; 37A:798.

Joyce JJ III, Harty M: The anatomical basis of the hip joint exposures. *Clin Orthop Rel Res* 1974; 98:27–31.

Kalamchi A, Schmidt TL, MacEwen GD: Congenital dislocation of the hip: open reduction by the medial approach. *Clin Orthop Rel Res* 1982; 169:127–132.

Light TR, Keggi KJ: Anterior approach to hip arthroplasty. *Clin Orthop Rel Res* 1980; 152:255–260.

Ludloff K: The open reduction of the congenital hip dislocation and anterior incision. *Am J Orthop Surg* 1913; 10:438.

Mau H, Dorr WM, Henkel L, Lutsche J: Open reduction of congenital dislocation of the hip by Ludloff's method. *J Bone Joint Surg* 1971; 53A:1281.

McFarland B, Osborne G: Approach to the hip. *J Bone Joint Surg* 1954; 36B:364.

Moore AT: The self-locking metal hip prosthesis. *J Bone Joint Surg* 1957; 39A:811.

Nachbur B, Meyer RP, Verkkala K, Zurcher R: The mechanisms of severe arterial injury in surgery of the hip joint. *Clin Orthop Rel Res* 1979; 141:122–133.

Netter FH: *The Ciba Collection: Musculoskeletal System.* Summit, NJ, Ciba-Geigy Corp, 1987.

Salter RB: Innominate osteotomy in the treatment of congenital dislocation and subluxation of the hip. *J Bone Joint Surg* 1961; 43B:518–539.

Smith-Petersen MN: A new supra-articular subperiosteal approach to the hip joint. *Am J Orthop Surg* 1917; 15:592.

Smith-Petersen MN: Approach to and exposure of the hip joint for mold arthroplasty. *J Bone Joint Surg* 1949; 31A:40.

Sutherland R, Rowe J Jr: Simplified surgical approach to the hip. *Arch Surg* 1944; 48:144.

Warren LF, Marshall JL, Girgis F: The prime static stabilizer of the medial side of the knee. *J Bone Joint Surg* 1974; 56A:665–674.

Watson-Jones R: Fractures of the neck of the femur. *Br J Surg* 1936; 23:787.

Wilson PD: Trochanteric arthroplasty in the treatment of ununited fractures of the neck of the femur. *J Bone Joint Surg* 1947; 29:313.

11

Knee

Frederick W. Reckling, M.D.
Stephen W. Munns, M.D.

ANATOMIC FEATURES OF THE KNEE

The knee is the largest joint in the body. It is also the most commonly injured due to its anatomy, exposure and the demands placed upon it. Function and stability of the knee depend upon a complex interrelationship of bony and soft tissue anatomy.

Bony Anatomy

The osseous structures of the knee are (1) the femoral condyles, (2) tibial plateaus, and (3) patella (Figs 11–1 and 11–2). The knee is considered a hinge joint, but in addition to flexion and extension it has some rotatory motion. The distal femur consists of the rounded condyles, which project only slightly in front of the body of the femur but markedly behind. Their long axes are not parallel but separated more widely posteriorly than anteriorly. The medial condyle projects about 0.5 cm below the lateral when the femur is held vertical. Anteriorly both condyles form the patellar articular surface, which is larger on the lateral than the medial condyle. Posteriorly the condyles are separated below the intercondylar line by the deep intercondylar fossa. The articular surfaces of the condyles differ: the articular surface of the lateral condyle is wide, but that of the medial condyle is longer. The medial condyle is more curved posteriorly than the lateral.

The region proximal to the condyle is called the epicondylar area. The medial epicondylar area is more prominent than the lateral. On its upper border it bears the adductor tubercle, which receives the lowest part of the insertion of the adductor magnus. Above and behind the lateral epicondyle is a depression for attachment of the lateral head of the gastrocnemius. Below the epicondyle is a depression marking the origin of the popliteus muscle. Adjacent to this is a well-marked groove (popliteal groove) for accommodation of the popliteus tendon.

The proximal end of the tibia is expanded and forms the tibial plateaus, which articulate with the femoral condyles. The tibial condyles are separated in the midline by the intercondylar eminence with its medial and lateral intercondylar tubercles. The cruciate ligaments and menisci attach anteriorly and posteriorly to the intercondylar eminence. The medial tibial plateau is flat whereas the posterior lip of the lateral tibial condyle is rounded. Both tibial plateaus slope posteriorly approximately 10 degrees. The articular surfaces of the knee are not totally congruent, and stability depends upon the ligaments and other soft tissues.

The patella is a somewhat triangular sesamoid bone. Its articular surface is divided by a vertical ridge, which creates a smaller medial and a larger lateral articulating facet. In extension the distal portion of the lateral patellar facet articulates with the lateral femoral condyle. Only in complete flexion does contact occur between the medial patellar facet and femoral condyle.

The fibula is the smaller of the two bones of the leg. Its proximal end (head) articulates with a facet

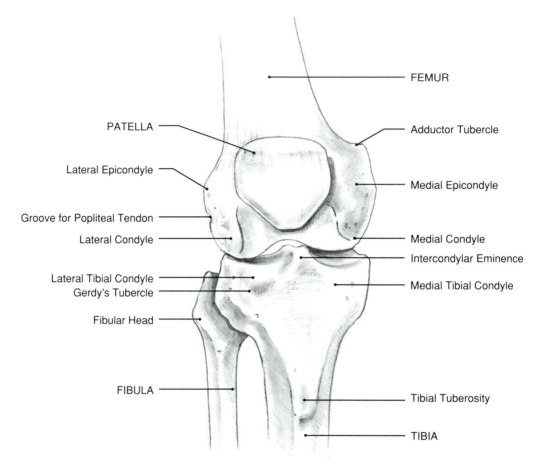

PATELLA

Lateral Epicondyle

Groove for Popliteal Tendon

Lateral Condyle

Lateral Tibial Condyle
Gerdy's Tubercle

Fibular Head

FIBULA

FEMUR

Adductor Tubercle

Medial Epicondyle

Medial Condyle

Intercondylar Eminence

Medial Tibial Condyle

Tibial Tuberosity

TIBIA

FIG 11–1.
Bony configuration of knee joint (frontal view).

on the undersurface of the lateral tibial condyle. The fibula does not provide an articulation for the knee joint per se, but it is the site of ligamentous and muscular structures pertinent to knee function.

Intraarticular Structures

The principal intraarticular structures are the medial and lateral menisci and the anterior and posterior cruciate ligaments (Fig 11–3). Each meniscus is a crescent-shaped fibrocartilaginous structure covering approximately the peripheral two thirds of the corresponding articular surface of the tibia. The menisci deepen the articular surfaces of the tibia to receive the condyles of the femur.

The medial meniscus is semicircular (Fig 11–4). In cross section it is triangular and wider posteriorly than anteriorly. It is firmly attached to the intercondylar fossa of the tibia posteriorly, but less firmly attached anteriorly to the intercondylar fossa. Peripherally the medial meniscus is attached to the capsule of the knee, which in turn is attached to the

tibia and femur. That part of the capsule which attaches to the tibia and medial meniscus is referred to as the coronary ligament.

The lateral meniscus covers a greater portion of the tibial articular surface than the medial meniscus and is nearly circular. The anterior horn of the lateral meniscus is attached to the intercondylar fossa lateral and posterior to the anterior cruciate ligament insertion. The posterior horn attaches to the intercondylar fossa anterior to the posterior end of the medial meniscus. Posterolaterally the lateral meniscus is grooved by the tendon of the popliteus muscle. In most knees some fibers of the popliteus insert into the periphery of the lateral meniscus. There are variable fibrous bands, the so-called posterior meniscofemoral ligaments (of Humphrey and Wrisberg), which run from the posterior attachment of the lateral meniscus to the medial condyle of the femur. In doing so they embrace the posterior cruciate ligament.

The anterior cruciate ligament is attached to the femur at the posterior part of the medial surface of

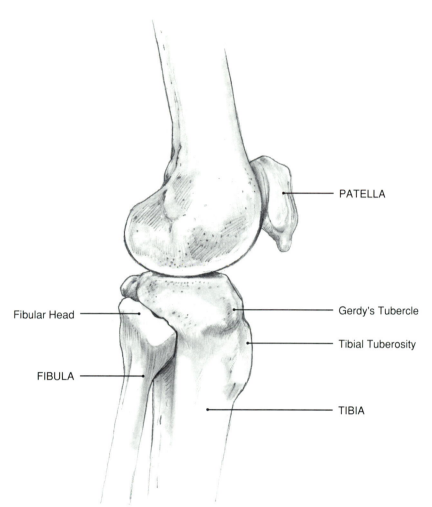

FIG 11–2.
Bony configuration of knee joint (lateral view).

PATELLA

Fibular Head

Gerdy's Tubercle

Tibial Tuberosity

FIBULA

TIBIA

the lateral femoral condyle. The general direction of the fibers is oblique. The tibial attachment is to a wide depressed area in front of the anterior tibial spine.

The posterior cruciate ligament is attached to the posterior part of the lateral surface of the medial condyle of the femur. It is vertical in its general direction. The tibial end attaches to a depression behind the intraarticular upper surface of the tibia. The attachment extends for a few millimeters onto the adjoining posterior surface of the tibia.

Extraarticular Ligamentous Structures

The capsule and collateral ligaments are the principal extraarticular static stabilizing structures of the knee. The capsule is a sleeve of fibrous tissue extending from the distal femur, patella, and patellar tendon to the tibia. The menisci are attached firmly to the periphery of this capsule, especially so medially and less so laterally. Posterolaterally the popli-

teus tendon courses by way of the popliteal hiatus to insert on the femoral condyle. This relationship produces a less secure lateral meniscal attachment than is present on the medial side of the knee. The medial portion of the capsule is more distinct and better defined than the lateral portion. The capsular structures, along with the medial and lateral extensor expansions of the powerful quadriceps muscle, are the principal stabilizing structures anterior to the transverse axis of the joint. Posterior to the transverse axis, the capsule is reinforced by the collateral ligaments and the medial and lateral hamstring muscles, as well as by the popliteus muscle and iliotibial band.

Supporting Structures on the Medial Side of the Knee

As described by Warren and Marshall, the supporting structures on the medial side of the knee can be divided into three layers (Fig 11–5). Layer one (superficial) is the first fascial plane beneath the

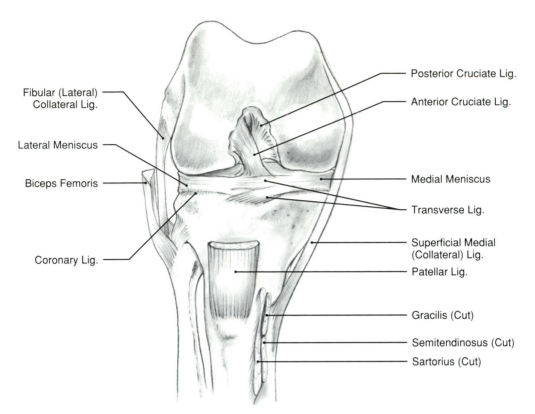

FIG 11–3.
Intraarticular structure of the knee joint (frontal view, patella removed).

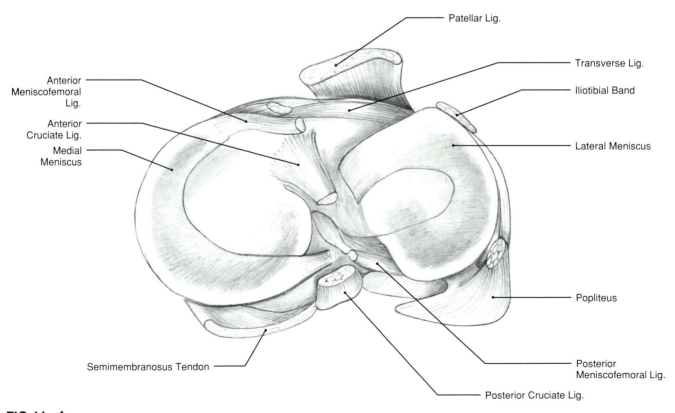

FIG 11–4.
Axial view of right knee joint with femur removed, showing the relationship of the menisci, cruciate ligaments, patellar ligament, popliteus tendon, and semimembranosus tendon.

ANTERIOR

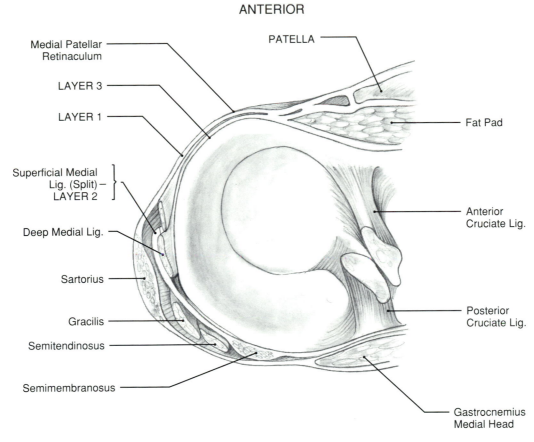

Medial Patellar Retinaculum

PATELLA

LAYER 3

LAYER 1

Fat Pad

Superficial Medial Lig. (Split) – LAYER 2

Deep Medial Lig.

Anterior Cruciate Lig.

Sartorius

Gracilis

Posterior Cruciate Lig.

Semitendinosus

Semimembranosus

Gastrocnemius Medial Head

FIG 11–5.
Supporting structures of the medial side of the right knee as seen from the axial view at the joint line with the femur removed. Layer one consists of the sartorius fascia, overlies the gracilis and semitendinosus tendons, and posteriorly overlies the two heads of the gastrocnemius and the structures of the popliteal fossa. Anteriorly layer one blends with the anterior part of layer two and the medial patellar retinaculum derived from the vastus medialis fascia. Layer two is the plane of the superficial medial (collateral) ligament. This ligament consists of parallel and oblique portions. The anterior fibers of layer 2 split vertically with the fibers anterior to the division going to the parapatellar retinaculum. The fibers posterior to the split run cephalad to the femoral condyle. Layer three is the joint capsule. The thickened portion of the capsule beneath the superficial medial ligament is known as the deep medial ligament. (Drawn after Warren LF, Marshall JL: The supporting structures and layers on the medial side of the knee: An anatomical analysis. *J Bone Joint Surg* 1979; 61A:56–62.)

skin, layer two (middle) is the plane of the superficial medial (collateral) ligament, and layer three (deep) is formed by the capsule of the medial side of the knee joint. The capsule includes the deep medial ligament of the knee, which, though it is referred to as a specific anatomical structure, is in reality a thickened portion of the knee capsule.

The superficial plane (Fig 11–6) is defined by the fascia that invests the sartorius muscle. The sartorius does not have a distinct tendon insertion as do the underlying gracilis and semitendinosus muscles, but instead inserts as an expansion of fascial fibers. From the sartorial fascia, layer one continues posteriorly as a fascial sheet and supports the gastrocnemius muscle heads and the neurovascular structures

in the popliteal region. In this area this fascial layer can be considered the "roof" of the popliteal fossa. In the posteromedial corner of the knee the tendons of the gracilis and semitendinosus are found in the layer of fatty tissue that lies between layer one and the deeper structures. Anteriorly the superficial layer blends with the anterior part of the middle layer and the medial patellar retinaculum. Only in its middle portion can layer one be readily separated from layer two (superficial medial ligament).

The plane of the superficial medial ligament constitutes layer two, the middle layer (Fig 11–7). This ligament has parallel (anterior) and oblique (posterior) portions. The anterior fibers are vertically oriented. These heavy fibers arise from the medial epi-

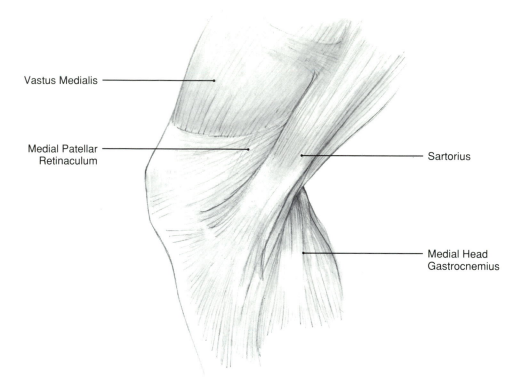

Vastus Medialis

Medial Patellar Retinaculum

Sartorius

Medial Head Gastrocnemius

FIG 11–6.
Layer one is defined by the fascia that invests the sartorius. Anteriorly it blends with the medial parapatellar retinaculum and posteriorly forms the superficial fascia of the popliteal fossa.

condyle of the femur and run distally to attach on the medial surface of the tibia approximately 5 cm below its articular surface and posterior to the pes anserinus. The posterior fibers course distally from femur to tibia in a slightly anterior oblique direction. They blend with the underlying deep or capsular layer to attach to the tibia below its posterior articular surface. Some of the fibers attach directly to the medial meniscus. Fibers from the semimembranosus tendon sheath join and strengthen the oblique portion of layer two near its insertion. According to Warren and Marshall, the anterior portion of layer two splits vertically. Anterior to the split, the more superior fibers proceed proximally to the vastus medialis and join layer one to form the so-called parapatellar retinacular fibers. Posterior to the split, fibers of layer two course proximally to attach to the femoral condyle. At the femoral condyle, a group of transverse fibers (the patellofemoral ligament, a continuation of the middle layer) courses anteriorly to the patella.

Layer three (deep layer) is formed by the capsule of the knee joint (Figs 11–5 and 11–8). It encompasses the entire medial aspect of the knee from the patella anteriorly to the midline of the popliteal space posteriorly. It consists of a thick central por-

tion of vertically oriented bands referred to as the deep medial ligament, as well as anterior and posterior components. The anterior portion of layer three is thin but can be easily separated from layer two, except near the margin of the patella.

The thicker central portion of layer three, the deep medial ligament, courses from the femur to insert in the midperipheral margin of the meniscus and rim of the tibial plateau. A bursa between the superficial and deep medial ligaments anteriorly allows easy separation of these structures. Posteriorly, however, the ligaments merge in their proximal (meniscofemoral) portion, making them more difficult to separate. Distally, the meniscotibial portion of the deep medial ligament is readily separated from the overlying superficial ligament.

The posterior portion of layer three blends with layer two to provide a strong posteromedial capsule, which encompasses the condyle of the femur.

Supporting Structures on the Lateral Side of the Knee

On the lateral side of the knee the supporting structures are also arranged in three layers (Fig 11–9). Layer one is the most superficial and consists of the lateral retinaculum of the knee and the iliotib-

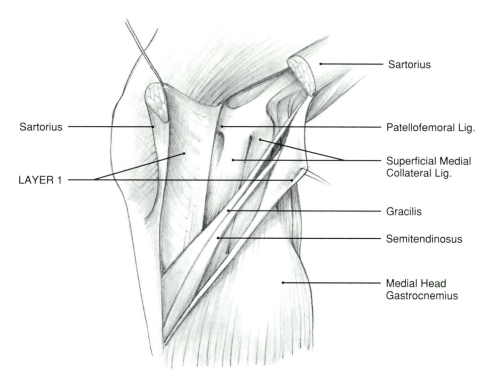

FIG 11–7.
Layer one has been opened. Transection and retraction of layer one exposes layer two, the superficial medial ligament. Note the tendons of the gracilis and semitendinosus which lie between layers one and two.

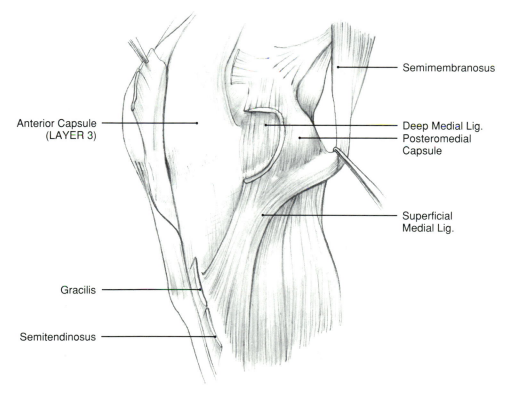

FIG 11–8.
A portion of the superficial medial ligament has been resected, exposing the deep medial ligament and posterior medial joint capsule (layer three).

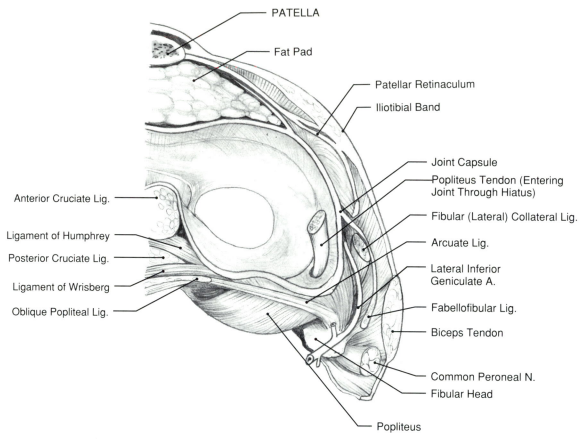

PATELLA

Fat Pad

Patellar Retinaculum

Iliotibial Band

Joint Capsule

Popliteus Tendon (Entering Joint Through Hiatus)

Fibular (Lateral) Collateral Lig.

Arcuate Lig.

Lateral Inferior Geniculate A.

Fabellofibular Lig.

Biceps Tendon

Common Peroneal N.

Fibular Head

Anterior Cruciate Lig.

Ligament of Humphrey

Posterior Cruciate Lig.

Ligament of Wrisberg

Oblique Popliteal Lig.

Popliteus

FIG 11–9.
Axial view of layers on the lateral side of the knee. Layer one consists of the lateral retinaculum and the iliotibial band. Layer two is the fibular (lateral) collateral, fabellofibular and arcuate ligaments. Layer three is the lateral joint capsule of the knee. (Modified from Seebacher JR, Inglis AE, Marshall JL, Warren RF: The structure of the posterolateral aspect of the knee. *J Bone Joint Surg* 1982; 64A:536–541).

ial band. The middle layer is the fibular (lateral) collateral, fabellofibular, and arcuate ligaments. The lateral capsule of the knee joint is the deep layer.

The lateral patellar retinaculum (layer one) (Fig 11–10) is a fibrous expansion of the vastus lateralis. Its longitudinally oriented fibers extend along the lateral border of the patella to merge distally with the patellar tendon. In addition, there are fibers that originate in the iliotibial band and course anteriorly to insert in the patellar tendon. These are known as the superficial oblique retinaculum. The posterior portion of the superficial layer is the iliotibial band, a distal continuation of the fascia lata, which descends along the lateral side of the knee to insert into Gerdy's tubercle on the tibia. Proximally the iliotibial band attaches to the femur via the lateral intermuscular septum. Posteriorly the iliotibial band merges into the biceps fascia and the fascia of the popliteal space.

The middle layer consists of the fibular (lateral) collateral, fabellofibular, and arcuate ligaments (Fig 11–11). The fibular collateral ligament forms a cord-like structure that originates on the lateral epicondyle of the femur and blends with the tendon of the biceps femoris as they insert on the fibular head. The fabellofibular ligament, when present, lies between the fibular collateral and arcuate ligaments. It arises from the region of the lateral head of the gastrocnemius and attaches to the styloid of the fibula. The arcuate ligament consists of a condensation of fibers of the posterolateral knee capsule. The most consistent fibers form a triangular sheet extending proximally from the fibular styloid. The strong, dense lateral edge of this sheet is attached to the femur and popliteus tendon. The medial side of the ligament is less dense. It arches over the popliteus muscle, extending proximally to attach to the posterior aspect of the lateral meniscus. The medial por-

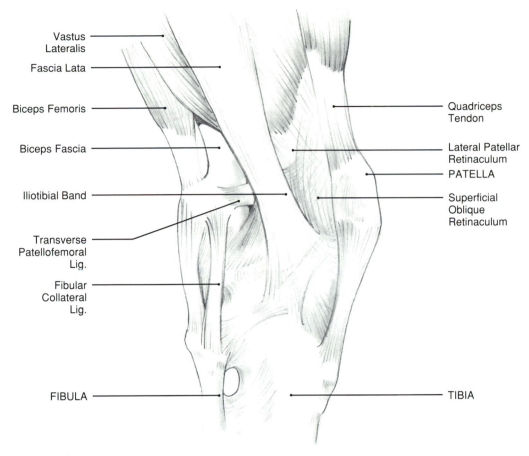

Vastus Lateralis

Fascia Lata

Biceps Femoris

Biceps Fascia

Iliotibial Band

Transverse Patellofemoral Lig.

Fibular Collateral Lig.

FIBULA

Quadriceps Tendon

Lateral Patellar Retinaculum

PATELLA

Superficial Oblique Retinaculum

TIBIA

FIG 11–10.
Superficial supporting structures (layer one) of the lateral side of the knee consist of the lateral patellar retinaculum, superficial oblique retinaculum, iliotibial band, biceps fascia, and transverse patellofemoral ligament.

tion of the arcuate ligament then continues proximally to insert diffusely on the posterior part of the joint capsule.

There is controversy over which attachment of the popliteus muscle should be considered its origin and which its insertion. The popliteus muscle attaches to the medial two thirds of a triangular surface proximal to the popliteal line on the posterior surface of the tibia. The tendon of this muscle inserts on a depression at the anterior part of the groove on the lateral condyle of the femur. In addition to its femoral attachment, at least in some knees, the tendon is also attached to the lateral meniscus and is joined by the lateral limb of the arcuate ligament.

The deep (third) layer is the capsule supporting the lateral side of the knee. It ensheathes the lateral knee joint with attachments on the tibia and femur. Where the capsule attaches to the outer edge of the lateral meniscus it is referred to as the coronary liga-

ment. A hiatus in the coronary ligament allows passage of the popliteus tendon as it courses proximally to attach to the femur (see Fig 11–9).

Muscles and Muscle Attachments

The movements of the knee are flexion, extension, and rotation. Flexion is performed by the hamstrings and biceps femoris and to a lesser extent the gastrocnemius and popliteus. Flexion is limited by soft tissues at the back of the knee. Extension is performed by the quadriceps (vastus lateralis, rectus femoris, vastus medialis, vastus intermedius) (Fig 11–12). Because of the shape of the articulation and the ligament attachments, the femur rotates medially on the tibia in terminal extension, the so-called "screw-home" mechanism that locks the joint. This movement is passive, as are other rotatory movements that occur during activity, except for lateral rotation of the femur. This latter movement, per-

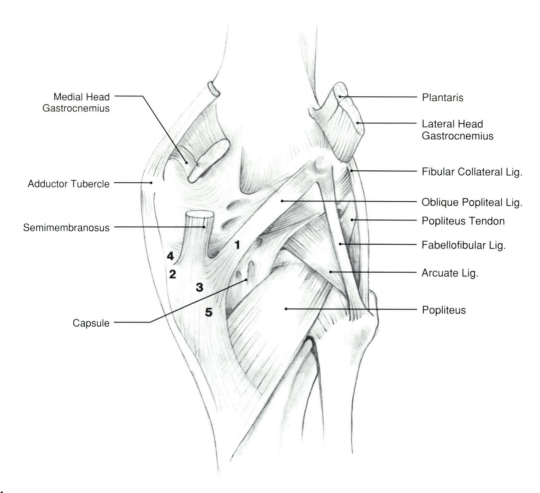

FIG 11–11.
Middle supporting structures (layer two) of the posterolateral side of the knee include the fibular collateral, fabellofibular (when present), and arcuate ligaments. The joint capsule is considered the deep layer (layer three). Also depicted is the distal expansion of the semimembranosus muscle of the posteromedial side of the knee. *1* = oblique popliteal ligament; *2* = tendinous attachment to the posterior capsule and posterior horn of the medial meniscus; *3* = deep head of the semimembranosus; *4* = direct head; *5* = fibrous expansions over the popliteus muscle.

formed by the popliteus, precedes flexion by "unlocking" the joint. The sartorius, gracilis, and hamstrings are weak rotators of the knee. The sartorius, gracilis, and semitendinosus medially, and the iliotibial tract laterally, serve as "guy ropes" to stabilize the pelvis.

The quadriceps tendon inserts into the proximal pole of the patella. The four components of the quadriceps mechanism form a trilaminar tendon to insert into the patella. The tendon of the rectus femoris flattens immediately above the patella and becomes the anterior lamina, which inserts at the anterior edge of the proximal pole. The tendon of the vastus intermedius continues downward as the deepest lamina of the quadriceps tendon and inserts into the posterior ridge of the proximal pole. The middle lamina is formed by the confluent edges of

the vastus lateralis and vastus medialis. The fibers of the medial retinaculum arise from the aponeurosis of the vastus medialis, insert directly into the side of the patella, and help prevent lateral displacement of the patella during flexion. The patellar tendon takes origin from the apex or distal pole of the patella and inserts distally into the tibial tuberosity.

The gastrocnemius is the most powerful calf muscle (Fig 11–13). It spans the posterior aspect of the knee. The two heads of the gastrocnemius arise from the posterior aspect of the medial and lateral femoral condyles. In addition to functioning as a powerful plantar flexor of the foot, it maintains the knee extended in midstance during gait. The so-called pes anserinus (goosefoot) is the name given the conjoined insertion of the sartorius, gracilis, and semitendinosus along the proximomedial aspect of

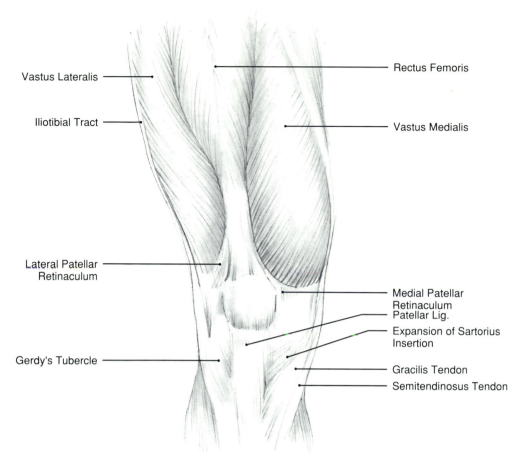

FIG 11–12.
Muscles, tendons and fascial expansions on the anterior aspect of the knee.

the tibia. As mentioned, these are primary flexors of the knee, but they also have a secondary internal rotational influence on the tibia. These muscles help protect the knee against rotatory as well as valgus stresses. Their counterpart on the lateral side of the knee is the strong biceps femoris insertion into the fibular head, lateral tibia, and posterolateral capsular structures. The biceps femoris is a flexor of the knee and a strong external rotator of the tibia. It provides rotatory stability by preventing forward dislocation of the tibia on the femur during flexion. By way of its contributions to the arcuate ligament complex of the posterolateral corner of the knee, it also provides lateral and rotatory stability. The iliotibial band, which is the distal, posterior third of the iliotibial tract, inserts proximally into the lateral epicondyle of the femur and distally into the lateral tibial tubercle, known as Gerdy's tubercle. The iliotibial band moves forward in extension and backward in flexion, but it is tense in all positions. During flexion the iliotibial band, popliteus tendon, and fibular collateral ligament cross each other, whereas the iliotibial

band and biceps tendon remain parallel to each other during flexion and extension. All serve to enhance lateral stability.

The semimembranosus muscle is especially important as a stabilizing structure about the posterior and posteromedial aspects of the knee. According to a number of anatomists, it has five distal expansions (see Fig 11–11). The first is the oblique popliteal ligament, which passes from the insertion of the semimembranosus on the posteromedial aspect of the tibia obliquely and laterally upward toward the insertion of the lateral gastrocnemius head. It acts as an important stabilizing structure on the posterior aspect of the knee. When the oblique popliteal ligament is pulled medially and forward it tightens the posterior capsule of the knee. This maneuver can be used to tighten the posterior capsule in the posteromedial corner of the knee during surgical repair. A second tendinous attachment is to the posterior capsule and, in some knees, the posterior horn of the medial meniscus. Some believe that this tendinous slip helps tighten the posterior capsule and pull the

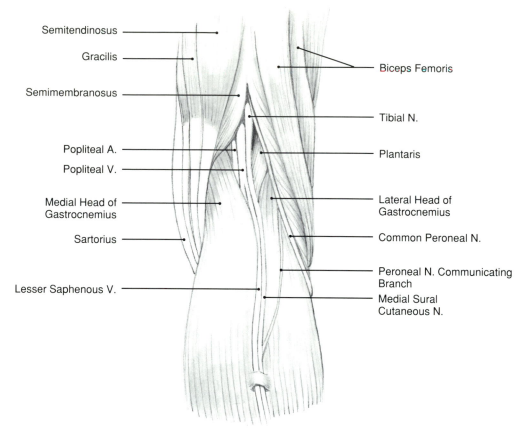

Semitendinosus

Gracilis

Semimembranosus

Popliteal A.

Popliteal V.

Medial Head of
Gastrocnemius

Sartorius

Lesser Saphenous V.

Biceps Femoris

Tibial N.

Plantaris

Lateral Head of
Gastrocnemius

Common Peroneal N.

Peroneal N. Communicating
Branch

Medial Sural
Cutaneous N.

FIG 11–13.
The fascia has been resected to show the muscles and tendons on the posterior aspect of the knee as well as the neurovascular structures of the popliteal fossa.

meniscus posteriorly during knee flexion. The anterior or deep head continues medially along the flare of the medial condyle and inserts beneath the superficial medial ligament just distal to the joint line. The direct head of the semimembranosus attaches to the tubercle on the posterior aspect of the medial condyle of the tibia, just below the joint line. This tendinous attachment provides a firm anchor in which sutures can be placed in posteromedial capsular repair. This distal portion of the semimembranosus tendon continues distally to form a fibrous expansion over the popliteus muscle and fuses with the periosteum of the medial tibia. The semimembranosus, through its muscle contraction, tenses the posterior capsule and posteromedial capsular structures to provide significant stability. Functionally it acts as a flexor of the knee and internal rotator of the tibia.

Vessels

The popliteal artery is a continuation of the femoral artery, which enters the knee through the hiatus in the adductor magnus (Fig 11–14). In the subsartorial (Hunter's) canal the femoral artery gives off the descending genicular artery. From this arises the superficial branch, which accompanies the saphenous nerve, as well as an articular branch. The popliteal artery runs vertically downward. It is separated from the femur by a thick pad of fat but comes into direct contact with the oblique popliteal ligament at the joint level. Below the knee joint the artery lies superficial to the popliteus muscle and ends by dividing into the anterior and posterior tibial arteries at the lower border of the popliteus muscle. Numerous muscular branches and five genicular branches arise from the popliteal artery.

The medial and lateral superior genicular arteries arise from the popliteal artery just above the femoral condyles and course anteriorly around the lower end of the femur. The middle genicular artery supplies the intraarticular structures and cruciate ligaments. It arises from the anterior aspect of the popliteal artery and enters the knee joint by piercing the oblique popliteal ligament.

The lateral inferior genicular artery courses ante-

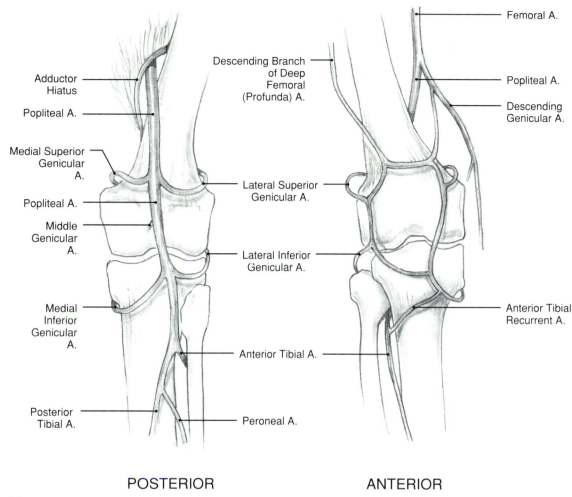

Adductor Hiatus

Popliteal A.

Medial Superior Genicular A.

Popliteal A.

Middle Genicular A.

Medial Inferior Genicular A.

Posterior Tibial A.

Descending Branch of Deep Femoral (Profunda) A.

Lateral Superior Genicular A.

Lateral Inferior Genicular A.

Anterior Tibial A.

Peroneal A.

Femoral A.

Popliteal A.

Descending Genicular A.

Anterior Tibial Recurrent A.

POSTERIOR

ANTERIOR

FIG 11–14.
Arteries of the knee region.

riorly at the level of the lateral joint line and thus is vulnerable to injury with surgery to the lateral aspect of the knee, particularly lateral meniscectomy and total joint replacement. The inferior medial genicular artery passes 2.5 cm distal to the medial joint line.

The five genicular arteries, the articular branch of the descending genicular artery, descending branch of the lateral circumflex femoral artery, and recurrent branches of the anterior tibial artery participate in an arterial anastomosis about the knee. This anastomosis provides communication between the femoral, deep femoral (profunda), and popliteal and anterior tibial arteries. A vascular circle around the patella gives rise to several nutrient arteries. Most of these arise at the lower pole of the patella and run proximally on its anterior surface.

In the popliteal fossa the popliteal vein lies superficial to the corresponding artery. Throughout its course in the fossa the vein lies between the

popliteal artery and tibial nerve, the nerve being most superficial in the fat beneath the deep fascia.

Nerves

The major nerves in the knee are two divisions of the sciatic nerve, the so-called tibial and common peroneal nerves, and the saphenous branch of the femoral nerve (see Fig 11–13). The tibial nerve arises from the sciatic nerve in the midportion of the thigh and courses distally through the popliteal fossa. At the lower end of the femur it lies deep in the interval between the two heads of the gastrocnemius. In the popliteal fossa the nerve crosses the popliteal vessels from lateral to medial, superficial to the vessels. The medial sural nerve, a cutaneous branch of the tibial nerve, descends on the surface of the gastrocnemius. The tibial nerve also gives off several muscular and articular branches.

Prior to entering the popliteal area, the common

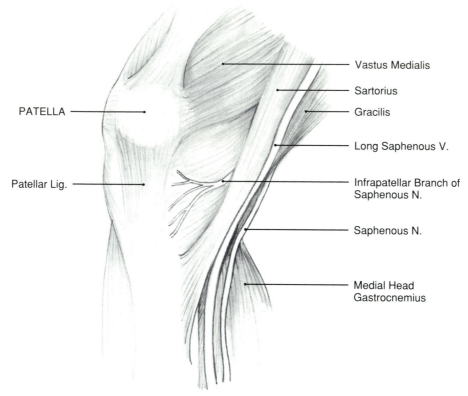

FIG 11–15.
Saphenous vein, saphenous nerve, and its infrapatellar branch.

peroneal nerve gives off a branch to the short head of the biceps femoris muscle. The common peroneal nerve enters the popliteal fossa just lateral to the tibial nerve and runs distally on the medial side of the biceps tendon. The common peroneal nerve passes superficial to the tendon of the lateral head of the gastrocnemius, coursing distally behind the fibular head. It courses around the lateral surface of the fibular neck, pierces the peroneus longus, and divides into the superficial and deep peroneal nerves. Three articular branches to the knee arise from the common peroneal nerve before it divides. The common peroneal nerve may give off the lateral sural cutaneous nerve, which supplies skin and fascia over the upper anterior aspect of the leg. It also gives off the peroneal communicating branch, which joins the medial sural cutaneous nerve.

The saphenous nerve (Fig 11–15) is a continuation of the femoral nerve, which emerges between the gracilis and sartorius. The nerve travels down the medial aspect of the leg with the saphenous vein to innervate the skin of the leg, medially, and the dorsum of the foot. The saphenous nerve is in jeopardy and must be protected in anteromedial surgical approaches to the knee. However, its infrapatellar

branch often must be divided because it crosses the operative field transversely.

SURGICAL APPROACHES TO THE KNEE AND SUPPORTING STRUCTURES

Skin Incisions

Wound breakdown and necrosis can be a major problem with surgery about the knee, particularly if there has been previous surgery in the area. Therefore the surgeon should bear in mind that the current surgical procedure may not be the last on that knee and plan the incision accordingly. Generally, a straight longitudinal incision is preferable to a curved one, because a straight incision can be reopened as many times as necessary. When the anteromedial or posteromedial aspect of the knee must be reached, a gently curving medial or lateral incision can be used. Sharply curved incisions about the knee should be avoided.

Except in some arthroscopic procedures, knee

surgery is usually carried out under tourniquet control. The entire extremity should be draped out to allow manipulation during the operative procedure. The tourniquet should generally be released prior to wound closure to assess for possible vascular damage and to obtain hemostasis.

Limited Approaches

A short oblique anteromedial or anterolateral approach to the knee can be used to perform a complete or partial meniscectomy, extract loose or foreign bodies, and manage such problems as osteochondritis dissecans of the medial and lateral femoral condyles (Fig 11–16). These approaches are carried out with the patient supine and the knee bent over the edge of the operating table with a bolster under the distal thigh. Placing the bolster under the distal thigh relieves tension on the capsule, allowing the vessels to displace posteriorly and keeping them out of harm's way. The anteromedial incision begins at the inferomedial corner of the patella and angles inferiorly and posteriorly, terminating approximately 1 cm below the joint line. Incisions continued further inferiorly put the infrapatellar branch of the saphenous nerve at risk as it traverses the upper leg approximately 1 cm below the joint line. The incision is carried down through the medial retinaculum, through the capsule, and into the synovium. It is best to begin the incision through the synovium proximally and work distally to avoid damage to the meniscus and coronary ligament.

A similar approach can be used on the lateral aspect of the knee. The skin incision begins at the inferolateral aspect of the patella and continues distally and posteriorly for approximately 5 cm. The fibular collateral ligament lies beneath a line drawn vertically from the lateral femoral epicondyle to the head of the fibula, and the entire incision should be anterior to this ligament to avoid injury to it. The incision should terminate proximal to the inferior lateral genicular artery, which courses around the upper part of the tibia next to the peripheral attachment of the lateral meniscus at the joint line. Injury to this artery may result in significant bleeding. The joint is entered proximally by incising the capsule and synovium in line with the skin incision. The incision is extended distally. Care is taken not to injure the meniscus or its attachments. The inferior lateral genicular artery may be damaged when the lateral meniscus is detached from the capsule during meniscectomy. If a tourniquet has been used, it should be deflated before the wound is closed to assess for the possibility of injury to this and other vessels.

Anteromedial Parapatellar Approach

This approach has been considered to be the standard utility incision to the anterior aspect of the knee. It can be used to carry out procedures such as medial meniscectomy, synovectomy, removal of loose bodies, patellectomy, and ligamentous reconstruction procedures, as well as total knee arthroplasty (Fig 11–17). The skin incision, which begins 3 to 5 cm above the superior border of the patella, is carried directly distally over the anteromedial surface of the patella and distally just medial to the patellar ligament. The quadriceps expansion is incised in line with the skin incision down to the superomedial aspect of the patella and then distally along the medial border of the patella. A cuff of tissue is left attached to the patella for subsequent repair.

The infrapatellar branch of the saphenous nerve is often cut. The major problem in cutting the nerve is the possibility that a painful neuroma will develop. The area of anesthesia produced is usually not troublesome, and the nerve should not be repaired if it is cut. Instead the cut ends of the nerve should be buried in the fat. A medial parapatellar capsular incision completes the deep dissection.

The incision can be extended superiorly in the intermuscular plane between the vastus medialis and rectus femoris. This is not an internervous plane because both muscles are supplied by the femoral nerve, but the nerve supply comes in well above the area of dissection. The exposure is completed by cutting through the joint capsule and along the patellar ligament distally and the quadriceps tendon proximally, in line with the original skin incision. The incision can be further extended distally and, if necessary, the pes anserinus as well as the insertion of the superficial medial collateral ligament can be lifted off the tibia with an elevator at the subperiosteal level. Eversion of the patella and flexion of the knee allows wide exposure to the total surface of the knee joint.

Straight Anterior Midline Approach

Insall has recommended modifying the anteromedial parapatellar approach, because it requires division of both the vastus medialis insertion on the patella and the medial retinaculum. He compares this to approaches to the hip that divide, and thus weaken, the abductor musculature. He also states

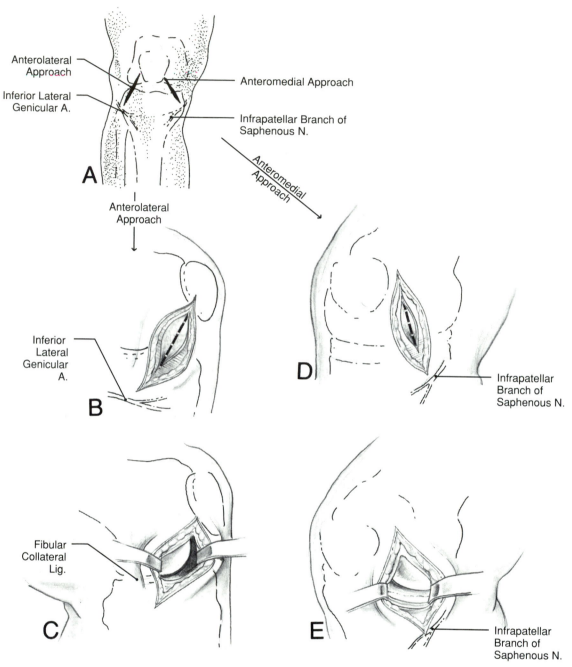

FIG 11–16.
Limited anteromedial and anterolateral approaches. **A,** skin incisions: note location of the infrapatellar branch of the saphenous nerve in relation to the anteromedial approach and the inferior lateral genicular artery in relation to the anterolateral approach. **B,** capsule and synovial incision for anterolateral approach. **C,** joint exposure. Note fibular collateral ligament. **D,** capsule and synovial incision for anteromedial approach. **E,** joint exposure.

that repair of the quadriceps muscle and medial retinaculum is never as sound as before surgery unless the knee is immobilized for a prolonged period. Instead of the anteromedial approach he advocates a straight anterior midline approach through the quadriceps mechanism, with dissection of the medial portion of the expansion directly off the patella.

A 10 to 12 cm midline skin incision is made directly over the anterior aspect of the knee (Fig 11–18). The subcutaneous tissue and fascia of the thigh are opened in line with the skin incision, and the extensor mechanism is exposed. A longitudinal incision is made through the quadriceps tendon and continued distally to the patella. The incision is ex-

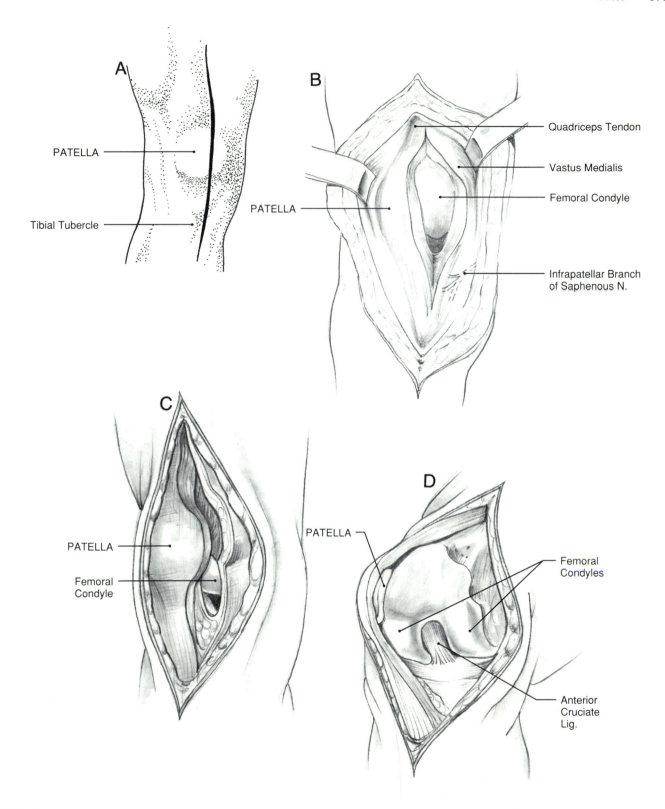

FIG 11–17.
Anteromedial parapatellar approach to the knee. **A,** skin incision. **B,** incision through vastus medialis and capsule. Note infrapatellar branch of saphenous nerve. **C,** proximal and distal extension of deep incision. **D,** eversion and dislocation of the patella allows wide exposure to the joint.

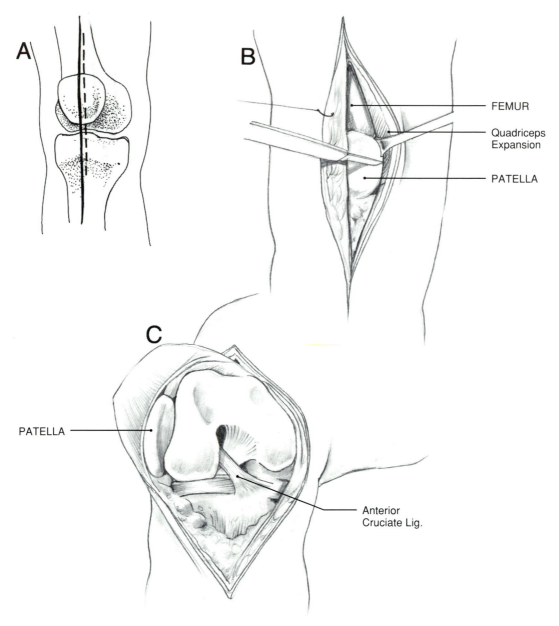

FIG 11–18.
Straight anterior midline approach. **A,** skin incision *(solid line);* deep incision *(dashed line).* **B,** incision of quadriceps tendon extended distally over the medial third of the patella and through the anterior capsule onto the subcutaneous surface of the tibia. The quadriceps expansion is peeled off the patella by sharp dissection. **C,** eversion and dislocation of the patella allows exposure to the joint.   *(Continued.)*

tended over the anterior surface of the medial third of the patella, through the anterior capsule, and onto the subcutaneous surface of the tibia. By sharp dissection the quadriceps expansion with attached vastus medialis is lifted from the anterior surface of the patella until the medial border of the patella is visualized. The joint is entered by incision of the joint capsule and synovium and splitting of the fat pad. The patella is everted and, as the knee is flexed, dislocated laterally.

For wider exposure, which may be required in cases such as total knee arthroplasty, the incision is carried distally several centimeters through the periosteum of the tibia. Maintaining the incision at least 1 cm medial to the tibial tubercle will allow for elevation of a cuff of thick periosteum from the anterior surface of the tibia along with a portion of the pes anserinus, and if necessary, a portion of the medial tibial attachment of the patellar ligament.

Closure is obtained by approximating the di-

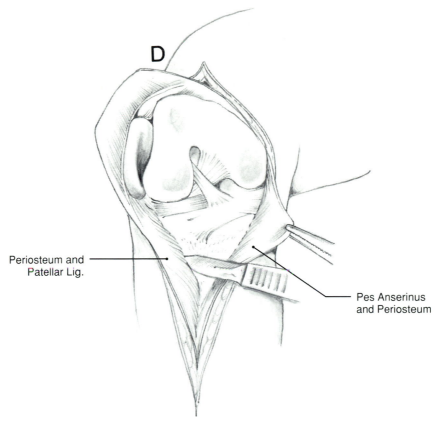

Periosteum and
Patellar Lig.

Pes Anserinus
and Periosteum

FIG 11–18 (cont.).
D, elevation of the pes anserinus and a small portion of the medial patellar ligament insertion. (Modified from Insall J: A midline approach to the knee. *J Bone Joint Surg* 1971; 53A:1584–1586).

vided quadriceps tendon and expansion side to side. Advantages of the straight midline approach are that it leaves a portion of the quadriceps expansion crossing the patella intact and that the closure is inherently stable, allowing early rehabilitation. The stability of this repair can be demonstrated on the operating table by flexing and extending the knee following closure of the quadriceps expansion and noting there is no tendency for the repair to separate.

Another advantage is that if avulsion of the patellar ligament insertion occurs, the ligament remains in continuity with the periosteum of the tibia, which anchors it to the tibia. This enhances the probability of success in reattachment.

The infrapatellar branch of the saphenous nerve may be cut during this approach. If so, the cut ends should be buried in fat.

Inverted V Approach

To deal with ankylosed knees and/or difficulty in achieving exposure, or cases in which contraction of the quadriceps imposes excessive tension on the patellar ligament insertion at the tibia, Coonse and Ad-

ams have described a procedure in which an inverted Y or V incision is made directly into the quadriceps tendon (Fig 11–19). The quadriceps incision is extended distally around the sides of the patella and patellar ligament to the level of the proximal tibia. The patella and patellar tendon are then reflected distally to expose the knee. This technic allows exposure of a knee with a contracted quadriceps expansion and prevents avulsion of the patellar ligament attachment to the tibia. However, it requires ligation of genicular arteries and may consequently compromise the blood supply to the patella.

Patellar Turndown Approach

To avoid avascular necrosis of the patella, Insall has modified the Coonse and Adams procedure for dealing with tight knees by developing a so-called patellar turndown approach (Fig 11–20). In the patellar turndown approach the skin is divided with a straight midline incision. The quadriceps incision crosses the medial third of the patella, and the expansion is dissected off the patella as described for the straight midline approach. A second incision in

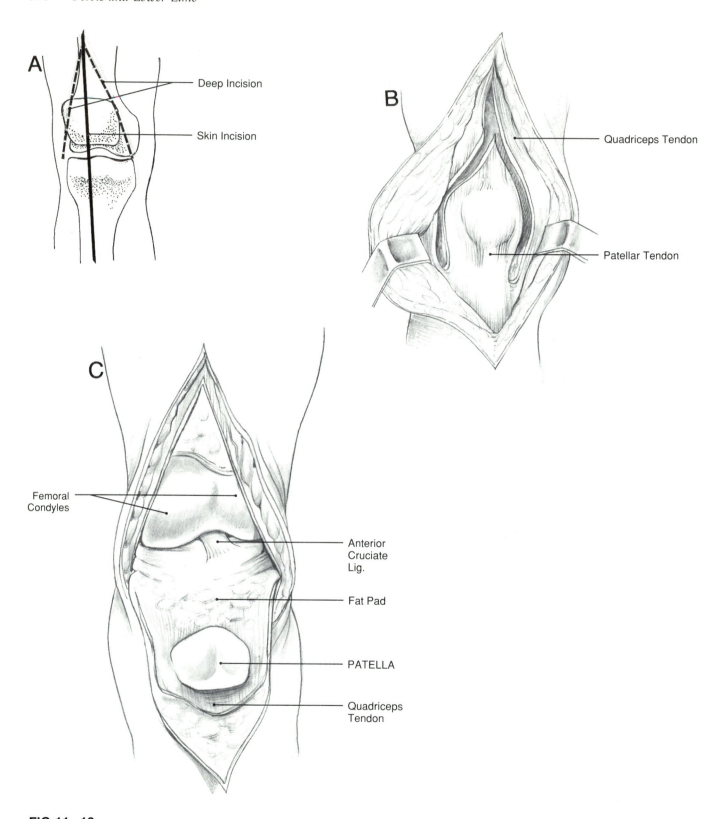

FIG 11–19.
Inverted V approach. **A,** skin incision *(solid line);* deep incision *(dashed line).* **B,** completed quadriceps incision. **C,** turndown of patella with portion of the quadriceps tendon. (Modified from Coonse K, Adams JD: A new operative approach to the knee joint. *Surg Gynecol Obstet* 1943; 77:344–347).

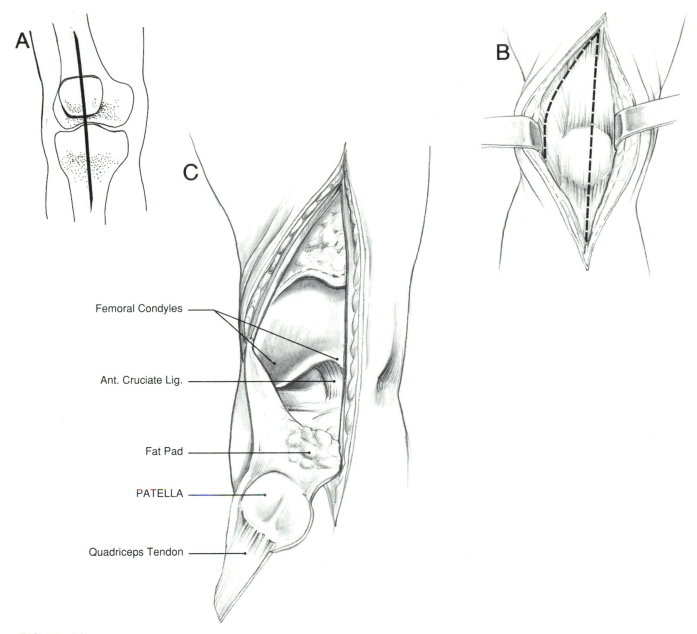

FIG 11–20.
Patellar turndown approach to the knee. **A,** skin incision. **B,** quadriceps incision. **C,** patellar turndown allows joint exposure. (Drawn after Insall JN: *Surgery of the Knee.* New York, Churchill Livingstone, Inc, 1984.)

the quadriceps tendon is begun at the proximal point of the midline incision and directed 45 degrees distally and laterally through the vastus lateralis and the upper portion of the iliotibial tract. This oblique incision ends proximal to the inferior lateral genicular artery and thus preserves its vascular supply to the patella. Another advantage of this approach over that of Coonse and Adams is that it does not transect the vastus medialis.

The midline incision is closed, but if excessive wound tension or patellar tracking problems are

present, the oblique limb of the quadriceps expansion may be left partially closed or open. This approach is increasingly employed in revision total knee arthroplasties. If this technic is utilized, knee flexion should be delayed for 2 weeks.

Utilitarian Anterolateral Approach to the Distal Femur, Knee Joint, and Proximal Tibia

An anterolateral approach to the knee joint can be extended proximally and distally to carry out almost any operation about the knee. This approach can be used to deal with any combination of femoral condyle, patella, and tibial plateau fractures, as well as anterior cruciate reconstruction, knee arthrodesis, and total knee arthroplasty. The approach avoids the infrapatellar branch of the saphenous nerve and preserves the vascularity of the skin flaps. Combined with osteotomy of the tibial tubercle and elevation of the menisci off the tibial plateau, the approach affords wide exposure to the entire anterior aspect of the knee joint, distal femur, and proximal tibia.

The approach is carried out under tourniquet control with the patient supine and the knee flexed to 60 degrees. A straight incision is begun approximately 1 cm lateral to the patella and extended proximally 10 cm and distally 15 cm (Fig 11–21). In the distal portion of the wound, the incision runs 2 cm lateral to the tibial tubercle. The lateral flap is developed subcutaneously as far as the anterior edge of the iliotibial band and the medial flap as far as the anterior edge of the medial collateral ligament. The iliotibial band is lifted off Gerdy's tubercle, or the tubercle itself can be elevated with an osteotome. Medially, the insertion of the pes anserinus is lifted off the tibia subperiosteally. A trapezoidal block of bone that includes the tibial tuberosity and measures approximately 5 cm in length, with a proximal width of 2 cm and a distal width of 1.5 cm, is cut with an osteotome. Before the bone block is raised, three equidistant screw holes are drilled. The bone block with the attached extensor mechanism is then raised and retracted proximally. Restrictive synovial attachments to the infrapatellar fat pad are incised. If the menisci obscure exposure to the tibial plateau, they may be raised after their anterior horns are incised and their capsular attachments judiciously released peripherally as far as required.

After the procedure, the menisci are carefully repaired (unless sacrificed as in total knee arthroplasty or arthrodesis). The tibial tubercle is secured with three screws, with care taken that secure purchase is obtained in the posterior tibial cortex. The iliotibial band and pes anserinus are carefully reattached to bone with interrupted sutures. The tourniquet is released prior to wound closure to assess for and deal with bleeding. Both intraarticular and extraarticular suction drainage are recommended.

Medial Approach

The medial approach to the knee is used for exploration and treatment of damage to the superficial medial collateral ligament and medial joint capsule, as well as for medial meniscectomy and complex ligamentous repairs (Fig 11–22). The patient is positioned supine on the operating table and the knee flexed approximately 60 degrees. The hip is abducted and externally rotated so that the foot of the operative leg rests on the opposite shin. A slightly curved incision is made, centered 3 cm medial to the patella border. The incision is extended proximally to the adductor tubercle and distally approximately 6 cm below the joint line. The flaps formed are raised enough to expose the knee from the midline anteriorly to the posteromedial corner. The saphenous nerve exits between the gracilis and sartorius and runs distally with the long saphenous vein. Both of these structures should be protected. The infrapatellar branch of the saphenous nerve is transected, and the cut ends are buried in the fat.

To expose the deep structures within the knee, incisions can be made anterior and posterior to the superficial medial collateral ligament. The anterior incision is utilized to expose the superficial medial ligament, the anterior portion of the medial meniscus, and the anterior cruciate ligament. An incision is made along the anterior border of the sartorius, beginning approximately 5 cm above the joint line and continuing to the muscle's attachment on the tibia. With flexion of the knee and posterior retraction of the components of the pes anserinus, the tibial insertion of the superficial medial ligament is identified.

At this point, if it is necessary to look at the most anterior aspect of the medial side of the knee joint, an accessory anterior incision can be made through the joint capsule in the medial parapatellar region. Wider posterior exposure can be obtained by separating the medial head of the gastrocnemius from the semimembranosus and the posterior capsule of the knee. This allows full exposure to the posteromedial corner of the capsule for inspection and repair.

In the proximal aspect of this deep posterior dissection, the popliteal artery is encountered where it lies on the posterior joint capsule, juxtaposed to the medial head of the gastrocnemius. If the medial head of the gastrocnemius is to be transected, the popliteal artery must be identified and protected. The posterior aspect of the joint can be inspected through a second arthrotomy placed just posterior to the superficial collateral ligament. In the distal portion of this wound, the medial inferior genicular artery may be at risk.

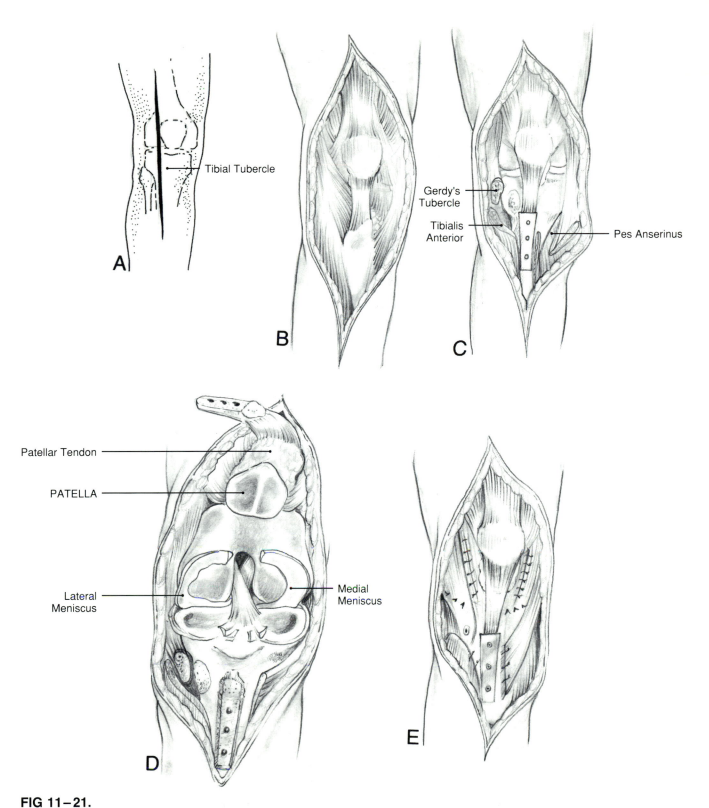

FIG 11–21.
Utilitarian anterolateral approach to the distal femur, knee joint, and proximal tibia. **A,** skin incision. **B,** development of subcutaneous flaps. **C,** screw holes placed in tibia and trapezoidal bone block outlined. Elevation of Gerdy's tubercle, anterior tibialis, and pes anserinus. **D,** proximal retraction of patella, patellar tendon, and bone block. Elevation of menisci from tibial plateaus. **E,** reattachment of menisci. Fixation of tibial bone block. Reattachment of Gerdy's tubercle and pes anserinus. (Drawn after Fernandez DL: Anterior approach to the knee with osteotomy of the tibial tubercle for bicondylar tibial fractures. *J Bone Joint Surg* 1988; 70A:208–219).

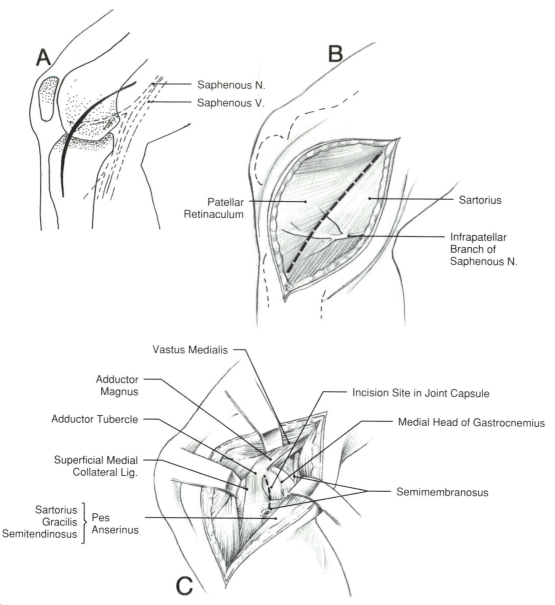

FIG 11–22.
Medial approach to the knee and supporting structures. **A,** skin incision. **B,** fascial incision along the anterior border of the sartorius. **C,** exposure of superficial medial collateral ligament, joint capsule, and medial head of gastrocnemius. Retraction of pes anserinus. *Dashed line:* location site for posterior joint capsule incision.　*(Continued.)*

Lateral Approach

The supporting structures on the lateral side of the knee, as well as the intraarticular structures, can be exposed by a lateral approach (Fig 11–23). The patient is placed supine on the operating table with a buttress under the affected side and the knee flexed to 90 degrees. A long, slightly curved incision is begun 3 cm lateral to the midpatella. The incision is extended 5 to 7 cm in a proximal direction, parallel with the distal femur, and distally over Gerdy's tu-

bercle, approximately 5 cm distal to the joint line. The skin flaps are mobilized and the fascia is incised in the interval between the iliotibial band and biceps femoris to avoid the common peroneal nerve, which is located at the posterior border of the biceps tendon. This is an internervous plane. The fibular collateral ligament is exposed by retraction of the iliotibial band anteriorly and the biceps femoris posteriorly.

The knee joint can be entered by incision of the capsule either in front of or behind the lateral collat-

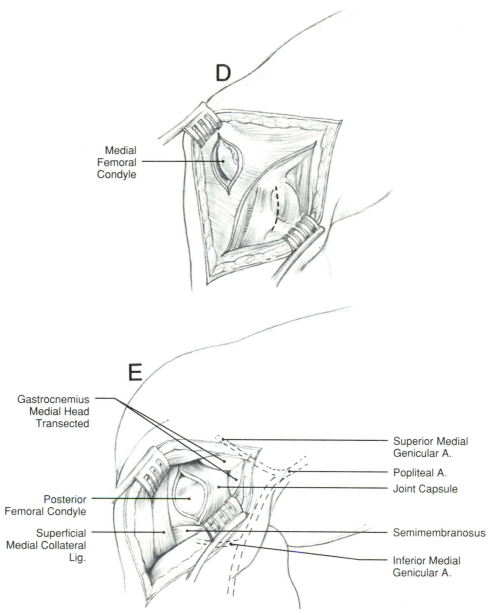

FIG 11–22 (cont.).
D, optional accessory incision in anteromedial joint capsule. **E,** transection of medial head of gastrocnemius and capsulotomy allows exposure to posteromedial corner of knee.

eral (fibular) ligament. If necessary to visualize the very anterior aspect of the lateral compartment of the knee, an incision is made in the lateral patellar retinaculum. To gain access to the posterior lateral aspect of the knee joint, a posterior arthrotomy is required. The arthrotomy site is found by dissection between the lateral head of the gastrocnemius at its origin on the posterior surface of the lateral femoral condyle and the posterolateral corner of the joint capsule. Care must be taken to identify the lateral superior and inferior genicular vessels, which will be

encountered in this region. They must be protected or ligated and divided. The posterior arthrotomy is made by a longitudinal incision in the capsule. It is best to start the capsular incision above the joint line and work distally to prevent injury to the popliteus tendon and/or lateral meniscus.

Posterior Approach

Access to the popliteal surface of the femur, the posterior capsule, and, when extended distally, the

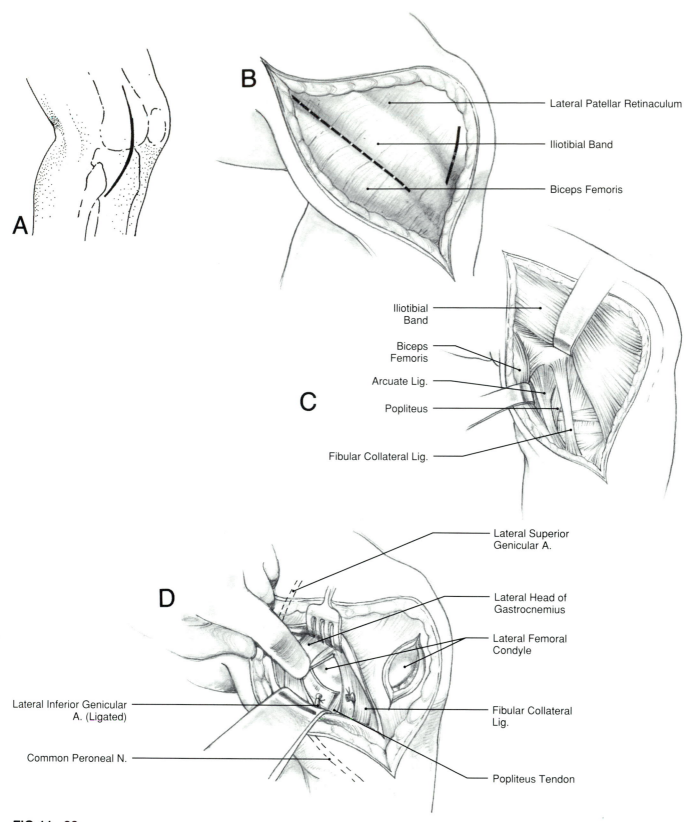

FIG 11–23.
Lateral approach to the knee and its supporting structures. **A,** skin incision. **B,** fascial incision in the interval between the iliotibial band and biceps femoris *(dashed line).* Another incision *(solid line)* can be made in the anterior capsule to expose the anterolateral aspect of the joint. **C,** retraction of the iliotibial band and biceps femoris reveals structures in the posterolateral aspect of the knee. **D,** a posterior arthrotomy is made by a longitudinal incision in the posterior capsule, allowing exposure to the posterior half of the lateral compartment of the knee. Note ligation and transection of lateral inferior genicular artery.

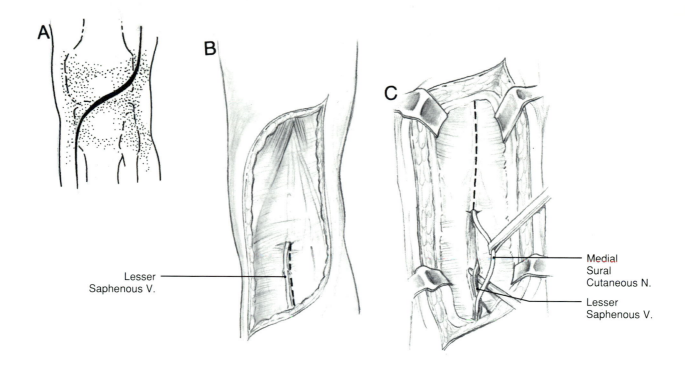

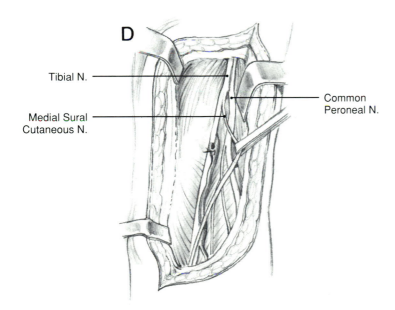

FIG 11–24.
Posterior approach to the knee and supporting structures. **A,** skin incision. **B,** identification of lesser saphenous vein and fascial incision to expose medial sural cutaneous nerve. **C,** extension of fascial incision, retraction of saphenous vein, and mobilization of medial sural cutaneous nerve. **D,** tracing medial sural cutaneous nerve to its origin from the tibial nerve in the popliteal fossa. *(Continued.)*

posterior aspect of the tibia, can be accomplished through this approach (Fig 11–24). It is most commonly used to provide access for repair of injury to the neurovascular structures behind the knee. It can also provide exposure for repair of avulsion fractures at the posterior cruciate ligament attachment to the tibia, release of gastrocnemius muscle origins in case of knee contractures, excision of popliteal cysts, and lengthening of hamstring tendons.

The approach is made with the patient lying prone on the operating table. Several skin incisions have been used. The most popular is a slightly curved incision, which is begun laterally over the biceps femoris, brought obliquely across the popliteal fossa, and extended downward into the medial calf. Alternatively the incision can begin on the medial side along the semitendinosus, curve across the back of the knee, and extend distally along the lateral calf. Following the incision, skin flaps are developed and the lesser saphenous vein, which lies superficial to the deep fascia of the calf, is identified. The fascia is incised just lateral to the vein. The medial sural cutaneous nerve is identified below the fascia and traced proximally to its source, the tibial nerve. The

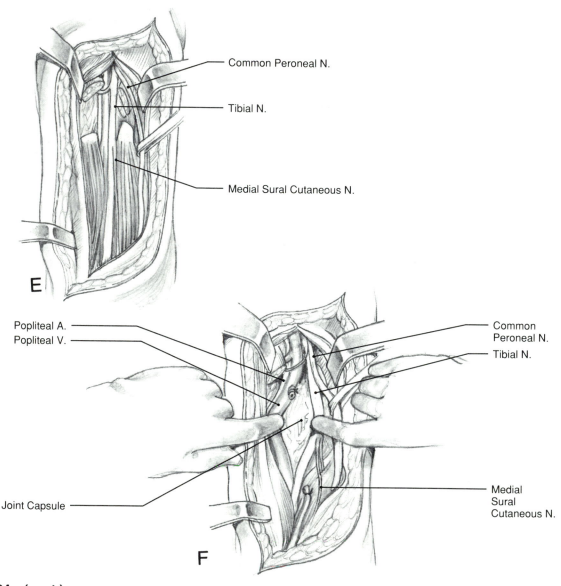

FIG 11–24   (cont.).
E, retraction of common peroneal nerve and resection of gastrocnemius heads and plantaris for wide exposure. **F,** wider exposure to the posterior aspect of the knee joint is facilitated by ligation of muscular branches of the tibial vessels. Retraction of vessels medially and nerves laterally.

tibial nerve lies between the twin heads of the gastrocnemius, and separation of the two heads allows identification of the muscular branches of the tibial nerve. In the popliteal fossa the popliteal vessels lie directly beneath the tibial nerve. Above the fossa the vessels are medial to the nerve and below the fossa they lie lateral to the nerve. If necessary, one or more of the genicular vessels can be ligated to increase exposure. Resecting and retracting the medial head of the gastrocnemius and plantaris origin and retracting the popliteal vessels and nerves will expose the posteromedial compartment. Elevation of the lateral head of the gastrocnemius will expose the posterolateral aspect of the knee. The central portion of the posterior knee capsule is most easily exposed by retraction of the vessels medially and the tibial nerve laterally. With this technic, only the nerve to the medial head of the gastrocnemius crosses the field.

If exposure below the knee joint is necessary, it can be carried out by transection of the popliteus and incision along its medial border in the direction of its vertical fibers, which pass distally from the semimembranosus expansion.

The structures that are vulnerable during this approach are the medial sural cutaneous nerve and the lesser saphenous vein, which serve as landmarks for entry to the popliteal space. The tibial nerve, common peroneal nerve, and popliteal vessels are also at risk and must be protected during this approach. Branches of the popliteal vessels may be judiciously ligated if necessary for wide exposure to the central portion of the posterior aspect of the knee joint.

ARTHROSCOPIC PORTAL ANATOMY

Diagnostic and operative arthroscopy have become major tools for dealing with problems of the knee. Although not a substitute for a thorough history, physical examination, and noninvasive studies (radiographs and magnetic resonance imaging), diagnostic arthroscopy has become the "gold standard" for complete diagnosis of intraarticular knee problems. Surgical arthroscopy is the treatment of choice for most intraarticular knee problems. The reader should consult other sources for descriptions of the intraarticular anatomy of the knee as viewed through the arthroscope. Discussion here is limited to arthroscopic portal anatomy with emphasis on an-

atomic structures at risk when diagnostic and/or surgical arthroscopy are carried out. Although many operative techniques exist, the portals of entry remain standard. In-depth knowledge of the three dimensional anatomy is necessary to carry out arthroscopy safely and efficaciously. This anatomical understanding is achieved by palpation of certain landmarks and correlation into a three-dimensional scheme.

Palpable Landmarks

The patella is the first landmark (Fig 11–25). Its superior border and quadriceps tendon attachment determine the sites of penetration for the two superior portals, its maximum width determines the lateral and medial midpatellar (Patel) portals, and its inferior pole determines the sites for the anterior infrapatellar portals and for location of the joint line. The patellar tendon (ligament) provides the second important landmark for determining the sites of routine anterior portals. Additional landmarks include the medial and lateral joint lines, medial and lateral collateral ligaments, fibular head, iliotibial band, medial hamstrings, and biceps femoris. Failure to appropriately identify these structures and correlate their three-dimensional relationships can result in injury to the articular surfaces, menisci, anterior and posterior cruciate ligaments, genicular vessels, popliteal artery, or peroneal and saphenous nerves. These complications will be discussed as they pertain to each portal or incision.

Portal Placement

Most arthroscopic surgery can be performed through three portals. One portal, usually suprapatellar, is used for fluid ingress-egress (depending on whether the arthroscope is used for ingress or egress), one portal for the arthroscope, and a third portal for surgical instruments. Occasionally, a fourth portal is required to complete a surgical procedure. Also, if meniscal repair is performed arthroscopically, an accessory posteromedial or posterolateral operative incision is mandatory. As discussed earlier in this chapter, longitudinal incisions are used. They are more easily incorporated into other incisions, are more accommodating to adjustment if not precisely placed initially, and heal in the lines of tension on the anterior surface of the knee. The knee should be distended with fluid before incisions are made to minimize the risk of inadvertent laceration of intraarticular structures.

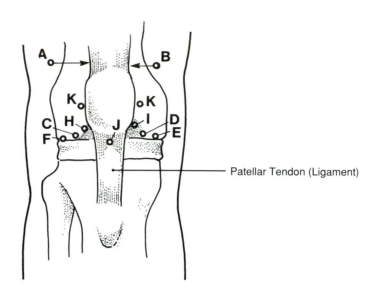

ANTERIOR

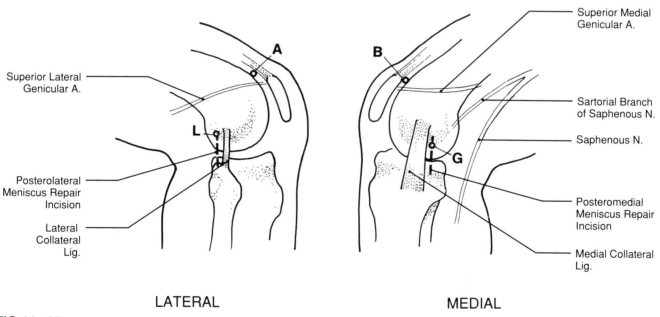

LATERAL   MEDIAL

FIG 11–25.
Arthroscopic portal sites, related anatomy, and accessory incisions for meniscal repair. *A* = lateral suprapatellar portal; *B* = medial suprapatellar portal; *C* = standard lateral infrapatellar portal; *D* = standard medial infrapatellar portal; *E* = accessory anteromedial portal; *F* = accessory anterolateral portal; *G* = posteromedial portal (seen on medial view); *H* = lateral paracentral portal; *I* = medial paracentral portal; *J* = central portal; *K* = midpatellar (Patel) portals; *L* = posterolateral portal.

Standard Portals

Lateral Suprapatellar Portal (Authors' Preference)

Placed 1 cm superior to the superior pole and 1 cm lateral to the lateral border of the patella, this portal is routinely used as an irrigation portal. It is used for fluid ingress by those who use the arthroscope for outflow, and it is used for fluid egress for those who use the arthroscope for inflow. This placement avoids penetration of the vastus lateralis muscle and potential injury to the superior lateral genicular artery.

Medial Suprapatellar Portal

Placed 1 cm proximal to the superior pole and 1 cm medial to the medial border of the patella, this portal is used by some as an irrigation portal and is often used as a fourth portal for synovectomy. In most patients it penetrates the inferior portion of the vastus medialis and may thus slow postoperative recovery.

Standard Lateral Infrapatellar Portal

Placed 1 cm lateral to the lateral border of the patellar tendon and along a horizontal line drawn at the inferior pole of the patella, this is the standard arthroscope portal. The incision should be made vertically on the distended knee with a No. 11 blade passed distal to proximal. The anterior horn of the lateral meniscus may be lacerated if the blade strays too far distally. Visualization of the posterior horn of the medial meniscus may be limited with this portal.

Standard Medial Infrapatellar Portal

Placed 1 cm medial to the medial border of the patellar tendon at the level of the inferior patellar pole, this is the standard instrumentation portal. As with the lateral portal, laceration of the medial meniscus by too distal placement of the incision should be avoided. This portal can also be used for visualization of blind spots not seen from the lateral portal.

Accessory Portals

Accessory Anteromedial Portal

This is the most common anterior accessory portal. It is positioned a minimum of 1 cm medial to the standard medial portal and as far medial as the anterior edge of the medial collateral ligament at the level of the joint line. To avoid laceration of the medial meniscus, the portal site is determined by preliminary placement of an 18-gauge spinal needle under direct visualization with the arthroscope from the lateral portal. On occasion the central portal (see below) is an alternative to this portal.

Accessory Anterolateral Portal

This portal site also should be determined by preliminary placement of a spinal needle above the lateral meniscus under direct visualization with the medially placed arthroscope. The portal must be at least 1 cm lateral to the standard lateral portal; however, greater than 2 cm makes it difficult to use due to the shape of the lateral condyle.

Posteromedial Portal

Used for visualizing the posterior compartment to retrieve loose bodies and perform synovectomies, this portal site is best determined by drawing the landmarks with a skin scribe. A "soft spot" can be palpated at the posterior border of the medial collateral ligament, where the posterior projection of the lateral femoral condyle and the posterior border of the tibia meet. With the knee fully distended to push the soft spot out and the knee flexed to 90 degrees, a small vertical skin incision is made 1 cm above the joint line. The sheath with sharp trocar inserted is advanced anteriorly and inferiorly to puncture the joint capsule. The sharp trocar is then withdrawn from the sheath and placement verified by the gush of fluid. The blunt trocar is used for further advancement. In the posterior aspect of the knee, plunging with the sharp trocar can result in neurovascular injury, as can careless use of power synovectomy blades.

Optional Portals

Lateral Parapatellar (or Paracentral) Portal
(Authors' Preference)

Placed at the inferior pole of the patella immediately adjacent to the lateral border of the patellar tendon, this is an alternative to the standard lateral infrapatellar portal. Advantages include better visualization of the posterior horn of the medial meniscus and posterior cruciate ligament. The primary disadvantage is the decreased distance to the medial infrapatellar portal. This increases anterior crowding of the instruments and makes triangulation of the instruments slightly more difficult.

Medial Parapatellar (or Paracentral) Portal
(Authors' Preference)

Placed at the inferior pole of the patella immediately adjacent to the medial border of the patellar tendon, this is usually used as the instrument portal when the arthroscope is in the lateral paracentral portal. All areas of the knee can usually be visualized with these two portals by use of both the 30- and 70-degree arthroscopes.

Central (Swedish or Gillquist) Portal

A small vertical skin incision is made 1 cm inferior to the inferior pole of the patella in the midline. The sharp trocar is advanced through the patellar tendon but not through the fat pad. Plunging can result in injury to the anterior cruciate ligament. Moving the sharp trocar proximally and distally within the patellar tendon creates a 1 cm split in the tendon in line with the fibers. The blunt trocar is then inserted and advanced into the intercondylar notch, then replaced with the arthroscope. This portal has the theoretical advantage of no intraarticular blind spots when both 30- and 70-degree arthroscopes are used. It also provides good instrument access to both sides of the knee when it is used as an instrument portal.

Midpatellar Medial and Lateral (Patel) Portals

After a line is drawn transversely across the maximum width of the patella, a 1 cm incision is made parallel to the medial or lateral border of the patella. These portals offer less instrument clutter when meniscal surgery is done anteriorly, but they have larger blind spots posteriorly than the more standard anterior portals.

Posterolateral Portal

Although it provides visualization of the posterolateral compartment, this portal is rarely used since other portals also demonstrate this area well. The borders of the posterior femoral condyle, fibular head, fibular collateral ligament, and biceps femoris are outlined with a skin scribe. A small vertical skin incision is placed 2 cm above the joint line, posterior to the fibular collateral ligament and anterior to the biceps femoris. The sharp trocar is advanced against the distended capsule distally and slightly anteriorly until the puncture is felt and verified by a gush of fluid with removal of the trocar from the sheath. As with the posteromedial portal, posterior plunging can result in neurovascular injury, as can careless use of power synovectomy tools. The sheath is further advanced with the blunt trocar.

Accessory Incisions for Meniscal Repair

Current instrumentation has made arthroscopic meniscus repair a viable alternative to open repair. An accessory incision is required to protect the neurovascular structures and ensure that the sutures are tied directly over the capsule. This avoids unnecessary tissue necrosis and suture loosening. These incisions are made in line with the posteromedial and posterolateral portal incisions.

Posteromedial Incision

Starting 2.5 cm proximal to the joint line and posterior to the medial collateral ligament, a 5 cm vertical incision is made. Only skin and subcutaneous tissue are incised, and care is taken to protect the saphenous nerve in the inferior portion of the wound. The knee is now flexed to 90 degrees. A smaller vertical incision is made at the posterior border of the medial femoral condyle, anterior to the gastrocnemius tendon. The gastrocnemius tendon is reflected posteriorly, and the posterior joint capsule is exposed with a right-angle retractor.

Posterolateral Incision

With the knee flexed 90 degrees and starting 3 cm proximal to the joint line, a 5 cm skin incision is made posterior to and parallel with the lateral collateral ligament. The posterior border of the iliotibial band is vertically incised anterior to the biceps femoris tendon and the gastrocnemius reflected posteriorly to expose the posterior capsule. The peroneal nerve is protected by retraction with the biceps femoris posteriorly. The popliteal artery is protected from puncture by direct observation and retrieval of the posteriorly exiting needles.

BIBLIOGRAPHY

Coonse K, Adams JD: A new operative approach to the knee joint. *Surg Gynecol Obstet* 1943; 77:344–347.

Crenshaw AH: *Campbell's Operative Orthopaedics,* ed 7. St Louis, CV Mosby Co, 1987.

Fernandez DL: Anterior approach to the knee with osteotomy of the tibial tubercle for bicondylar tibial fractures. *J Bone Joint Surg* 1988; 70A:208–219.

Grant JCB: *Grant's Atlas of Anatomy,* ed 5. Baltimore, Williams & Wilkins Co, 1962.

Gray H: *Anatomy of the Human Body,* ed 30. Philadelphia, Lea & Febiger, 1973.

Guyot J: *Atlas of Human Limb Joints.* New York, Springer-Verlag, New York, 1981.

Highgenboten CL: Arthroscopic synovectomy. *Orthop Clin North Am* 1981; 13:399–405.

Hollinshead WH: *The Back and Limbs,* Philadelphia, Harper & Row, 1982.

Hoppenfeld S, deBoer P: *Surgical Exposures in Orthopaedics: The Anatomic Approach.* Philadelphia, JB Lippincott Co, 1984.

Insall J: A midline approach to the knee. *J Bone Joint Surg* 1971; 53A:1584–1586.

Insall JN: *Surgery of the Knee.* New York, Churchill Livingstone, Inc, 1984.

Jakob RP: The arthroscopic meniscal repair: Techniques and clinical experience. *Am J Sports Med* 1988; 16B:137–142.

Johnson LL: *Diagnostic and Surgical Arthroscopy: The Knee and Other Joints,* ed 2. St Louis, CV Mosby Co, 1981.

Kaplan EB: The fabellofibular and short lateral ligaments of the knee joint. *J Bone Joint Surg* 1961; 43A:169–179.

Lindenfeld TN: Arthroscopically aided meniscal repair. *Am J Knee Surg* 1988; 1A:146–149.

Metcalf RW, Rosenberg TD: *Arthroscopic Surgery of the Knee.* Salt Lake City, Arthroscopic Surgery, 1984.

Moore KL: *Clinically Oriented Anatomy*, ed 2. Baltimore, Williams & Wilkins Co, 1985.

Muller W: *The Knee: Form, Function, and Ligament Reconstruction.* New York, Springer-Verlag New York, 1983.

Netter FH: *The Ciba Collection of Medical Illustrations: Musculoskeletal System*, vol 8. Summit, NJ, Ciba-Geigy Corp, 1987.

Nicholas JA, Hershman EB: *The Lower Extremity and Spine in Sports Medicine.* St Louis, CV Mosby Co, 1986.

Patel D: Superior lateral-medial approach to arthroscopic meniscectomy. *Orthop Clin North Am* 1982; 13:299–305.

Scapinelli R: Blood supply of the human patella: Its rela-tion to ischaemic necrosis after fracture. *J Bone Joint Surg* 1967; 49B:563–570.

Seebacher JR, Inglis AE, Marshall JL, Warren RF: The structure of the posterolateral aspect of the knee. *J Bone Joint Surg* 1982; 64A:536–541.

Warren LF, Marshall JL, Girgis F: The prime static stabilizer of the medial side of the knee. *J Bone Joint Surg* 1974; 56A:665–674.

Warren LF, Marshall JL: The supporting structures and layers on the medial side of the knee: An anatomical analysis. *J Bone Joint Surg* 1979; 61A:56–62.

12

Leg

Frederick W. Reckling, M.D.
Melvin P. Mohn, Ph.D.

ANATOMIC FEATURES OF THE LEG

The leg transmits forces from the foot and ankle to the knee and, in addition, provides attachment for muscles that stabilize the knee and move the foot and ankle.

Bony Anatomy

The bones of the leg are the tibia and fibula. The tibia is much larger than the fibula and transmits most of the stress of walking. It is a long bone with expanded extremities, especially above the point at which it widens to receive the condyles of the femur (Fig 12–1). The proximal articular surface of the tibia is divided into medial and lateral condyles. The superior articular surface has two facets. The medial facet is oval and slightly concave; the lateral facet is nearly round and is concave from side to side but convex from front to back. The central parts of these facets receive the condyles of the femur. The rims give attachment to the menisci of the knee joint. Between the two articular facets is an intercondylar eminence, which contains a medial and a lateral intercondylar tubercle (see Knee chapter).

Anteriorly, the proximal portion of the tibia has a tuberosity for insertion of the patellar ligament. Lateral to this area is another prominence known as Gerdy's tubercle, where the iliotibial band inserts on the tibia. Posteriorly, on the medial condyle, there is a groove for insertion of the semimembranosus tendon. On the posteroinferior surface of the lateral condyle is a nearly circular facet for articulation with the head of the fibula.

The shaft of the tibia is triangular in cross section with medial, lateral, and posterior surfaces, and anterior, medial, and interosseous borders. The anteromedial surface of the proximal shaft of the tibia is smooth and provides for attachment of the sartorius, gracilis, and semitendinosus muscles (pes anserinus). For the most part the medial surface is subcutaneous. The lateral surface of the tibia provides the origin of the tibialis anterior.

On the proximoposterior aspect of the tibia is a prominence known as the soleal line. This line begins behind the facet for the head of the fibula and runs down obliquely to the medial border of the tibia at the junction of the upper and middle thirds of the shaft. The area proximal to the soleal line gives attachment for the popliteus muscle. The soleal line itself gives origin to the soleus muscle. The very distal portion of the medial surface of the tibia becomes the medial malleolus, which forms a subcutaneous prominence at the ankle joint. The medial malleolus has a groove posteriorly to accommodate the tibialis posterior and flexor digitorum longus tendons. In some instances there is another more lateral groove for the tendon of the flexor hallucis longus muscle. On the lateral surface of the inferior aspect of the tibia is a triangular notch to accommodate the distal fibula. The borders of the notch are quite prominent to allow attachments of the anterior and posterior tibiofibular ligaments.

The cartilaginous surface at the distal end of the tibia articulates with the body of the talus. This sur-

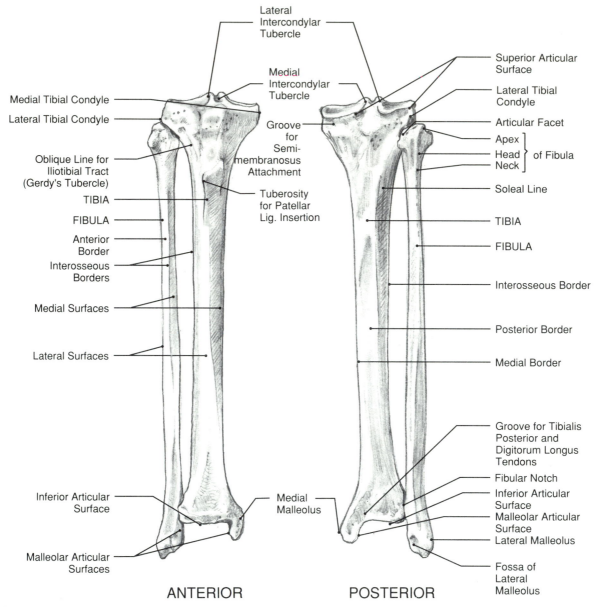

FIG 12-1.
Bones of the leg.

face is wider anteriorly than posteriorly and is concave anteroposteriorly. It is continuous with the malleolar articular surface on the internal aspect of the medial malleolus.

The fibula lies parallel to the tibia. It plays a significant role in ankle stability and provides for some weight bearing. Except at its distal end it is covered by muscles and has extensive muscle attachments. The proximal portion of the fibula is known as the head. It is almost circular and articulates with the undersurface of the lateral condyle of the tibia. The fibular collateral ligament and biceps tendon attach

to the fibular head. The neck of the fibula is that area just distal to the head. It is here that the common peroneal nerve passes around the lateral side of the fibula and here that the nerve is vulnerable to injury. The long slender body of the fibula is described as having three borders (interosseous, anterior, and posterior), and three surfaces (medial, lateral, and posterior). The expanded lower end of the fibula, the so-called lateral malleolus, is subcutaneous and extends distally approximately 1.5 cm beyond the tip of the medial malleolus. Its medial surface is largely occupied by the malleolar articular surface for the talus. Behind and below this is the roughened malleolar fossa into which the posterior talofibular ligament attaches. There may be a groove on the posterior surface of the lateral malleolus for passage of the peroneus brevis tendon.

Joints and Ligaments

The tibia and fibula are united to each other proximally by the tibiofibular synovial joint and distally by the tibiofibular syndesmosis. The shafts of these bones are connected by the interosseous membrane (Fig 12–2).

The proximal tibiofibular synovial articulation is between the head of the fibula and the posterolateral part of the lower surface of the lateral tibial condyle. At times this cavity communicates with the knee joint proper through the subpopliteal recess. The capsule of this joint is reinforced anteriorly and posteriorly by ligaments that run from the head of the fibula upward and medially to the tibia.

The shafts of the tibia and fibula are connected by a heavy fibrous structure called the interosseous membrane, which separates the anterior and posterior compartments of the leg and gives origin to muscles of both areas. The fibers of this membrane pass from the tibia laterally and inferiorly to the fibula. The upper margin does not reach the tibiofibular articulation. Instead, there is an oval aperture above the upper end of the membrane for passage of the anterior tibial vessels to the front of the leg. Close to the lower end of the interosseous membrane is a smaller aperture for the perforating branch of the peroneal artery. Between the closely adjacent lower ends of the tibia and fibula the membrane becomes much thicker. In this area it is known as the interosseous ligament.

The distal ends of the tibia and fibula are connected by fibrous structures, which are collectively referred to as the tibiofibular syndesmosis (Fig 12–3). Three ligaments are involved in this articulation: the interosseous ligament and anterior and posterior tibiofibular ligaments. The interosseous ligament is continuous with the interosseous mem-

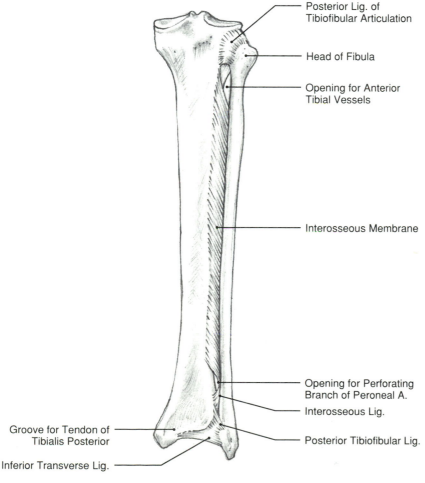

Posterior Lig. of
Tibiofibular Articulation

Head of Fibula

Opening for Anterior
Tibial Vessels

Interosseous Membrane

Opening for Perforating
Branch of Peroneal A.

Interosseous Lig.

Groove for Tendon of
Tibialis Posterior

Posterior Tibiofibular Lig.

Inferior Transverse Lig.

FIG 12–2.
Tibia and fibula and interconnecting ligamentous structures, posterior view.

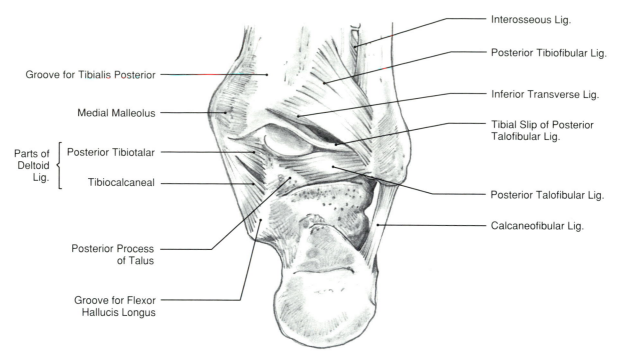

FIG 12-3.
Tibiofibular syndesmosis.

brane above and consists of short, strong fibrous bands uniting the two bones. The anterior and posterior tibiofibular ligaments pass respectively from the borders of the fibular notch of the tibia to the anterior and posterior surfaces of the lateral malleolus of the fibula. Another structure known as the inferior transverse tibiofibular ligament is located deep to the posterior tibiofibular ligament. It arises from the whole inferior border of the tibia posteriorly and attaches to the upper portion of the malleolar fossa of the fibula, actually forming part of the articulating fossa for the talus. There is a recess in the roof of the articular cavity of the ankle joint where the synovial membrane extends upward between the tibia and fibula to the lower end of the interosseous ligament.

Fascia and Fibro-osseous Compartments

The investing layer of the deep fascia of the leg is referred to as the crural fascia. It is a continuation of the fascia lata of the thigh. In the proximal aspect of the leg the crural fascia has numerous attachments (Fig 12-4). These include attachments to the patella, patellar ligament, condyles of the tibia, tibial tuberosity, and head of the fibula, as well as the medial and lateral patellar retinaculum. On the proximomedial aspect of the leg the fascia is reinforced by

the expansions of the sartorius, gracilis, and semitendinosus (pes anserinus). On the proximal lateral aspect of the leg the fascia is reinforced by the insertion of the biceps femoris muscle.

In the midportion of the leg the crural fascia gives origin to superficial muscle fibers and blends with the periosteum of the subcutaneous border of the tibia. Just above the ankle it blends with the periosteum of the lower lateral shaft of the fibula, and distally it attaches to the medial and lateral malleoli and calcaneus.

Deep partitions, or septa, of the crural fascia, together with the surfaces of the tibia and fibula and the interosseous membrane between them, divide the leg into compartments. These contain groups of related muscles and vessels, as well as nerves supplying the muscles (Fig 12-5). Clinically, these arrangements are important in that certain injuries can lead to increased pressure and cause necrosis of the contents of these compartments. The result can be significant morbidity.

The anterior intermuscular septum represents a deep extension of the crural fascia. It runs from the superficial aspect of the leg medially and posteriorly to attach to the anterior border of the fibula. The posterior intermuscular septum arises from the crural fascia and runs anteriorly and medially to attach

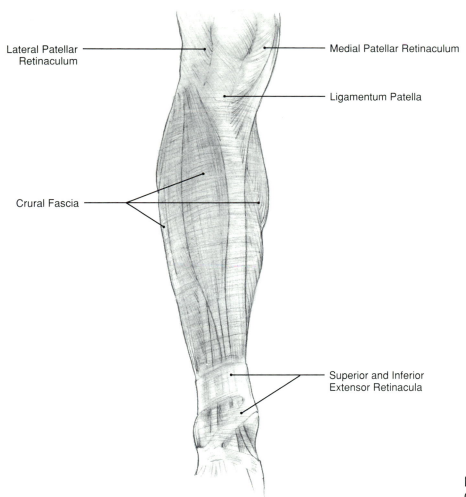

Lateral Patellar Retinaculum

Medial Patellar Retinaculum

Ligamentum Patella

Crural Fascia

Superior and Inferior Extensor Retinacula

FIG 12–4.
Crural fascia and attachments.

to the posterior border of the fibula. This area, bordered by the anterior and posterior intermuscular septa and the fibula, as well as the crural fascia superficially, is known as the lateral compartment.

A compartment bordered by the interosseous membrane posteriorly, the tibia medially, the anterior interosseous membrane laterally, and the crural fascia superficially is referred to as the anterior compartment.

The posterior compartment consists of two separate components, the deep and superficial posterior compartments. The borders of the deep posterior compartment consist of the interosseous membrane, tibia, and fibula anteriorly and the transverse intermuscular septum posteriorly. The transverse intermuscular septum runs from the posterior intermuscular septum adjacent to the fibula, extends medially superficial to the flexor hallucis longus and flexor digitorum longus, and ends on the tibia and the crural fascia just behind the tibia. The superficial poste-

rior compartment of the leg is bounded by the posterior and transverse intermuscular septa anteriorly and the crural fascia medially, posteriorly, and laterally.

Muscles

Anterior Compartment

The tibialis anterior, extensor hallucis longus, extensor digitorum longus, and peroneus tertius muscles occupy the anterior compartment of the leg (Figs 12–5 and 12–6). These muscles are all innervated by the deep peroneal nerve, and their arterial blood supply is from the anterior tibial artery. They function to dorsiflex the foot and extend the toes. In addition, the tibialis anterior inverts the sole of the foot.

The tibialis anterior muscle has an extensive origin from the proximal lateral surface of the tibia. Some fibers arise from the interosseous membrane

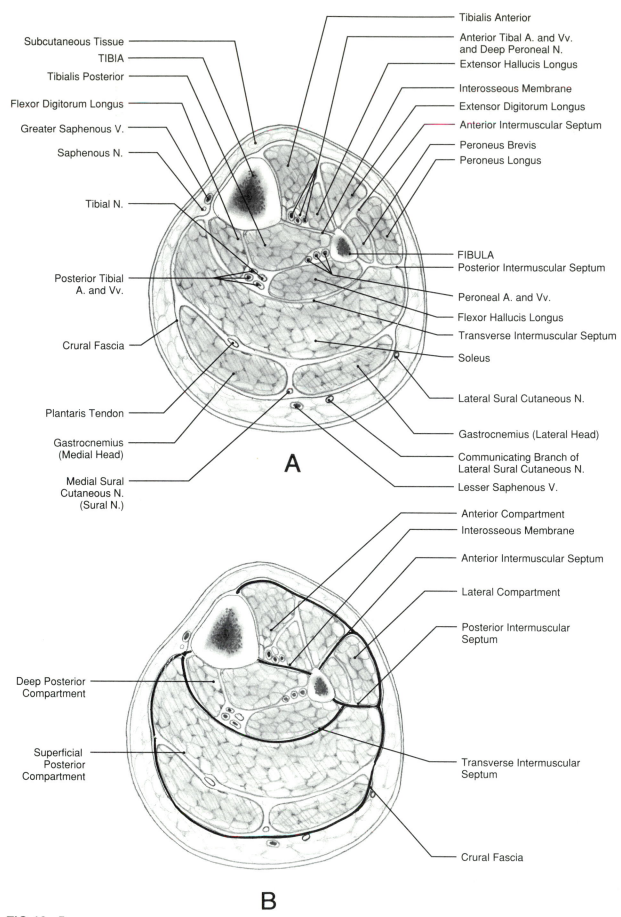

Subcutaneous Tissue

TIBIA

Tibialis Posterior

Flexor Digitorum Longus

Greater Saphenous V.

Saphenous N.

Tibial N.

Posterior Tibial A. and Vv.

Crural Fascia

Plantaris Tendon

Gastrocnemius (Medial Head)

Medial Sural Cutaneous N. (Sural N.)

Tibialis Anterior

Anterior Tibal A. and Vv. and Deep Peroneal N.

Extensor Hallucis Longus

Interosseous Membrane

Extensor Digitorum Longus

Anterior Intermuscular Septum

Peroneus Brevis

Peroneus Longus

FIBULA

Posterior Intermuscular Septum

Peroneal A. and Vv.

Flexor Hallucis Longus

Transverse Intermuscular Septum

Soleus

Lateral Sural Cutaneous N.

Gastrocnemius (Lateral Head)

Communicating Branch of Lateral Sural Cutaneous N.

Lesser Saphenous V.

A

Anterior Compartment

Interosseous Membrane

Anterior Intermuscular Septum

Lateral Compartment

Posterior Intermuscular Septum

Deep Posterior Compartment

Superficial Posterior Compartment

Transverse Intermuscular Septum

Crural Fascia

B

FIG 12–5.
A, cross-section of the midleg. **B,** fibro-osseous compartments at the midleg level.

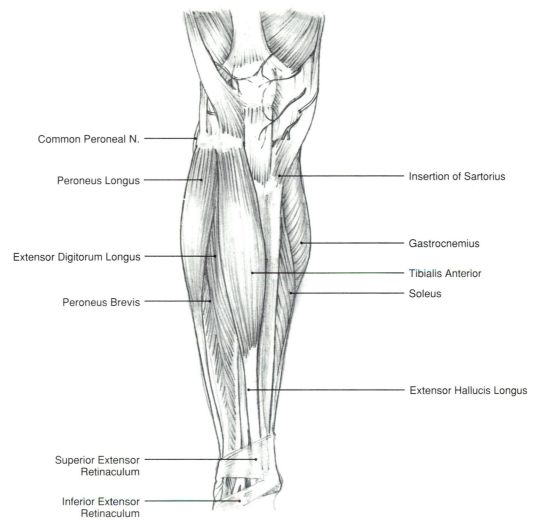

Common Peroneal N.

Peroneus Longus

Extensor Digitorum Longus

Peroneus Brevis

Superior Extensor
Retinaculum

Inferior Extensor
Retinaculum

Insertion of Sartorius

Gastrocnemius

Tibialis Anterior

Soleus

Extensor Hallucis Longus

FIG 12–6.
Muscles of the anterior aspect of the leg. Note the peroneus tertius, which lies deep to the flexor digitorum longus, is not shown.

and the crural fascia as well. The tendon passes under the superior and inferior extensor retinaculum, near the ankle, and inserts on the medial surface of the medial cuneiform and the base of the first metatarsal.

The extensor hallucis longus muscle arises from the middle half of the anterior surface of the fibula and from the interosseous membrane. Its tendon passes under the two extensor retinacula at the ankle and inserts into the base of the distal phalanx of the great toe.

The extensor digitorum longus muscle has an extensive origin from the fibula and lateral condyle of the tibia, with a few fibers arising from the crural fascia. Its tendon begins at about the middle of the leg. Beneath the superior extensor retinaculum the tendon divides into two parts, which pass under the

inferior extensor retinaculum; at this point each tendon divides again, and thus four tendons cross the dorsum of the foot to the lateral four toes.

The peroneus tertius muscle in reality represents a lateral slip of the extensor digitorum longus muscle. It arises from the distal third of the anterior surface of the fibula, descends under the extensor retinacula in the ankle, and inserts on the dorsum of the shaft of the fifth metatarsal.

Lateral Compartment

The lateral compartment contains the peroneus longus and brevis muscles (Figs 12–5 and 12–7). The more superficial peroneus longus muscle arises in the proximal leg from the head and upper two thirds of the lateral surface of the body of the fibula, as well as from the anterior and posterior intermus-

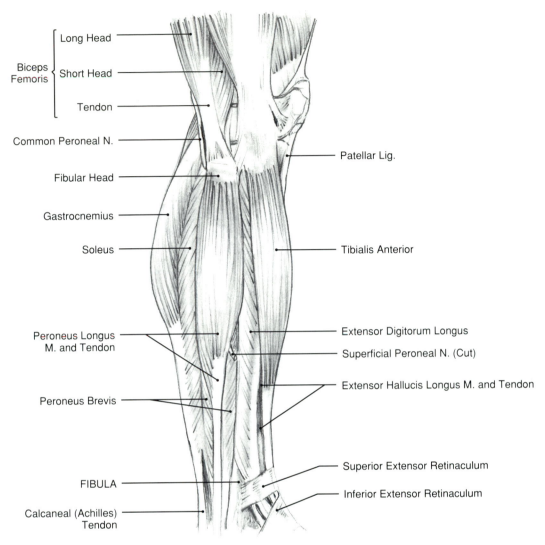

FIG 12–7.
Muscles of the lateral aspect of the leg.

cular septum and the crural fascia. At the ankle the tendon runs behind the lateral malleolus and beneath the superficial peroneal retinaculum in a common sheath with the tendon of the peroneus brevis. It wraps around the cuboid, then crosses the sole of the foot, and inserts on the inferolateral surface of the medial cuneiform and the base of the first metatarsal.

The peroneus brevis muscle lies deep to the peroneus longus, arising from the lateral surface of the shaft of the fibula. Its tendon shares a common sheath with the tendon of the peroneus longus behind the lateral malleolus and deep to the superficial peroneal retinaculum. At this location the peroneus brevis tendon lies anterior to the peroneus longus tendon in the groove on the posterior surface of the

lateral malleolus. The tendon of the peroneus brevis inserts in the foot on the dorsolateral surface of the fifth metatarsal.

The peroneus longus and brevis are innervated by the superficial peroneal nerve. The peroneus longus frequently also receives a branch from the common or deep peroneal nerve. There is no major artery in the lateral compartment. The peroneal muscles receive blood supply from perforating branches of the peroneal artery, which is located in the posterior compartment.

Superficial Posterior Compartment

The muscles of the superficial posterior compartment of the leg are the gastrocnemius, soleus, and plantaris (Figs 12–5 and 12–8). They are innervated

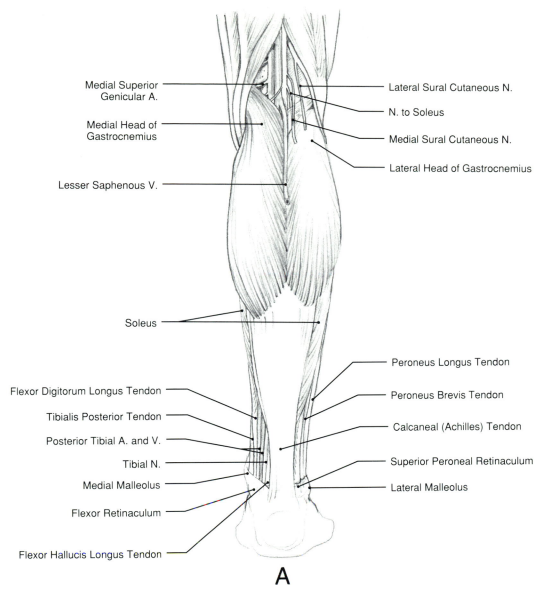

Medial Superior Genicular A.

Medial Head of Gastrocnemius

Lesser Saphenous V.

Soleus

Flexor Digitorum Longus Tendon

Tibialis Posterior Tendon

Posterior Tibial A. and V.

Tibial N.

Medial Malleolus

Flexor Retinaculum

Flexor Hallucis Longus Tendon

Lateral Sural Cutaneous N.

N. to Soleus

Medial Sural Cutaneous N.

Lateral Head of Gastrocnemius

Peroneus Longus Tendon

Peroneus Brevis Tendon

Calcaneal (Achilles) Tendon

Superior Peroneal Retinaculum

Lateral Malleolus

A

FIG 12–8.
A, superficial structures of the posterior aspect of the leg.
(Continued.)

by the tibial nerve. The gastrocnemius arises from two heads from the popliteal surface of the distal femur. The fibers of both heads converge and meet in the middle of the leg. Just distal to this point the gastrocnemius fuses with the tendon of the soleus muscle to form the calcaneal tendon.

The soleus muscle arises entirely below the knee joint from the posterior surface of the fibula, a tendinous arch from the fibula to the tibia, the soleal line of the posterior tibia, and the transverse intermuscular septum. The two heads of the gastrocnemius and the soleus are collectively referred to as the triceps surae. The calcaneal tendon (gastrosoleus tendon) is

approximately 15 cm in length. It inserts on the posterosuperior aspect of the calcaneal tuberosity.

The plantaris is essentially vestigial and arises from the posterolateral aspect of the femur proximal to the lateral head of the gastrocnemius. Its long, slender tendon runs between the gastrocnemius and soleus muscles and usually attaches to the medial border of the superior aspect of the calcaneus.

Deep Posterior Compartment
The muscles in the deep posterior compartment are the popliteus, flexor digitorum longus, tibialis posterior and flexor hallucis longus (Figs 12–5 and

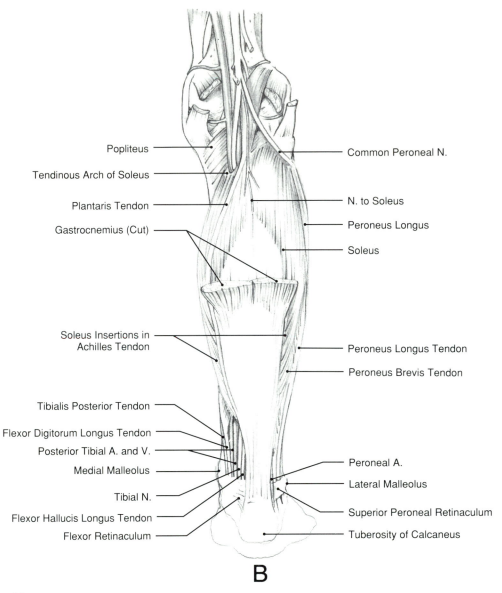

Popliteus

Tendinous Arch of Soleus

Plantaris Tendon

Gastrocnemius (Cut)

Soleus Insertions in
Achilles Tendon

Tibialis Posterior Tendon

Flexor Digitorum Longus Tendon

Posterior Tibial A. and V.

Medial Malleolus

Tibial N.

Flexor Hallucis Longus Tendon

Flexor Retinaculum

Common Peroneal N.

N. to Soleus

Peroneus Longus

Soleus

Peroneus Longus Tendon

Peroneus Brevis Tendon

Peroneal A.

Lateral Malleolus

Superior Peroneal Retinaculum

Tuberosity of Calcaneus

B

FIG 12–8 (cont.).
B, gastrocnemius has been resected to show the soleus muscle and plantaris tendon.

12–9). These muscles are also innervated by the tibial nerve. The popliteus muscle occupies the floor of the lower part of the popliteal fossa. Because the tendinous portion of the muscle is proximal to the distal fleshy part of the muscle, there is some controversy over which end is the origin and which is the insertion. Most anatomists consider that the muscle arises from a stout cord from the anterior end of the groove of the lateral surface of the lateral femoral condyle, quite close to the articular margin. The tendon passes between the lateral meniscus and the capsule of the knee joint. The muscle inserts by fleshy fibers into the triangular area on the back of the tibia. Some fibers of this muscle arise from the

arcuate popliteal ligament (see Knee chapter). In most limbs there are also muscle attachments to the lateral meniscus of the knee joint. There is some question as to the precise function of the popliteus muscle. There is evidence that in early knee flexion it provides for rotation of the femur, thus unlocking the knee; in standing on the flexed knee, the popliteus resists anterior displacement of the femur. Based on cadaver dissections, Tria et al. have challenged the long-held concept that the popliteus tendon retracts, and thus protects, the lateral meniscus.

The flexor digitorum longus muscle arises from the medial side of the posterior surface of the middle three fifths of the tibia and from the intermuscular

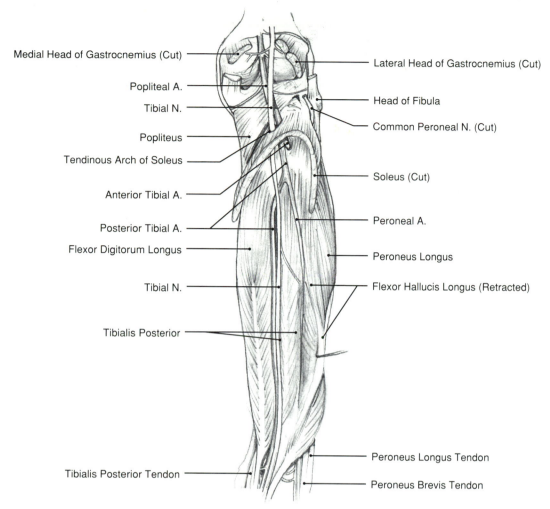

Medial Head of Gastrocnemius (Cut)

Popliteal A.

Tibial N.

Popliteus

Tendinous Arch of Soleus

Anterior Tibial A.

Posterior Tibial A.

Flexor Digitorum Longus

Tibial N.

Tibialis Posterior

Tibialis Posterior Tendon

Lateral Head of Gastrocnemius (Cut)

Head of Fibula

Common Peroneal N. (Cut)

Soleus (Cut)

Peroneal A.

Peroneus Longus

Flexor Hallucis Longus (Retracted)

Peroneus Longus Tendon

Peroneus Brevis Tendon

FIG 12–9.
Gastrocnemius and soleus muscles have been resected to show the relationship of structures in the deep posterior compartment of the leg.

septum. As the tendon of the flexor digitorum longus passes the ankle joint it lies posterior to the tendon of the tibialis posterior. Its relationship to structures in the foot is somewhat complex (see Foot chapter), but it eventually inserts into the distal phalanges of the second, third, fourth, and fifth toes.

The tibialis posterior is the deepest muscle in the posterior compartment. It lies between the flexor digitorum longus and flexor hallucis longus muscles. Its origin is from the interosseous membrane and the posterior surfaces of the tibia and fibula. At the ankle joint its tendon passes just behind the medial malleolus, anterior to the flexor digitorum longus tendon. The tendon inserts into the tuberosity of the navicular and the underside of the medial cuneiform, with expansions to the remaining cuneiforms.

The flexor hallucis longus arises from the lower two thirds of the posterior shaft of the fibula and

from the posterior intermuscular septum. It passes into the foot as a tendon that grooves the posterior aspect of the talus, crosses the sole of the foot, and inserts on the base of the distal phalanx of the great toe.

Arteries

There is considerable variation in the arterial pattern of the leg. For the most part the arterial supply of the leg is provided by the anterior tibial, posterior tibial, and peroneal arteries and their branches (Fig 12–10).

Anterior Tibial Artery and Branches

The anterior tibial artery begins at the bifurcation of the popliteal artery at the distal border of the popliteus muscle. It passes anteriorly between the

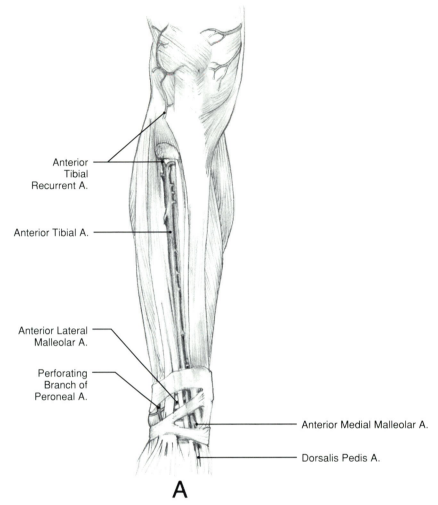

Anterior
Tibial
Recurrent A.

Anterior Tibial A.

Anterior Lateral
Malleolar A.

Perforating
Branch of
Peroneal A.

Anterior Medial Malleolar A.

Dorsalis Pedis A.

A

FIG 12–10.
Arteries of the leg. **A,** anterior tibial artery and branches.
(Continued.)

two heads of the tibialis posterior and through the aperture above the proximal border of the interosseous membrane to reach the anterior compartment of the leg. In the proximal portion of the leg the artery lies close to the medial side of the neck of the fibula. As it descends on the anterior surface of the interosseous membrane it gradually approaches the tibia. In the distal part of the leg it lies on the dorsal surface of the tibia. Distal to the ankle it becomes known as the dorsalis pedis artery.

Although somewhat variable, the most common branches of the anterior tibial artery include the posterior tibial recurrent, anterior tibial recurrent, circumflex fibular, anterior medial malleolar, lateral malleolar, and muscular arteries.

The posterior tibial recurrent artery is an inconstant branch that is given off from the anterior tibial

artery before it passes through the interosseous space. The posterior tibial recurrent artery ascends deep to the popliteus muscle, which it supplies, and then anastomoses with the lateral inferior genicular branch of the popliteal artery, giving a branch to the tibiofibular joint.

The anterior tibial recurrent artery arises from the anterior tibial as soon as it has passed through the interosseous space. The anterior tibial recurrent artery ascends in the tibialis anterior muscle, then ramifies on the front and sides of the knee joint. It assists in the formation of the patellar plexus by anastomosing with the genicular branches of the popliteal and with the descending genicular artery (see Knee chapter).

The fibular circumflex artery usually is a branch of the anterior tibial artery, but in some instances it

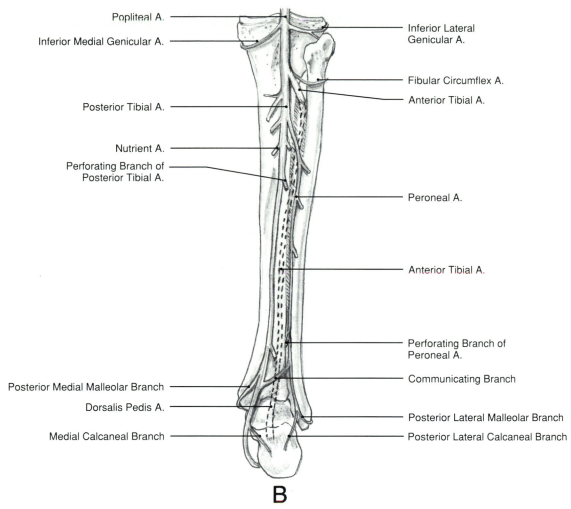

Popliteal A.

Inferior Medial Genicular A.

Posterior Tibial A.

Nutrient A.

Perforating Branch of
Posterior Tibial A.

Posterior Medial Malleolar Branch

Dorsalis Pedis A.

Medial Calcaneal Branch

Inferior Lateral
Genicular A.

Fibular Circumflex A.

Anterior Tibial A.

Peroneal A.

Anterior Tibial A.

Perforating Branch of
Peroneal A.

Communicating Branch

Posterior Lateral Malleolar Branch

Posterior Lateral Calcaneal Branch

B

FIG 12–10   (cont.).
B, posterior tibial and peroneal arteries and branches.
(Continued.)

arises from the posterior tibial or peroneal artery. It arises in the posterior compartment of the leg, passes laterally around the neck of the fibula through the soleus muscle, which it supplies, and ends in the substance of the peroneus longus.

The anterior medial malleolar artery arises about 5 cm proximal to the ankle joint and passes deep to the tendons of the flexor hallucis longus and tibialis anterior to the medial side of the ankle. The anterior lateral malleolar artery passes deep to the tendons of the extensor digitorum longus and peroneus tertius and supplies the lateral side of the ankle, anastomosing with the perforating branch of the peroneal artery and with ascending twigs from the lateral tarsal artery of the foot.

The muscular branches are distributed to the

muscles that lie on either side of the anterior tibial artery as it descends in the leg.

Posterior Tibial Artery and Branches

The posterior tibial artery begins at the distal border of the popliteus muscle opposite the interval between the tibia and fibula. It descends obliquely and then approaches the tibial side of the leg, lying superficial to the tibialis posterior muscle and just posterior to the tibia in the lower part of the leg. At the ankle it is situated midway between the medial malleolus and the medial process of the calcaneal tuberosity.

The branches of the posterior tibial artery include the peroneal artery, a nutrient artery to the tibia, a communicating branch to the peroneal ar-

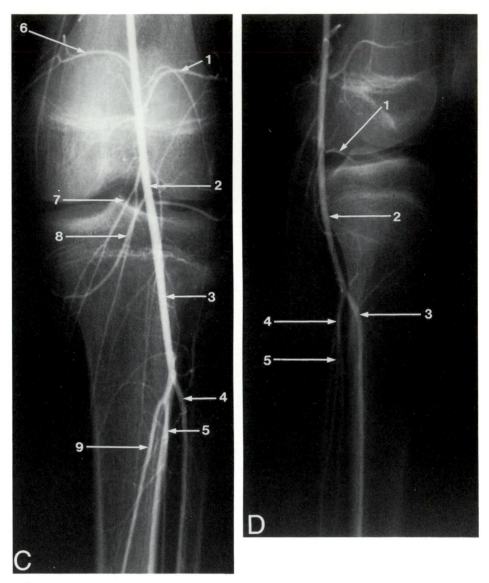

FIG 12–10 (cont.).
C, arteriogram of left leg, frontal view. *1* = lateral superior genicular artery; *2* and *3* = popliteal artery; *4* = anterior tibial artery; *5* = peroneal artery; *6* = medial superior genicular artery; *7* = middle genicular artery; *8* = medial inferior genicular artery; *9* = posterior tibial artery. **D,** arteriogram of left leg, sagittal view. *1* = middle genicular artery; *2* = popliteal artery; *3* = anterior tibial artery; *4* = posterior tibial artery; *5* = peroneal artery.

tery, the posterior medial malleolar branch, a medial calcaneal branch, and branches to the muscles of the posterior compartments. In the foot, the posterior tibial artery divides into the medial and lateral plantar arteries.

Peroneal Artery and Branches

The peroneal artery is the largest branch of the posterior tibial artery. It is located in the posterior compartment of the leg. It supplies the muscles of the lateral side of the leg and is important for collateral circulation via its communicating branch to the

posterior tibial artery and its perforating branch to the anterior tibial artery. It generally arises 2 to 3 cm beyond the origin of the posterior tibial artery and descends near the fibula within the substance of the flexor hallucis longus muscle or between the flexor hallucis longus and tibialis posterior muscles.

A nutrient branch enters the nutrient foramen of the fibula. Muscular branches are provided to the tibialis posterior, flexor hallucis longus, and the peroneus longus and brevis in the lateral compartment of the leg. The perforating branch of the peroneal artery passes forward at the distal border of the interosseous membrane to enter the anterior compartment of the leg. This artery supplies the joints at the ankle and anastomoses with the anterior lateral malleolar branch of the anterior tibial artery and with the lateral tarsal and arcuate branches of the dorsalis pedis artery. The communicating branch arises below the perforating branch, runs medially deep to the tendon of the flexor hallucis longus, and joins the communicating branch of the posterior tibial artery. The posterior lateral malleolar branch gives off twigs to the lateral malleolus and anastomoses with the anterior lateral malleolar branch of the anterior tibial artery.

Veins

The deep veins of the leg generally follow the arteries. They are typically two in number for each artery and take the name of the artery they accompany.

The superficial veins of the leg begin in the foot and form two main channels, the greater (long) saphenous vein and the lesser (small) saphenous vein (Fig 12–11). The greater saphenous vein originates on the medial side of the dorsum of the foot. It passes in front of the medial malleolus and along the medial side of the leg, accompanied by the saphenous nerve.

The lesser saphenous vein begins along the lateral side of the dorsum of the foot, passes upward behind the lateral malleolus and along the lateral border of the tendo Achillis. In the lower part of the calf it is accompanied by the sural (medial sural cutaneous) nerve. The nerve usually lies directly beneath the vein, but this relationship is variable.

Nerves

The major nerves to the leg are the tibial nerve and the common peroneal nerve, which divides into

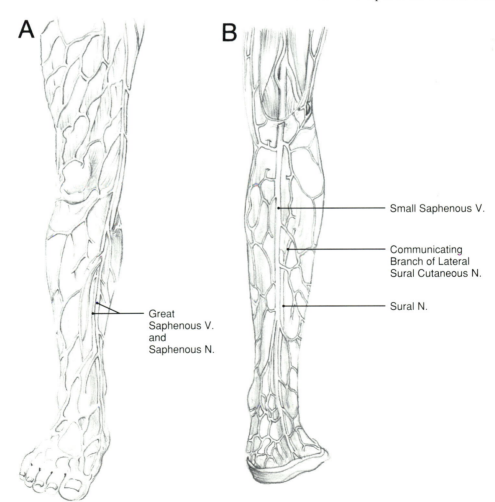

FIG 12–11.
Superficial veins of the leg. **A,** anterior view. **B,** posterior view.

superficial and deep branches. In addition, the saphenous branch of the femoral nerve provides cutaneous innervation to the medial aspect of the leg and dorsum of the foot.

Tibial Nerve

The tibial nerve is the largest terminal branch of the sciatic nerve (Fig 12–12). Its fibers are derived from the anterior divisions of the ventral rami of L4, L5, S1, S2, and S3. The tibial nerve extends directly in line with the sciatic nerve through the popliteal fossa and into the leg. From the popliteal fossa the tibial nerve enters the leg by disappearing into the gap between and beneath the heads of the gastrocnemius and plantaris muscles. It passes superficial to the popliteus muscle but under the tendinous arch of the soleus muscle to lie on the medial side of the posterior tibial vessels. It then descends between the gastrocnemius and soleus muscles posteriorly and the upper part of the tibialis posterior muscle anteriorly. Continuing down the leg it crosses over the posterior tibial vessels to reach their lateral side, lying between the flexor digitorum longus and flexor hallucis longus muscles. In the distal third of the leg the nerve is covered only by skin and fascia as it descends toward the ankle region. Here it curves anteroinferiorly into the sole of the foot behind the medial malleolus. Throughout its course in the leg the nerve supplies branches to the muscles of the posterior compartment, including the gastrocnemius, plantaris, popliteus, soleus, tibialis posterior, flexor digitorum longus, and flexor hallucis longus. It also provides one cutaneous branch known as the medial sural cutaneous nerve (see Cutaneous Nerves).

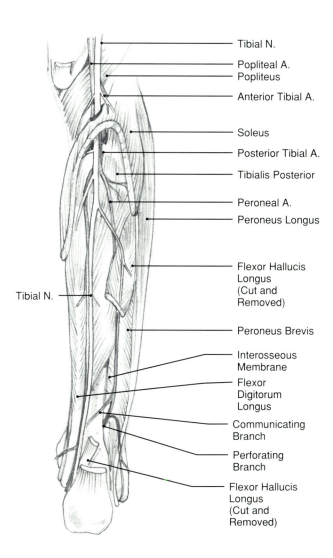

FIG 12–12.
Tibial nerve and branches.

Common Peroneal Nerve

The common peroneal nerve is the smaller lateral terminal division of the sciatic nerve (Fig 12–13). Its fibers are derived from posterior divisions of the ventral rami of L4, L5, S1, and S2. In the distal thigh the nerve supplies the short head of the biceps femoris. It descends along the lateral side of the popliteal fossa, overlapped by the medial margin of the biceps femoris, and then passes between the biceps tendon and the lateral head of the gastrocnemius to reach the back of the fibular head. Finally it winds around the back and outer surface of the neck of the fibula between the two heads of the peroneus longus and divides into the superficial and deep peroneal nerves. The common peroneal nerve gives off articular branches to the knee and the lateral sural cutaneous nerve.

Deep Peroneal Nerve

The deep peroneal nerve passes obliquely forward and downward around the fibular neck between the peroneus longus and extensor digitorum longus muscles to the front of the interosseous membrane. As it descends in the leg with the anterior tibial artery and vein, it lies lateral to the tibialis anterior muscle. In the leg the deep peroneal nerve supplies motor branches to the tibialis anterior, extensor digitorum longus, extensor hallucis longus, and peroneus tertius muscles, along with an articular branch to the ankle. It also supplies the extensor digitorum brevis on the dorsum of the foot and gives a cutaneous branch to the web between the hallux and second toe.

Superficial Peroneal Nerve

The superficial peroneal branch of the common peroneal nerve descends between the extensor digitorum longus and peroneus longus muscles. It supplies the peroneus longus and peroneus brevis muscles before piercing the deep fascia at or about the junction of the middle and lower thirds of the leg. There it divides into the medial and intermediate dorsal cutaneous nerves of the foot.

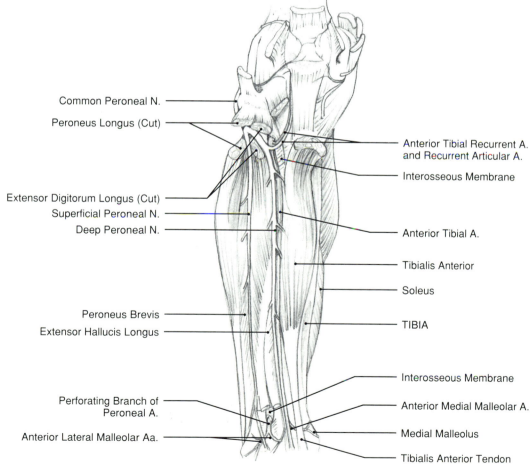

FIG 12–13.
Common, superficial, and deep peroneal nerves and branches.

Cutaneous Nerves

Several cutaneous nerves in the leg are vulnerable to injury during surgical approaches (Fig 12–14). The saphenous nerve is the largest continuation of the femoral nerve. Its course in the thigh has been described (see Hip and Thigh chapter). It pierces the fascia lata in the lower thigh between the tendons of the sartorius and gracilis above the knee. It runs down the medial side of the leg along the medial border of the tibia, accompanied by the long saphenous vein. In the lower third of the leg it divides into two branches, one of which ends at the ankle while the other passes in front of the ankle to supply the skin on the dorsomedial aspect of the foot.

The sural (medial sural cutaneous) nerve arises from the posterior aspect of the tibial nerve and courses downward superficially between the two heads of the gastrocnemius and along the superficial surface of this muscle deep to the crural fascia. It pierces the crural fascia in the middle of the upper part of the leg, where it is joined by the sural communicating branch of the common peroneal nerve. At this point the nerve is referred to as the sural nerve, which then passes down the leg along the lateral margin of the tendo Achillis in the interval between the lateral malleolus and calcaneus. It supplies the skin of the lateral and posterior parts of the lower third of the leg.

The lateral sural cutaneous nerve arises from the common peroneal nerve and supplies the skin of the posterior and lateral surface of the calf. A communicating ramus arises from the lateral sural cutaneous nerve near the head of the fibula, crosses superficial to the lateral head of the gastrocnemius, and, in the middle of the leg, joins the medial sural cutaneous nerve to form the sural nerve, as mentioned above.

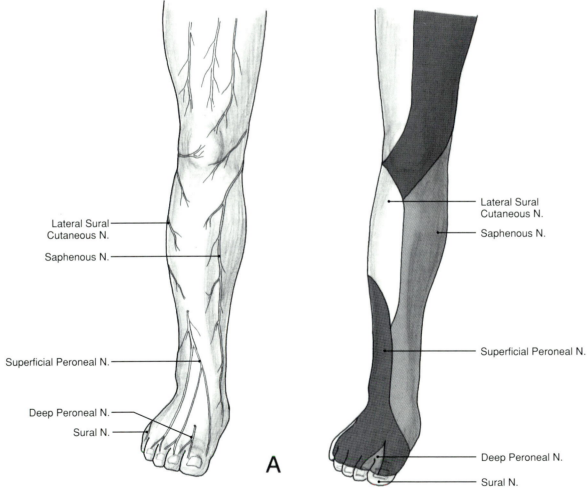

FIG 12–14.
Cutaneous nerves and dermatome patterns of the leg. **A,** anterior.
(Continued.)

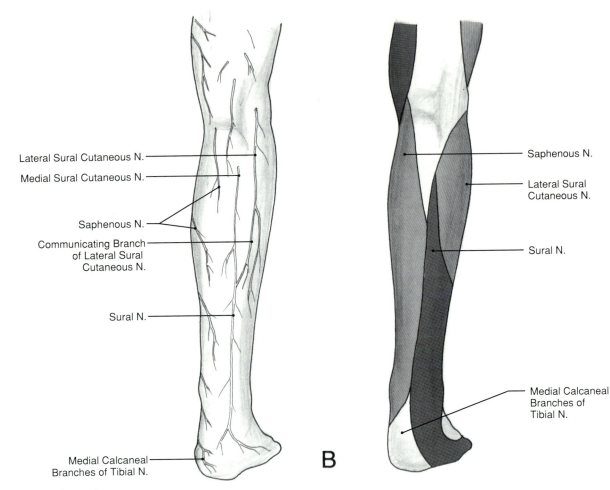

FIG 12-14　(cont.).
B, posterior.

The superficial peroneal nerve pierces the fascia in the lateral aspect of the distal third of the leg and subsequently divides into medial and lateral branches. The medial branch passes in front of the ankle and divides into digital nerves. The lateral branch passes along the dorsolateral aspect of the foot and divides into digital branches.

SURGICAL APPROACHES TO THE LEG

Skin Incisions

Skin incisions in the leg must be carefully planned in elective surgical procedures, as well as in acute trauma situations. If possible, skin incisions should not be placed over the subcutaneous surface of the tibia. The skin in this area is poorly vascular-ized and breakdown is common. However, if there are scars on the leg from previous surgery or injury, they should be utilized as incision sites rather than risk the possibility of creating a vascularly impaired flap that is apt to necrose. If fixation devices are used, they should not be placed on the bone directly underneath the skin incision.

Approach to the Lateral Tibial Plateau

Several surgical approaches requiring the formation of skin flaps, incision of the coronary ligament, or lateral meniscectomy to repair depressed lateral tibial plateau fractures have been described. Perry et al. have reported excellent results using an incision that divides the anterior horn of the lateral meniscus and allows the plateau fracture to be opened like a book. This in turn provides exposure for accurate assessment of the fracture pattern (Fig 12-15). This approach does not require skin flaps, incision of

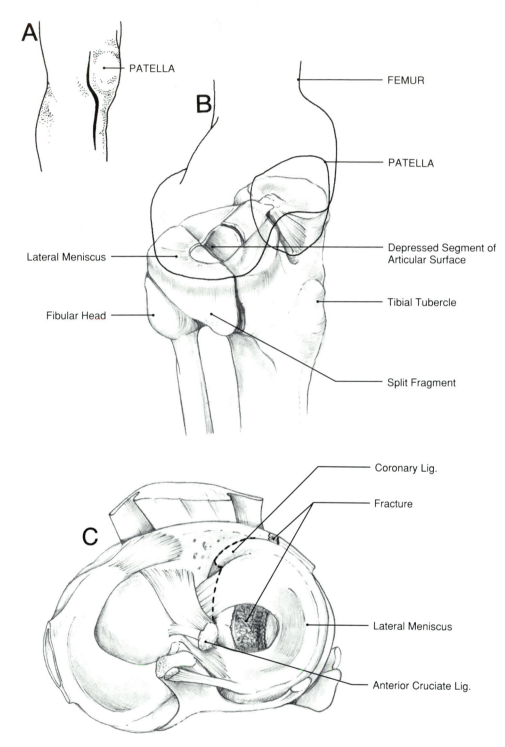

FIG 12–15.
Approach to the lateral tibial plateau. **A,** skin incision. **B,** depressed fracture of the lateral tibial plateau with associated central depression fracture of the articular surface. **C,** division of anterior horn of the lateral meniscus and coronary ligament *(dashed line).*
(Continued.)

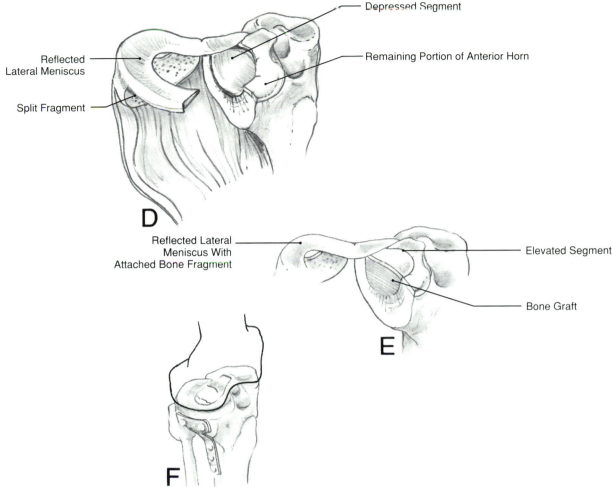

Reflected
Lateral Meniscus

Split Fragment

Depressed Segment

Remaining Portion of Anterior Horn

D

Reflected Lateral
Meniscus With
Attached Bone Fragment

Elevated Segment

Bone Graft

E

F

FIG 12–15 (cont.).

D, plateau fracture has been opened like a book. **E,** central depression fracture has been elevated and supported with bone graft. **F,** fixation accomplished with buttress plate. (Drawn after Perry CR, Evans LG, Rice S, et al: A new surgical approach to fractures of the lateral tibial plateau. *J Bone Joint Surg* 1984; 66A:1236–1240.)

much of the coronary ligament, or lateral meniscectomy.

Under tourniquet control a skin incision is begun just lateral to the proximal pole of the patella, curved slightly medially to a point just lateral to the patellar tendon, and then extended distally along the lateral crest of the tibia approximately 6 to 10 cm. The knee joint is opened with a lateral parapatellar capsular incision, the synovium incised in line with the capsular incision, and as much fat pad removed as needed to expose the anteromedial attachment of the lateral meniscus. The fracture in the lateral cortex of the tibia is exposed by an incision through the crural fascia and subperiosteal elevation of the muscles. The recurrent anterior tibial artery is cauterized to prevent bleeding and compartment syndrome. The anterior horn of the lateral meniscus is divided along with that portion of the coronary ligament which remains attached to the tibia medial to the fracture fissure. The fracture is then opened like a book, the depressed articular surface elevated, and bone graft placed in the subarticular defect. The fracture is reduced and secured with a buttress plate, and the meniscus and coronary ligament are repaired. Hemovac drainage and postoperative continuous passive knee motion are recommended. When 90 degrees of knee flexion has been obtained, a long leg plaster cast is applied and maintained for 6 to 8 weeks.

Insertion Site for Tibial Intermedullary Nailing

Closed tibial nailing has become a popular and effective method of managing certain unstable tibial fractures. A 3 to 4 cm longitudinal skin incision is

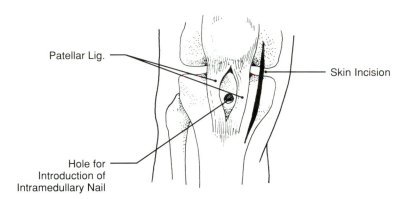

FIG 12–16.
Insertion site for tibial intermedullary nailing.

placed just medial to the tibial tubercle (Fig 12–16). In most instances the nail can be inserted through the tibial cortex at this site. If necessary, the patellar tendon can be split longitudinally to centralize the entry site in the proximal tibia.

Anterior Extensile Exposure of the Tibia

The entire length of the tibia from the knee to the ankle can be approached through a so-called anterior extensile exposure. All or part of this approach can be utilized for procedures such as open reduction and internal fixation of tibial fractures, debridement of osteomyelitis, and biopsy or excision of bone tumors. The skin incision is placed 1 cm lateral to the subcutaneous border of the tibia (Fig 12–17). Either the medial or lateral surface of the tibia may be approached through this incision. In the more common exposure to the medial surface of the tibia, it is important that the subcutaneous tissue be raised with the skin and undermined as little as possible to avoid injury to the precarious blood supply.

The lateral surface of the tibia can be exposed by resection of the tibialis anterior muscle off the bone. If this dissection is developed deep enough to expose the interosseous membrane, the anterior tibial artery and vein and deep peroneal nerve will be in the vicinity. Care must be exercised to avoid their injury.

In approaching the tibia the periosteum is pre-

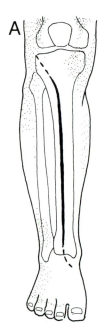

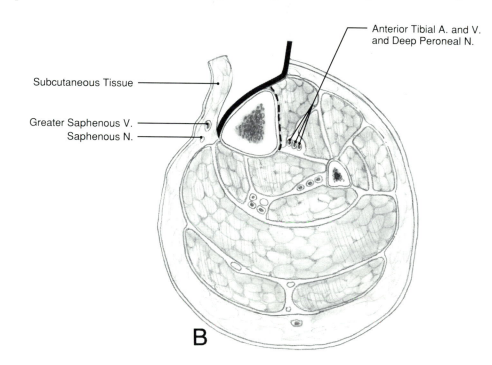

FIG 12–17.
Anterior extensile exposure of the tibia. **A,** skin incision *(solid line)* with proximal and distal extensions *(dashed line)*. **B,** cross section of leg depicting exposure of the medial surface of the tibia *(solid line)*, or alternatively, the lateral surface of the tibia *(dashed line)*.

served, along with bone fragments and their soft tissue attachments. Proximally, the dissection can be extended to expose the lateral tibial plateau. At the ankle the incision can be directed medially or laterally to expose the tibial articular surface and ankle joint itself, if necessary. Distally the incision should curve just medial to the anterior tibial tendon. The anterior tibial tendon sheath should be preserved, if possible, or carefully repaired so the anterior tibial tendon does not lie directly under the skin incision.

Posteromedial Approach to the Tibia

A posteromedial approach to the tibia may be used to decompress the deep posterior compartment of the leg or to carry out a limited bone-grafting procedure. On rare occasions it may be used to perform open reduction of a tibial fracture.

The incision is placed 1 cm posterior to the medial border of the tibia. Care must be taken to avoid the saphenous vein and nerve (Fig 12–18). The crural fascia is incised, and the flexor digitorum longus and tibialis posterior muscles are stripped off the posterior surface of the tibia.

Posterolateral Approach to the Tibia

The posterolateral approach to the tibia has been effectively used to treat such problems as nonunions and infected nonunions of the tibia. It is particularly appropriate when there are problems in the anterior or anteromedial aspect of the leg, because it avoids the old wounds, scars, and draining sinuses that often occur after extensive soft-tissue damage associated with tibial fractures. When an infection is present, it is usually confined to the anterior compartment of the leg, and this compartment is not violated by the posterolateral approach to the tibia. Furthermore, this approach takes advantage of the nearby musculature of the posterolateral aspect of the leg, which has the rich blood supply necessary to heal fractures and incorporate bone grafts. Another advantage is that the space available for placement of bone grafts is larger than with other approaches. If there has been significant bone loss of the tibia, tibiofibular synostosis above and below the fracture will stabilize the leg.

The procedure is carried out with the patient in prone or lateral decubitus position. A tourniquet is used routinely. The skin incision is made longitudinally on the posterolateral aspect of the leg approximately 1 to 2 cm posterior and parallel to the fibula (Fig 12–19). The length of the incision is determined by the extent needed to expose 4 or 5 cm of tibia above and below the fracture site. After the subcutaneous tissue is divided, the internervous fascial plane between the gastrocnemius-soleus muscle group and the peroneal muscles is identified and de-

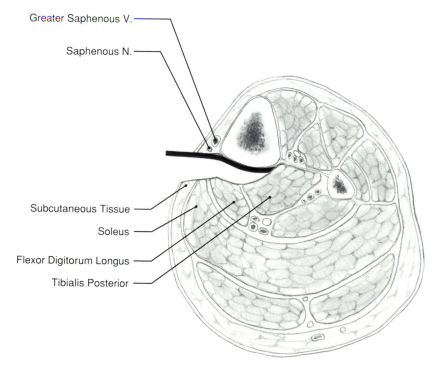

Greater Saphenous V.

Saphenous N.

Subcutaneous Tissue

Soleus

Flexor Digitorum Longus

Tibialis Posterior

FIG 12–18.
Cross section of leg showing posteromedial approach to the tibia. *Solid line* indicates skin incision and exposure of the tibia.

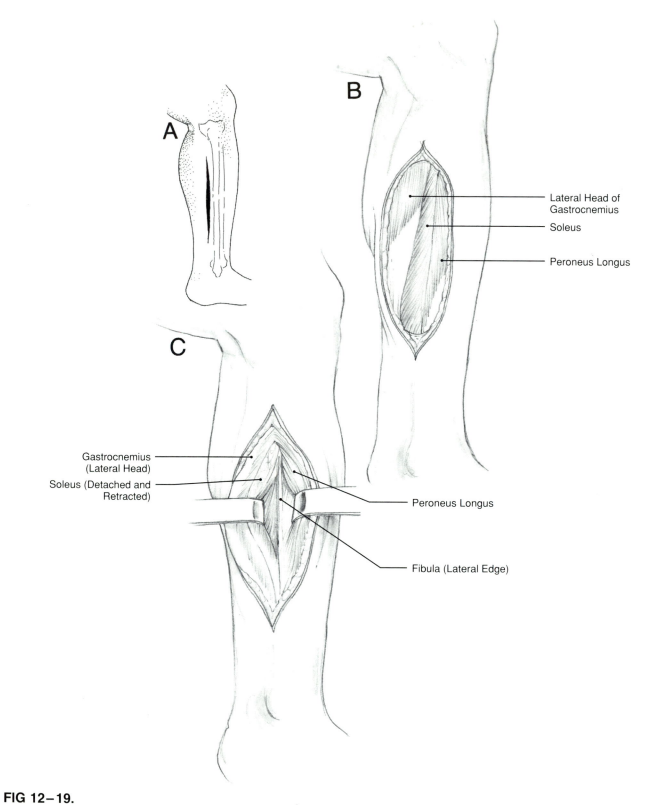

FIG 12–19.
Posterolateral approach to the tibia. **A,** skin incision. **B,** fascial incision exposing peroneus longus and gastrosoleus. **C,** dissection in the plane between the peroneus longus anteriorly and the gastrosoleus group posteriorly.

(Continued.)

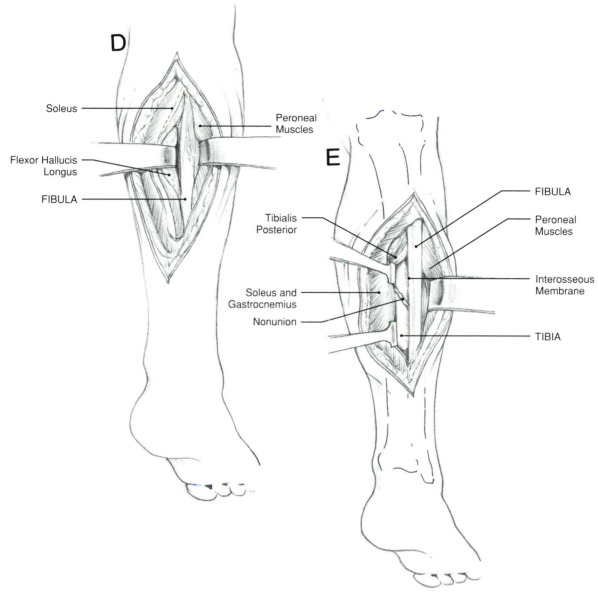

FIG 12–19 (cont.).
D, resection of flexor hallucis longus from posterolateral surface of the fibula. **E,** interosseous membrane and posterior surface of the tibia are exposed by dissecting the tibialis posterior muscle off of these structures at the level of the nonunion.

(Continued.)

veloped by dissection. The fibular origins of the flexor hallucis longus and soleus muscles are reflected subperiosteally. The posterior and medial surfaces of the fibula are carefully exposed subperiosteally. If the dissection strays into the substance of the flexor hallucis longus, the peroneal vessels may be injured. Dissection is continued, and the origin of the tibialis posterior muscle is reflected from the interosseous membrane. It is very important to keep the dissection directly on the interosseous membrane. This keeps the tibial nerve and posterior tibial

vessels out of harm's way because they lie superficial to the tibialis posterior muscle. The tibia is then exposed for the desired length by dissection of the remainder of the tibialis posterior origin from the tibia. During this procedure care must be taken to avoid injury to the lesser (short) saphenous vein. Branches of the peroneal artery that cross the intermuscular plane between the gastrocnemius and peroneus brevis should be ligated or coagulated to reduce postoperative bleeding, but care must be taken to maintain an adequate vascular supply to the per-

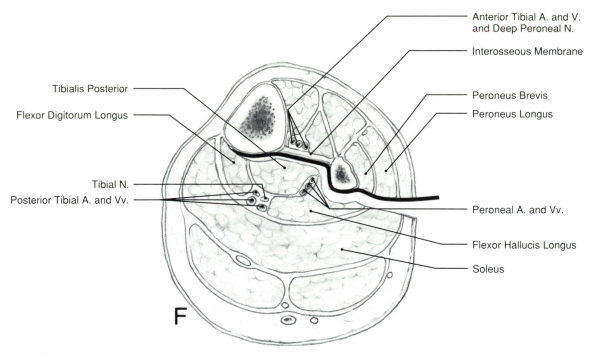

Anterior Tibial A. and V.
and Deep Peroneal N.

Interosseous Membrane

Peroneus Brevis

Peroneus Longus

Peroneal A. and Vv.

Flexor Hallucis Longus

Soleus

Tibialis Posterior

Flexor Digitorum Longus

Tibial N.

Posterior Tibial A. and Vv.

F

FIG 12–19   (cont.).
F, cross section of the leg depicting the path of dissection to expose the tibia from the posterolateral approach.

oneal muscles. The posterior tibial artery and tibial nerve are safe as long as dissection is carried out on the interosseous membrane and not in the substance of the tibialis posterior or flexor hallucis longus muscles. In the proximal aspect of the wound the posterior tibial artery and tibial nerve are at risk; therefore this approach cannot be utilized to approach the very proximal portion of the tibia. However, if desired, the approach can be extended distally by developing the dissection between the posterior aspect of the lateral malleolus and the calcaneal tendon.

Extensile Approach to the Fibula

An extensile approach to the fibula can be used to obtain a large portion of this bone when required for extensive bone-grafting procedures. However, to avoid ankle instability, the distal 7 cm of fibula should be preserved in most instances.

The procedure is carried out with the patient in the lateral decubitis position. A tourniquet is optional. The incision commences approximately a hand-breadth proximal to the head of the fibula in line with the biceps tendon, curves anteriorly over the head and neck of the fibula, and continues distally, ending just behind the lateral malleolus (Fig 12–20). The actual length of the incision depends upon the amount of fibular resection required. The

dissection is carried out in the internervous plane between the peroneal muscles, which are supplied by the superficial peroneal nerve, and the flexor muscles, which are supplied by the tibial nerve.

The fibular head and neck are exposed by a fascial incision in line with the skin incision. Dissection in the posterior aspect of the biceps femoris tendon allows exposure of the common peroneal nerve, which is identified and protected. The nerve is traced around the neck of the fibula and carefully mobilized by cutting of some fibers of the peroneus longus and gentle retraction of the nerve forward over the fibular head. In the proximal portion of the leg the plane between the peroneal muscles and the soleus is developed.

The midshaft of the fibula is exposed by subperiosteal stripping of the muscles that originate from the fibula, both anteriorly and posteriorly. The interosseous membrane is incised immediately adjacent to its attachment on the medial surface of the fibula. Care must be taken in carrying out this part of the procedure to avoid injury to the peroneal artery, which lies close to the deep surface of the shaft of the fibula. Branches of this artery must be ligated or cauterized as dissection is carried out. The small saphenous vein should be identified in the distal portion of the wound and may be ligated if necessary. If a tourniquet has been utilized, it should be

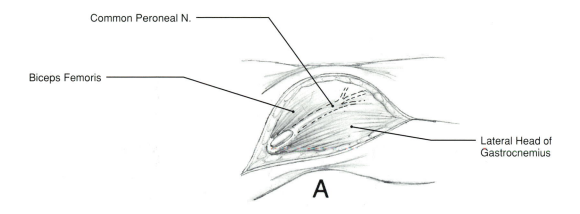

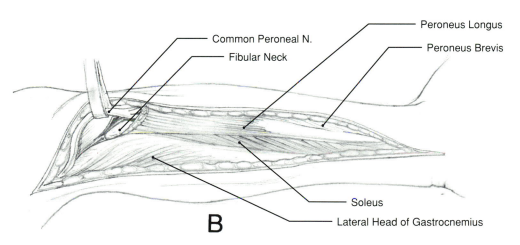

FIG 12–20.
Extensile approach to the fibula. **A,** skin and fascial incision and exposure of common peroneal nerve in proximal portion of dissection. **B,** extension of skin and fascial incision distally, exposing the lateral leg muscles.

(Continued.)

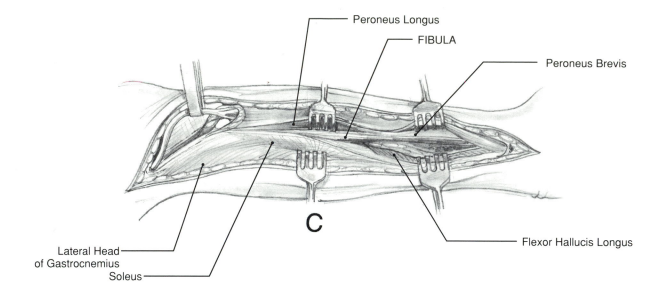

Peroneus Longus

FIBULA

Peroneus Brevis

C

Lateral Head of Gastrocnemius

Soleus

Flexor Hallucis Longus

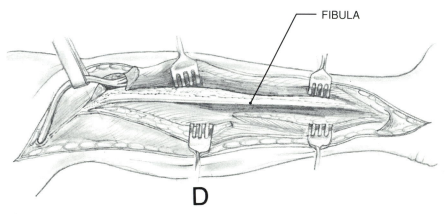

FIBULA

D

FIG 12–20   (cont.).
C, development of plane between the peroneus longus anteriorly and gastrosoleus group posteriorly and resection of muscle attachments from fibula. **D,** exposure of almost entire length of fibula.

(Continued.)

released prior to wound closure to enable identification and cauterization of any bleeding vessels.

Fasciotomy of the Leg

Posttraumatic or postoperative compartment syndromes of the leg require extensive fasciotomy to prevent damage to the tissues within these fibro-osseous enclosures and resultant morbidity. Most surgeons prefer two separate fasciotomy incisions to prevent compartment syndromes. These can be carried out with the patient in a prone, supine, or lateral position. The anterior and lateral compartments can be approached by a lateral longitudinal skin incision beginning one finger-breadth anterior to the fibula, or by two short skin incisions, one proximal and one distal (Fig 12–21). The crural fascia of the anterior compartment is split, and after the skin is retracted posteriorly, the lateral compartment is exposed. The posterior compartments can be fasciotomized through a second incision placed over the medial aspect of the leg, close to the posteromedial border of the tibia. The long saphenous vein and saphenous nerve are avoided. With retraction of the skin posteriorly, the superficial posterior compartment is entered directly. Deeper dissection through the intermuscular septum and over the posteromedial bony surface of the tibia allows entry to the deep posterior compartment.

Another method of decompressing the compartments of the leg is parafibular decompression. The skin incision runs the whole length of the fibula. Di-

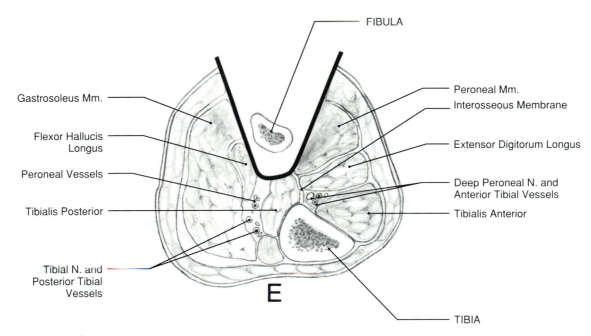

FIBULA

Gastrosoleus Mm.

Flexor Hallucis
Longus

Peroneal Vessels

Tibialis Posterior

Tibial N. and
Posterior Tibial
Vessels

Peroneal Mm.

Interosseous Membrane

Extensor Digitorum Longus

Deep Peroneal N. and
Anterior Tibial Vessels

Tibialis Anterior

TIBIA

E

FIG 12–20   (cont.).
E, cross section of the leg depicting plane of dissection. (Modified from Hoppenfeld S, deBoer P: *Surgical Exposures in Orthopaedics: The Anatomic Approach.* Philadelphia, JB Lippincott Co, 1984.)

rectly underneath, the lateral compartment is opened. The anterior compartment can be entered by retraction of the skin anteriorly. The superficial posterior compartment is reached by retraction of the skin posteriorly or through the posterior wall of

the lateral compartment. After the peroneal muscles and posterior border of the lateral compartment are freed and retracted posteriorly, the posterior septum of deep fascia attached to the fibula will be stretched and can be split along the dorsal edge of the fibula.

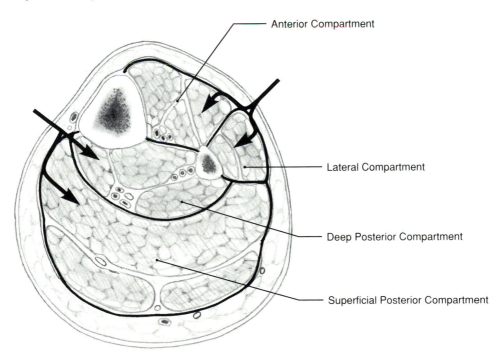

Anterior Compartment

Lateral Compartment

Deep Posterior Compartment

Superficial Posterior Compartment

FIG 12–21.
Cross section of the leg showing decompression fasciotomy *(arrows)* of the four compartments.

During this dissection the peroneal artery and both the superficial and deep peroneal nerves must be identified and protected.

BIBLIOGRAPHY

Crenshaw AH: *Campbell's Operative Orthopaedics*, ed 7. St Louis, CV Mosby Co, 1987.

Grant JCB: *Grant's Atlas of Anatomy*, ed 5. Baltimore, Williams & Wilkins Co, 1962.

Gray H: *Anatomy of the Human Body*, ed 30. Philadelphia, Lea & Febiger, 1973.

Hollinshead WH: *The Back and Limbs*, Philadelphia, Harper & Row, 1982.

Hoppenfeld S, deBoer P: *Surgical Exposures in Orthopaedics: the Anatomic Approach*. Philadelphia, JB Lippincott Co, 1984.

Lambert KL: The weight-bearing function of the fibula: A strain gauge study. *J Bone Joint Surg* 1971; 53A:507–513.

Moore KL: *Clinically Oriented Anatomy*, ed 2. Baltimore, Williams & Wilkins Co, 1985.

Netter FH: *The Ciba Collection of Medical Illustrations: Musculoskeletal System*, vol 8. Summit, NJ, Ciba-Geigy Corp, 1987.

Perry CR, Evans LG, Rice S, et al: A new surgical approach to fractures of the lateral tibial plateau. *J Bone Joint Surg* 1984; 66A:1236–1240.

Reckling FW, Waters CH: Treatment of non-unions of fractures of the tibial diaphysis by posterolateral cortical cancellous bone-grafting. *J Bone Joint Surg* 1980; 62A:936–941.

Schatzker J, Tile M: *The Rationale of Operative Fracture Care*, New York, Springer-Verlag New York, 1987.

Tria AJ, Johnson CD, Zawadsky JP: The popliteus tendon. *J Bone Joint Surg* 1989; 71A:714–715.

Youdas JW, Wood MB, Cahalan TD, Chao EYS: A quantitative analysis of donor site morbidity after vascularized fibula transfer. *J Orthop Res* 1988; 6:621–629.

13

Ankle and Foot

Brad W. Olney, M.D.

ANATOMIC FEATURES OF THE ANKLE AND FOOT

The human foot is a specialized structure that sets humans apart from the other members of the animal kingdom. The foot has two main functions: support and propulsion. Some joints of the foot actually receive more load per unit area than the knee or hip. In the past, the study of the anatomy and function of the foot always took a back seat to other areas of the human body, particularly the hand. It is only relatively recently that we are finding out what an anatomically and biomechanically complex structure the human foot really is.

Bony Anatomy

The bones of the foot include seven closely articulated tarsal bones firmly interlocking with five metatarsals, which in turn articulate with the five proximal phalanges of the toes (Fig 13–1). The foot can be divided into the hindfoot (talus and calcaneus), midfoot (navicular, cuboid, and cuneiforms), and forefoot (metatarsals and phalanges). The division between the hindfoot and midfoot is often called Chopart's transverse tarsal joint. The articulation between the midfoot and the forefoot is known as Lisfranc's joint.

Hindfoot

In the hindfoot, the talus connects the foot to the leg through its articulation with the tibia and fibula at the ankle joint. The body of the talus is cov-ered superiorly by the trochlear articular surface, which supports most of the body weight. Medially and laterally the articular cartilage extends distally down the sides of the body to articulate with the respective malleoli. The neck of the talus is roughened by vascular foramina and ligamentous attachments and is the area of the bone most vulnerable to fracture. Fractures through the neck of the talus can disrupt the blood supply to the body of the talus, leading to avascular necrosis. Distally the rounded head of the talus articulates with the navicular. On the plantar aspect of the talus are three cartilaginous surfaces that articulate with the calcaneus (Fig 13–2). The talus is unusual in that it has no muscle attachments; its only connection to adjacent structures is through the synovial membrane and joint capsule. Since the blood supply of the talus depends upon these structures, trauma associated with capsular tears may lead to avascular necrosis of the talus.

The calcaneus is the largest tarsal bone. It carries most of the body weight transmitted by the tibia and fibula through the talus. It articulates with the talus through two or three facets (Fig 13–3). For anatomic consideration the calcaneus can be divided into anterior, middle, and posterior thirds. The posterior third of the calcaneus does not articulate with the talus, but provides an effective lever for the insertion of the triceps surae. The middle third contains the large posterior facet, which articulates with the body of the talus. On the anterior third of the calcaneus, just in front of the posterior facet, is the groove that forms the floor of the sinus tarsi. Projecting medially from the anterior third of the calcaneus is the sus-

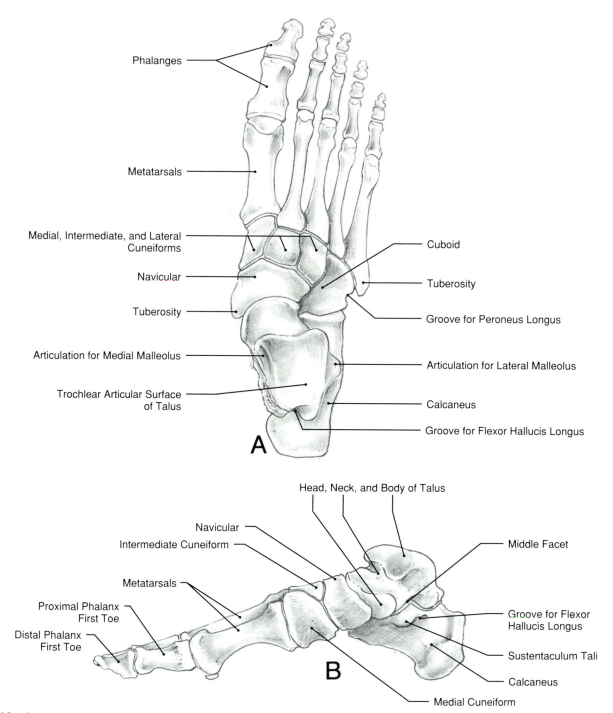

FIG 13–1.
Bony anatomy of the right foot. **A,** dorsal view. **B,** medial view.
(Continued.)

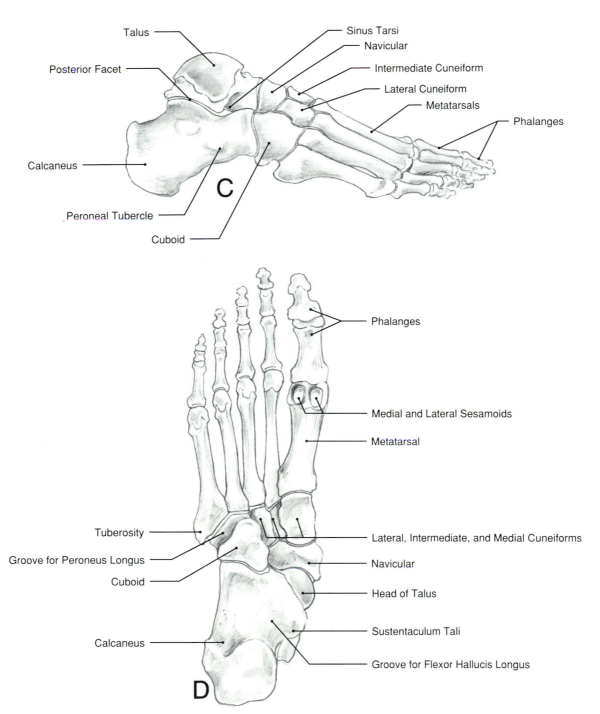

FIG 13–1 (cont.).
C, lateral view. **D,** plantar view.

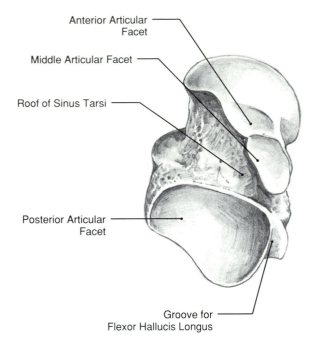

Anterior Articular Facet

Middle Articular Facet

Roof of Sinus Tarsi

Posterior Articular Facet

Groove for Flexor Hallucis Longus

FIG 13–2.
Plantar (inferior) view of the right talus. Note extensive articular surfaces.

tentaculum tali. The inferior surface of the sustentaculum contains a groove for the flexor hallucis longus tendon. The superior surface contains the articular surface of the middle facet. The middle talocalcaneal facet articulation is a common site of a tarsal coalition. The anterior facet is supported by the beak of the calcaneus and is often confluent with the middle

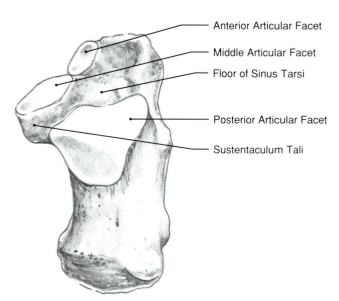

Anterior Articular Facet

Middle Articular Facet

Floor of Sinus Tarsi

Posterior Articular Facet

Sustentaculum Tali

FIG 13–3.
Right calcaneus (dorsal view). Note arrangement of articular facet surfaces.

facet. The distal articular surface of the calcaneus articulates with the cuboid. The calcaneus has a high proportion of cancellous to cortical bone, making it susceptible to compression fractures.

Midfoot

The midfoot is made up of five tarsal bones: the navicular, cuboid, and three cuneiforms. The navicular varies in size and shape more than any other tarsal bone and is the last bone in the foot to ossify. It articulates with the talus proximally and the cuneiforms distally and has a small facet for articulation with the cuboid laterally. Medially the navicular has a tuberosity that is the primary insertion site of the tibialis posterior tendon. Occasionally an accessory navicular can be found on the medial aspect of the navicular or in the tibialis posterior tendon itself.

The cuboid articulates with the calcaneus proximally, the fourth and fifth metatarsals distally, and the lateral cuneiform medially. The plantar surface of the cuboid contains a groove for the peroneus longus tendon. The three cuneiforms articulate with the navicular proximally and the first through third metatarsals distally. The cuneiforms can be identified as medial, intermediate, and lateral, or first, second, and third, respectively. The medial and lateral cuneiforms project farther distally than the intermediate, creating a recess for the base of the second metatarsal. This anatomical arrangement provides stability between the midfoot and forefoot. However, it can also result in a fracture of the base of the second metatarsal, sometimes associated with fracture dislocations through Lisfranc's joint.

Forefoot

The five metatarsals articulate with the cuneiforms and cuboid proximally and the phalanges distally. The first metatarsal is the shortest and strongest. Distally it has two plantar articular surfaces for the sesamoid bones, and it is the only metatarsal with a proximal epiphysis. The second metatarsal is the longest and least mobile because it is held firmly in the recess formed by the cuneiforms. Because of this immobility the second metatarsal is the axis through which adduction and abduction of the other rays are related. This differs from the hand, in which the axis is through the third ray. The base of the fifth metatarsal has a lateral prominence, known as the tuberosity, or styloid, which serves as the insertion site for the peroneus brevis tendon. This insertion is often involved in avulsion fractures of the fifth metatarsal base, which occur as a result of inversion injuries. The phalanges are identical in num-her to those in the hand, with two in the hallux and three in each of the lesser toes.

Ligaments and Supporting Structures

Ankle (Talocrural) Joint

The ankle is a uniaxial joint. Because the superior articular surface of the talus is wider anteriorly than posteriorly, the ankle joint is more stable in dorsiflexion than plantar flexion. Stability of this articulation is provided by the bony configuration as well as by the fibrous capsule and ligaments. The ankle mortise itself is stabilized by three major ligaments; the anterior tibiofibular, interosseous, and posterior tibiofibular (Fig 13–4). The anterior tibiofibular ligament originates from the anterior border of the lateral malleolus and inserts on the anterolateral aspect of the distal tibia. The interosseous ligament is a thickening of the distal portion of the interosseous membrane. The third ligamentous stabilizer of the ankle mortise is the posterior tibiofibular ligament, which is composed of superior and inferior portions. The inferior fibers are also called the transverse ligament.

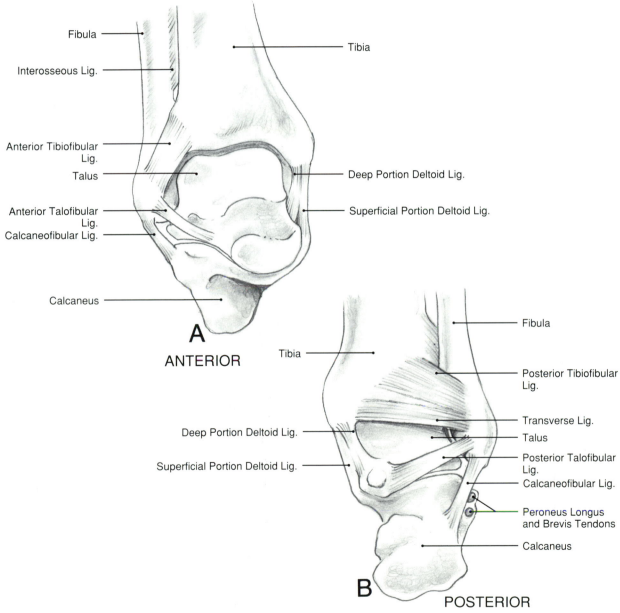

FIG 13–4.
Ligamentous structures of the ankle and hindfoot. **A,** anterior view. **B,** posterior view.

The primary medial stabilizer of the ankle joint is the deltoid ligament, which has superficial and deep portions. The superficial portion is composed of the anterior tibiotalar, tibionavicular, tibiocalcaneal, and posterior tibiotalar ligaments (Fig 13–5). The anterior tibiotalar and tibionavicular ligaments have a common origin on the medial malleolus. The deeper fibers insert on the dorsum of the talar neck and the more superficial fibers on the dorsomedial aspect of the navicular. The tibiocalcaneal ligament crosses the talocalcaneal joint to help stabilize the subtalar and ankle joints. The deep portion of the deltoid ligament is composed of a small anterior and a large posterior tibiotalar component. The latter stabilizes the ankle mortise by keeping the talus close to the medial malleolus.

The lateral collateral ligamentous complex of the ankle consists of the anterior talofibular, calcaneofibular, and posterior talofibular ligaments (Fig 13–6). Like the tibiocalcaneal ligament on the medial side of the ankle, the calcaneofibular ligament also helps stabilize the subtalar joint. The anterior talofibular ligament is the structure most often injured in the common lateral ankle sprain.

Subtalar (Talocalcaneal) Joint

The subtalar joint is formed by the posterior facet on the plantar surface of the talus and its corresponding articulation on the superior aspect of the calcaneus. The subtalar joint is surrounded by a thin capsule and does not communicate with other joints. This joint derives stability from thickenings of the capsule designated as the posterior, medial, and lateral talocalcaneal ligaments. Further stability is provided by the interosseous, cervical, tibiocalcaneal, and calcaneofibular ligaments. The interosseous talocalcaneal ligament crosses the sinus tarsi, while the cervical ligament covers the lateral entrance to the sinus tarsi (see Fig 13–6).

Talocalcaneonavicular Joint

The talocalcaneonavicular joint is a multiaxial joint complex formed by the head of the talus, concavity of the navicular, and middle and anterior facets of the calcaneus. This common articular cavity is enclosed by a thin capsule, which thickens dorsally to form the dorsal talonavicular ligament (Fig 13–7). The joint complex is supported below by the thick plantar calcaneonavicular (spring) ligament, which extends from the sustentaculum tali to the inferior surface of the navicular (Figs 13–7 and 13–8). Laterally, stability of the talocalcaneonavicular joint is provided by the calcaneonavicular portion of the bifurcate ligament (see Fig 13–6).

Calcaneocuboid Joint

The calcaneocuboid joint, along with the talocalcaneonavicular joint, creates the midtarsal (Chopart's) joint. The joint capsule thickens dorsally to form the dorsal calcaneocuboid ligament, which, along with the calcaneonavicular ligament, forms the bifurcate ligament (see Fig 13–6). Inferiorly the plantar calca-

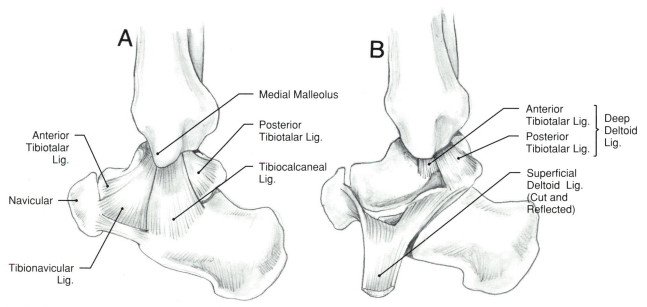

FIG 13–5.
Deltoid ligament (primary medial stabilizer of the ankle joint). **A,** superficial portion. **B,** deep portion.

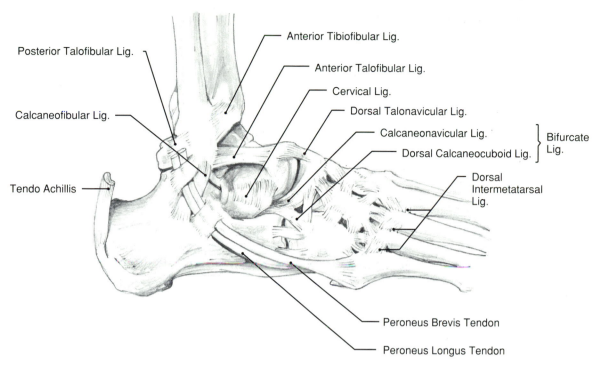

FIG 13–6.
Ligaments of the ankle and foot (lateral view).

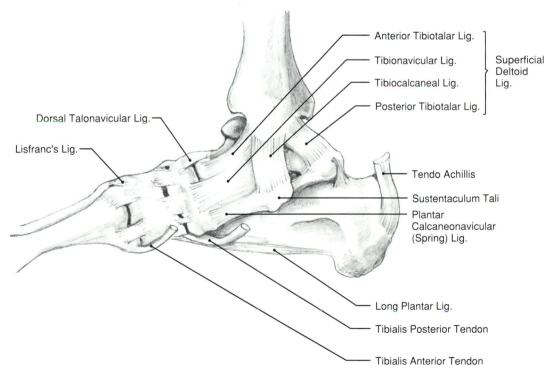

FIG 13–7.
Ligaments of the ankle and foot (medial view).

neocuboid (short plantar) ligament extends from the plantar surface of the calcaneus to the cuboid (see Fig 13–8). The deeper fibers of the long plantar ligament stretch from in front of the calcaneal tuberosity to the underside of the cuboid. The more superficial fibers spread forward to the bases of the second through fifth metatarsals. The two plantar ligaments help maintain the longitudinal arch of the foot.

Tarsometatarsal (Lisfranc's) Joint

The tarsometatarsal joints of the lateral four rays are synovial joints that communicate with each other. The first ray has a separate joint capsule and synovial cavity. The second metatarsal base projects more proximally, making its articulation with the intermediate cuneiform approximately 3 mm off line with the rest of the tarsometatarsal joints. All the tarsometatarsal joints are stabilized by dorsal, plantar, and interosseous cuneometatarsal ligaments.

The bases of the lateral four metatarsals are connected to each other by dorsal, plantar, and interosseous intermetatarsal ligaments (see Figs 13–6 and 13–8). The base of the second metatarsal is connected to the medial cuneiform by the strong Lisfranc's ligament (see Fig 13–7). The base of the first metatarsal is not connected to the second by any ligaments. This permits more dorsal and plantar flexion at the tarsometatarsal joint of the hallux than at the joint of the lateral four rays.

Metatarsophalangeal and Interphalangeal Joints

The metatarsophalangeal (MP) joints are similar to the metacarpophalangeal joints in the fingers in that each joint is enclosed by its own articular capsule and reinforced by collateral and plantar ligaments. The plantar ligament is a dense, fibrocartilaginous plate attached to the proximal phalanx; it serves as part of the weight-bearing surface for the

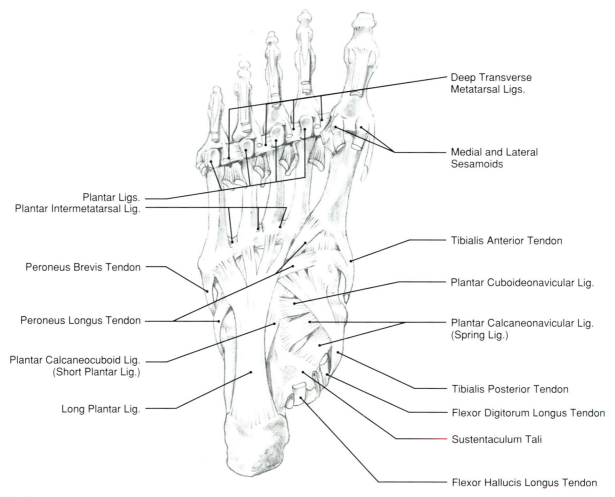

FIG 13–8.
Ligaments of the plantar aspect of the foot.

metatarsal head. The plantar ligaments of all the metatarsal heads are interconnected by the deep transverse metatarsal ligament (see Fig 13–8). The interphalangeal (IP) joints are similar to the MP joints in that each has an articular capsule with collateral and plantar ligaments. The proximal IP joints have a greater degree of flexion than the distal IP joints, although extension is limited in both.

Plantar Aponeurosis

The plantar aponeurosis is a strong, longitudinally oriented, fibrous structure on the plantar aspect of the foot. It has three portions: medial, lateral, and central (Fig 13–9,A). The central portion is the largest, arising as a thick band from the calcaneal tuberosity and extending distally into five processes. At the level of the metatarsophalangeal joints these

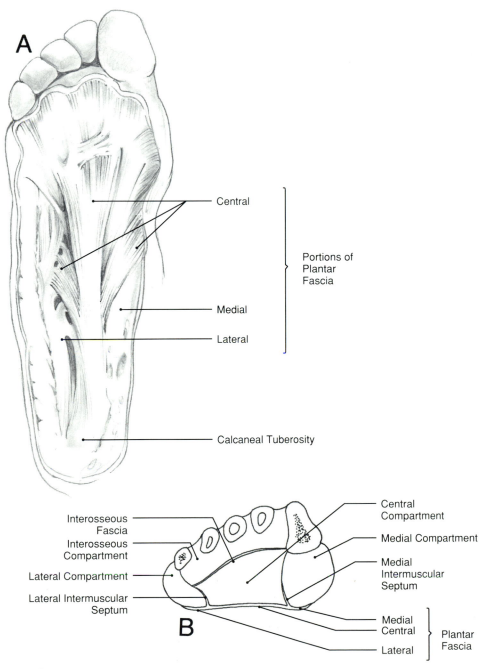

FIG 13–9.
A, plantar aponeurosis. **B,** intermuscular septa and compartments.

five processes divide into a superficial portion that attaches to the skin of the toes and a deeper portion that blends with the fibrous sheaths for the flexor tendons. The medial and lateral portions of the plantar aponeurosis are thinner. They give rise to vertical intermuscular septa where they connect with the central portion of the aponeurosis. These intermuscular septa divide the plantar muscles of the foot into medial, lateral, and central compartments (Fig 13–9,B).

Retinacula of the Foot and Ankle

Since many of the extrinsic muscles of the foot have tendons that cross the ankle at near 90-degree angles, retaining retinacular systems are necessary to prevent bowstringing of the tendons. These retinacula are formed from thickenings of the investing crural fascia of the leg. The three main retinacular systems of the foot are the extensor, flexor, and peroneal retinacula.

The extensor retinacular system is made up of superior and inferior components (Figs 13–10 and 13–11). The superior extensor retinaculum is a transverse aponeurotic band located proximal to the ankle joint. It extends from the crest of the fibula laterally, across the anterior aspect of the distal tibia, to attach to the anterior crest of the tibia and medial malleolus. The fibers are continuous with the superior peroneal retinaculum laterally and the flexor retinaculum medially. The muscles of the anterior compartment of the leg (extensor digitorum longus, peroneus tertius, extensor hallucis longus, and tibialis anterior) are contained by the superior extensor retinaculum. The superior and inferior borders of this retinacular system are often difficult to delineate.

The inferior extensor retinaculum is a Y-shaped retaining structure containing the same tendons as the superior extensor retinaculum. It is located across the anterior aspect of the ankle joint and talus. The inferior extensor retinaculum is made up of three main components: the stem or frondiform ligament, the oblique superomedial band, and the oblique inferomedial band. The stem blends with the inferior peroneal retinaculum laterally and contains the extensor digitorum longus and peroneus tertius tendons against the talus and calcaneus. It divides into the oblique superomedial and oblique inferomedial bands. The superomedial band passes over the extensor hallucis longus and tibialis anterior tendons to insert on the anterior aspect of the medial malleolus. The inferomedial band passes over the extensor hallucis longus tendon laterally. The medial fibers divide to form a fibrous tunnel for the tibialis anterior tendon. The terminal medial fibers of the oblique inferomedial band envelop the abductor hallucis muscle and attach to the navicular and medial cuneiform.

The peroneal retinaculum is also made up of superior and inferior components (see Fig 13–10). The superior peroneal retinaculum extends from the lat-

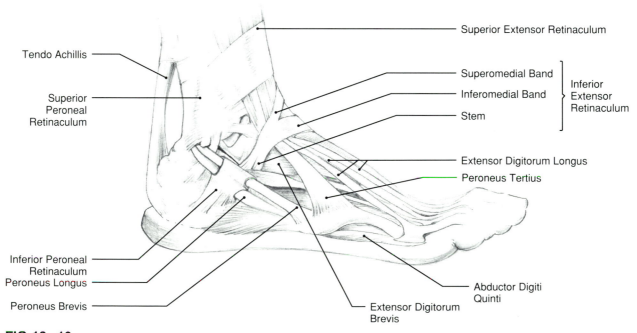

FIG 13–10.
Muscles, tendons, and retinacula of the ankle and foot (lateral view).

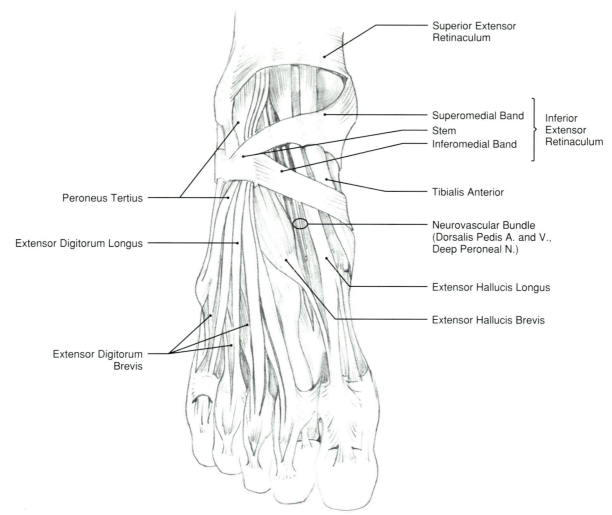

Superior Extensor Retinaculum

Superomedial Band ⎤
Stem   ⎬ Inferior Extensor Retinaculum
Inferomedial Band   ⎦

Tibialis Anterior

Neurovascular Bundle (Dorsalis Pedis A. and V., Deep Peroneal N.)

Extensor Hallucis Longus

Extensor Hallucis Brevis

Peroneus Tertius

Extensor Digitorum Longus

Extensor Digitorum Brevis

FIG 13–11.
Muscles, tendons, and retinacula of the ankle and foot (dorsal view).

eral malleolus, passing over the peroneal tendons, to insert on the tendo Achillis (tendo calcaneus) and posterolateral aspect of the calcaneus. The inferior peroneal retinaculum originates from the lateral rim of the sinus tarsi to insert on the lateral aspect of the calcaneus. The inferior retinaculum also passes over the peroneus longus and brevis tendons but forms two separate fibrous tunnels.

The tarsal (tibiotalocalcaneal) tunnel is enclosed by the triangular flexor retinaculum (Fig 13–12). The apex of the retinaculum inserts on the anteromedial aspect of the medial malleolus. The retinaculum then fans out over the contents of the tarsal tunnel to insert on the medial aspect of the calcaneus. The order of the structures in the tarsal tunnel, from anterior to posterior, can be remembered by the mnemonic "Tom, Dick, and never Harry" (*T*, tibialis posterior tendon; *D*, flexor digitorum longus tendon; *A*,

posterior tibial artery; *N*, tibial nerve; and *H*, flexor hallucis longus tendon) (Fig 13–13).

Muscles

The muscles of the foot and ankle can be divided into extrinsic and intrinsic groups. The extrinsic muscles originate in the four compartments of the leg, and all have tendinous portions that cross the ankle joint and insert on the foot. The intrinsic muscles originate and insert in the foot, distal to the ankle joint.

The extrinsic muscles of the lateral leg compartment include the peroneus longus and brevis. The tendons of these muscles pass posterior to the lateral malleolus under the superior peroneal retinaculum (see Fig 13–10). The peroneus longus tendon runs posterior to the brevis tendon in a groove behind the

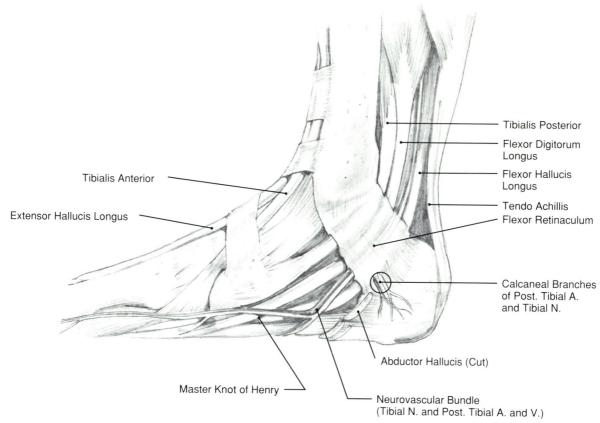

Tibialis Posterior

Flexor Digitorum
Longus

Flexor Hallucis
Longus

Tendo Achillis

Flexor Retinaculum

Tibialis Anterior

Extensor Hallucis Longus

Calcaneal Branches
of Post. Tibial A.
and Tibial N.

Abductor Hallucis (Cut)

Master Knot of Henry

Neurovascular Bundle
(Tibial N. and Post. Tibial A. and V.)

FIG 13–12.
Muscles, tendons, and retinacula of the ankle and foot (medial view).

lateral malleolus, and then courses obliquely under the cuboid to insert on the first metatarsal base and the medial cuneiform (Fig 13–14). Due to its transverse course, the peroneus longus tends to pull the medial and lateral borders of the foot together, as well as plantar flexing the first metatarsal. In addition, the peroneus longus is a weak evertor of the foot. Dysfunction of the peroneus longus caused by trauma or paralysis may lead to a dorsal bunion deformity because of the unopposed pull of the tibialis anterior. The peroneus brevis inserts on the base of the fifth metatarsal and acts as an evertor of the foot and plantar flexor of the ankle.

In the anterior compartment of the leg are four muscles whose tendons pass under the superior and inferior extensor retinacula to insert on the foot (see Fig 13–11). The tibialis anterior tendon courses medially after passing under the inferior extensor retinaculum to insert on the base of the first metatarsal and first cuneiform (see Fig 13–12). It acts as a dorsal flexor of the ankle and invertor of the foot. Under the superior extensor retinaculum, the extensor digitorum longus tendon divides into two tendons,

each of which divides into two additional tendons just distal to the inferior extensor retinaculum. These four tendons course over the dorsum of the foot to insert on the corresponding lateral four toes. The extensor digitorum longus tendons form a trifurcation over the dorsum of the middle phalanx of the lateral four toes. The central slip inserts on the dorsum of the middle phalanx, while the lateral slips rejoin to insert on the dorsum of the distal phalanx (Fig 13–15). The extensor digitorum longus acts primarily as an extensor of the MP and IP joints of the lateral four toes but is also a weak dorsiflexor of the ankle. The extensor hallucis longus tendon is lateral to the tibialis anterior tendon at the level of the ankle. After passing under the inferior extensor retinaculum it travels in its own fibrous tunnel over the dorsum of the first metatarsal to insert on the base of the distal phalanx of the first toe (see Fig 13–11). The extensor hallucis longus acts as an extensor of the first MP joint and a dorsiflexor of the ankle. The fourth muscle in the anterior compartment is the peroneus tertius, the muscle belly of which shares the same compartment as the extensor digitorum

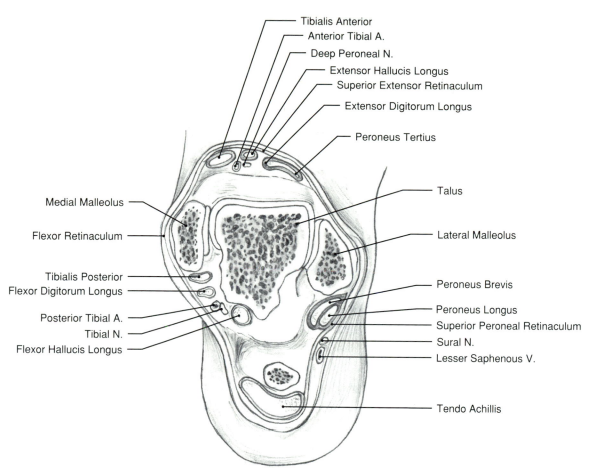

FIG 13–13.
Cross section through ankle.

longus. The tendon of the peroneus tertius runs lateral to the extensor digitorum longus and inserts on the fifth metatarsal (see Fig 13–10) to act as a dorsiflexor of the ankle and evertor of the foot.

There are three muscles in the deep posterior compartment of the leg, all of which cross the ankle under the flexor retinaculum in a shallow groove behind the medial malleolus (see Fig 13–12). The tibialis posterior tendon passes closest to the medial malleolus to reach the plantar aspect of the foot. There it inserts on the navicular, the first and second cuneiforms, and the bases of the second through fourth metatarsals (see Fig 13–14). The tibialis posterior acts as an invertor of the foot and a plantar flexor of the ankle. Loss of function of this muscle can lead to a progressive flatfoot deformity. The flexor digitorum longus tendon passes behind the medial malleolus, just posterior to the tibialis posterior tendon. The flexor digitorum longus tendon enters the central compartment of the foot where it runs superfi-

cial to the tendon of the flexor hallucis longus and then divides into four diverging tendons. The area in which the tendons of the flexor hallucis longus and flexor digitorum longus cross is known as the master knot of Henry (see Figs 13–12 and 13–18). Each of the four tendons of the flexor digitorum longus, with its accompanying flexor digitorum brevis tendon, enters a fibrous tunnel to each of the lesser toes. The flexor digitorum brevis tendons are more plantar and bifurcate at the level of the proximal phalanges (see Fig 13–17). The flexor digitorum longus tendons pass through these bifurcations to insert on the bases of the distal phalanges. The flexor digitorum longus flexes the IP and MP joints of the lesser toes and assists with plantar flexion of the ankle. The flexor hallucis longus tendon is the most posterior tendon passing behind the medial malleolus. It passes under the sustentaculum tali and progresses along the medial aspect of the sole to insert on the base of the distal phalanx of the hallux.

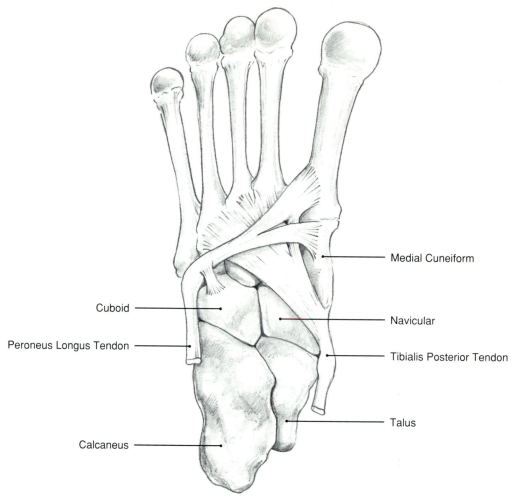

FIG 13–14.
Insertion of the peroneus longus and tibialis posterior tendons (plantar view).

The flexor hallucis longus flexes the MP and IP joints of the first toe and assists in plantar flexing the ankle.

In the superficial posterior compartment of the leg the soleus and gastrocnemius muscles form the triceps surae, which inserts on the posterior aspect of the calcaneus by means of the tendo Achillis (see Fig 13–12). The tendon fibers rotate 90 degrees, with the fibers located on the medial side proximally becoming posterior at their insertion on the calcaneus. The triceps surae is the primary plantar flexor of the ankle. The plantaris is a small muscle in the superficial compartment that arises from the lateral femoral condyle. The plantaris has a long slender tendon that runs between the gastrocnemius and soleus to course along the medial border of the tendo Achillis and insert on the calcaneus.

The intrinsic muscles of the plantar surface of the foot, together with associated extrinsic muscle tendons, are classically described in four layers (Fig 13–16). The first layer, which is the most plantar, contains three muscles, all of which arise from the calcaneal tuberosity and insert on the phalanges (Fig 13–17). The abductor hallucis is the most medial of the three muscles and inserts on the medial side of the base of the first proximal phalanx. It abducts the first toe away from the second at the MP joint. The flexor digitorum brevis has four tendons, each of which divides into medial and lateral slips that insert into the middle phalanges of the lesser toes. The tendons of the flexor digitorum longus pass between these slips to insert on the distal phalanges. The flexor brevis tendon to the fifth toe is frequently absent. The flexor digitorum brevis flexes the MP and IP joints of the lesser toes and helps maintain the longitudinal arch of the foot. The abductor digiti minimi is the most lateral muscle in the first layer and inserts on the lateral side of the proximal pha-

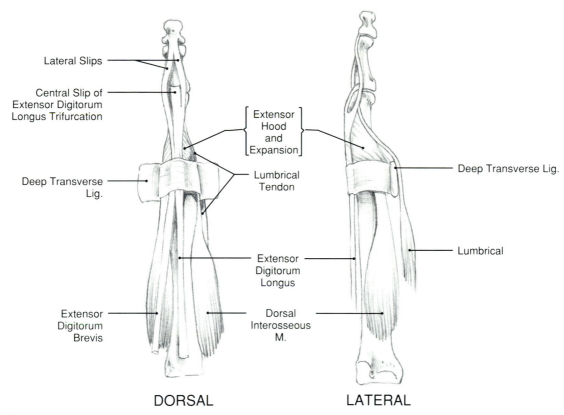

FIG 13–15.
Extensor mechanism of lesser toes.

lanx of the fifth toe. It acts to abduct the fifth toe at the MP joint.

The second layer consists of the quadratus plantae and the four lumbrical muscles together with the tendons of the flexor hallucis longus and flexor digitorum longus (Fig 13–18). The plantar nerves and arteries are also located in this layer. The quadratus plantae has medial and lateral heads that arise from their respective sides of the calcaneal tuberosity. The heads converge and insert on the long flexor tendons to the lesser toes. The quadratus plantae acts to assist in flexing the toes at the same time it brings

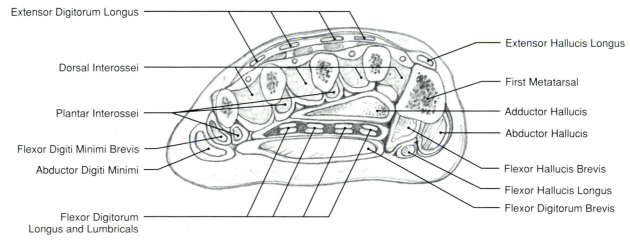

FIG 13–16.
Cross section of foot through forefoot at the base of the metatarsals.

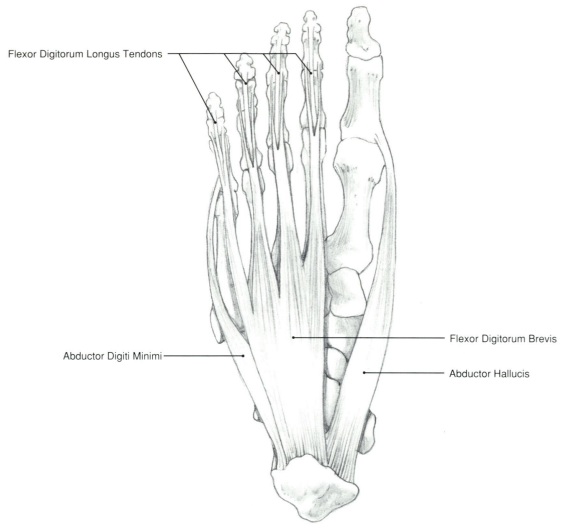

Flexor Digitorum Longus Tendons

Flexor Digitorum Brevis

Abductor Digiti Minimi

Abductor Hallucis

FIG 13–17.
Muscles of the first layer of the foot (plantar aspect).

the tendons of the flexor digitorum longus in line with the digits. The lumbricales are four small muscles that arise from the flexor digitorum longus tendons and insert on the tibial side of the extensor hoods of the lesser toes. These muscles assist in flexion of the MP joints and extension of the IP joints (see Fig 13–15).

The third layer contains three short intrinsic muscles of the first and fifth toes (Fig 13–19). The flexor hallucis brevis has a Y-shaped origin. The lateral arm originates from the plantar aspect of the cuboid and lateral cuneiform, and the medial arm originates from the insertion of the tibialis posterior tendon. The muscle then divides into two separate tendons. Each tendon contains a sesamoid bone and inserts on the medial and lateral sides of the base of the first proximal phalanx. The flexor hallucis brevis flexes the MP joint of the first toe. The flexor digiti

minimi brevis arises from the plantar aspect of the fifth metatarsal and inserts on the base of the fifth proximal phalanx to assist in flexion of the MP joint. The adductor hallucis has an oblique and a transverse head. The oblique head arises from the base of the second through fourth metatarsal heads. The smaller transverse head originates from the deep transverse metatarsal ligaments between the second through fifth metatarsal heads. Both heads of the adductor hallucis insert into the lateral tendon of the flexor hallucis brevis, which in turn inserts into the lateral aspect of the proximal phalanx of the first toe. The adductor hallucis adducts and flexes the MP joint of the first toe.

The plantar and dorsal interossei are the only muscles in the fourth layer, which also contains the tibialis posterior and peroneus longus tendons. The interossei arise from and lie between the metatar-

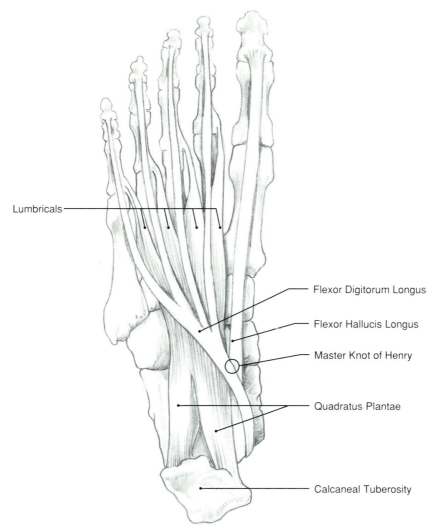

Lumbricals

Flexor Digitorum Longus

Flexor Hallucis Longus

Master Knot of Henry

Quadratus Plantae

Calcaneal Tuberosity

FIG 13–18.
Muscles and tendons of the second layer of the foot (plantar aspect).

sals. The three plantar interossei arise from the medial side of the third, fourth, and fifth metatarsals and insert on the medial sides of the proximal phalanges of the same toes (Fig 13–20). The four dorsal interossei are bipinnate, arise from adjacent metatarsals, and lie in the four intermetatarsal spaces (Fig 13–21). They send tendons to insert on the base of the proximal phalanges and the extensor hoods. The first dorsal interosseous inserts on the medial side of the second toe, while the second, third, and fourth dorsal interossei insert on the lateral aspect of each respective toe. The plantar interossei adduct the lateral three toes to the axis of the foot (second metatarsal). The dorsal interossei abduct the middle three toes away from the axis and assist in flexion of the MP joints.

The only intrinsic muscle on the dorsum of the foot is the extensor digitorum brevis, which arises from the superolateral surface of the distal calcaneus (see Fig 13–10). The muscle terminates in four tendons. The lateral three tendons insert on the tendons of the extensor digitorum longus to the second, third, and fourth toes (see Fig 13–11). The most medial tendon inserts on the dorsum of the first proximal phalanx. Along with its usually distinct muscle belly, this tendon is sometimes referred to as the extensor hallucis brevis. The extensor digitorum brevis assists in extension of the MP and IP joints of the medial four toes.

Arteries

The main arterial supply to the foot is derived from the anterior and posterior tibial arteries. The larger posterior tibial artery is accompanied by the tibial nerve and posterior tibial vein, forming the

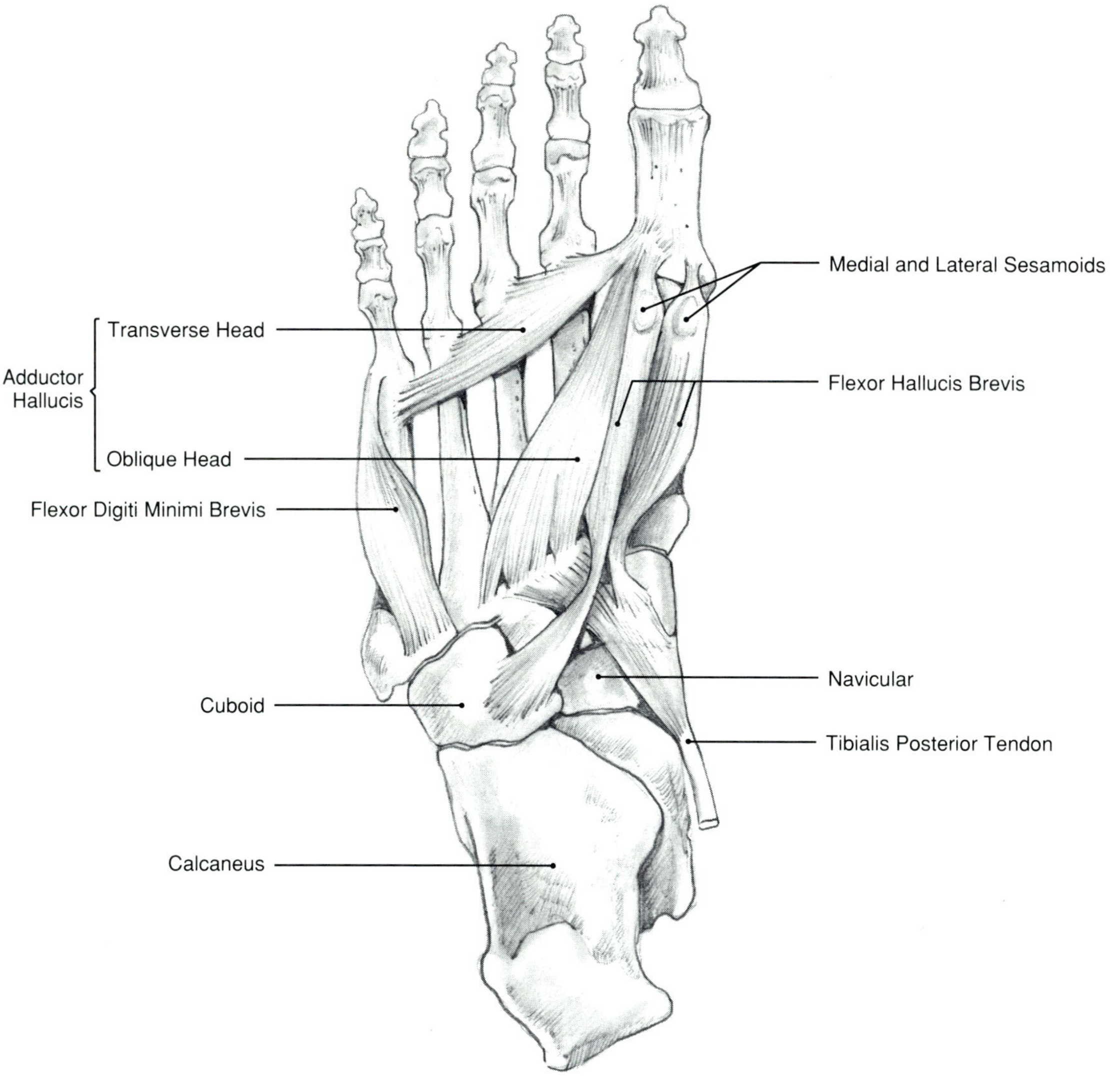

FIG 13–19.
Muscles of the third layer of the foot (plantar aspect).

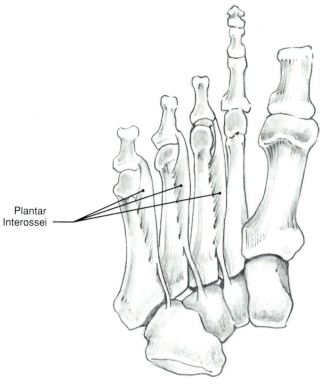

Plantar
Interossei

FIG 13–20.
The plantar interossei in the fourth muscle layer (plantar view).

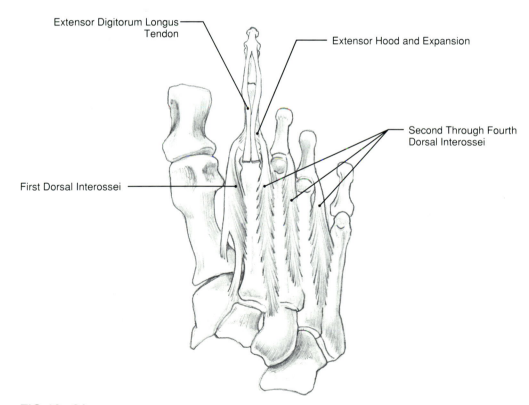

Extensor Digitorum Longus
Tendon

Extensor Hood and Expansion

Second Through Fourth
Dorsal Interossei

First Dorsal Interossei

FIG 13–21.
The dorsal interossei in the fourth muscle layer (dorsal view).

neurovascular bundle which passes deep to the flexor retinaculum behind the medial malleolus (Fig 13–22). The posterior tibial artery gives off a medial calcaneal branch and divides into the medial and lateral plantar arteries.

The medial plantar artery runs along the medial aspect of the foot beneath the abductor hallucis muscle and continues deep to the flexor digitorum brevis (Fig 13–23). It divides near the base of the first metatarsal to supply the medial three inner metatarsal spaces and portions of the first through fourth toes.

The lateral plantar artery courses under the fascia of the quadratus plantae muscle to the base of the fifth metatarsal. There it gives off the superficial fibular plantar artery to the little toe and courses medially to anastomose with the perforating branch of the dorsalis pedis artery. This anastomosis forms the deep plantar arch, which gives off three to four metatarsal branches to the lateral four toes. The deep plantar arch is a significant source of blood supply of the foot. If one of the major arteries is injured, the other artery will supply the foot through the anastomotic connections.

The anterior tibial artery passes beneath the superior and inferior extensor retinacula and continues on the dorsum of the foot as the dorsalis pedis artery (Fig 13–24). As the anterior tibial artery passes beneath the superior extensor retinaculum it lies between the anterior tibial and extensor hallucis longus tendons. After passing under the inferior extensor retinaculum, the extensor hallucis longus crosses over the artery. The artery emerges on the dorsum of the foot between the extensor digitorum longus and extensor hallucis longus tendons. Prior to becoming the dorsalis pedis artery, the anterior tibial artery gives off anteromedial and anterolateral malleolar arteries, which pass deep to the extensor tendons to supply the respective malleoli.

The dorsalis pedis artery continues on the dor-

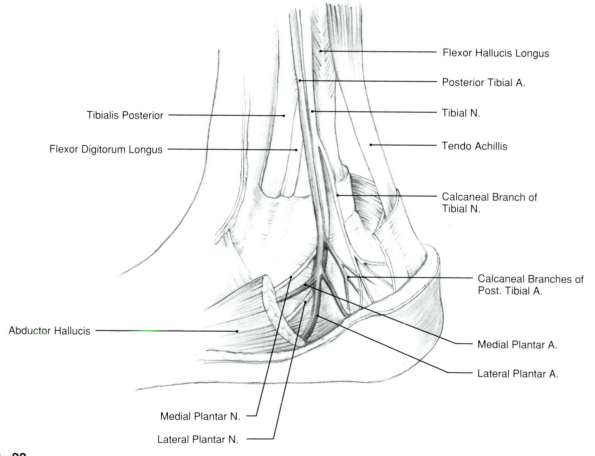

FIG 13–22.
Neurovascular structures of the medial aspect of the ankle and foot. Note arrangement of structures passing behind the medial malleolus.

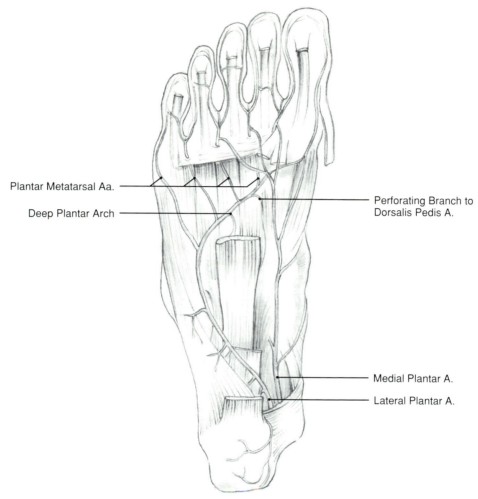

Plantar Metatarsal Aa.

Deep Plantar Arch

Perforating Branch to
Dorsalis Pedis A.

Medial Plantar A.

Lateral Plantar A.

FIG 13–23.
Arteries in the plantar aspect of the foot.

sum of the foot deep to the extensor tendons. While on the dorsum of the foot it gives off branches to form the arcuate and first dorsal metatarsal arteries. The dorsalis pedis artery then enters the plantar aspect of the foot between the first and second metatarsals to anastomose with the lateral plantar artery.

The peroneal artery is the smallest artery contributing to the blood supply of the foot. It is a branch of the posterior tibial artery of the leg that runs along the medial crest of the fibula between the tibialis posterior and flexor hallucis longus muscles. The peroneal artery terminates posterior to the distal tibiofibular syndesmosis. It gives off numerous calcaneal branches to the lateral and posterior aspects of the hindfoot and a perforating branch that anastomoses with the anterior tibial artery. Occasionally this perforating branch of the peroneal artery is large and actually forms or continues as the dorsalis pedis

artery. The calcaneal branches of the peroneal artery anastomose with branches of the lateral malleolar artery, also connecting the peroneal artery blood flow to the anterior tibial artery system.

There is extensive superficial and deep venous drainage in the foot. The deep venous system parallels the arterial system of the foot. The superficial veins of the foot primarily drain into the greater and lesser saphenous veins (Fig 13–25). The greater saphenous vein runs anterior to the medial malleolus, while the lesser saphenous vein courses posterior to the lateral malleolus.

Nerves

The motor and sensory innervation of the foot is primarily from the common peroneal and tibial branches of the sciatic nerve. The peroneal portion

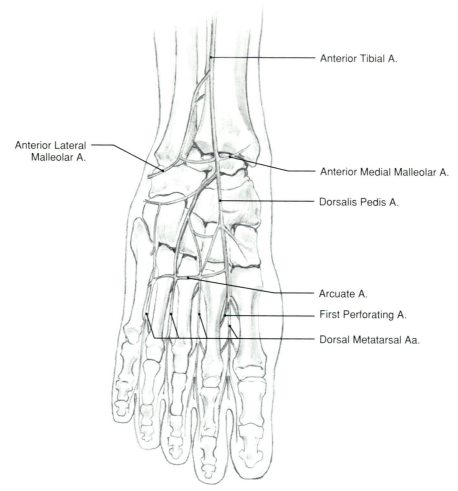

Anterior Tibial A.

Anterior Lateral
Malleolar A.

Anterior Medial Malleolar A.

Dorsalis Pedis A.

Arcuate A.

First Perforating A.

Dorsal Metatarsal Aa.

FIG 13–24.
Arterial supply of the dorsum of the foot.

of the sciatic nerve arises from nerve roots L4 to S1 and the tibial portion from L4 to S3.

Five nerves supply sensation and motor function to the foot and ankle. The largest is the tibial nerve, which runs beneath the flexor retinaculum with the posterior tibial vessels (see Fig 13–22). The tibial nerve gives off a medial calcaneal branch that pierces the retinaculum to supply sensation to the medial aspect of the heel. The tibial nerve can be compressed where it passes under the retinaculum, and the result is the so-called tarsal tunnel syndrome. After emerging from under the flexor retinaculum, the tibial nerve divides into the medial and lateral plantar nerves.

The medial plantar nerve passes into the plantar aspect of the foot in the interval between the abductor hallucis and flexor digitorum brevis (Fig 13–26). At the base of the first metatarsal it divides into ter-

minal medial and lateral branches. The smaller medial branch ends as the medial plantar digital nerve to the hallux. The larger lateral branch forms the first, second, and part of the third common digital nerves. The common digital nerves pass between the metatarsal heads, where interdigital neuromas (Morton's neuroma) occasionally form. The third common digital nerve is formed by branches of both the lateral and medial plantar nerves, making it larger and less mobile. It is speculated that this anatomical arrangement makes the third common digital nerve more subject to trauma and for that reason the most common site of interdigital neuromas. The medial plantar nerve supplies sensation to the medial and plantar aspects of the first toe as well as plantar sensation of the second, third, and part of the fourth toes (Fig 13–27). The medial plantar nerve also provides motor innervation to the flexor

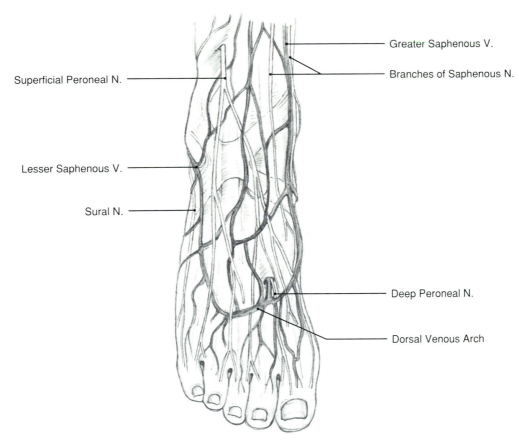

Superficial Peroneal N.

Lesser Saphenous V.

Sural N.

Greater Saphenous V.

Branches of Saphenous N.

Deep Peroneal N.

Dorsal Venous Arch

FIG 13–25.
Superficial nerves and veins on the dorsal aspect of the foot.

hallucis brevis, abductor hallucis, flexor digitorum brevis, and first lumbrical muscles.

The lateral plantar nerve crosses the sole of the foot between the quadratus plantae and flexor digitorum brevis to divide into its terminal branches at the base of the fifth metatarsal (see Fig 13–26). The terminal branches include the lateral collateral nerve of the fifth toe, the fourth common digital nerve, and a communicating branch to the third common digital nerve. Through its branches the lateral plantar nerve provides sensation to the lateral plantar aspect of the foot as well as the plantar surface of the fifth toe and the lateral half of the fourth toe (see Fig 13–27). The lateral plantar nerve supplies motor innervation to the quadratus plantae, abductor digiti minimi, flexor digiti minimi, adductor hallucis, all plantar and dorsal interossei, and the second through fourth lumbrical muscles.

In the leg the common peroneal nerve divides into the superficial and deep peroneal nerves at the level of the neck of the fibula. After supplying motor innervation to the muscles of the lateral compart-

ment of the leg, the superficial peroneal nerve divides into medial and lateral branches that pass anterior to the ankle joint, superficial to the extensor retinaculum in the subcutaneous tissue (see Fig 13–25). The medial branch passes in front of the ankle joint and divides into two dorsal digital nerves, which supply sensation to the medial aspect of the first toe and the dorsum of the second and third toes. The lateral branch of the superficial peroneal nerve supplies sensation to the lateral side of the ankle and then passes along the lateral aspect of the dorsum of the foot. There it divides into dorsal digital branches, which supply sensation to the fourth and fifth toes.

The deep peroneal nerve supplies motor innervation to the muscles of the anterior compartment of the leg and then descends with the anterior tibial artery deep to the extensor retinaculum (see Fig 13–25). Distal to the retinaculum the nerve runs with the dorsalis pedis artery, terminating in cutaneous branches that supply sensation to the lateral side of the hallux, the medial side of the second toe,

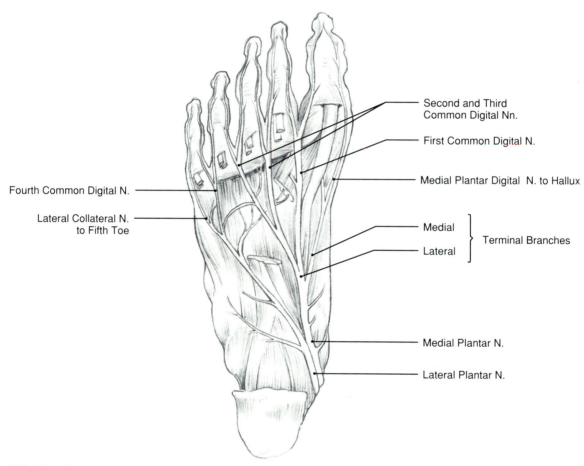

FIG 13–26.
Nerves in the plantar aspect of the foot.

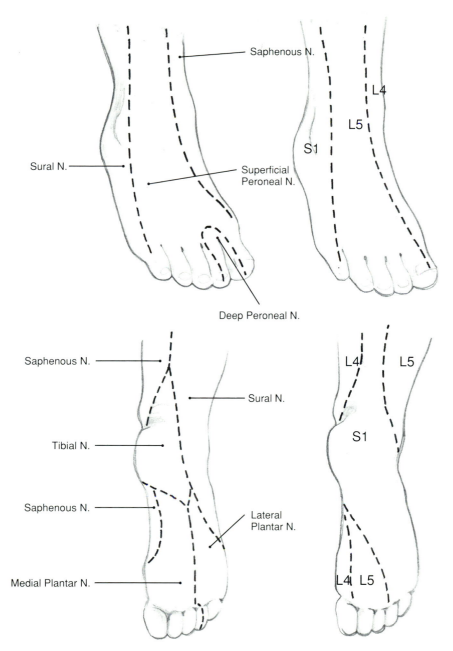

FIG 13–27.
Cutaneous nerve supply and dermatome pattern of the ankle and foot.

and the web space between them (see Fig 13–27). The deep peroneal nerve also provides motor innervation to the extensor digitorum brevis muscle.

The sural nerve is formed by both the peroneal and tibial nerves. It descends with the small saphenous vein in the leg, courses along the lateral edge of the tendo Achillis, and passes posterior to the lateral malleolus (see Fig 13–25). The sural nerve provides cutaneous sensation to the lateral malleolar area and the lateral aspect of the foot (see Fig 13–27).

The saphenous nerve arises from the femoral

nerve in the thigh. It is the only source of innervation for the foot that is not derived from the sciatic nerve or its branches. In the distal third of the leg the saphenous nerve runs along the medial border of the tibia, accompanied by the long saphenous vein, and divides into two terminal branches (see Fig 13–25). One terminal branch continues along the medial border of the tibia to end just distal to the ankle joint. The other branch passes superficial to the extensor retinaculum to continue along the medial side of the foot and anastomose with branches of the superficial peroneal nerve. This second terminal branch of the saphenous nerve supplies sensation to the medial aspect of the foot.

SURGICAL APPROACHES TO THE ANKLE

Anterior Approach

The anterior approach to the ankle provides excellent exposure of the ankle mortise, including both malleoli. It is often used for ankle arthrodesis.

The patient is placed in supine position and the skin incision is begun 7 to 10 cm proximal to the ankle over the anterior aspect of the tibia (Fig 13–28). The incision is extended distally midway between the malleoli, ending approximately 5 cm distal to the joint. The deep fascia, including the extensor retinaculum, should be incised in line with the skin incision. Care must be taken to avoid injury to branches of the superficial peroneal nerve, which cross the ankle joint in the subcutaneous tissue. After the retinaculum is divided, the plane between the extensor hallucis longus and extensor digitorum longus is developed. The neurovascular bundle (the anterior tibial artery and vein, and deep peroneal nerve) must be identified and protected. Proximal to the ankle the neurovascular bundle runs between the tibialis anterior and extensor hallucis longus. The extensor hallucis longus then crosses in front of the bundle at the level of the ankle joint. The neurovascular structures (dorsalis pedis artery and vein, and deep peroneal nerve) continue on the dorsum of the foot between the extensor hallucis longus and extensor digitorum longus. Once they are identified, the extensor hallucis longus and neurovascular bundle are retracted medially and the extensor digitorum longus laterally. The periosteum, capsule, and synovium are incised in the same line as the deep fascia. The entire width of the ankle joint can then be exposed by sharp dissection of the capsule off the distal tibia and the talus. The anterior approach can also be performed between the tibialis anterior and extensor hallucis longus. The incision can be extended proximally by developing the plane between the tibial crest and tibialis anterior muscle.

Anterolateral Approach

The anterolateral approach also provides good exposure to the ankle joint, although it does not expose the medial aspect of the talus as readily as the

anterior approach. The main advantage of the anterolateral approach is that it can be extended distally to expose the talocalcaneal, talonavicular, and calcaneocuboid joints. All or part of this incision can be used for ankle fusion, talectomy, triple arthrodesis, and even pantalar arthrodesis. Since numerous operations can be performed on the structures exposed with this approach, it is often referred to as the universal approach to the foot and ankle.

The patient is placed in supine position on the operating table with a large bolster under the ipsilateral hip. The incision begins 5 cm proximal to the ankle joint and 2 cm anterior to the fibula (Fig 13–29). It gently curves across the ankle joint and over the lateral aspect of the talus and calcaneocuboid joint, ending at the base of the fourth metatarsal. The deep fascia and extensor retinaculum are incised in line with the skin incision. Care is taken to protect branches of the superficial peroneal nerve located in the subcutaneous tissue. The peroneus tertius and extensor digitorum longus are retracted medially to expose the periosteum of the tibia and the ankle joint capsule. The ankle joint and distal tibia can be exposed by sharp division and reflection of the periosteum and capsule. This dissection usually divides the anterolateral malleolar and lateral tarsal arteries, both of which must be cauterized to prevent postoperative hematoma. The incision can be extended distally by splitting of the fibers of the extensor digitorum brevis or by detachment of its fibers and distal reflection of the muscle. This exposes the fat in the sinus tarsi, which can be excised to expose the talocalcaneal joint. However, when possible, it is preferable to leave this fat in place to prevent an unsightly depression postoperatively and to maintain blood supply for wound healing. The talonavicular and calcaneocuboid articulations can be exposed by sharp subperiosteal dissection. This approach can be extended proximally in the anterior compartment of the leg and distally to expose the subcutaneous tarsometatarsal joints of the lateral aspect of the foot.

Medial Approach

The medial approach to the ankle requires osteotomy of the medial malleolus but provides excellent exposure of the talus and medial ankle joint. It is useful for removal of loose bodies of the ankle and osteochondral fragments of the medial aspect of the talus, as well as for reduction of fractures of the talus.

The patient is positioned supine with a bolster under the contralateral hip. A 10 cm curved incision

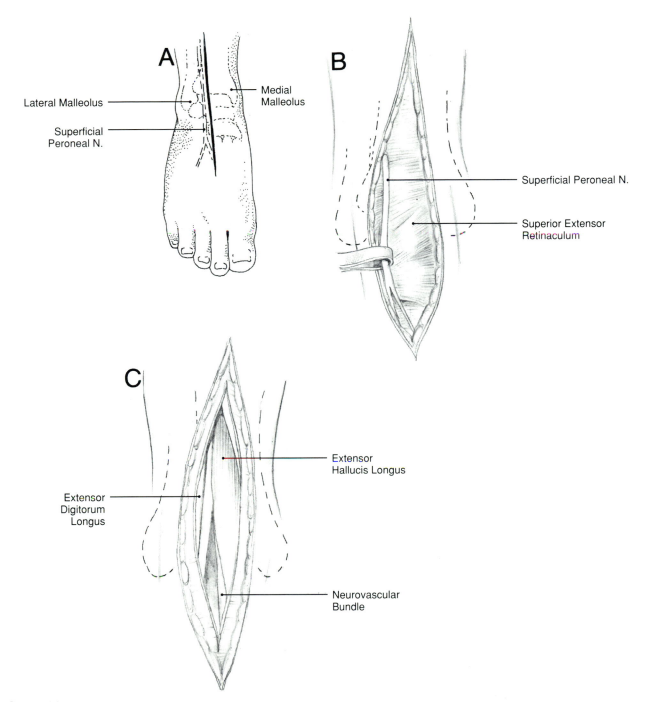

FIG 13–28.
Anterior approach to the ankle. **A,** the skin incision is made with care to protect the superficial peroneal nerve in the subcutaneous tissue. **B,** the superficial peroneal nerve is retracted laterally while the deep fascia and superior extensor retinaculum are incised. **C,** the neurovascular bundle is identified in front of the ankle between the extensor hallucis longus and extensor digitorum longus.
(Continued.)

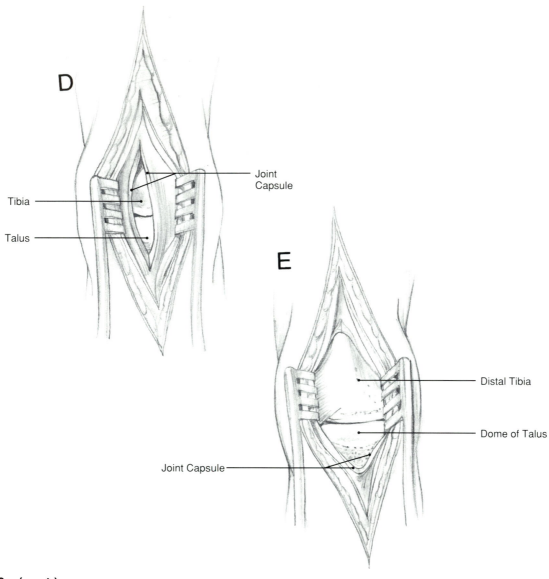

FIG 13–28   (cont.).
D, the neurovascular bundle and extensor hallucis longus are retracted medially and the extensor digitorum longus laterally to expose the ankle joint capsule. **E,** the capsule is incised and sharply dissected off the distal tibia and talus.

is centered over the tip of the medial malleolus, ending distally over the medial cuneiform (Fig 13–30). The skin flaps are elevated to expose the medial malleolus and distal tibia. Care is taken to protect the saphenous nerve and greater saphenous vein, which lie just anterior to the medial malleolus. The tip of the malleolus is identified, and a small anterior arthrotomy is made in the ankle joint to determine the point at which the medial malleolus joins the shaft of the tibia. The flexor retinaculum is incised to identify the tibialis posterior tendon so as to avoid injuring it during the osteotomy. The malleolus is predrilled and tapped for later reattachment with a screw and then osteotomized obliquely from top to bottom. The osteotomy should end at the point, previously identified, at which the malleolus joins the tibial shaft. Score marks perpendicular to the osteotomy site help maintain anatomic alignment when the malleolus is reattached. The medial malleolus is reflected downward on its attached deltoid ligament, and the foot is everted to expose the talar dome.

Posteromedial Approach

The posteromedial approach exposes the posterior aspect of the ankle and subtalar joint. It is useful for posterior ankle release and fixation of posterior

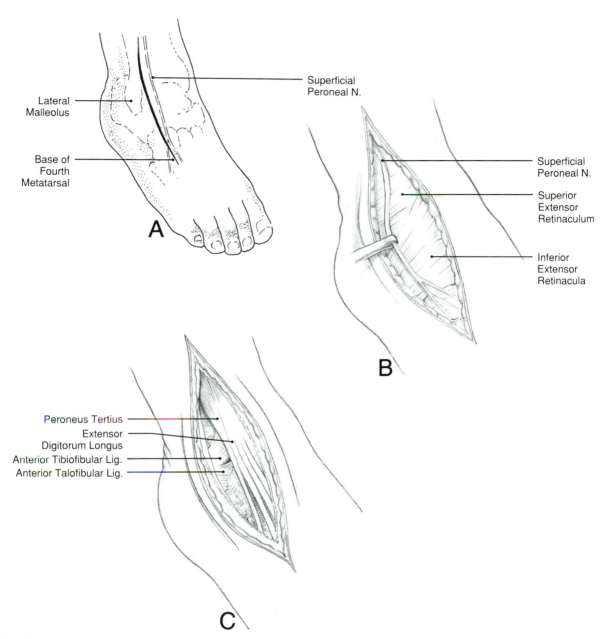

FIG 13–29.
Anterolateral approach to the ankle and hindfoot. **A,** the skin incision is made anterior to the fibula. Care is taken to protect the superficial peroneal nerve and its branches. **B** and **C,** the superior and inferior extensor retinacula are incised to expose the extensor digitorum longus and peroneus tertius. *(Continued.)*

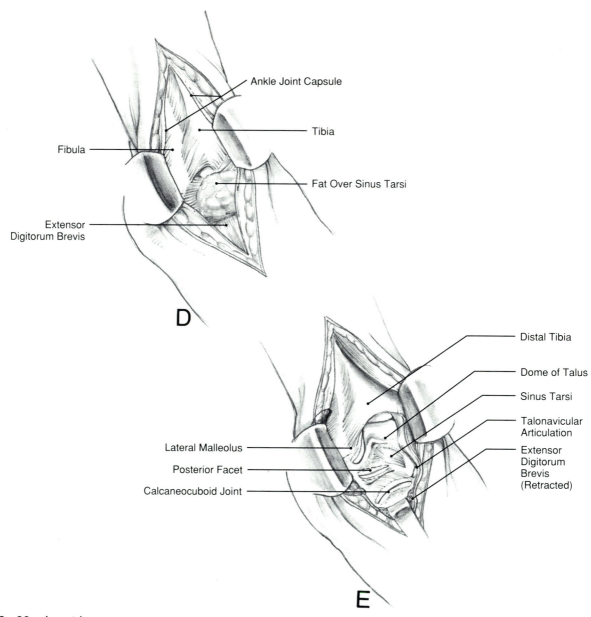

FIG 13–29   (cont.).
D, the extensor digitorum longus and peroneus tertius are retracted medially to expose the ankle capsule and sinus tarsi fat pad. **E,** the ankle joint is exposed by splitting of the capsule. The fat pad is excised to expose the posterior facet of the subtalar joint and sinus tarsi. The extensor digitorum brevis is incised sharply off the calcaneus to expose the calcaneocuboid and talonavicular articulations.

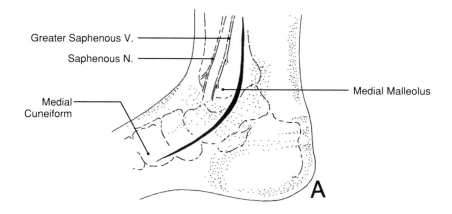

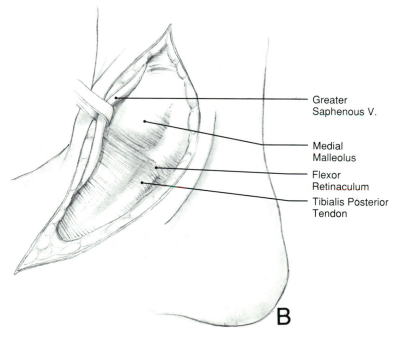

FIG 13–30.
Medial approach to the ankle. **A** and **B,** the skin incision is located over the medial malleolus. Care is taken to avoid damage to the greater saphenous vein and saphenous nerve.
(Continued.)

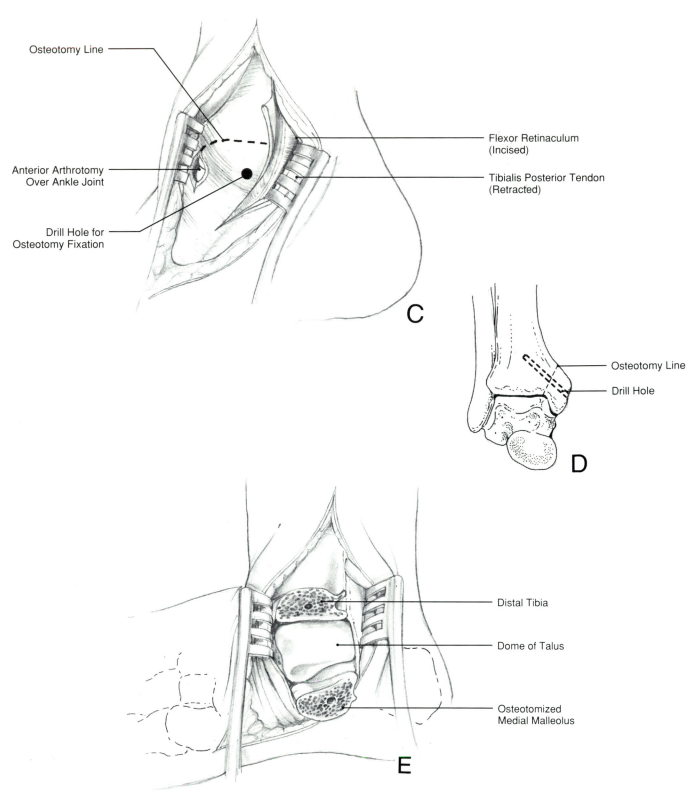

FIG 13-30   (cont.).
C and **D,** the ankle capsule is opened anteriorly while the tibialis posterior tendon is exposed and protected posterior to the malleolus. The medial malleolus is osteotomized from proximal to distal. **E,** the malleolus is retracted distally and the foot inverted to expose the ankle joint and dome of the talus. (Modified from Hoppenfeld S, deBoer P: *Surgical Exposures in Orthopaedics: The Anatomic Approach.* Philadelphia, JB Lippincott Co, 1984.)

malleolar fractures. When used for clubfoot soft-tissue release, the exposure can be extended medially over the talocalcaneonavicular joint.

The patient may be placed in either of two positions for this approach. Prone position is best if just a posterior capsulotomy and elongation of the tendo Achillis are planned; however, if medial release of the talocalcaneonavicular joint is also required, supine position with the leg externally rotated is preferred. The incision is made along the medial border of the tendo Achillis, continuing beyond the medial malleolus (Fig 13–31). If necessary the incision can be extended along the medial border of the foot to the insertion of the tibialis anterior. The tendo Achillis is dissected free and transected with a Z-cut in either the frontal or sagittal plane. Complete visualization of the posterior ankle and subtalar joint requires transection of the tendo Achillis. However, this is

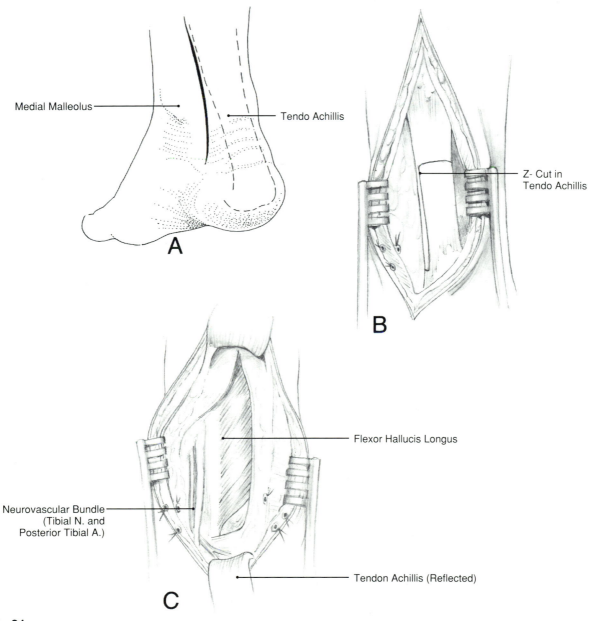

FIG 13–31.
Posteromedial approach to the ankle. **A,** the skin incision is just medial to the tendo Achillis. **B,** if necessary, the tendo Achillis is transected with a Z-cut. **C,** the muscle fibers of the flexor hallucis longus are identified beneath the tendo Achillis. Care is taken not to damage the tibial nerve and posterior tibial artery, which lie medial to the flexor hallucis longus.

(Continued.)

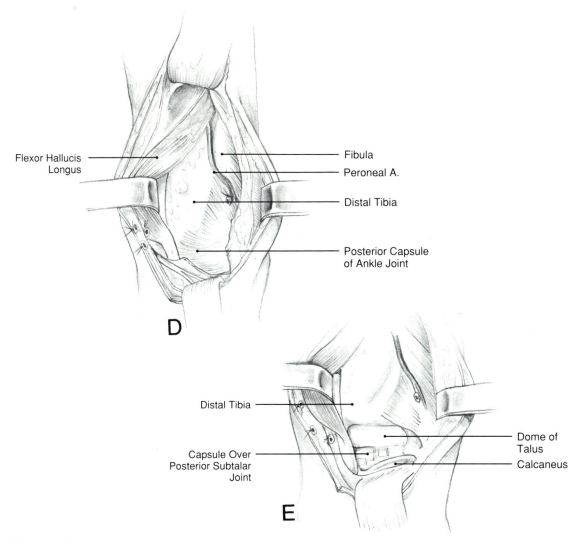

FIG 13–31   (cont.).
D, the flexor hallucis longus and neurovascular bundle are retracted medially to expose the posterior capsule of the ankle. The peroneal artery may have to be ligated. **E,** the posterior aspect of the ankle and subtalar joint can be exposed by incision of their respective capsules.

not necessary if exposure of the posteromedial aspect of the joint is all that is required. The flexor hallucis longus tendon, which still has muscle fibers at this level, and the neurovascular bundle (tibial nerve and posterior tibial artery), are identified and retracted medially to expose the ankle and subtalar joints. Care must be taken in releasing the subtalar joint medially to avoid damage to the flexor hallucis longus tendon. When release is done laterally, care is necessary to avoid injuring the peroneal tendons.

Posterolateral Approach

The posterolateral approach can also be used to expose the posterior ankle joint, but the exposure is not as good as with the posteromedial approach. The posterolateral approach does provide good exposure of the peroneal tendons, and it can be extended distally to reach the lateral aspect of the calcaneus.

The patient is placed in the prone position, and a longitudinal incision is made halfway between the lateral border of the fibula and the tendo Achillis (Fig 13–32). The incision is begun at the level of the tip of the fibula and extended proximally about 10 cm. Care must be taken to protect the lesser saphenous vein and sural nerve; these are located in the subcutaneous tissue, usually anterior to the skin incision. The deep fascia is incised in line with the skin incision, and the peroneal tendons are located.

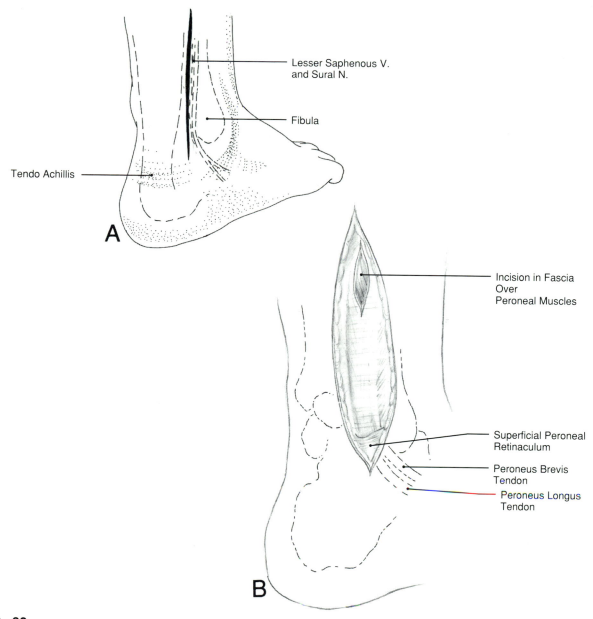

Lesser Saphenous V. and Sural N.

Fibula

Tendo Achillis

Incision in Fascia Over Peroneal Muscles

Superficial Peroneal Retinaculum

Peroneus Brevis Tendon

Peroneus Longus Tendon

A

B

FIG 13–32.
Posterolateral approach to the ankle. **A,** the skin incision is made posterior to the fibula. Care is taken to protect the lesser saphenous vein and sural nerve in the subcutaneous tissue. **B,** fascial incision. *(Continued.)*

The peroneus brevis lies anterior to the longus and at this level still contains some muscle fibers. The proximal portion of the peroneal retinaculum is incised, and the peroneal tendons are retracted laterally. The fibers of the flexor hallucis longus muscle, which are attached to the fibula in the proximal aspect of the wound, are sharply dissected off the fibula and retracted medially. The peroneal artery lies deep to the flexor hallucis longus and should be protected, although several small branches may have to be cauterized. The posterior aspect of the tibia and the ankle capsule are now exposed, and the ankle joint is entered by transverse incision of the capsule.

Approach to the Lateral Malleolus

This is a relatively safe approach, since the distal fibula is a subcutaneous bone. The approach is primarily used for fractures of the lateral malleolus but also for ligament reconstruction and repair of dislocating peroneal tendons.

The patient is placed in supine position with a

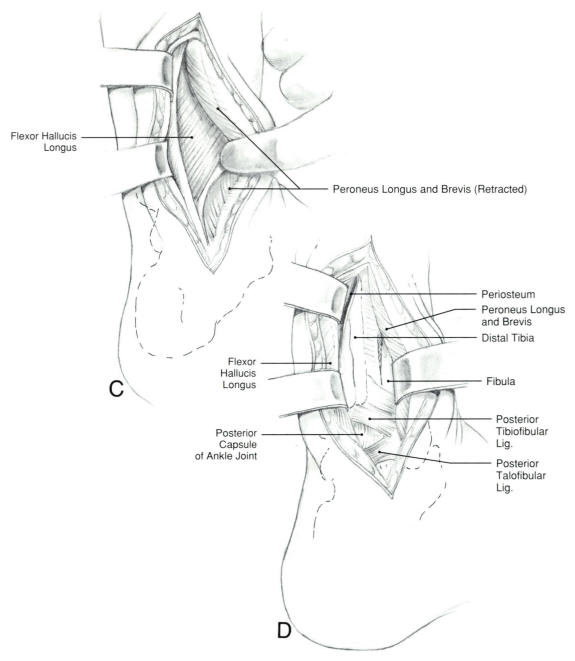

FIG 13–32   (cont.).
C, the fascia over the peroneal tendons has been incised and the tendons retracted laterally. This exposes the fibers of the flexor hallucis longus. **D,** the flexor hallucis longus is dissected off the fibula to expose the posterior capsule of the ankle joint.

bolster under the ipsilateral hip. The incision is made along the posterior margin of the fibula, curving slightly anterior distally to end below the tip of the lateral malleolus (Fig 13–33). The skin flaps are elevated carefully to protect the lesser saphenous vein and sural nerve, which lie posterior to the malleolus, and the superficial peroneal nerve, which lies anterior to the malleolus. The deep fascia and peri-

osteum are incised over the lateral aspect of the fibula to expose as much of the bone as required.

Approach to the Medial Malleolus

Approaches to the medial malleolus are used primarily for reduction and fixation of fractures. Either an anterior or posterior skin incision can be

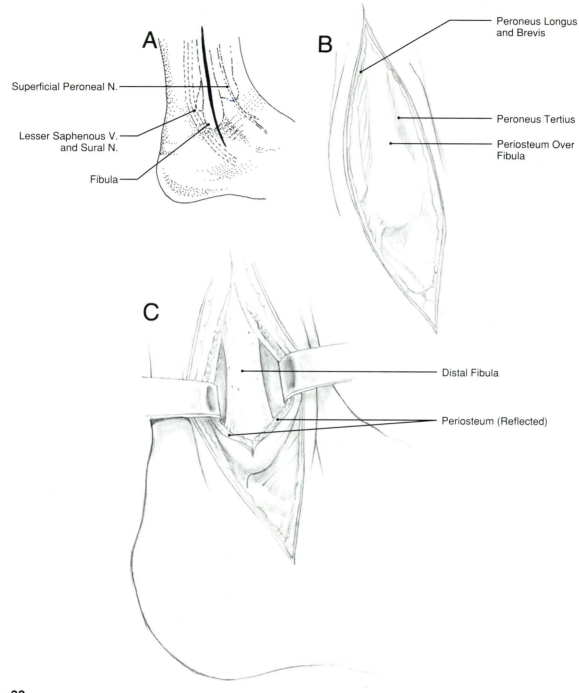

FIG 13–33.
Approach to the lateral malleolus. **A,** the skin incision is made directly over the fibula. **B** and **C,** since the fibula is a subcutaneous bone, the deep fascia and periosteum can be split in line with the skin incision to expose the bone.

used. The anterior incision allows inspection of the anteromedial ankle joint, while the posterior incision permits visualization of the posterior margin of the tibia.

With either incision the patient is positioned in supine position with a bolster under the contralat-

eral hip. The anterior incision is longitudinally curved over the anterior third of the malleolus, with its midpoint at the tip of the malleolus (Fig 13–34). The skin flaps are mobilized with care to identify and protect the saphenous nerve and greater saphenous vein located anterior to the malleolus. The sa-

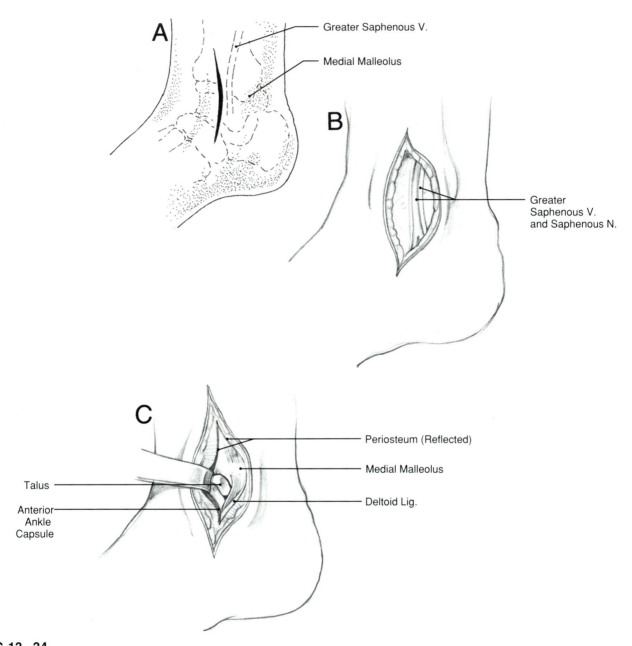

FIG 13–34.
Approach to the medial malleolus with an anterior incision. **A** and **B,** the skin incision is made anterior to the medial malleolus. Care is taken to protect the greater saphenous vein and branches of the saphenous nerve. **C,** the periosteum over the malle- olus is split to expose the bone. The anterior capsule of the ankle joint is incised to expose the talus.

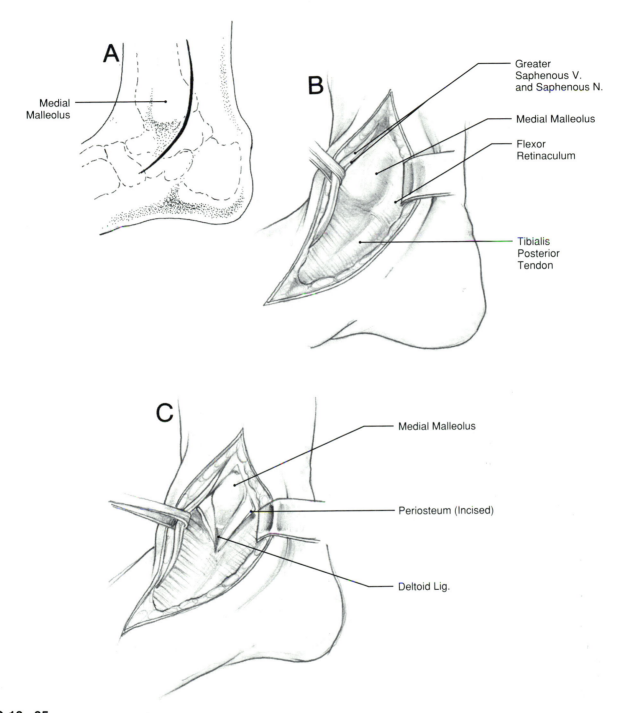

FIG 13—35.
Approach to the medial malleolus with a posterior incision. **A** and **B,** the skin incision is curved posterior to the medial malleolus. The anterior flap is elevated. Care is taken to protect the greater saphenous vein and saphenous nerve. **C,** the periosteum over the medial malleolus is split to expose the bone. If dissection is carried out posterior to the malleolus, the tibialis posterior tendon and neurovascular bundle must be protected.

phenous nerve is small and often in two branches closely bound to the vein. The periosteum over the malleolus is split longitudinally to expose the bone. A small incision in the anterior joint capsule can be made through which to inspect the joint or check the reduction of a fracture. If internal fixation is to be placed through the tip of the malleolus, the fibers of the deltoid ligament can be split longitudinally.

The posterior incision starts 5 cm proximal to the malleolus at the posterior border of the tibia (Fig 13–35). It then curves distally behind the tip of the malleolus to end approximately 5 cm distal to the malleolus. The skin flaps are elevated and the periosteum over the malleolus incised to expose the bone. Care must be taken not to injure the tibialis posterior tendon, which lies immediately posterior to the malleolus. If greater exposure of the posterior aspect of the malleolus is required, it is best to incise the flexor retinaculum and retract the tibialis posterior tendon anteriorly. The dissection posterior to the malleolus should be carried out close to the bone to avoid injury to the flexor digitorum longus tendon, posterior tibial artery, or tibial nerve.

SURGICAL APPROACHES TO THE FOOT

Lateral Approach to the Talocalcaneonavicular Joint

Several incisions can be used for exposure of the hindfoot, two of which will be described here. These approaches are primarily used to perform corrective osteotomy or triple arthrodesis.

The patient is positioned supine with a bolster under the ipsilateral hip. The incision starts 2 cm distal and posterior to the lateral malleolus and extends across the dorsum of the foot to the talocalcaneonavicular joint (Fig 13–36). Care is taken to protect the sural nerve in the posterior aspect of the wound and branches of the superficial peroneal nerve in the anterior portion of the wound. The sheaths of the peroneal tendons are opened and the tendons retracted in a plantar direction. The tendons of the extensor digitorum longus and the peroneus tertius are retracted dorsally to expose the fat in the sinus tarsi. Excision of this fibrofatty tissue exposes the lateral aspect of the talocalcaneonavicular joint. The origin of the extensor digitorum brevis can be elevated off the calcaneus with sharp dissection to expose the talonavicular and calcaneocuboid articulations.

A second incision for lateral exposure of the talo-

calcaneonavicular joint starts at the level of the ankle joint, 1 cm anterior to the lateral malleolus, and extends to the cuboid–fifth metatarsal joint (Fig 13–37). The deep fascia and inferior extensor retinaculum are incised and the tendons of the extensor digitorum longus and peroneus tertius retracted dorsally. Branches of the superficial peroneal nerve are also protected and retracted. The fatty tissue is removed from the sinus tarsi to expose the talocalcaneonavicular joint. The extensor digitorum brevis is sharply dissected off the calcaneus to expose the talonavicular and calcaneocuboid articulations. It is often unnecessary to expose the peroneal tendons with this approach. Although this alternative incision seems to heal better than the previously described approach, it provides less exposure of the posterior talocalcaneal articulation. It is useful for an in situ or inlay triple arthrodesis for which removal of a wedge of bone from the posterior subtalar joint is not required.

Lateral Approach to the Talocalcaneal Joint

This approach allows complete exposure of the subtalar joint, including the posterior facet. It is used primarily for subtalar arthrodesis when exposure of the talocalcaneonavicular joint complex is unnecessary.

The patient is placed in supine position with a bolster under the ipsilateral hip. The incision starts just distal and posterior to the tip of the lateral malleolus and extends distally over the sinus tarsi (Fig 13–38). The deep fascia is incised in line with the skin incision. Care is taken not to injure the peroneal tendons in the proximal aspect of the incision or the peroneus tertius and extensor digitorum longus tendons in the distal aspect. The tendons of the peroneus tertius and extensor digitorum longus are retracted dorsally to expose the fat in the sinus tarsi and the origin of the extensor digitorum brevis. The fat is excised or retracted dorsally to expose the sinus tarsi and the anterior aspect of the subtalar joint. If more distal exposure is required, the origin of the extensor digitorum brevis can be sharply dissected off the calcaneus and reflected distally. To expose the posterior facet of the talus the peroneal retinaculum is incised and the peroneal tendons retracted dorsally. This exposes the capsule over the posterior facet, which can then be incised to expose the joint.

Lateral Approach to the Calcaneus

The lateral approach to the calcaneus is used primarily for osteotomies and fixation of calcaneal frac-

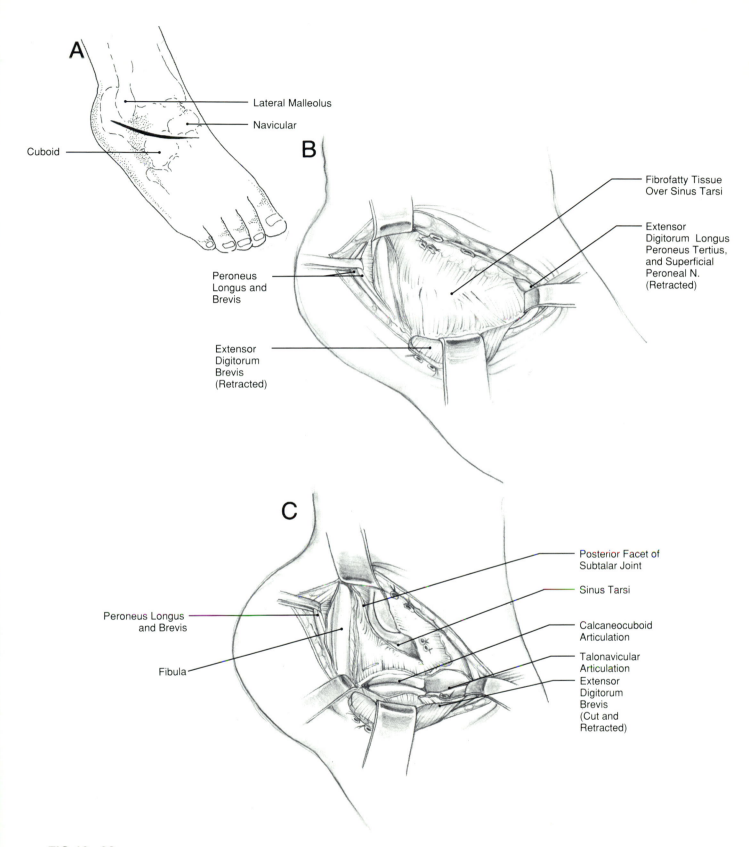

FIG 13–36.
Lateral approach to the talocalcaneonavicular joint. **A,** the skin incision starts distal to the fibula and extends obliquely over the midfoot. **B,** the superficial peroneal nerve and extensor tendons are retracted medially. The peroneal tendon sheaths are opened and the tendons retracted laterally along with the sural nerve. **C,** the fatty tissue is excised from the sinus tarsi to expose the posterior facet of the talocalcaneal (subtalar) joint. The extensor digitorum brevis is elevated sharply off the calcaneus and retracted distally to expose the calcaneocuboid and talonavicular articulations.

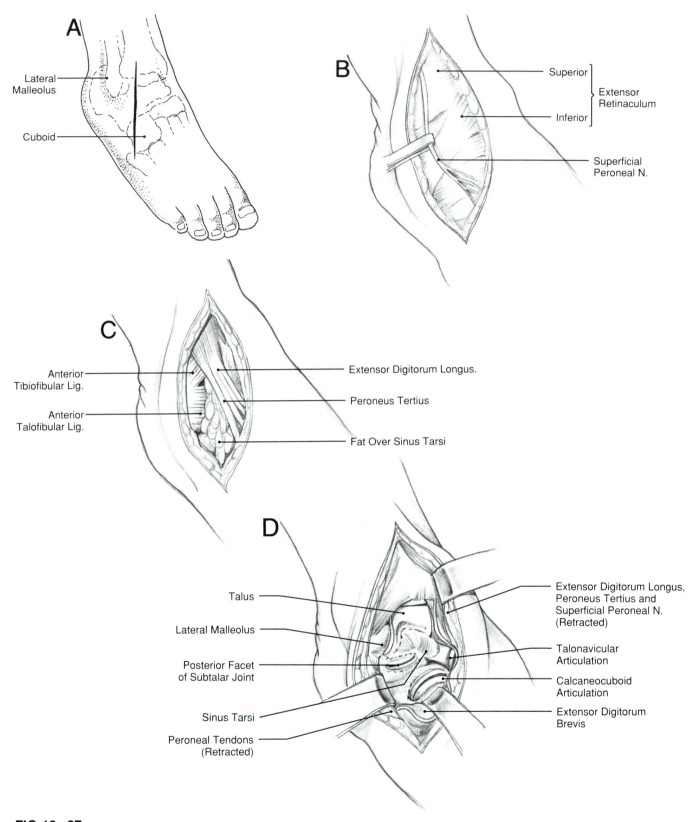

FIG 13–37.
Alternative incision for lateral approach to the talocalcaneonavicular joint. **A,** the incision starts anterior to the fibula and extends to the base of the fifth metatarsal. **B,** the superficial peroneal nerve is identified. **C,** the extensor retinaculum is incised to expose the extensor digitorum longus and peroneus tertius. **D,** the extensor digitorum longus, peroneus tertius, and superficial peroneal nerve are retracted dorsally. The fat is removed from the sinus tarsi to expose the talocalcaneal (subtalar) joint. The talonavicular and calcaneocuboid articulations are exposed by elevation and retraction of the extensor digitorum brevis distally.

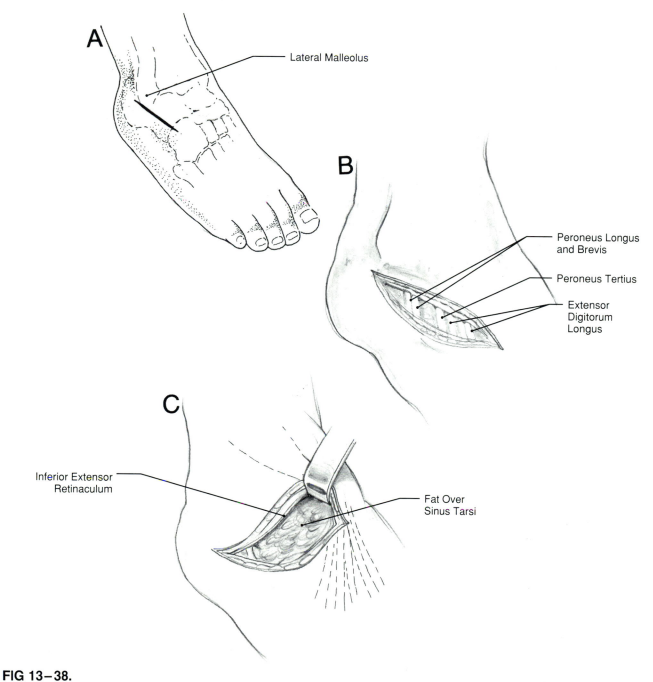

FIG 13–38.
Lateral approach to the talocalcaneal joint. **A,** the incision starts distal to the fibula and extends over the sinus tarsi. **B** and **C,** the extensor digitorum longus and peroneus tertius are retracted dorsally to expose the fat over the sinus tarsi.

(Continued.)

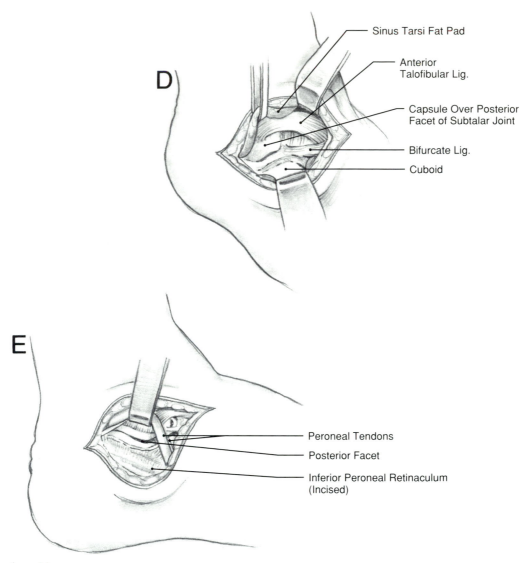

FIG 13–38 (cont.).
D, the fat over the sinus tarsi is elevated to expose the capsule of the subtalar joint and sinus tarsi. **E,** to expose the entire aspect of the posterior facet, the peroneal tendons are retracted dorsally.

tures. If a limited osteotomy is planned, only the center of the incision is utilized. The whole incision is used to visualize the entire lateral aspect of the calcaneus, which may be necessary for reduction of complex fractures.

The patient is placed in supine position with a bolster under the ipsilateral hip. The incision starts proximal to the ankle joint and posterior to the peroneal tendons (Fig 13–39). It is curved over the tuberosity of the calcaneus and continued along the inferior aspect of the calcaneus to the calcaneocuboid joint. If only limited exposure of the calcaneus is required, the incision is less curved and more oblique. The skin flaps are elevated carefully to protect the lesser saphenous vein and sural nerve, which are usually located anterior to the skin incision. The

deep fascia and periosteum are split in line with the incision to expose the calcaneus. If more exposure is needed, the anterior flap (including the peroneal tendons and their sheaths) is elevated off the lateral calcaneus with sharp subperiosteal dissection. This will expose the calcaneus as far dorsally as the posterior facet and as far distally as the calcaneocuboid joint. The large anterior skin flap should be kept as broad and thick as possible to prevent skin necrosis.

Approach to the Talocalcaneal Middle Facet

This approach is used for exploration of the middle facet or excision of a talocalcaneal middle facet coalition.

The patient is placed supine with a bolster

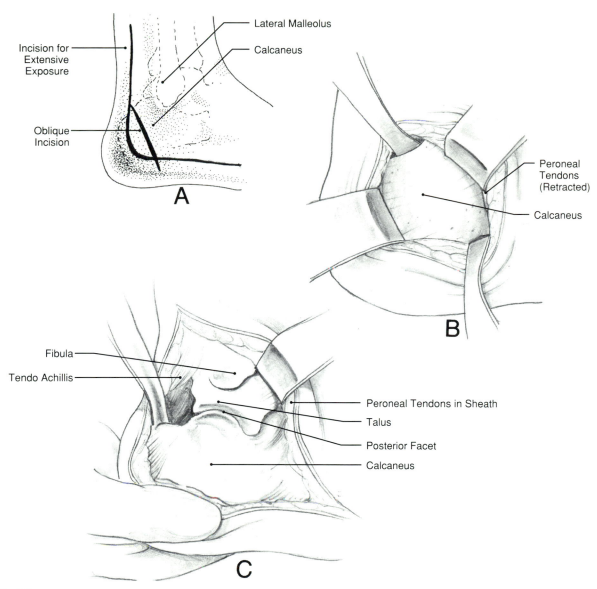

FIG 13–39.
Lateral approach to the calcaneus. **A,** for limited exposure a short oblique incision is used. A long curved incision is used for more extensive exposure. **B,** with the short oblique incision, dissection can be carried down to the calcaneus. The peroneal tendons are retracted anteriorly. **C,** for extensile exposure the anterior flap, including the peroneal tendons in their sheaths, is elevated from the calcaneus. The flap can be elevated off the entire lateral aspect of the calcaneus, but must be retracted gently to prevent skin necrosis.

under the contralateral hip. The skin incision is approximately 6 cm long, centered over the sustentaculum tali (Fig 13–40). The abductor hallucis is reflected plantarward from its calcaneal origin and the flexor retinaculum incised. The flexor digitorum longus tendon and neurovascular bundle (posterior tibial artery and tibial nerve) are identified and protected. The middle facet of the talocalcaneal joint is located between these structures and can be visualized by incision of the capsule and periosteum. The sustentaculum tali, with the flexor hallu-

cis longus tendon running below it, is located inferior to the middle facet.

Medial Approach to the Midtarsal Joints

The approach to the medial aspect of the midfoot is used primarily for capsulorrhaphy, arthrodesis, and medial release of metatarsus adductus. The skin incision can be an extension of the medial approach to the ankle or the Cincinnati clubfoot incision (see below).

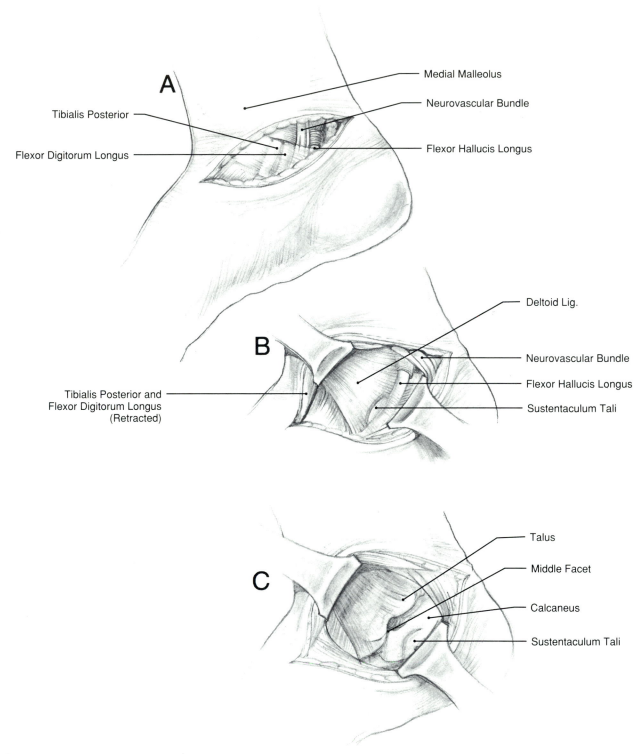

FIG 13–40.
Approach to the talocalcaneal middle facet. **A,** incision through the skin and subcutaneous tissue is made distal to the medial malleolus. The flexor digitorum longus and neurovascular bundle are identified. **B,** the flexor digitorum longus is retracted dorsally and the neurovascular bundle plantarward. The middle facet is located in this interval just superior to the sustentaculum tali. The flexor hallucis longus tendon can be identified where it passes under the sustentaculum. **C,** the periosteum and joint capsule are elevated to expose the talocalcaneal middle facet joint.

The patient is placed in supine position with the leg externally rotated. The incision starts posterior and distal to the medial malleolus, extends distally over the navicular and along the medial aspect of the first metatarsal, and ends at the level of the first MP joint (Fig 13–41). The skin flaps are elevated and the abductor hallucis muscle is released from its origin on the calcaneus and reflected plantarward. This exposes the tendon sheaths of the flexor digitorum longus and flexor hallucis longus, along with the reinforcing ligament (the master knot of Henry) that binds them together. The tendon sheaths and reinforcing ligament can be incised if exposure of these tendons is necessary. Care must be taken to identify and protect the medial plantar nerve, which runs between the abductor hallucis and flexor hallucis brevis. To expose the midtarsal joints, the muscle belly of the flexor hallucis brevis is also reflected

plantarward and the tendon of the tibialis posterior identified where it inserts on the navicular. The navicular-cuneiform and first tarsometatarsal joints are located just distal to this and are exposed by incision of the joint capsules. To expose the talonavicular articulation it may be necessary to tenotomize the tendon of the tibialis posterior with a Z-shaped cut. This exposes the capsule of the talonavicular joint, which can then be incised.

Cincinnati Incision

The Cincinnati incision provides excellent exposure of the posterior, medial, and lateral aspects of the hindfoot, as well as the medial and lateral aspects of the midfoot. It is used primarily for soft-tissue release of clubfoot deformities.

The patient is placed in prone position on the

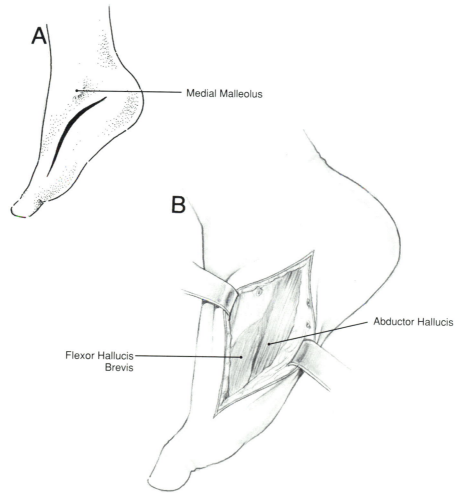

FIG 13–41.
Medial approach to the midtarsal joints. **A** and **B**, the skin incision is made over the medial aspect of the foot, and the abductor hallucis muscle is identified.
(Continued.)

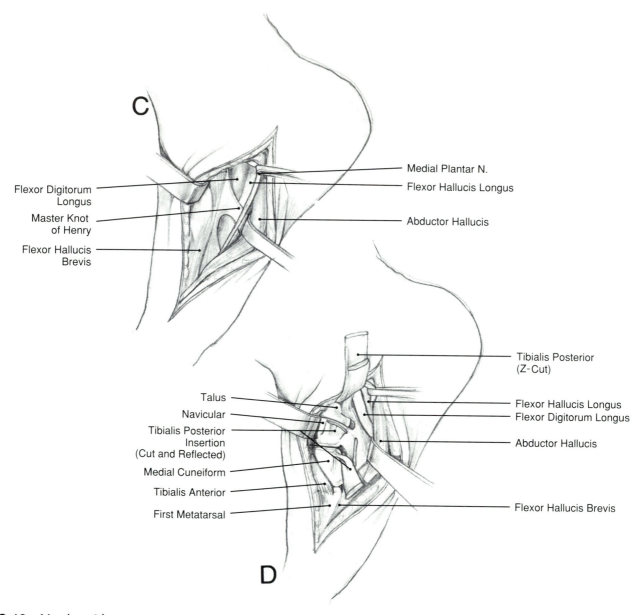

FIG 13–41 (cont.).
C, the abductor hallucis is retracted plantarward to expose the flexor digitorum longus and flexor hallucis longus. Care must be taken to protect the medial plantar nerve, which runs between the abductor hallucis and the flexor hallucis brevis. **D,** to expose the midtarsal joints, the flexor hallucis brevis is also retracted plantarward. The tibialis posterior tendon is tenotomized to increase the exposure.

operating table. The skin incision starts on the medial aspect of the first MP joint and extends proximally along the medial side of the foot parallel to the sole (Fig 13–42). The incision continues around the posterior aspect of the hindfoot, just proximal to the heel crease. It continues along the lateral side of the foot to end at the level of the calcaneocuboid joint. It may be extended across the cuboid if necessary.

The dissection is done perpendicular to the skin incision. Care is taken to avoid undermining the

skin flaps. The tendo Achillis is exposed first and a Z-shaped tenotomy performed. This exposes the capsules of the posterior ankle and subtalar joints, which then may be incised to allow visualization of the joints. The dissection is continued on the lateral aspect of the hindfoot, where the sural nerve and peroneal tendons are identified. The entire lateral capsule of the subtalar joint can be visualized and incised. The peroneal tendon sheaths are adherent to this lateral capsule, and if they also have to be in-

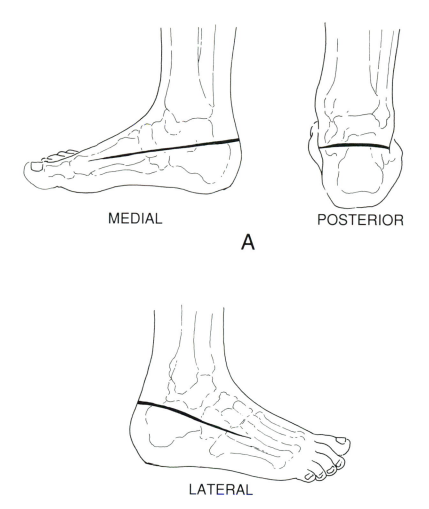

MEDIAL   POSTERIOR

A

LATERAL

FIG 13–42.
The Cincinnati incision. **A,** the incision starts over the first metatarsal and extends around the posterior aspect of the foot just distal to the medial and lateral malleoli. The incision can be extended across the cuboid, if necessary.

(Continued.)

cised the tendons are protected by lateral retraction.

On the medial side of the foot the neurovascular bundle (tibial nerve and posterior tibial artery) is identified as it courses behind the medial malleolus. The sheaths of the tibialis posterior and flexor digitorum longus are identified anterior to the neurovascular bundle, and the tendon of the flexor hallucis longus is identified posterior to it. The tendon sheaths are opened to expose the tendons, which can be tenotomized with a Z-shaped cut to increase the exposure or for lengthening. Retraction of the flexor hallucis longus tendon and neurovascular bundle anteriorly allows exposure of the posteromedial corner of the ankle and subtalar joints. If incision of the capsule of the subtalar joint in this area is necessary, care must be taken to not injure the tendon of the flexor hallucis longus, which courses very close to the capsule as it runs under the sustentaculum tali. After tenotomy of the tibialis posterior and

flexor digitorum longus are performed, the talonavicular and talocalcaneal articulations can be exposed on the medial side of the foot. Release and retraction of the origin of the abductor hallucis plantarward allow the flexor digitorum longus tendon to be followed to the point at which it crosses the tendon of the flexor hallucis longus (master knot of Henry). Care must be taken with dissection in this area to protect the medial plantar nerve, which runs parallel to the flexor digitorum longus tendon. Further dissection just inferior to the talonavicular joint exposes the medial aspect of the calcaneocuboid joint.

The skin incision can be extended down to the level of the first MP joint. Continued plantar retraction of the abductor hallucis and flexor hallucis brevis exposes the first tarsometatarsal and cuneonavicular joints. If these joints are to be released, the tendon of the tibialis anterior, which inserts on the first cuneiform and base of the first metatarsal, must

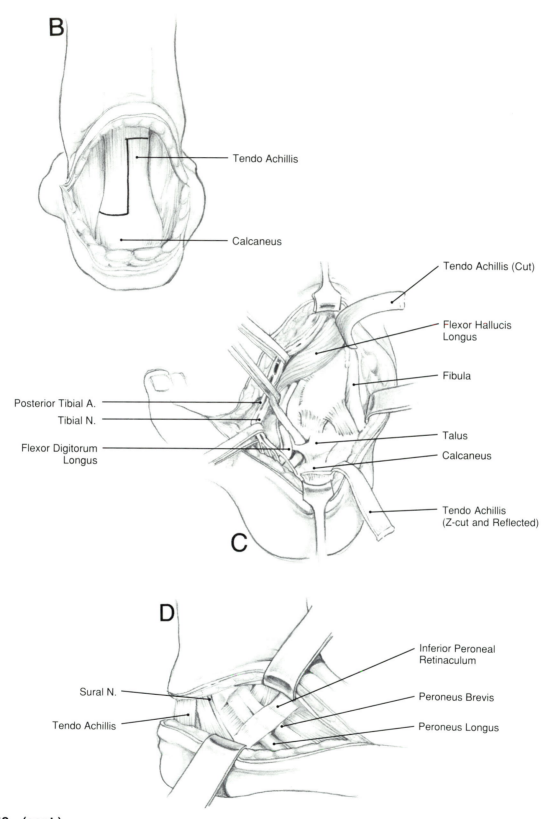

FIG 13–42 (cont.).
B, posteriorly, the tendo Achillis is cut with a Z-shaped incision. **C,** retracting the ends of the tendo Achillis will expose the posterior ankle and subtalar joints. If the subtalar joint is to be released, care is taken not to injure the tendon of the flexor hallucis longus. **D,** the dissection is continued around the lateral aspect of the foot, first exposing the peroneal tendons and sural nerve.

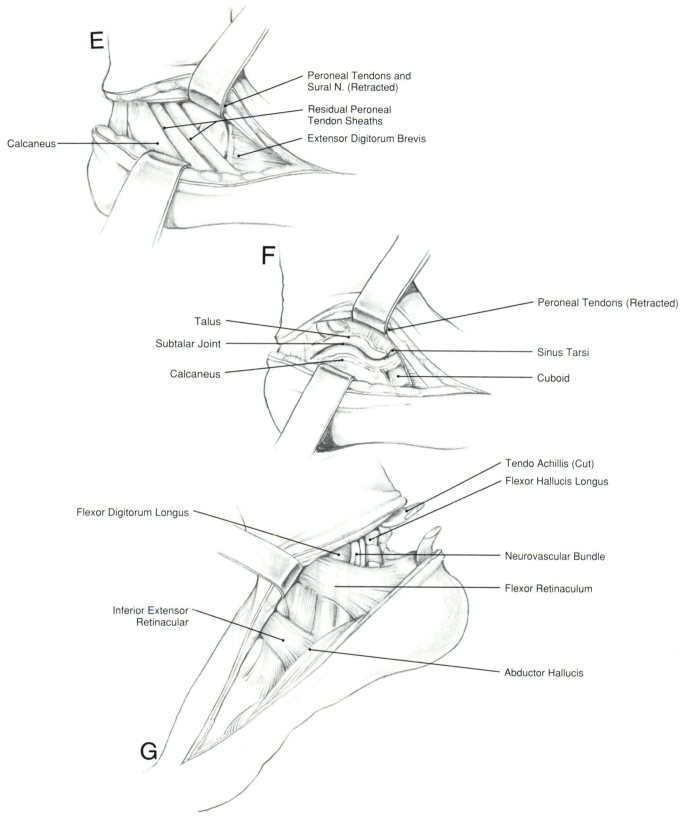

FIG 13–42 (cont.).
E and **F,** the peroneal tendons and sural nerve are retracted dorsally to expose the entire lateral aspect of the subtalar joint and sinus tarsi. **G,** the dissection is continued along the medial aspect of the foot. First the neurovascular bundle and flexor tendons are identified.

(Continued.)

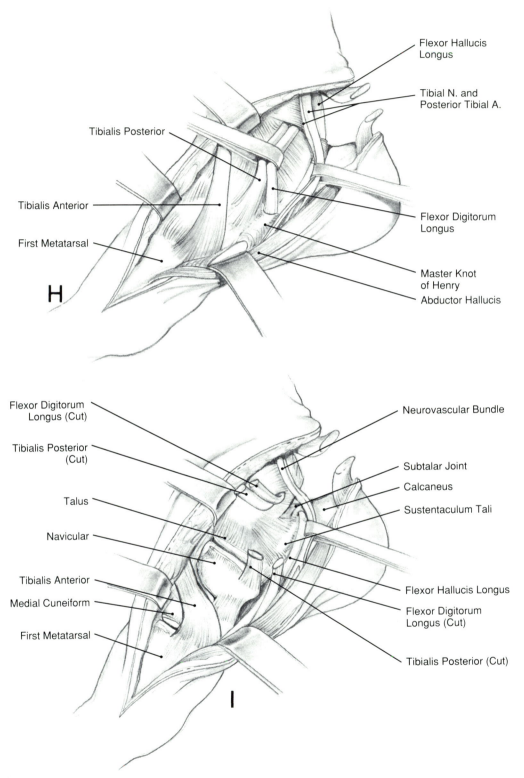

FIG 13–42 (cont.).
H, the abductor hallucis is retracted plantarward, exposing the master knot of Henry. **I,** the tibialis posterior and flexor digitorum longus tendons can be tenotomized to increase the exposure and reattached later. All of the midtarsal joints can be exposed by incision of their respective joint capsules.

be protected. In the distal aspect of the incision the tendinous portion of the abductor hallucis can be identified.

Dorsal Approach to the Midfoot

This approach is utilized to expose the tarsal joints of the midfoot and the tarsometatarsal joints. It is used primarily for midfoot osteotomies and treatment of foot fracture-dislocations. The trans-

verse incision is described here, although two longitudinal incisions over the medial and lateral dorsal aspect of the foot may be used.

The patient is positioned supine and a transverse incision is made over the cuneiforms (Fig 13–43). The branches of the superficial peroneal nerve, as well as the greater saphenous vein and nerve, which are located in the medial aspect of the incision, are protected. The deep fascia is incised in line with the skin incision, and the deep peroneal

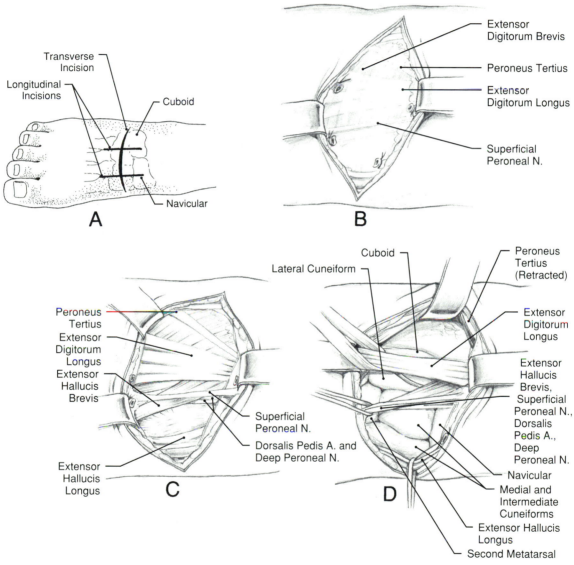

FIG 13–43.

Dorsal approach to the midfoot. **A,** the midfoot can be approached by either a transverse or two longitudinal incisions. **B** and **C,** if the transverse incision is used, the extensor digitorum longus and peroneus tertius are retracted laterally while the extensor hallucis longus, saphenous nerve and, if possible, the greater saphenous vein are retracted medially. The branches of the superficial peroneal nerve, along with the extensor hallucis brevis, dorsalis pedis artery, and deep peroneal nerve, are identified in the center of the wound and elevated. **D,** the periosteum and capsule are elevated off the joints that are to be exposed. (Modified from Bauer R, Kerschbaumer F, Poisel S: *Operative Approaches in Orthopedic Surgery and Traumatology.* New York, Thieme Medical Publishers, 1987.)

nerve and dorsalis pedis artery are located as they run along the medial border of the extensor hallucis brevis. The muscle belly of the extensor digitorum brevis and the tendon of the peroneus tertius are retracted laterally. The tendon of the extensor hallucis longus and the saphenous nerve and vein are retracted medially. The extensor hallucis brevis, dorsalis pedis artery, and deep peroneal nerve are retracted as a group, either medially or laterally. The tendons of the extensor digitorum longus can also be retracted in either direction to allow complete exposure of the periosteum of the midtarsal bones. The periosteum and joint capsules are incised to expose the bones and joints as necessary. The lateral tarsal artery is often encountered crossing the operative field and can be ligated.

Dorsomedial Approach to the First Metatarsophalangeal Joint

The dorsomedial approach to the MP joint of the first toe can be used for most operations on this joint. This approach is used primarily in the treatment of hallux valgus and hallux rigidus and for arthrodesis of the first MP joint. In the treatment of hallux valgus the approach is often combined with a

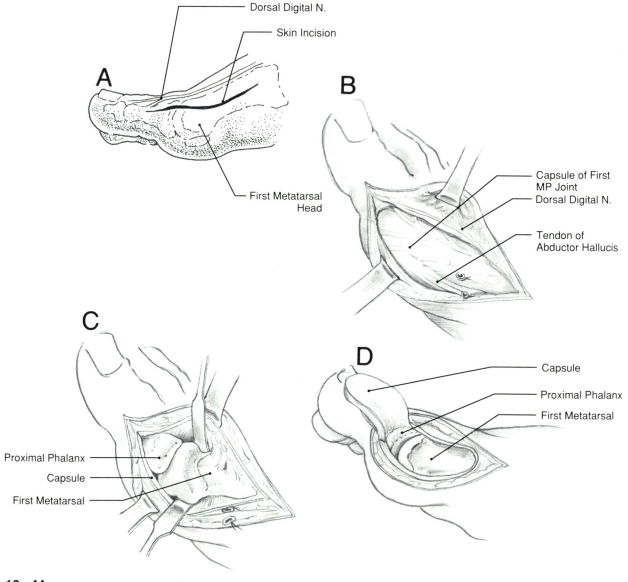

FIG 13–44.
Dorsomedial approach to the first metatarsophalangeal joint. **A,** the skin incision is made over the dorsomedial aspect of the first MP joint. Care is taken to protect the dorsal digital nerve. **B,** the incision is made directly down to the joint capsule to keep the skin flaps as thick as possible. **C,** the capsule can be opened in line with the skin incision or as a distally based flap **(D).**

separate incision over the first dorsal web space.

The patient is placed in the supine position. The skin incision extends approximately 6 cm over the dorsomedial aspect of the MP joint (Fig 13–44). To keep the flaps as thick as possible, dissection is car-ried down to the joint capsule before the skin flaps are elevated. Care is taken to protect the dorsal dig-ital nerve under the dorsal skin flap. The joint cap-sule can be incised transversely, longitudinally, or as a distally based flap, depending upon the operation.

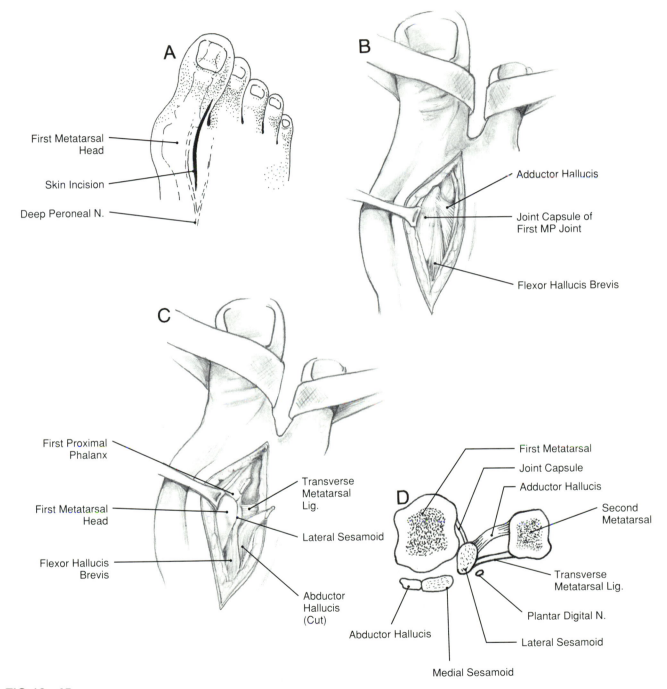

FIG 13–45.
Dorsal approach to the first web space. **A,** the skin incision is made over the first web space. Care is taken not to injure the dorsal digital nerves. **B,** dissection is carried down between the metatarsal heads, and the tendon of the adductor hallucis is identified. **C,** the adductor tendon can be detached from the proximal phalanx and the joint capsule opened to expose the MP joint. **D,** deep to the adductor tendon is the deep transverse metatarsal ligament which is incised with care to protect the un-derlying plantar digital nerve. (Modified from Goldstein LA, Dickerson RC: *Atlas of Orthopaedic Surgery.* ed 2. St Louis, CV Mosby Co, 1981.)

This will completely expose the MP joint. The skin incision can be extended proximally along the first metatarsal if a proximal osteotomy is planned.

Dorsal Approach to the First Web Space

This approach is used to expose the lateral capsule of the first MP joint and the adductor hallucis muscle. It is often used in combination with the dorsomedial approach in the treatment of hallux valgus.

The patient is placed in the supine position. A dorsal incision is made in the first intermetatarsal space (Fig 13–45). If a dorsomedial incision is also to be used, an adequate skin bridge should be planned to prevent skin necrosis. Dissection is carried down between the metatarsal heads. The branches of the

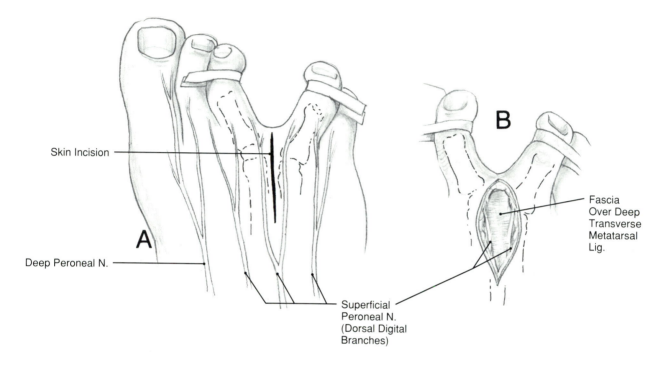

Skin Incision

Deep Peroneal N.

A

B

Fascia Over Deep Transverse Metatarsal Lig.

Superficial Peroneal N. (Dorsal Digital Branches)

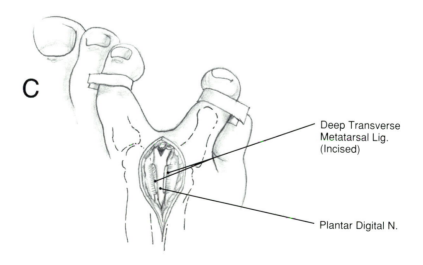

C

Deep Transverse Metatarsal Lig. (Incised)

Plantar Digital N.

FIG 13–46.
Dorsal approach to the second through fourth web spaces. **A** and **B**, the skin incision is made over the appropriate web space. Care is taken to avoid injury to the dorsal digital branches of the peroneal nerves. The deep transverse ligament is located between the metatarsal heads. **C**, the ligament is carefully incised to expose the underlying plantar digital nerve. (Modified from Hoppenfeld S, deBoer P: *Surgical Exposures in Orthopaedics: The Anatomic Approach.* Philadelphia, JB Lippincott Co, 1984.)

deep peroneal nerve, located on either side of the incision, are protected. The tendon of the adductor hallucis is located where it attaches to the capsule of the first MP joint and the base of the proximal phalanx. The tendon may be released to expose the lateral joint capsule, which may be incised to release or expose the MP joint. The transverse metatarsal ligament, which connects the fibular sesamoid to the second metatarsal head, is located deep to the adductor hallucis. If the ligament is to be incised, care

must be taken to protect the underlying plantar digital nerve and vessel.

Dorsal Approach to the Second Through Fourth Web Spaces

This approach is primarily used for excision of an interdigital neuroma. It can also be used for exploration and drainage of a web space infection.

The patient is placed in supine position with a

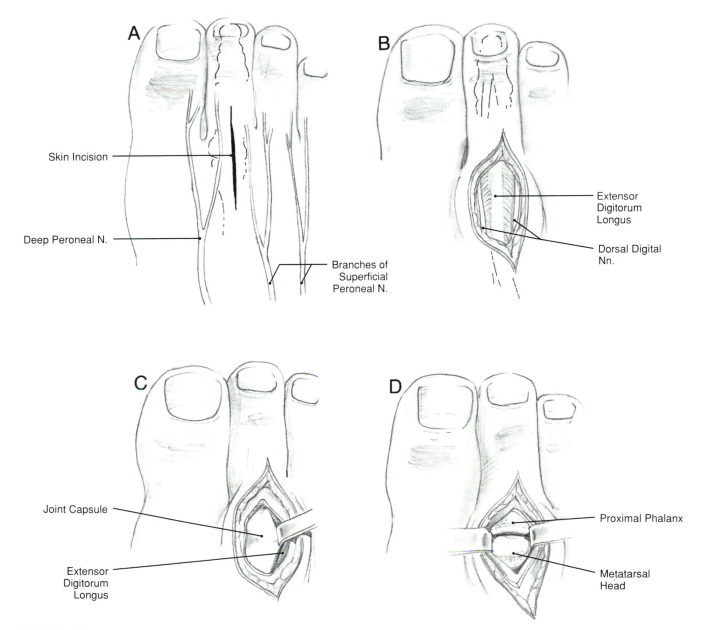

FIG 13–47.
Dorsal approach to the metatarsophalangeal joints of the lesser toes. **A** and **B,** the skin is incised over the selected MP joint. Care is taken to protect the superficial cutaneous nerves. **C** and **D,** the extensor digitorum longus tendon is retracted to the side and the joint capsule opened transversely. (Modified from Hoppenfeld S, deBoer P: *Surgical Exposures in Orthopaedics: the Anatomic Approach.* Philadelphia, JB Lippincott Co, 1984.)

bolster under the knee to allow the foot to lie with its plantar surface on the table. A dorsal incision is centered over the web space starting at the distal end of the web and continuing proximally about 3 cm (Fig 13–46). Dissection is carried down to the transverse metatarsal ligament. Care is taken to protect any dorsal cutaneous nerves. The metatarsal heads are retracted apart, and the transverse metatarsal ligament is incised in line with the skin incision to expose the underlying plantar digital nerve.

Dorsal Approach to the Metatarsophalangeal Joints of the Lesser Toes

This approach is used for exposure or release of the MP joints of the lesser toes. It can also be used for excision of the metatarsal heads or partial proximal phalangectomy.

The patient is placed in supine position with a bolster under the knee. A 2 to 3 cm incision is made over the affected metatarsal head just lateral to the extensor digitorum longus tendon (Fig 13–47). The deep fascia is incised and the extensor digitorum longus tendon retracted. If the dissection is centered over the metatarsal head, the digital nerves and vessels should be on either side of the approach. The dorsal capsule of the MP joint is located deep to the extensor tendon and incised longitudinally to expose the joint.

ANKLE ARTHROSCOPY

Stephen W. Munns, M.D.
Frederick W. Reckling, M.D.

Although diagnostic and operative ankle arthroscopy are still in the developmental stages, when properly performed they can allow direct visualization of intraarticular and intracapsular structures without the need for a wide arthrotomy. Arthroscopy has been advocated for evaluation of the persistently symptomatic traumatic ankle; ankle impingement syndromes; evaluation, debridement, or curettage of chondral or osteochondral defects of the talus or tibial plafond; removal of loose bodies; excision of osteophytes from the medial or lateral malleoli, distal tibia, or talus; partial synovectomy for chronic inflammatory disorders; and lysis of adhesions. Because of the close proximity of tendons and superficial and deep neurovascular structures, the placement of ankle arthroscopy entry portals has a greater potential to cause injury than in other joints.

Ankle arthroscopy can be carried out with the patient under local, spinal, epidural, or general anesthesia. Patient positioning is a matter of the surgeon's preference. Most procedures can be carried out without use of a tourniquet, unless profuse bleeding obscures the operative field. Guhl has developed an ankle holder-distraction technique that greatly facilitates arthroscopic visualization by increasing the space between the talus and tibia. The technic of ankle arthroscopy is much the same as for other joints.

The most commonly used entry sites in ankle arthroscopy are the anterolateral, anteromedial, and anterocentral portals. In addition, posterolateral, posteromedial, and more recently, trans–tendo Achillis portals have been described. Regardless of the entry site utilized, the surgeon must be familiar with the local anatomy. The initial incision should be made vertically just through the skin itself, and the underlying subcutaneous tissue, which contains the cutaneous nerves, should be gently spread apart with a hemostat. Careful visual inspection must be done to ensure that deeper neurovascular structures are not injured, although proper attention to the area of portal placement should avoid these structures. Care must be exercised in penetrating the joint capsule to prevent injury to the articular cartilage.

Anterolateral Portal

The anterolateral portal is placed, according to standard technique, at the level of the joint line just lateral to the well-defined tendon of the peroneus tertius (Fig 13–48). However, the intermediate dorsal cutaneous nerve may be vulnerable to injury with this approach. The lateral branch of the superficial peroneal nerve divides into the intermediate and lateral dorsal cutaneous nerves just proximal to the ankle joint. The lateral dorsal cutaneous nerve generally lies out of the way of the arthroscope, over the anterior aspect of the lateral malleolus. The intermediate branch, however, is vulnerable to injury as it courses just anterior to the malleolus, close to the peroneus tertius tendon. It can usually be palpated or visualized by plantar flexion and eversion of the foot. Injury to this nerve may result in a painful neuroma and/or hypesthesia over the dorsal as-

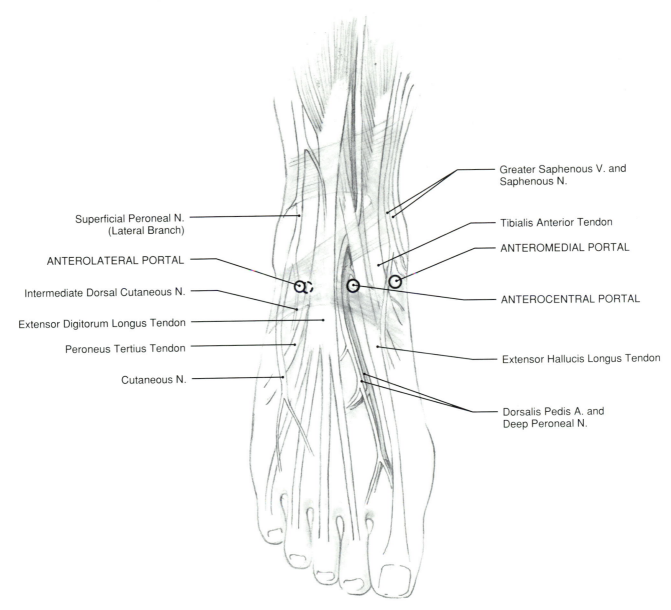

Superficial Peroneal N. (Lateral Branch)

ANTEROLATERAL PORTAL

Intermediate Dorsal Cutaneous N.

Extensor Digitorum Longus Tendon

Peroneus Tertius Tendon

Cutaneous N.

Greater Saphenous V. and Saphenous N.

Tibialis Anterior Tendon

ANTEROMEDIAL PORTAL

ANTEROCENTRAL PORTAL

Extensor Hallucis Longus Tendon

Dorsalis Pedis A. and Deep Peroneal N.

FIG 13–48.
Anterior arthroscopic portals. Note modification of anterolateral portal *(dashed circle)* advocated by Voto.

pect of the lateral toes. Because of this anatomical arrangement, and based upon cadaver studies, Voto has challenged the standard technique. Voto advises placing the anterolateral portal just medial to the peroneus tertius tendon to avoid injury to the intermediate dorsal cutaneous branch of the superficial peroneal nerve.

Anteromedial Portal

The anteromedial portal is placed at the level of the ankle joint line just medial to the tibialis anterior tendon (see Fig 13–48). Care must be taken when

this portal is established to avoid injury to the greater saphenous vein and nerve, which traverse the ankle joint along the anterior edge of the medial malleolus.

Anterocentral Portal

The anterocentral portal is placed just lateral to the tendon of the extensor hallucis longus at the level of the ankle joint (see Fig 13–48). Branches of the superficial peroneal nerve must be avoided in the superficial dissection. The dorsalis pedis artery and deep peroneal nerve are located deep in the interval between the extensor hallucis longus tendon and the medial border of the extensor digitorum longus tendon. This arrangement is somewhat variable. In some individuals the dorsalis pedis artery and deep peroneal nerve lie directly under the extensor hallucis longus at the joint line. Care must be taken to avoid injury to these structures when the antero-central portal is placed. If a tourniquet is to be used, the dorsalis pedis artery should be located by palpation and the skin marked before the tourniquet is inflated.

Posterolateral Portal

The posterolateral portal is placed immediately lateral to the border of the tendo Achillis, slightly proximal to the joint line (Fig 13–49). The short saphenous vein and branches of the sural nerve located in this area must be avoided. The peroneal

tendons are anterior to this portal entry site and should not be in jeopardy.

Posteromedial Portal

The posteromedial portal is placed just medial to the tendo Achillis, slightly proximal to the joint line (see Fig 13–49). The neurovascular bundle (posterior tibial vessels and tibial nerve) lie medial to this point. The flexor hallucis longus and flexor digitorum longus tendons lie directly anterior to the neurovascular bundle. In some individuals the medial calcaneal nerve may separate from the tibial nerve proximal to the ankle joint and run in the interval between the tibial nerve and tendo Achillis. Voto describes a constant communicating branch of the posterior tibial artery that is also in danger with this entry portal. With improved visualization anterior portals with distraction devices, or the trans-tendo

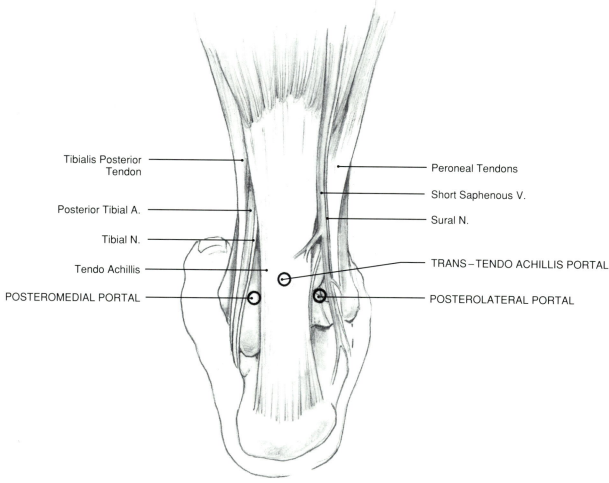

Tibialis Posterior Tendon

Posterior Tibial A.

Tibial N.

Tendo Achillis

POSTEROMEDIAL PORTAL

Peroneal Tendons

Short Saphenous V.

Sural N.

TRANS–TENDO ACHILLIS PORTAL

POSTEROLATERAL PORTAL

FIG 13–49.
Posterior arthroscopic portals.

Achillis portal described below, the posteromedial portal may become less commonly used.

Trans—Tendo Achillis Portal

A trans-tendo Achillis portal that allows visualization of the posterior aspect of the ankle joint has been described. (see Fig 13–49). It is much like the transpatellar tendon approach to the knee. A longitudinal incision is placed in the tendo Achillis at the level of the joint line. The fibers are split to allow central placement of the arthroscope. This portal appears to be safe based on cadaver studies, but the biomechanical implications for possible weakening of the tendo Achillis have not been established.

BIBLIOGRAPHY

Andrews JR, Previte WJ, Carson WG: Arthroscopy of the ankle: Technique and normal anatomy. *Foot Ankle* 1985; 6:29–33.

Banks SW, Laufman H: *An Atlas of Surgical Exposures of the Extremities.* Philadelphia, WB Saunders Co, 1953.

Bauer R, Kerschbaumer F, Poisel S: *Operative Approaches in Orthopedic Surgery and Traumatology.* New York, Thieme Medical Publishers Inc, 1987.

Berquist TH: *Radiology of the Foot and Ankle.* New York, Raven Press, 1989.

Carson WG, Andrews JR: Arthroscopy of the ankle. *Clin Sports Med,* 1987, 6:503–512.

Colonna PC, Ralston EL: Operative approaches to the ankle joint. *Am J Surg* 1951; 82:44–54.

Crawford AH, Marxen JL, Osterfeld DL: The Cincinnati incision: A comprehensive approach for surgical procedures of the foot and ankle in childhood. *J Bone Joint Surg* 1982; 64A:1355–1358.

Crenshaw AH: *Campbell's Operative Orthopaedics,* ed 7. St Louis, CV Mosby Co, 1987.

Drez D, Guhl JF, Gollehon DL: Ankle arthroscopy: Technique and indications. *Foot Ankle* 1981; 2:138–144.

Ferkel RD, Fischer SP: Progress in ankle arthroscopy. *Clin Orthop Rel Res* 1989; 240:210–220.

Giannestras NJ: *Foot Disorders: Medical and Surgical Management,* ed 2. Philadelphia, Lea & Febiger, 1973.

Goldstein LA, Dickerson RC: *Atlas of Orthopaedic Surgery,* ed 2. St Louis, CV Mosby Co, 1981.

Gould JS: *The Foot Book.* Baltimore, Williams & Wilkins Co, 1988.

Grant JCB: *Grant's Atlas of Anatomy,* ed 6. Baltimore, Williams & Wilkins Co, 1962.

Guhl JF: New concepts (distraction) in ankle arthroscopy. *Arthroscopy* 1988; 4:160–167.

Hackenbroch M, Witt AN (eds): *Surgery of the Lower Leg and Foot,* Philadelphia, WB Saunders Co, 1980.

Helal B, Wilson D: *The Foot,* New York, Churchill Livingstone, Inc, 1988.

Henry AK: *Extensile Exposure,* ed 2. New York, Churchill Livingstone, Inc, 1963.

Hollinshead WH: *The Back and Limbs,* Philadelphia, Harper & Row, 1982.

Hoppenfeld S, deBoer P: *Surgical Exposures in Orthopaedics: The Anatomic Approach,* Philadelphia, JB Lippincott Co, 1984.

Jahss MH: *Disorders of the Foot,* Philadelphia, WB Saunders Co, 1982.

Johnson LL: *Arthroscopic Surgery: Principles and Practice,* ed 3. St Louis, CV Mosby Co, 1986.

Kelikian H, Kelikian AS: *Disorders of the Ankle,* Philadelphia, WB Saunders Co, 1985.

Klenerman L: *The Foot and its Disorders,* ed 2. Oxford, Blackwell Scientific Publications, 1982.

Mann RA (ed): *Surgery of the Foot,* ed 5. St Louis, CV Mosby Co, 1986.

Martin DF, Baker CL, Curl WW, et al: Operative ankle arthroscopy: Long-term followup. *Am J Sports Med* 1989; 17:16–23.

Mitchell CL, Fleming JL, Allen R, et al: Osteotomy-bunionectomy for hallux valgus. *J Bone Joint Surg* 1958; 40A:41–60.

Moore KL: *Clinically Oriented Anatomy,* ed 2. Baltimore, Williams & Wilkins Co, 1985.

Netter FH: *The Ciba Collection of Medical Illustrations: Musculoskeletal System,* vol 8. Summit, NJ, Ciba-Geigy Corp, 1987.

Olney BW, Asher MA: Excision of symptomatic coalition of the middle facet of the talocalcaneal joint. *J Bone Joint Surg* 1987; 69A:539–544.

Parisien JS: Diagnostic and operative arthroscopy of the ankle: Technique and indications. *Bull Hosp J Dis Orthop Inst* 1985; 45:38–47.

Parisien JS, Shereff MJ: The role of arthroscopy in the diagnosis and treatment of disorders of the ankle. *Foot Ankle* 1981; 2:144–149.

Pritsch M, Horoshovski H, Farine I: Arthroscopic treatment of osteochondral lesions of the talus. *J Bone Joint Surg* 1986; 68A:862–864.

Romanes GJ: *Cunningham's Manual of Practical Anatomy, vol 1: Upper and Lower Limbs,* ed 14. New York, Oxford University Press, 1976.

Sarrafian SK: *Anatomy of the Foot and Ankle: Descriptive, Topographic, Functional.* Philadelphia, JB Lippincott Co, 1983.

Tachdjian MO: *The Child's Foot,* Philadelphia, WB Saunders Co, 1985.

Voto SJ, Ewing JW, Fleissner PR, et al: Ankle arthroscopy: Neurovascular and arthroscopic anatomy of standard and trans-achilles tendon portal placement. *Arthroscopy* 1989; 5:41–46.

Warwick R, Williams PL: *Gray's Anatomy,* ed 35. Philadelphia, WB Saunders Co, 1973.

PART V

Anatomy and Musculoskeletal Oncology

Overview

James R. Neff, M.D.

Neoplasms arising within the extremities, shoulder and pelvic girdle, axillary skeleton, and retroperitoneum comprise a broad spectrum of pathological entities. Knowledge of the natural history and growth characteristics of these lesions is required to properly understand the appropriate staging, biopsy, and management techniques for these patients. The first step in management is to establish a differential diagnosis. With the use of a thorough knowledge of three-dimensional compartmental anatomy and information obtained from the history, family history, physical, and radiographic findings, a biopsy can usually be planned and performed without contaminating vital structures or interfering with reconstruction options. However, if the surgeon is unfamiliar with the growth characteristics of the lesion and the concepts of compartmental anatomy, a simple error in biopsy incision placement or the injudicious exposure of neurovascular structures can render the limb or operative site unsuitable for definitive operative management or limb-preserving surgery.

A careful patient interview may elicit a history that will be helpful in describing the rapidity of growth of the lesion as well as its general location. The majority of soft tissue masses are painless unless they involve underlying neural structures or are in close proximity to underlying joints where capsular invasion may lead to a reactive synovitis. Physical examination may provide useful information about the location of the lesion, as well as its relationship and attachment to deep structures. Occasionally it will elucidate the structures of origin of the primary tumor (e.g., a neurogenic tumor arising within a major peripheral nerve).

For those primary tumors arising within bone, no obvious soft tissue mass may be evident; how-

ever, careful questioning may elicit a history of low-grade, poorly-localized pain, usually worse at night. Neoplasms that arise in bones of the upper extremity frequently are recognized by either local pain and tenderness, or the presence of a mass. Lesions arising in the axial and weight-bearing skeleton often erode and thin the cortex. When subjected to repeated stress, microfractures within the thinned cortex result, and a pathological fracture may ensue with minimal trauma. The occurrence of a displaced pathological fracture may have a detrimental effect on the course of the disease (contaminating multiple adjacent compartments) and thus profoundly alter management options.

Bone tumors metastasize primarily by vascular invasion, with pulmonary metastases being most common. Local lymph node involvement is less frequent unless the skin is involved by either direct extension or by surgical contamination of a biopsy incision. However, soft tissue tumors such as synovial sarcoma, epithelioid sarcoma, and clear cell sarcoma of the tendon sheath are known to produce a disproportionately high incidence of lymph node involvement. Thus, thorough physical examination of local lymph nodes should be performed as part of the preoperative staging evaluation.

RADIOGRAPHIC, SCINTIGRAPHIC, AND MAGNETIC RESONANCE (MR) IMAGING

As an integral part of the preoperative evaluation, a variety of imaging techniques are available to evaluate the location, extent, and possible metastatic spread of neoplasms arising in nonepithelioid structures. Plane radiographs may show the presence of a soft tissue mass in the extremity but are usually only helpful if the lesion is of a markedly different density than the surrounding tissue (e.g., lipoma), or if it produces calcifications (e.g., phlebolith formation in a hemangioma) that can be identified within the lesion. The most common radiographic finding related to neoplasms arising in bone is loss of trabeculation. Furthermore, some lesions produce a matrix that can be identified using conventional x-ray. Magnification techniques and polytomes may be used to enhance visualization of loss of trabeculation or identification of tumor matrix mineralization.

Bone scintigraphy may provide information about the primary lesion and assist in detection of metastatic disease. Early blood pool images may be helpful to evaluate the vascularity of the lesion, and later static studies commonly reveal the presence or absence of skeletal involvement. Although extraordinarily sensitive, bone scans are relatively nonspecific and commonly only localize areas of interest where other imaging techniques can be utilized to better understand the underlying process.

Computed axial tomography (CT/T) is helpful in evaluating soft tissue as well as bone lesions. For those lesions of soft tissue not isodense with muscle, or in lesions where calcifications are evident (i.e., hemangiomas, enchondromas, chondrosarcomas), CT/T may provide cross-sectional (axial) information about the lesion. Also, CT/T is the most efficacious method of evaluation for pulmonary metastases. When used in the dynamic mode, CT/T may provide useful information regarding the vascularity of the lesion. For soft tissue lesions isodense with muscle and for evaluation of extremity lesions in children where sufficient development of fatty soft tissue planes has not yet occurred, magnetic resonance is a superior imaging technique. When visualizing structures (e.g., retroperitoneal lymph nodes) in regions where breathing and peristaltic artifacts cannot be avoided, CT/T remains the study of choice.

Although originally thought to contribute mainly to imaging of the central nervous system, MR has proven to be exceptionally useful in imaging the skeletal system. Because of its increased contrast capabilities, in many circumstances MR imaging has surpassed CT/T in evaluating some bone and the majority of soft tissue neoplasms. However, CT/T is superior to MR in demonstrating punctate calcifications and some pathological fractures. MR has been shown to be superior to CT/T in evaluating and demonstrating the relationship of normal tissue to tumor (including neural structures), in evaluating the involvement of the medullary canal of long bones, and in documenting local recurrence. Because of the reactive edematous tissue surrounding most malignant soft tissue neoplasms, the pseudocapsule may often be delineated better with MR than with CT/T. Also, because of the additional ability to reconstruct images in the coronal as well as sagittal planes and with extraordinary contrast, the proximal and distal extent of the lesion can be better appreciated (e.g., lesions arising within the supraclavicular region).

Magnetic resonance imaging has also proven to be superior when monitoring for local recurrence in patients in whom *nonferromagnetic* fixation devices and implants have been used. Artifactual degradation of the image around such implants may be less bothersome with MR imaging than with CT/T.

BIOPSY GUIDELINES

The biopsy may be the most important procedure in managing patients with bone and soft tissue tumors.[1, 2, 3] In most instances, by using a combination of the historical, physical, and radiographic findings combined with a thorough knowledge of the natural history of the suspected lesion, the surgeon should be able to obtain sufficient tissue for diagnosis without rendering the patient inoperable for limb-preservation procedures. It is advisable to discuss the anticipated biopsy with the consulting radiologist and pathologist prior to the procedure. Biopsy incision placement should be carefully planned so that the surrounding skin and contaminated soft tissues can be excised en bloc with the lesion at the time of definitive surgery.

There are many methods by which tissue and/or fluid can be obtained for evaluation. Fine-needle aspiration biopsy is appropriate only for those surgeons and pathologists who are comfortable with this technique. Needles of larger caliber can be used for bone biopsies in special anatomic regions (e.g., vertebral bodies, iliac crest); however, sampling errors become more likely when using these techniques. In most instances a small, appropriately-placed, open biopsy is preferred for obtaining several samples of tissue. Many bone and soft tissue le-

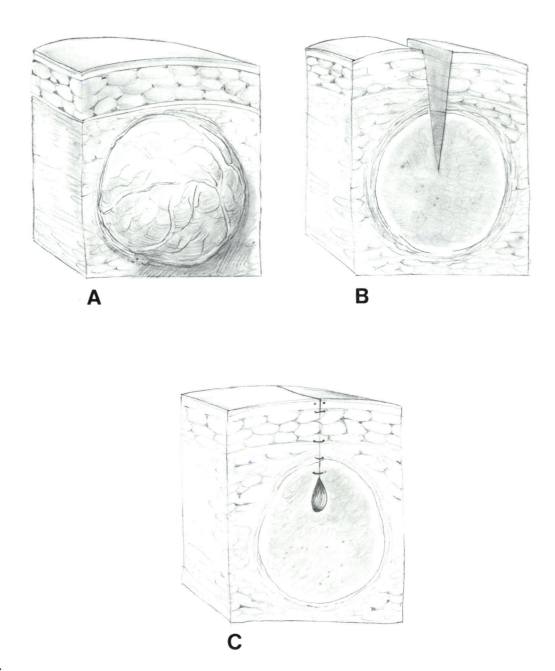

A

B

C

FIG V−1.
A, illustration depicts a tumor arising in a muscle beneath the deep fascia. The compressed and displaced muscle fibers and the adjacent reactive tissue and neovascularity representing the outer surface of the pseudocapsule are shown. **B,** the biopsy incision is directed down through the skin, subcutaneous tissue, and fascia *without* lateral dissection. Tissue and fluid for biopsy have been obtained by directly incising the superficial border of the tumor pseudocapsule, leaving the deep and lateral tumor margins completely undisturbed. **C,** wound and pseudocapsular structures are closed. A hemostatic agent is placed within the biopsy defect, followed by multiple deep layer closure, and a subcuticular suture is then used to approximate the skin edges.

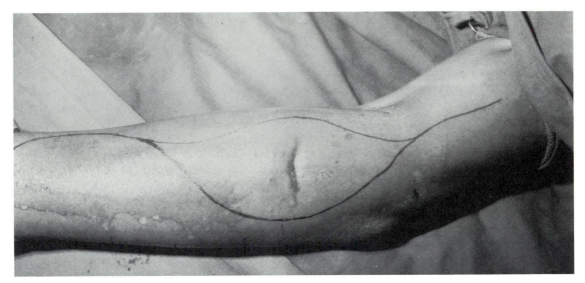

FIG V–2.
Preoperative photograph shows the nondominant upper extremity of a patient referred for management of a subtotally excised alveolar soft part sarcoma. The transverse biopsy scar can be seen with persistent tumor growing within the incision (transverse incisions should be avoided). The patient was managed with an en bloc resection of the adjacent soft tissues (as drawn with a marking pencil) and resection of the underlying soft tissues, including the motor branch of the radial nerve, and the proximal radius.

sions are not homogeneous; therefore, several areas of the lesion, including the interface between the lesion and reactive tissue, should be evaluated histologically.

Many surgeons recommend excisional biopsy when the lesion is small (<3 cm) and favorably located, and when excision of the lesion and cuff of surrounding tissue will not result in significant morbidity (e.g., ribs, skin lesions, expendable bones). When a choice is available, however, most oncologic surgeons prefer an incisional technique where the deep or critical margins are *not* disturbed [Fig V–1]. Then, if appropriate management of the lesion requires a compartmental resection, the surgeon may proceed after the biopsy without extending the margins of resection beyond those usually required. Consequently, *longitudinal* incisions are preferable and should be placed in a manner that permits subsequent wide en bloc excision of the tumor. Figures V–2, V–3, and V–4 depict *transverse* biopsy incisions which necessitated very wide tissue resection to obtain appropriate margins.

Spillage of tumor cells associated with postoperative hematoma formation can render a previously resectable lesion unresectable. Techniques that will diminish the likelihood of hematoma formation include the use of a tourniquet (after gravity exsanguination), thrombogenic agents, methylmethacrylate, and hemostatic wound closure. The tourniquet should be *deflated* prior to closure in order to obtain absolute hemostasis. Presumably, anatomic planes dissected by hematoma should be considered contaminated and therefore should be included within the subsequent surgical margins.

Once tissue is obtained for evaluation, proper handling of the specimens is mandatory. The operating surgeon must be certain that sufficient material has been obtained for multiple analyses (culture, cell markers, cytogenetics, use of different fixatives, etc.) to permit full evaluation of the previously entertained diagnosis and to provide sufficient information for differentiating one lesion from another. Tissue for electron microscopy should be *routinely obtained* and fixed; if not required, it can then be disposed of after the definitive diagnosis is made.

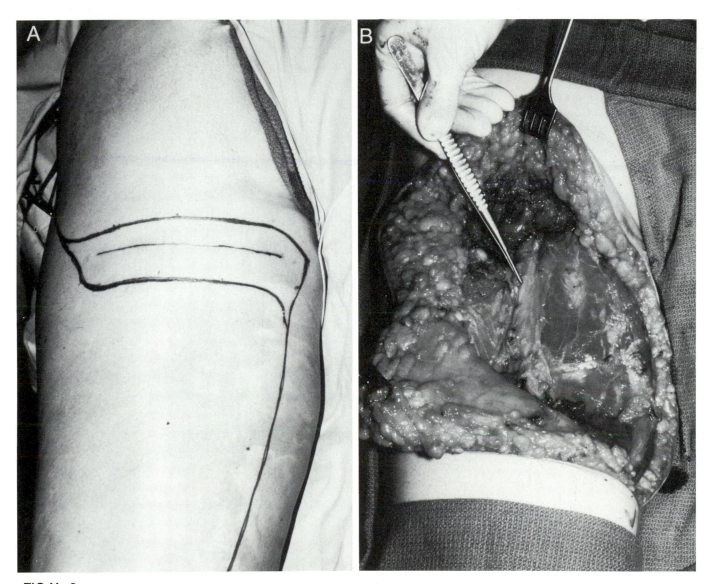

FIG V–3.
A, photograph shows the posterior aspect of the left thigh with a subtotally excised liposarcoma. The intended incision for resection is shown, as well as the original transverse incision site (transverse incisions should be avoided). **B,** completed resection with the forceps pointing to the sciatic nerve.

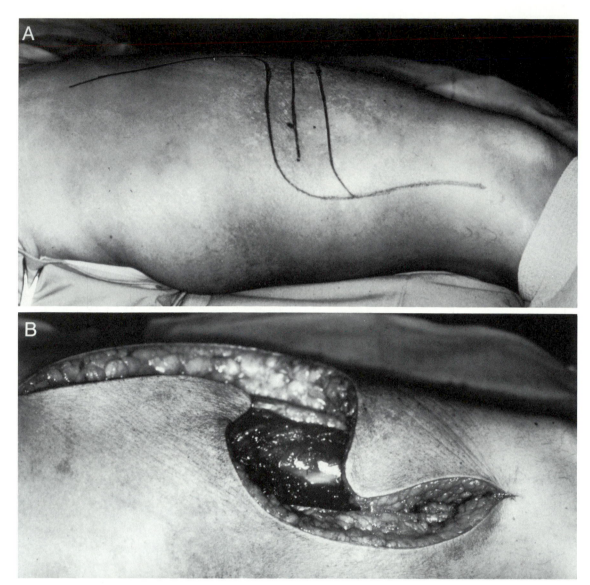

FIG V–4.
A, photograph of a patient who was referred for further management of a subtotally excised malignant fibrous histiocytoma of the right lateral thigh. **B,** the soft tissue deficit for closure is shown after completion of the resection and utilization of intraoperative radiation therapy. (Transverse incisions should be avoided.)

TUMOR STAGING AND GRADING

Staging and grading of bone and soft tissue sarcomas provide information regarding prognosis, planning, and evaluation of therapeutic modalities.

Staging provides information regarding the extent or state of disease at a given point in time, and is based on data obtained from history, physical examination, and imaging techniques. It usually includes information about the size and location of the lesion and the presence or absence of distant metastases (e.g., distant organs, lymph nodes, "skip" metastases). Anatomic location is of prognostic significance in staging (i.e., distal tumors in general have a favorable prognosis; patients with superficial tumors tend to do better than those with lesions more deeply seated).

Grading is determined by the degree of cellularity, anaplasia or pleomorphism, mitotic activity, infiltrative growth, and necrosis. Ideally these parameters should be *reproducible*. Unfortunately, not all sarcomas easily lend themselves to accurate grading because of the variation and degree of differentiation of separate foci within the tumor. In general, the overall grade of the tumor is determined by the grade of the least differentiated foci within the tumor.

Grading requires representative, appropriately managed tissue, usually obtained by open biopsy, to provide an accurate histopathologic diagnosis. Although needle biopsy may provide diagnostic information in some obviously malignant or benign tumors, it may not provide sufficient tissue for accurate grading in nonhomogeneous tumors, and attempts to use flow cytometry to provide consistent grading information from needle biopsy samples have been only partially successful.

REFERENCES

1. Enneking WF: Editorial: The issue of the biopsy. *J Bone Joint Surg* 1982; 64-A(8):1119–1120.
2. Mankin HJ, Lange TA, Spanier SS: The hazards of biopsy in patients with malignant primary bone and soft-tissue tumors. *J Bone Joint Surg* 1982; 64-A(8):1121–1127.
3. Simon MA: Current Concepts Review: Biopsy of musculoskeletal tumors. *J Bone Joint Surg* 1982; 64-A(8):1253–1257.

14

Anatomic Considerations for Biopsy in Orthopaedic Oncologic Management

James R. Neff, M.D.

Consideration of anatomical factors in diagnosis and treatment of musculoskeletal tumors is crucial for optimum management of such lesions at the time of initial biopsy, as well as for carrying out extensive reconstruction procedures. The Musculoskeletal Tumor Society has developed a surgical staging system, based upon extensive correlative clinical and histopathologic data, to incorporate significant prognostic factors, provide guidelines for adjunctive therapy, and provide a stratification for surgical management.[1]

SURGICAL STAGING SYSTEM

The staging system adopted by the Musculoskeletal Tumor Society conveniently integrates tumor grade and stage with surgical concepts derived from knowledge of the histopathology and growth and spread of sarcomas.[2, 3] In general, sarcomas grow by expansion and flattening (compression) of normal surrounding tissues which are usually confined by a surrounding anatomic barrier (fascia) to tumor growth. This *zone of compression* (see Fig V–1, Overview) is, in turn, surrounded by condensed, atrophic, and edematous tissue, usually defined best on MR and usually containing the neovascularity seen on conventional and digital angiography. This surrounding area is designated as the *reactive zone*. The zone of compression and the reactive zone comprise

the *pseudocapsule*. Furthermore, note should be made of the infiltrative longitudinal growth of tumors, usually in the planes of least resistance between muscle fibers. In general, the proximal and distal extent of the tumor is often less well defined both pathologically and radiographically. Even with excellent MR data, the proximal and distal infiltrative margins are difficult to accurately predict, and therefore resections that do not include generous proximal and distal margins (myectomy) may be incomplete.

By recognition and imaging of the precise anatomic location of the tumor and pseudocapsule (CT/T, MR, angiography, etc.), and by applying a definable system of surgical margins (intralesional, marginal, wide, and radical), it is possible to combine the concepts of stage and grade with definable surgical procedures.

Grading of Tumors

The number of grades in other staging systems varies from two to four depending upon the system and the tumor. In an effort to consolidate grades, in this surgical staging system tumors are divided into three grades: benign (G_0), low-grade malignant (G_1), and high-grade malignant (G_2). Low-grade lesions (G_1) are comprised of Broder's I and II lesions, and have a low probability of metastasis (25%). In general, these lesions can be managed by relatively conservative surgical procedures. High-grade lesions (G_2) are comprised of Broder's III and IV tumors with a significantly higher incidence of local persistence and metastases requiring more radical surgical procedures and possibly adjuvant therapy. Table 14–1 shows a representative grouping of the low- and high-grade tumors.

Anatomical Sites of Tumor Presentation

Anatomic fascial compartments may serve as anatomic barriers to infiltrative tumor growth. Based upon this knowledge, the anatomic setting or topography (T_0, T_1, and T_2) in which the tumor presents may be utilized to define surgical margins and to design procedures to render the patient locally tumor-free (local control). Lesions confined within the capsule and that do not extend beyond the fascial compartment of origin are considered T_0 lesions. Lesions

with extracapsular extension into the reactive zone, either by direct extension or by lobulation (satellites), but contained within the anatomic compartment of origin, are considered T_1 lesions. Lesions extending beyond compartmental barriers are considered T_2 lesions. Table 14–2 lists surgical sites for the staging of lesions, separated by columns into recognized anatomic compartments (intracompartmental) and anatomic regions without well defined fascial margins (extracompartmental).

Metastases

Metastatic spread of the lesion evident from the clinical staging studies is designated as M. In general, metastatic disease present in either the lung, lymph nodes, or as a "skip" lesion has the same ominous prognostic significance and is designated M_1 while those patients without evidence of metastatic disease are designated as M_0.

Surgical Stages

The surgical staging system (Table 14–3) combines both bone and soft tissue tumors by grade (G_0, G_1 and G_2), anatomic setting (T_0, T_1 or T_2), and the presence or absence of metastases (M_0 or M_1). The *surgical stage* combines the grade and metastatic status, and is subdivided into A and B depending upon

TABLE 14–1.
Surgical Grade (G)*

Low (G_1)	High (G_2)
Parosteal osteosarcoma	Classic osteosarcoma
Periosteal osteosarcoma	Radiation sarcoma
Low-grade central osteosarcoma	Paget's sarcoma
Secondary chondrosarcoma	Primary chondrosarcoma
	Dedifferentiated chondrosarcoma
Fibrosarcoma, Kaposi's sarcoma	Fibrosarcoma
Atypical malignant fibrous histiocytoma	Malignant fibrous histiocytoma
	Undiff. primary sarcoma
Giant cell tumor, bone	Giant cell sarcoma, bone
Hemangioendothelioma	Angiosarcoma
Hemangiopericytoma	Hemangiopericytoma
Myxoid liposarcoma	Pleomorphic liposarcoma
	Neurofibrosarcoma (Schwannoma)
	Rhabdomyosarcoma
	Synovial sarcoma
Clear cell sarcoma	
Epithelioid sarcoma	
Chordoma	
Adamantinoma	
Alveolar cell sarcoma	Alveolar cell sarcoma
Other and undifferentiated	Other and undifferentiated

*Adapted from Enneking WF, Spanier SS, Goodman MA: A system for the surgical staging of musculoskeletal sarcoma. *Clin Orthop* 1980; 153:108.

TABLE 14–2.
Surgical Sites (T)*

Intracompartmental (T_1)	Extracompartmental (T_2)
Intraosseous	Soft tissue extension
Intra-articular	Soft tissue extension
Superficial to deep fascia	Deep fascial extension
Parosseous	Intraosseous or extrafascial
Intrafascial compartments	Extrafascial planes or spaces
Ray of hand or foot	Mid- and hindfoot
Anterolateral leg	Popliteal "space"
Posterior leg	Groin-femoral triangle
Middle thigh	Intrapelvic (retroperitoneal)
Posterior thigh	Midhand
Buttocks	Antecubital fossa
Dorsal forearm	Axilla
Volar forearm	Periclavicular
Anterior arm	Paraspinal
Posterior arm	Head and neck
Periscapular	

*Adapted from Enneking WF, Spanier SS, Goodman MA: A system for the surgical staging of musculoskeletal sarcoma. *Clin Orthop* 1980; 153:110.

TABLE 14–3.

Surgical Stages*

Stage	Grade	Site	Metastasis
IA	Low (G_1)	Intracompartmental (T_1)	M_0
IB	Low (G_1)	Extracompartmental (T_2)	M_0
IIA	High (G_2)	Intracompartmental (T_1)	M_0
IIB	High (G_2)	Extracompartmental (T_2)	M_0
III	Any (G)	Any (T)	M_1
		(With regional or distant metastasis)	

*Adapted from Enneking WF, Spanier SS, Goodman MA: A system for the surgical staging of musculoskeletal sarcoma. *Clin Orthop* 1980; 153:111.

the anatomic setting of the tumor (A = intracompartmental, B = extracompartmental). Therefore, a low grade (G_1) intracompartmental (T_1) tumor without metastases (M_0) would be designated as stage IA while a high-grade (G_2) extracompartmental (T_2) tumor without recognizable metastases (M_0) would be defined as stage IIB.

Surgical Margins

Surgical margins (Table 14–4) may be described as intralesional, marginal, wide, or radical, depending upon their relationship to the plane of dissection and the pseudocapsule. Intralesional margins are accomplished by an incisional biopsy or curettage of a presumed benign tumor. Marginal margins are evident when the plane of dissection passes through the reactive zone or pseudocapsule. Marginal excisional margins occur when the surgeon "shells out" a malignant neoplasm, leaving viable tumor at the periphery, and *will* result in local recurrence. Marginal margins are generally *not sufficient* for adequate local control when managing *malignant lesions* (G_1 or

G_2). Wide margins are accomplished when the plane of dissection passes only through absolutely normal tissues, providing a generous cuff of normal tissue surrounding the pseudocapsule. This margin does not always require removal of the entire length of the muscle. Radical margins are achieved when the plane of dissection passes entirely outside of the involved compartment outside of the investing fascia from its origin to insertion. Radical margins will generally provide adequate local control for most high-grade malignant neoplasms when an adjuvant such as neoadjuvant chemotherapy or preoperative radiation therapy is *not* utilized. Wide margins may be sufficient to control high-grade intracompartmental lesions when a good preoperative therapeutic response has been achieved by using neoadjuvant therapy (either chemotherapy or radiation therapy).

Surgical Procedures

Surgical procedures (Table 14–5) may be integrated with the surgical staging system whereby in the majority of cases, if correctly applied, will render

TABLE 14–4.

Surgical Margins*

Surgical Margin	Plane of Dissection	Result
Intralesional	Debulking or curettage	Leaves macroscopic disease
Marginal	Shell out through pseudocapsule or reactive zone	May leave either "satellite" or "skip" lesions
Wide	Intracompartmental en bloc with cuff of normal tissue	May leave "skip" lesions
Radical	Extracompartmental en bloc entire compartment	No residual

*Adapted from Enneking WF, Spanier SS, Goodman MA: A system for the surgical staging of musculoskeletal sarcoma. *Clin Orthop* 1980; 153:111.

TABLE 14–5.
Surgical Procedures*

Margin	Local	Amputation
Intralesional	Curettage or debulking	Debulking amputation
Marginal	Marginal excision	Marginal amputation
Radical	Radical local resection	Radical disarticulation

*Adapted from Enneking WF, Spanier SS, Goodman MA: A system for the surgical staging of musculoskeletal sarcoma. *Clin Orthop* 1980; 153:112.

the patient locally free of disease. The surgical staging system, as defined, has been clinically tested and found to be useful. Present criticisms are primarily concerned with the apparent lack of sensitivity of the system (i.e., 95% of all conventional osteosarcomas are Stage IIB) when evaluating some patient populations. The system, as described, remains under intensive investigation while other staging systems for patients with sarcomas of bone and soft tissue are also being reviewed.

BIOPSY CONSIDERATIONS FOR THE UPPER EXTREMITY AND PARASPINOUS REGION

Hand and Wrist

The hand and wrist, anatomically comprised of 14 phalanges, 5 metacarpals and 8 carpal bones, have numerous osseous compartments but relatively few soft tissue anatomic compartments. The dorsum of the hand is comprised primarily of tendons, vessels, and subcutaneous tissues while the palmar structures include numerous small intrinsic muscles and tendons primarily contained by the palmar interosseous fascia. Since the majority of muscles in the forearm arise from the distal humerus and cross the wrist into the hand, involvement of the tendons or tendon sheaths with tumor tissue may allow for longitudinal spread of tumor, thereby requiring special consideration as to the extent of the tumor involvement. If primary tumors arise within bones of the phalanges and metacarpals they may often be managed by ray amputation. If there is a question of soft tissue involvement, then MR of the hand using surface coils to improve spacial resolution, and detail should be obtained. If tissues contained within the central palmar compartment (flexor profundus tendons, flexor digitorum superficialis tendons, etc.)

are involved, having transgressed the palmar interosseous fascia, then an amputation through the distal forearm proximal to the termination and extent of the synovial sheaths should be used.

Forearm

The forearm is comprised of two compartments on either side of the centrally located interosseous membrane (Fig 14–1, Cross Section 1). When possible, the ulna should be approached through the subcutaneous border of the forearm. The distal two-thirds of the radius may also be biopsied through the most direct route, avoiding the radial vessels and sensory branch of the radial nerve.

Special reference to the course of the motor branch of the radial nerve should be considered when biopsying the proximal radius (Cross Section 2). In general, however, reconstruction for the functional loss of the motor branch of the radial nerve is less complex than reconstruction for loss of flexor motor function. Therefore, when a choice is available, biopsy through the extensor compartment is preferred over biopsy through the flexor compartment. Primary tumors involving the proximal radius and extending into the extensor compartment may be managed by resection of the proximal radius in continuity with the adjacent extensor compartment. A synostosis between the retained distal radius and ulna may be used to maintain length and the distal radio-ulnar joint while extensor function can be restored with appropriate tendon transfers. In general, the function of a one bone forearm is far superior to the function of any amputation. Presently there is no satisfactory prosthetic replacement comparable to a sensate, painless, functioning hand.

Antecubital Fossa

Soft tissue lesions arising within the antecubital fossa frequently require amputation because of the

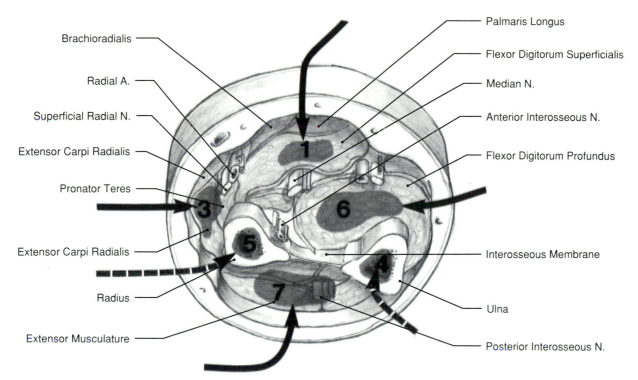

Brachioradialis

Radial A.

Superficial Radial N.

Extensor Carpi Radialis

Pronator Teres

Extensor Carpi Radialis

Radius

Extensor Musculature

Palmaris Longus

Flexor Digitorum Superficialis

Median N.

Anterior Interosseous N.

Flexor Digitorum Profundus

Interosseous Membrane

Ulna

Posterior Interosseous N.

CROSS SECTION 1.

Middle third of forearm (refer to Fig 14–1 for orientation to cross section levels). **Tumors presenting in bone** (*dashed arrows*). Tumors presenting in either the radius or ulna in the middle and distal third of the forearm should be approached directly through the subcutaneous tissues. When the bone cannot be approached without contaminating a muscle belly, the major nerves and vessels must be avoided with the biopsy incision. Therefore, the biopsy incision is most often placed on the extensor side of the interosseous membrane. In general, extensor function is easier to reconstruct than flexor function. **Tumors presenting in soft tissue** (*solid arrows*). The hypothetical tumor (1) arises within the flexor digitorum superficialis. The recommended biopsy incision avoids the median nerve which lies adjacent but deep to the muscle. If only the muscle is involved, a myectomy would provide potentially wide curative margins. If, however, the adjacent fascia is infiltrated with tumor, the median nerve and surrounding tissue would be involved, possibly requiring amputation. Similar arguments could be made for tumor 3. Lesions arising within the extensor musculature (7) may lend themselves to radical resection (en bloc removal of all extensor musculature) with or without a portion of either the adjacent radius or ulna. If both bones are contaminated, then amputation should strongly be considered.

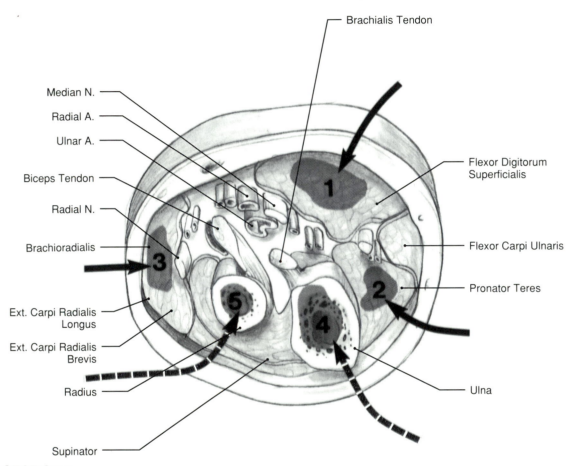

Brachialis Tendon

Median N.

Radial A.

Ulnar A.

Biceps Tendon

Radial N.

Brachioradialis

Ext. Carpi Radialis Longus

Ext. Carpi Radialis Brevis

Radius

Supinator

Flexor Digitorum Superficialis

Flexor Carpi Ulnaris

Pronator Teres

Ulna

CROSS SECTION 2.
Proximal third of forearm. Tumors presenting in bone *(dashed arrows)*. Tumors represented by *4* can usually be approached through the subcutaneous border of the ulna. Tumors arising within the proximal radius *(5)*, however, may require biopsy through the extensor musculature as mentioned in Cross Section 1 (also see Fig V–2, Overview). *Only* longitudinal incisions should be used. **Tumors presenting in soft tissue** *(solid arrows)*. Tumors represented by *1, 2,* and *3* should all be approached directly, *avoiding* mobilization of fascial planes or exposure of vessels or nerves, and without disturbing the deep tumor margins or fascial planes. Only when the diagnosis is known can the surgical and therapeutic options be explored. Absolute hemostasis must be obtained with the tourniquet deflated prior to fascial and skin closure to prevent hematoma dissection.

and local control, the specimen should include the epitrochlear nodes in continuity with the surgical specimen.

Arm

The arm is divided into anterior and posterior compartments by the medial and lateral intermuscular septum (Cross Section 3). The medial septum arises and is contiguous with the pectoralis major tendon and attaches to the medial supracondylar ridge ending at the medial epicondyle. The medial septum is pierced by the ulnar nerve and the superior ulnar collateral artery passing together into the posterior compartment within the midarm. The lateral intermuscular septum begins below the deltoid muscular insertion on the humerus. It lies between the brachialis and brachioradialis muscles, and extends and attaches to the lateral epicondyle. The radial nerve and the anterior descending branch of the profunda brachii artery pierce the lateral septum in the midarm, and may be identified deep to the brachioradialis muscle near the elbow joint. Care should be exercised to carefully evaluate tumors arising within regions where the respective nerves and accompanying vessels pierce the septae. Tumor tissue involving the compartments may grow through the foramina into the adjacent compartment along the course of the vessels and nerves.

When considering biopsy of the middle to distal one-third of the humerus, the biopsy should in general pass through the triceps musculature, avoiding either the medial or lateral intermuscular septum and the radial and the ulnar nerves (Cross Section 4). In many instances the triceps muscle can be resected in continuity with the underlying distal humerus and overlying brachialis muscle, leaving the biceps for elbow flexion and gravity to assist passive extension of the elbow in the upright position. In this instance, the triceps is said to be "silent" or expendable.

Lesions involving the proximal one-third of the humerus are most commonly approached anteriorly within the most *medial* extent of the deltoid muscle just immediately *lateral* to the deltopectoral groove (Fig 14–2). In this way, the contaminated tissue and biopsy tract are positioned within the most medial muscle edge. If resection is required, the medial portion of the deltoid muscle can be resected en bloc along with the proximal humerus without defunctionalizing the remaining, posteriorly-enervated deltoid muscle (Fig 14–3).

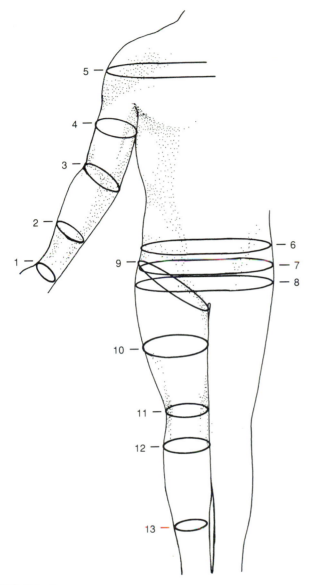

FIG 14–1.
Cross section level orientation. Each of the planes depicted in this figure shows the orientation (viewed from distal to proximal) and level of a cross section illustration (see cross section illustrations throughout remainder of this chapter). These illustrations are used to demonstrate the appropriate anatomic planes for biopsy. The cross section illustrations should be used in conjunction with the appropriate figures to show the correct orientation and position of the biopsy incision.

ill-defined borders of this anatomic compartment. Small lesions reasonably well-confined may on occasion be resected after an appropriate preoperative response to neoadjuvant therapy (either preoperative chemotherapy or radiation therapy). If an above elbow amputation is required for surgical therapy

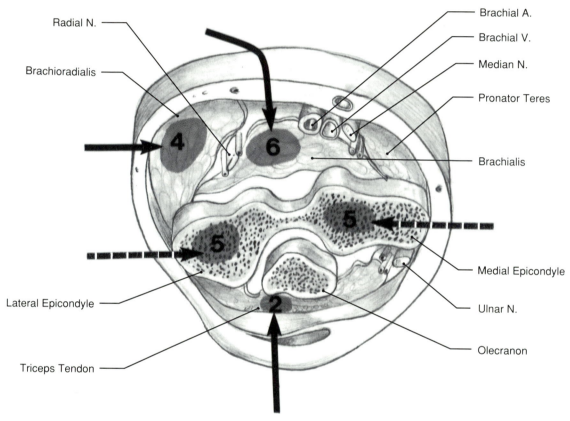

Radial N.

Brachioradialis

Brachial A.

Brachial V.

Median N.

Pronator Teres

Brachialis

Medial Epicondyle

Ulnar N.

Olecranon

Lateral Epicondyle

Triceps Tendon

CROSS SECTION 3.
Distal third of arm. Tumors presenting in bone *(dashed arrows).* Lesions presenting in either the medial or lateral epicondyle may be biopsied directly through the subcutaneous tissues. Care should be taken *not* to penetrate the anterior or posterior surface of the distal humerus to prevent contamination of the anterior or posterior compartments and possibly the ulnar nerve. **Tumors presenting in soft tissues** *(solid arrows).* Hypothetical lesions *2, 4,* and *6* should be approached directly. Note that the incisions into the brachioradialis *(4)* and brachialis *(6)* are performed in such a way as to prevent mobilization and exposure of the radial nerve, which may lead to its contamination. Also, care should be taken to avoid contamination of the more medial brachial vessels and median nerve. Special care should be exercised when biopsying lesions located in area 2 to prevent contamination of the elbow joint or the ulnar nerve.

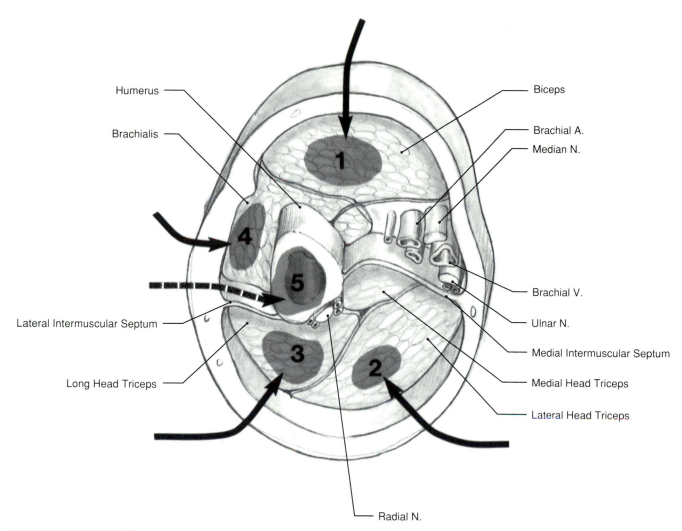

Humerus

Brachialis

Lateral Intermuscular Septum

Long Head Triceps

Biceps

Brachial A.

Median N.

Brachial V.

Ulnar N.

Medial Intermuscular Septum

Medial Head Triceps

Lateral Head Triceps

Radial N.

CROSS SECTION 4.

Middle of arm. Tumors presenting in bone *(dashed arrow).* Because of the spiraling nature of the radial nerve about the humerus, special attention should be given when performing an open biopsy of the humerus. In the lower third of the arm, an anterolateral brachialis-splitting incision should be used, thereby avoiding the radial nerve and the medial neurovascular bundle. If one dissects along the lateral septum however, the area contaminated by the biopsy can be easily included in the subsequent resection in that the septum and the adjacent soft tissue can be included and the exact anatomic location of the contaminated area is known and can be readily identified by the operating surgeon. **Tumors presenting in soft tissues** *(solid arrows).* Every effort should be made to sample the tumor without surgical contamination of either the vessels or nerves. In the upper extremity, triceps function can be mimicked by gravity extension of the elbow. Lesions presenting within the triceps *(2 and 3)* may be completely resected, using compartmental surgical margins, resulting in little functional deficit. Minimal functional deficit would also be associated with resection of lesions involving only the biceps musculature *(1).*

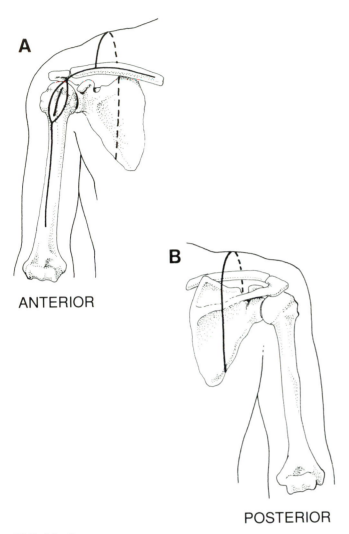

ANTERIOR

POSTERIOR

FIG 14–2.
Illustration shows the comprehensive exposure for lesions presenting around the shoulder and proximal humerus. **A,** anterior biopsy incision. **B,** biopsies can be performed at any point along the potential comprehensive incision line.

Shoulder and Paraspinous Region

The scapula is essentially encased within muscle, and lesions arising within the scapula commonly produce an adjacent soft tissue mass (Cross Section 5). The general principles are to obtain diagnostic tissue with as direct approach as possible, but in the general overall path of the comprehensive shoulder strap incision over the shoulder (see Fig 14–2).[4] In some instances a small window can be made within the scapula to approach lesions arising within the confines of the subscapularis muscle. This approach avoids contamination of the interscapulothoracic plane. If the margin between the scapula and thorax is not involved, the lesion could then be managed

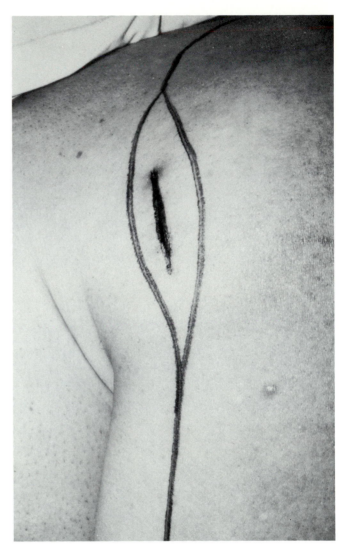

FIG 14–3.
Photograph shows the anterior aspect of the left shoulder and the vertical biopsy incision placement immediately lateral to the deltopectoral groove. The biopsy incision, orientation, and placement allowed for the en bloc resection of the proximal humerus for chondrosarcoma, followed by prosthetic replacement through the comprehensive incision shown.

by a scapular resection, thereby preserving a functioning useful upper extremity.[5]

Malignancies presenting within and involving the supraclavicular tissues often require a forequarter amputation for local control. In many instances the ill-defined margins of the supraclavicular fossa do not lend themselves to compartmental surgery without the use of sophisticated oncologic techniques.[6–9] If there is a question as to appropriate management, a musculoskeletal oncologic surgeon should be consulted *prior* to the biopsy.

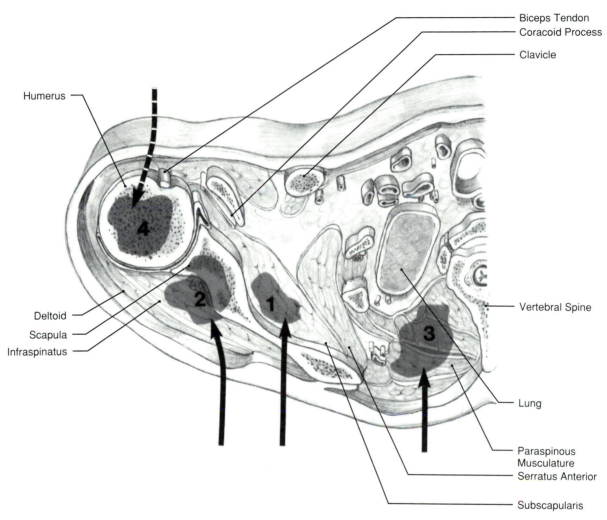

CROSS SECTION 5.

Shoulder. Tumors presenting in bone *(dashed arrow)*. Lesions presenting within the clavicle may be approached directly through the subcutaneous tissues. The proximal humerus, however, should be approached through a specific incision placed just *lateral* to the deltopectoral groove (tumor *4*) (see Fig 14–2). with the biopsy tract coursing through the most *medial* portion of the posteriorly enervated deltoid muscle. The bone biopsy tract should be placed *lateral* to the insertion of the pectoralis major tendon to prevent contamination of the deep axillary tissues and vessels. The scapula should be approached posteriorly in line with the comprehensive shoulder incision (see Fig 14–2) through the spine of the scapula where possible. If it is necessary to contaminate a muscle belly, the infraspinatus is preferred over the supraspinatus where possible. **Tumors presenting in soft tissue** *(solid arrows)*. Tumors presenting in the paraspinous musculature may be sampled through a longitudinal incision paralleling but *not* exposing the osseous structures (tumor *3*) (see Fig 14–4). Lesions within the subscapularis (tumor *1*) should be sampled by making a small window through the thin membranous portion of the body of the scapula just below the scapular spine and in line with the comprehensive incision. A similar soft tissue approach should be used to sample tumors arising within the infraspinatus and the teres major and minor muscles (tumor *2*).

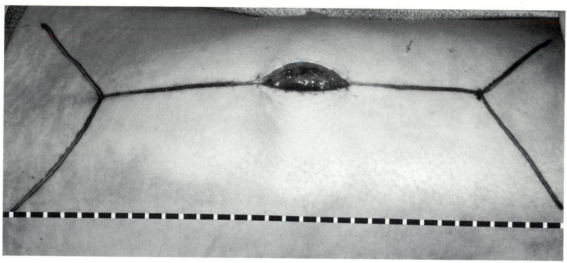

FIG 14–4.
This intraoperative photograph demonstrates a large left paraspinous mass of a patient positioned prone for biopsy. The intended resection incision has been drawn on the skin with the pelvis to the left (*dashed line* indicates spinous processes). The biopsy incision (as shown) is in line with the intended resection incision and can easily be re-excised at the time of the definitive procedure.

Tumors arising within the paraspinous musculature are best sampled through a longitudinal incision directly over the lesion, *not* exposing the adjacent osseous structures Fig 14–4 and Cross Section 5, Tumor 3). In some instances, small lesions may be resected with wide margins when appropriately managed, sparing the adjacent osseous structures.

BIOPSY CONSIDERATIONS FOR THE LOWER EXTREMITY

Pelvis

Tumors presenting within the pelvis should be subcategorized into intrapelvic, intraosseous, and extrapelvic to better understand the methods of resection and reconstruction. The biopsy tract should be positioned in such a way that the incision can be resected en bloc with the primary lesion. The biopsy incision placement and orientation is critical for appropriate oncologic management.

In general, the majority of pelvic tumors are resected through an exposure gained by the utilitarian incision, which begins at the posterior iliac spine, courses along the crest of the ilium, and curves distally to end at the level of the midthigh (Fig 14–5).[10–12] The gluteus maximus musculature is

taken down laterally, exposing the ilium and the attached musculature while detachment of the abdominal wall exposes the retroperitoneal structures. The majority of pelvic resection procedures may be performed through this incision. Therefore, lesions arising within the pelvis (intrapelvic and intraosseous lesions) should be biopsied through incisions made *in line with* the utilitarian incision (Fig 14–6).

Intrapelvic tumors are often approached by taking down the abdominal wall attachment to the ilium and dissecting beneath the iliacus muscle and

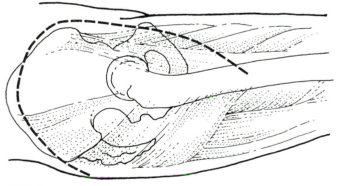

FIG 14–5.
Illustration shows the position and anatomic landmarks of the utilitarian incision for the comprehensive exposure of the right hemipelvis and proximal femur. Resection of the ilium, proximal femur, and acetabulum with or without the pubis or ischium may be performed through this incision.

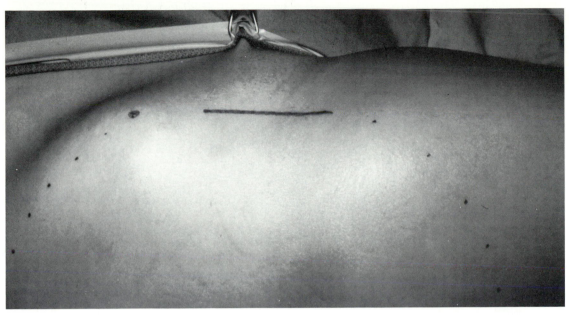

FIG 14–6.
This patient presented with a radiographically identifiable mass originating within the direct head of the right rectus femoris muscle. The photograph shows the intended biopsy incision in line with intended utilitarian resection incision shown as the *dotted line.* This patient eventually required an internal hemipelvectomy for synovial sarcoma.

psoas fascia, avoiding the femoral nerve and vessels (Cross Sections 6, 7, and 8). Intraosseous lesions of the ilium can be approached in several ways: first by anterior exposure between the inner and outer tables of the cortex just superior to the anterior *inferior* iliac spine, secondly through the dome of the iliac crest between the inner and outer cortex, and finally posteriorly through the subcutaneous border of the posterior spine of the ilium (Fig 14–7). Frequently either CT/T or MR imaging studies will better define the best approach to biopsy.

Extrapelvic lesions arising within soft tissues will often require biopsy through incisions compatible with the utilitarian incision in order to turn an appropriate flap for exposure and closure (Fig 14–8). Other lesions confined to the gluteus maximus muscle may be biopsied, followed immediately by resection of the gluteus maximus muscle (buttockectomy) and closure.[13–16]

Thigh

Lesions arising within the proximal femur are difficult to biopsy without significant contamination of tissues beneath the fascia lata. When the lesion appears entirely confined to bone, an approach to the intramedullary canal through the tip of the greater trochanter may prove beneficial (see Cross Section 8). With the patient in the lateral position and utilizing image intensification, limited exposure through a small incision in the gluteus medius tendon and through a small defect in the greater trochanter will provide access to the upper half of the medullary canal, and specimens may be obtained using long biopsy forceps (Fig 14–9). In this manner, the tissues surrounding the femur are *not* contaminated and the shaft may be resected and reconstructed using a variety of techniques. When this technique is not appropriate, a direct approach through the vastus lateralis, near but not through the lateral septum, may be utilized.

Lesions arising within the anterior thigh may be directly approached surgically to minimize soft tissue contamination (Cross Sections 9, 10, and 11). The femoral vessels and nerves should *not* be exposed and should be avoided by biopsying the involved muscle compartment directly. Using these principles, the femoral sheath may provide a sufficient fascial barrier to preserve the vascular integrity to the lower extremity and still provide adequate (wide to compartmental) margins. If the vessels are involved, however, and the femoral nerve preserved, then consideration should be given to resecting the vessels in continuity with the tumor and then reconstructing the vasculature. If the femoral nerve is involved, resection of the nerve may well be

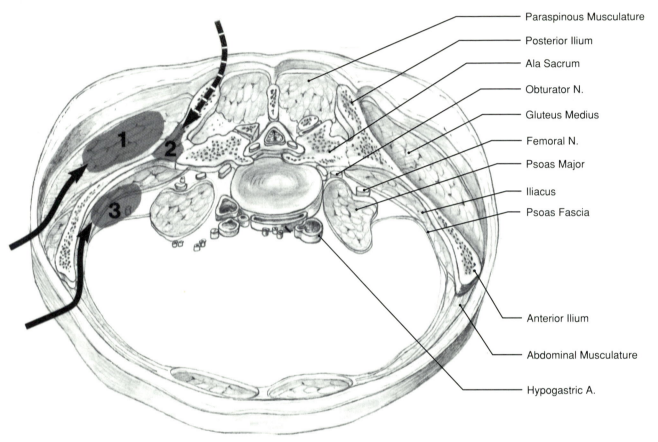

Paraspinous Musculature

Posterior Ilium

Ala Sacrum

Obturator N.

Gluteus Medius

Femoral N.

Psoas Major

Iliacus

Psoas Fascia

Anterior Ilium

Abdominal Musculature

Hypogastric A.

CROSS SECTION 6.

Upper portion of pelvis. **Tumors presenting in bone** *(dashed arrow)*. Malignant lesions arising within the ilium (tumor 2) may be approached either anteriorly or posteriorly, or along the dome of the iliac crest through the adjacent subcutaneous borders *but remaining in line* with the utilitarian incision (Fig 14–5). Frequently either CT/T or MR will be helpful in localizing the lesions to be biopsied. **Tumors presenting in soft tissues** *(solid arrows)*. Intrapelvic tumors arising in retroperitoneal structures are frequently large at the time of diagnosis. Every effort must be made to prevent contamination of the peritoneum or other retroperitoneal structures (vessels, nerves, etc.). The biopsy tract shown to tumor 3 begins in line with the utilitarian incision, courses immediately medial to the ilium through the substance of the iliacus muscle beneath the psoas muscle and adjacent femoral nerve to the lesion. The iliacus and psoas fascia should not be compromised, thereby leaving this plane for dissection during subsequent surgical procedures. Extrapelvic lesions arising within the gluteus medius muscle (tumor 1) should be biopsied through a small incision in line with the utilitarian incision and then directly into the tumor. In many instances, the adjacent ilium will also require en bloc removal and therefore one may choose to expose the lesion through a subperiosteal exposure of the outer table *only*.

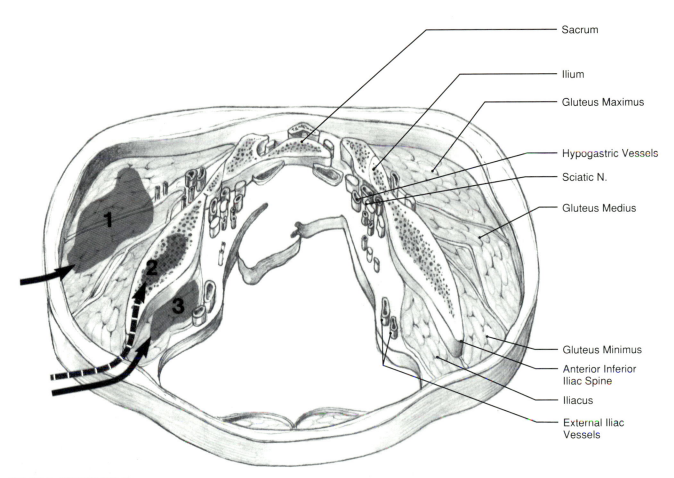

Sacrum

Ilium

Gluteus Maximus

Hypogastric Vessels

Sciatic N.

Gluteus Medius

Gluteus Minimus

Anterior Inferior
Iliac Spine

Iliacus

External Iliac
Vessels

CROSS SECTION 7.

Mid pelvis. Tumors presenting in bone *(dashed arrow).* The supra-acetabular lesion depicted as tumor *2* is best biopsied through an anterior skin incision (Fig 14–6) in line with the utilitarian incision. A cortical window is made *superior* to the anterior inferior spine and the lesion sampled *between* the inner and outer tables. **Tumors presenting in soft tissues** *(solid arrows).* Lesion *3* may also be biopsied through a limited skin incision in line with the utilitarian incision. Exposure is gained along the inner table of the ilium, leaving the limiting iliacus fascia, vessels, and nerves uncompromised. The lesion depicted as tumor *1* does *not* involve the ilium and only in this instance is a more direct approach utilized. A lesion arising in this area will require a buttockectomy, preserving the ilium and sparing the sciatic nerve.

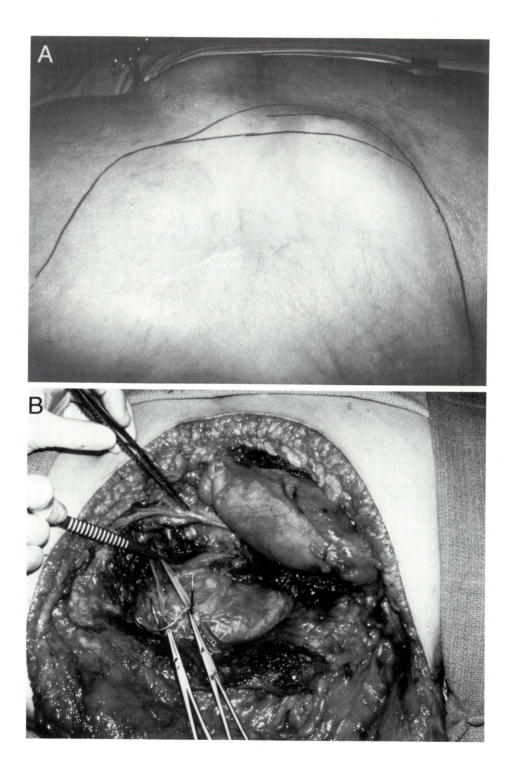

FIG 14–7.
A, lateral photograph of the left hemipelvis (patient is lying supine) shows the intended utilitarian incision planned for resection of a biopsy-proven malignant fibrous histiocytoma of the left acetabulum. Note the placement of the previous longitudinal biopsy incision oriented in line with the comprehensive utilitarian incision required for the procedure. **B,** intraoperative photograph shows the completion of the resection (internal hemipelvectomy) with the upper forceps demonstrating the femoral nerve. The heavy sutures have been passed through drill holes in the ischium to secure the proximal femur to the ischium.

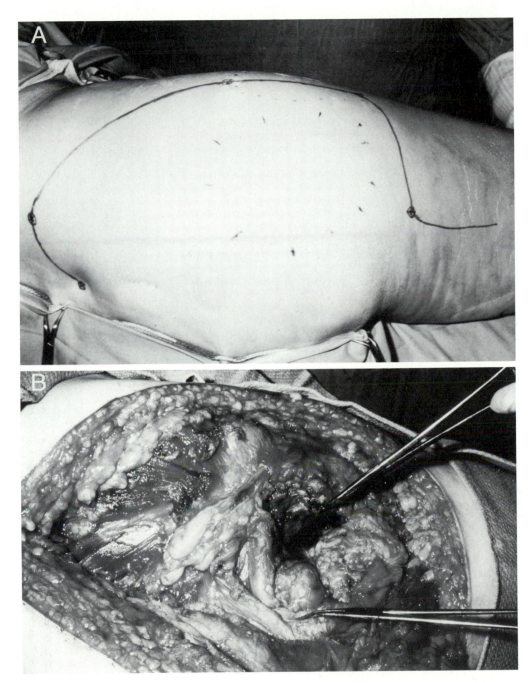

FIG 14–8.
A, photograph shows the incision required to expose and remove the lesion beneath the right gluteus maximus muscle. A biopsy incision through the middle of the large flap could have jeopardized this procedure (see Cross Section 8). **B,** the medially based flap has provided sufficient exposure for resection of the tumor. The sciatic nerve can be seen just inferior to the bottom clamp. Tumors presenting in this region are demanding to biopsy and manage (see Cross Section 9, tumor 3).

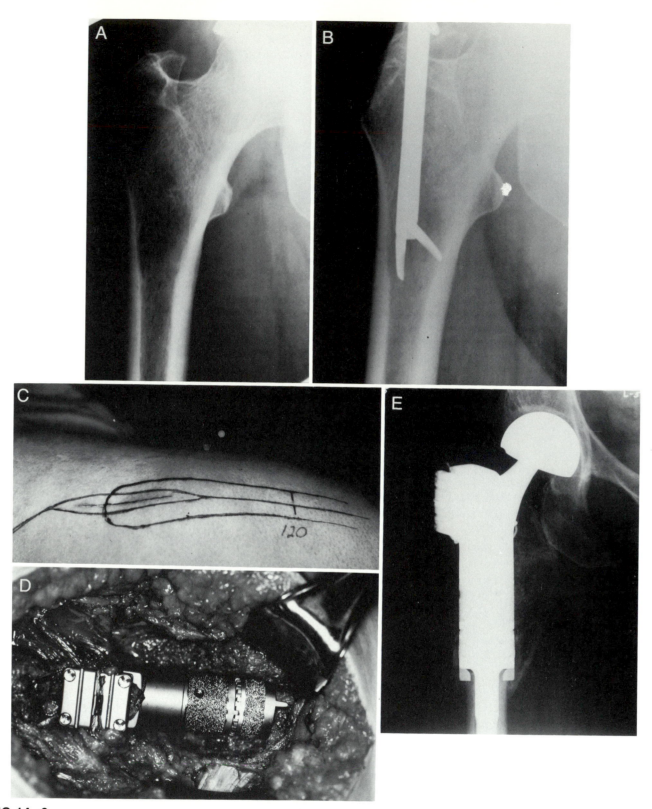

FIG 14–9.
A, this AP x-ray reveals a destructive lesion with loss of trabeculations within the subtrochanteric and trochanteric region of the right proximal femur. Staging procedures revealed no evidence of disease outside of the proximal femur. **B,** with the patient in the lateral position and under fluoroscopic control, a limited open biopsy was performed using a pituitary rongeur through a small round osseous window in the greater trochanter. **C,** the stage IB chondrosarcoma was managed surgically by resection of the proximal 120 cm of the right femur. The healed biopsy incision can be identified in line with the incision planned for resection. The palpable "image" of the underlying proximal femur planned for resection is also shown. **D,** this intraoperative photograph demonstrates the 120-cm modular titanium tumor prosthesis used to reconstruct the osseous defect with the abductor musculature secured in the titanium clamp (shown on the left). As in this case, the transtrochanteric biopsy used for truly intraosseous lesions of the proximal femur provides a method for direct tissue examination without extensive soft tissue contamination. **E,** this x-ray shows the final result after the press-fit insertion of the modular titanium prosthesis. A mixture of autograft and allograft provided medial augmentation of the extracortical fixation.

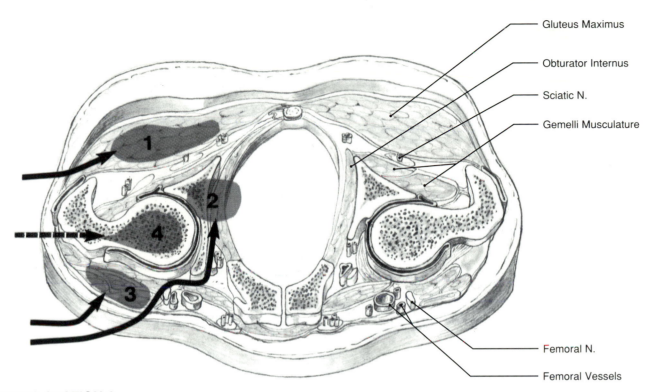

Gluteus Maximus

Obturator Internus

Sciatic N.

Gemelli Musculature

Femoral N.

Femoral Vessels

CROSS SECTION 8.

Through hips. Tumors presenting in bone *(dashed arrow)*. Lesions presenting within the proximal half of the femur (tumor *4*) may be biopsied using a limited exposure through the greater trochanter, just anterior to the trochanteric bursa. This approach minimizes contamination of peritrochanteric tissues beneath the fascia lata. Pituitary forceps can then be used to sample the intramedullary contents of the bone (Fig 14–9, B). **Tumors presenting in soft tissues** *(solid arrows)*. Tumor *2* should be sampled as shown, but alternatively may be approached more superiorly on the ilium with subperiosteal dissection down the inner table until the lesion is encountered. The lesion depicted as *1* may be managed by buttockectomy if the deep margins do *not* involve adjacent structures. If, however, the sciatic nerve is involved along with additional soft tissues, then a hemipelvectomy may be required to render the patient locally free of disease.

Postoperative function using either a hamstring transfer or no reconstruction still provides a stable, sensate extremity that is preferred to amputation.

Tumors presenting within the adductor musculature can usually be biopsied directly over the mass, once again avoiding the vascular sheath. If vascular reconstruction is contemplated, the biopsy incision should be positioned in such a way as to provide for later exposure of the vein to be used as a graft, but to *prevent* contamination at the time of biopsy. Very little recognizable functional deficit will occur after resection of all of the adductor musculature along with the obturator nerve.

Tumor involving the posterior compartment of the thigh should be carefully evaluated prior to biopsy using either CT/T or MR. The exact position of the sciatic nerve should be identified prior to biopsy and the incision then placed to avoid contamination of the sciatic nerve. As previously mentioned, the vascular integrity of the extremity may be reliably reconstructed; however, reconstruction of major nerves remains unpredictable.

When the nerve is involved, the entire contents of the posterior compartment may be resected, along with the sciatic nerve, and still retain a serviceable limb. The absence of protective sensation over the plantar aspect of the foot requires constant observation for pressure-related problems. However, the presence of active extension of the knee will usually allow ambulation with a cane and an ankle/foot orthosis to control the loss of active dorsiflexion of the ankle.

Leg

Tumors arising within the tibia may be sampled through a small anteriorly placed incision in line with the "Mercedes" incision (Figs 14–10 to 14–12 and Cross Section 12).[17] The periosteum should *not* be stripped except in the exact location of the intended biopsy tract to prevent subperiosteal hematoma dissection. The medullary contents may be sampled over a considerable distance, using a pituitary rongeur or suction/aspiration techniques (Cross

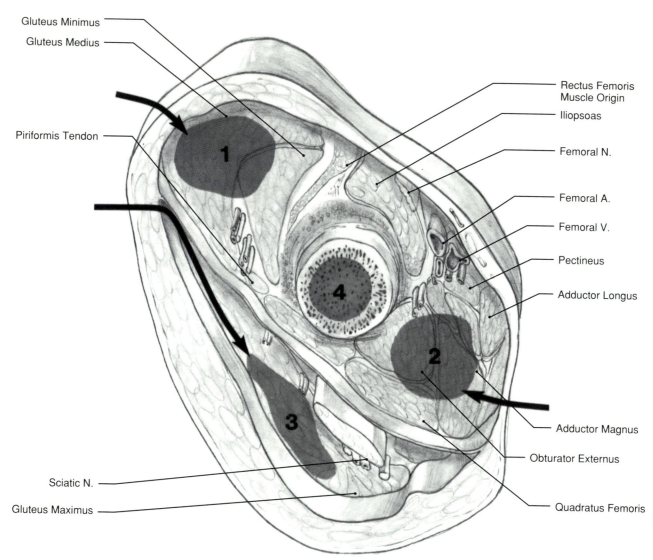

Gluteus Minimus

Gluteus Medius

Piriformis Tendon

Rectus Femoris Muscle Origin

Iliopsoas

Femoral N.

Femoral A.

Femoral V.

Pectineus

Adductor Longus

Adductor Magnus

Obturator Externus

Sciatic N.

Gluteus Maximus

Quadratus Femoris

CROSS SECTION 9.

Proximal thigh. Tumors presenting in bone. Intramedullary tumor as depicted by *4* is best sampled from above using the techniques described in Cross Section 8 and Fig 14–9, B. **Tumors presenting in soft tissues** *(solid arrows).* Soft tissue tumors arising in position *1* and not involving either the proximal femur or the ilium may be locally resected. Frequently, however, the lesion will involve one or both of these bones, requiring an internal hemipelvectomy. Lesions arising in the adductor region *(2)* may be approached directly. However, tumors arising within the gluteus maximus *(3)* or deeper, may require exposure through the lateral portion of the muscle (Fig 14–8, A). Both CT/T and MR are invaluable adjuncts to therapy in these anatomically demanding areas.

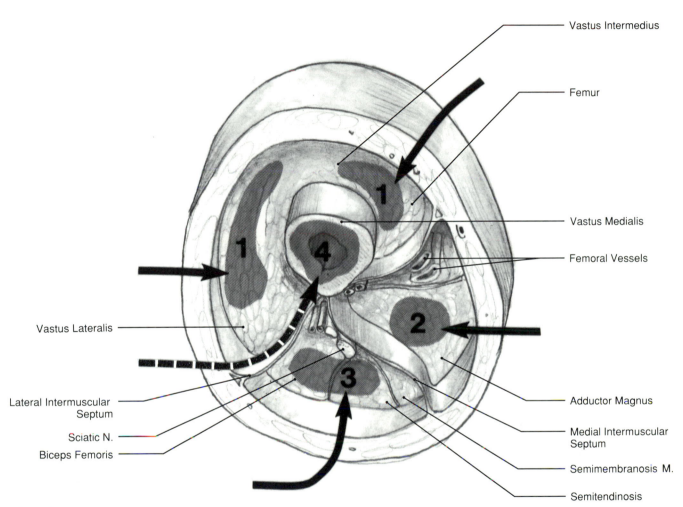

Vastus Intermedius

Femur

Vastus Medialis

Femoral Vessels

Adductor Magnus

Medial Intermuscular Septum

Semimembranosis M.

Semitendinosis

Vastus Lateralis

Lateral Intermuscular Septum

Sciatic N.

Biceps Femoris

CROSS SECTION 10.

Mid thigh. Tumors presenting in bone *(dashed arrow)*. The midshaft of the femur is best surgically approached laterally through the most posterior portion of the vastus lateralis, with the incision coursing anterior to the lateral septum *(4)*. If a femoral resection is oncologically feasible, then the en bloc planes of dissection will pass through the posterior compartment and through the medial half of the vastus lateralis, thereby encompassing all biopsy contaminated tissue. **Tumors presenting in soft tissues** *(solid arrows)*. Malignant lesions arising within the quadriceps musculature *(1)* may be approached directly followed by complete resection including either the medial or lateral or both intermuscular septae. Adductor lesions may be similarly managed *(2)*. Tumors arising within the muscles of the posterior compartment *(3)* are more demanding, requiring careful imaging (CT/T or MR) to evaluate possible sciatic nerve involvement. When biopsying these lesions the deep surface of the tumor and the investing fascia of the muscle should remain undisturbed.

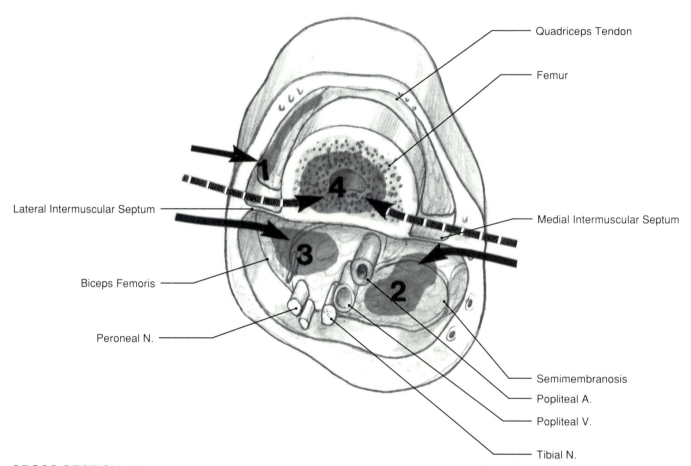

CROSS SECTION 11.

Distal third of thigh. Tumors presenting in bone *(dashed arrows).* Because of the small amount of surrounding muscle and the close proximity of the vessels to the femur posteriorly, biopsy of osseous lesions involving the distal femur should avoid contamination of the joint and tendinous tissues and should closely approximate either the medial or lateral intermuscular septae *(4).* **Tumors presenting in soft tissues** *(solid arrows).* Every effort should be made to avoid exposure of the neural and vascular structures. Therefore, the deep surface of the tumor and investing muscular fascia should remain undisturbed until the time of definitive therapy. Cross sectional and sagittal imaging with CT/T and MR is mandatory to plan the biopsy and to identify important structures to be avoided.

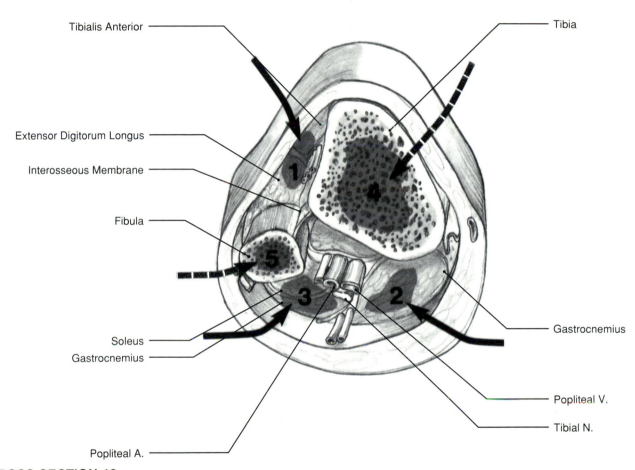

Tibialis Anterior

Tibia

Extensor Digitorum Longus

Interosseous Membrane

Fibula

Gastrocnemius

Soleus

Gastrocnemius

Popliteal V.

Tibial N.

Popliteal A.

CROSS SECTION 12.

Proximal portion of leg. Tumors presenting in bone *(dashed arrows).* A direct approach to the subcutaneous borders of either the tibia or proximal fibula will often result in diagnostic tissue. Incision orientation and placement is important, however, to accommodate the planned resection incision (see Figs 14–10 to 14–12). **Tumors presenting in soft tissues** *(solid arrows).* Once again, every effort should be made to avoid contaminating any major nerves or vessels. A direct approach to the affected muscle commonly results in the best overall outcome.

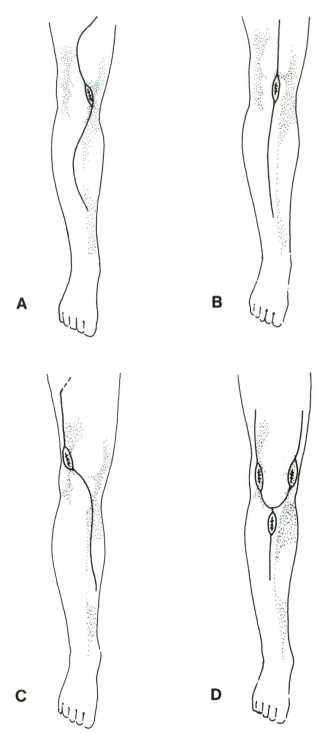

FIG 14–10.
This illustration shows various biopsy incisions about the region of the knee and the variations of incisions that may be utilized for the subsequent exposure required for definitive therapy. Incision B should be reserved only for those lesions superficial to the quadriceps tendon or lesions involving the patella. Incision D shows three separate biopsy incisions about the knee that may be incorporated into the "Mercedes" incision.

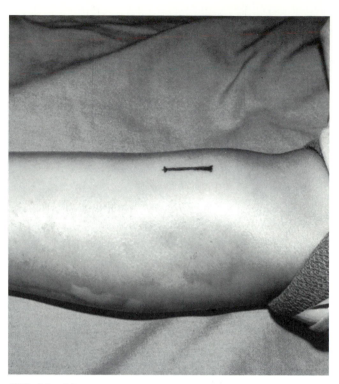

FIG 14–11.
This adolescent patient presented with pain and a tender soft tissue mass immediately below the left tibial apophysis. The biopsy incision placement will allow for the application of the "Mercedes" incision shown in Fig 14–10, D for management of the subsequently biopsy-proven osteosarcoma of the proximal tibia.

Section 13). Once the sample has been obtained, a hemostatic material may be placed within the canal and the periosteal defect sealed using a plug of cotton Oxycel or methylmethacrylate. The tourniquet should always be deflated prior to skin closure to be certain that *absolute hemostasis* has been obtained.

In general, drains are contraindicated in biopsy wounds. If, for some reason, they are deemed necessary, then a closed suction drain placed only within the biopsy tract may be used. The exit point of the drainage tubing should be in line with the biopsy incision and approximately 1 cm to either end. By positioning the drain tract in line with the incision, the entire biopsy incision and drain tract can easily be excised en bloc at the time of the definitive procedure.

Malignant tumors involving the proximal tibia and managed by surgery are often difficult to close surgically. The small loss of skin associated with the en bloc excision of the biopsy tract and tumor frequently requires that a gastrocnemius flap and skin graft be used to achieve primary closure. Therefore, it is mandatory that the posterior compartment or

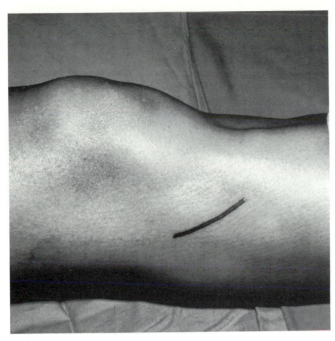

FIG 14–12.
This patient presented with an intraosseous lesion within the lateral plateau of the right tibia. This orientation of the biopsy incision allows for sampling of the lesion without contamination of the knee joint, the proximal fibula, and the peroneal nerve. Yet it allows flexibility in selection of exposures about the knee, as shown in Fig 14–10.

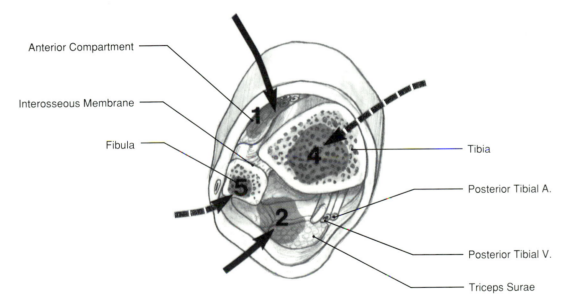

Anterior Compartment

Interosseous Membrane

Fibula

Tibia

Posterior Tibial A.

Posterior Tibial V.

Triceps Surae

CROSS SECTION 13.
Distal leg. Tumors presenting in bone *(dashed arrows)*. Both the distal tibia and fibula present subcutaneous borders that may be used for a limited exposure and biopsy. Minimal skin and soft tissue contamination can be tolerated, however, for skin closure after definitive resection may be very difficult or impossible. **Tumors presenting in soft tissues** *(solid arrows)*. Soft tissues within the distal leg are primarily composed of tendinous structures and like the forearm and hand, tumors arising in these areas frequently stream longitudinally up and down the tendons making local resection and reconstruction very difficult. The majority of lesions arising in this area require amputation.

the gastrocnemius musculature *not* be contaminated at the time of biopsy. The injudicious placement of the biopsy scar may require a more radical procedure, or perhaps amputation, if the biopsy is not planned in conjunction with the anticipated surgical procedure.

Foot and Ankle

The foot is comprised of four ill-defined soft tissue compartments and in many respects mirrors the difficulties previously discussed with respect to biopsies of the hand. Only longitudinal incisions in line with the underlying metatarsals should be used. Where possible, the incision should be placed on the dorsum of the foot or on either the medial or lateral side, thereby avoiding incisions in the plantar skin. Many tumors arising within the foot mimic abscess formation or osteomyelitis and therefore both microbiologic cultures *and* tissue for histopathologic examination should be obtained at the time of diagnostic biopsy. Soft tissue tumors arising within the plantar aspect of the foot are rarely managed by local resection, and most will require either a Syme or a below-knee amputation.

CONCLUSION

This chapter was included to provide the current concepts of musculoskeletal oncologic imaging, staging, and management of patients presenting with musculoskeletal lesions. Special reference to the anatomy involved and biopsy techniques along with incision placement have been reviewed. There are no hard and fast rules, but only general principles and guidelines to follow. The material presented in no way provides the fund of knowledge necessary for the management of such patients presenting with bone and soft tissue malignancies. In general, if the operating surgeon does not feel comfortable and confident in managing the patient *after* the biopsy, then the surgeon should strongly consider referral *before* the biopsy.

REFERENCES

1. Enneking WF, Spanier SS, Goodman MA: A system for the surgical staging of musculoskeletal sarcoma. *Clin Orthop* 1980; 153:106–120.
2. Bowden L, Booher RJ: The principles and technique of resection of soft parts for sarcoma. *Surgery* 1958; 44:963–977.
3. Simon MA, Enneking WF: The surgical management of soft-tissue sarcomas of the extremities. *J Bone Joint Surg* 1976; 58A:317–327.
4. Linberg BE: Interscapulothoracic resection for malignant tumors of the shoulder joint region. *J Bone Joint Surg* 1928; 10:344–349.
5. Syme J: *Excision of the Scapula.* Edinburgh, Edmonston and Douglas, 1864.
6. Littlewood H: Amputation at the shoulder and at the hip. *Br Med J* 1922; 1:381–383.
7. Nadler SH, Phelan JT: A technique of interscapulothoracic amputation. *Surg Gynecol Obstet* 1966; 122:359–364.
8. Wurlitzer FP: Improved technique for radical transthoracic forequarter amputation. *Ann Surg* 1973; 177:467–471.
9. Mansour KA, Powell RW: Modified technique for radical transmediastinal forequarter amputation and chest wall resection. *J Thorac Cardiovasc Surg* 1978; 76:358–363.
10. Enneking WF, Dunham WK: Resection and reconstruction for primary neoplasms involving the innominate bone. *J Bone Joint Surg* 1978; 60A(6):731–746.
11. Banks SW, Coleman S: Hemipelvectomy: Surgical techniques. *J Bone Joint Surg* 1956; 38:1147–1155.
12. Frey C, Matthews LS, Benjamin H, et al: A new technique for hemipelvectomy. *Surg Gynecol Obstet* 1976; 143:753–756.
13. Sugarbaker PA, Chretien PA: A surgical technique for buttockectomy. *Surgery* 1982; 91:104–107.
14. Mnaymneh W, Temple W: Modified hemipelvectomy utilizing a long vascular myocutaneous thigh flap. *J Bone Joint Surg* 1980; 62A:1013–1015.
15. Steel HH: Partial or complete resection of the hemipelvis. *J Bone Joint Surg* 1978; 60A:719–730.
16. Sugarbaker PH, Chretien PA: Hemipelvectomy for buttock tumors utilizing an anterior myocutaneous flap of quadriceps femoris muscle. *Ann Surg* 1983; 197:106–115.
17. Muller ME, Allgower M, Schneider R, et al: *Manual of Internal Fixation. Techniques Recommended by the AO Group,* ed 2. New York, Springer-Verlag, 1979; pp 256–257.

Index